U0332465

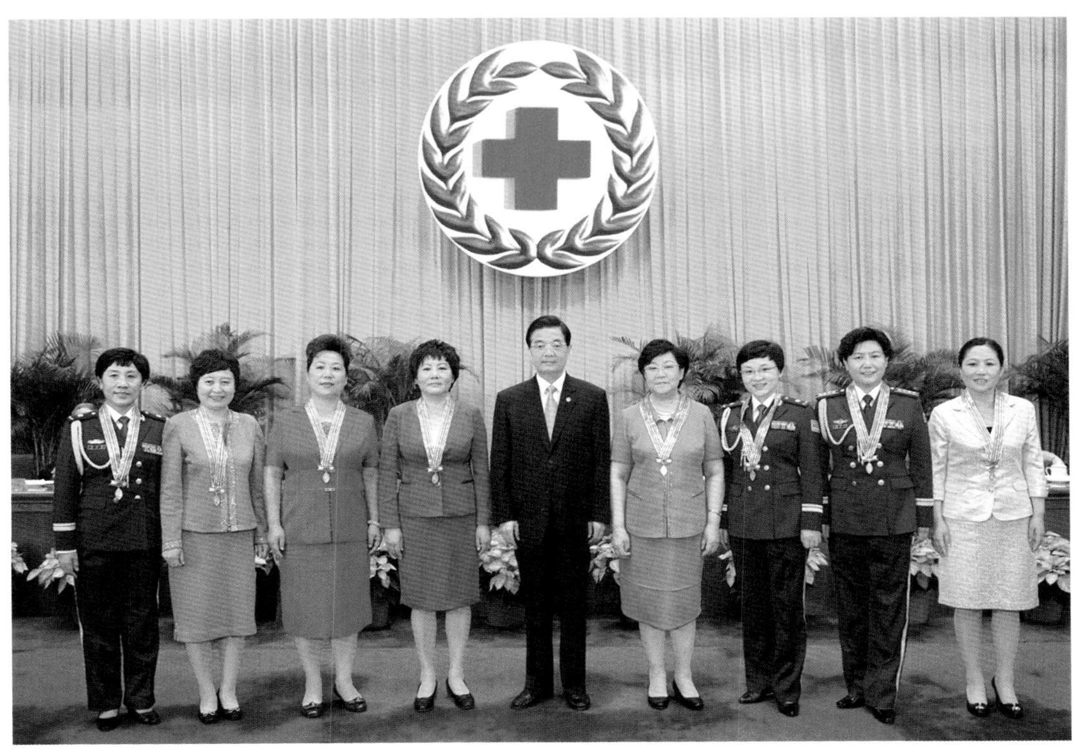

The 43rd Prize-Giving Ceremony for Nightingale Medal was held, August 26, 2011. Chinese President Hu Jintao was pictured with eight Chinese prize-winners.

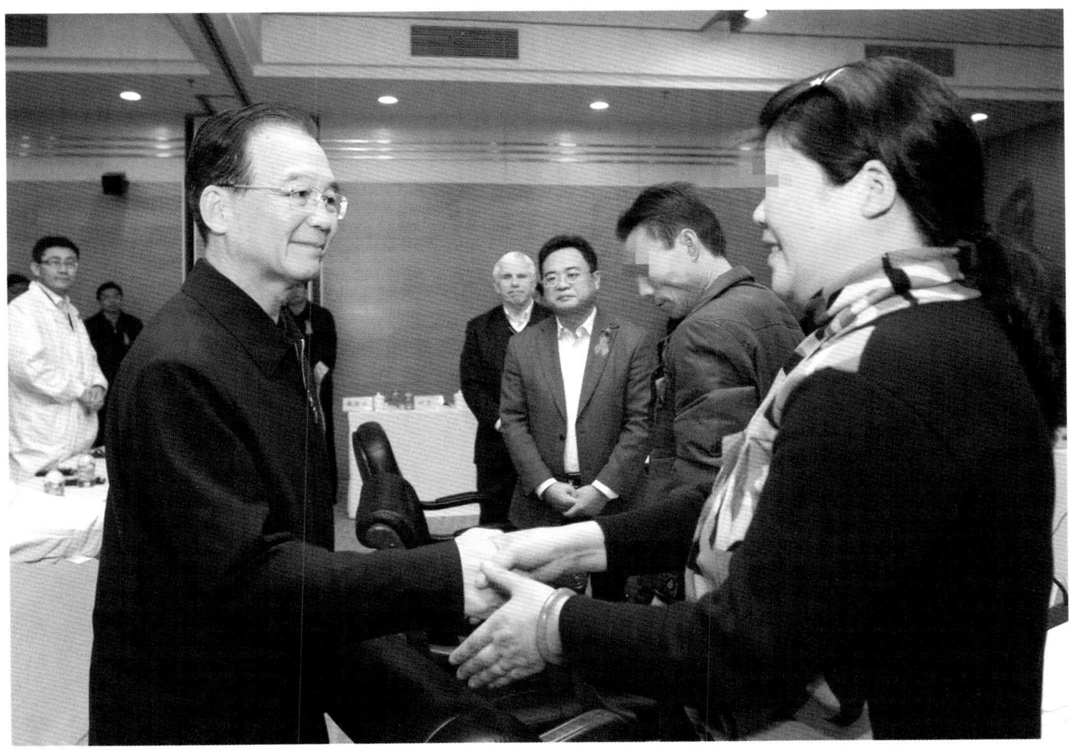

Premier Wen Jiabao paid an inspection visit to Chinese Center for Disease Control and Prevention (China-CDC) December 1, 2011. Wen Jiabao was pictured with one of the HIV-infected patients for hand–shake.

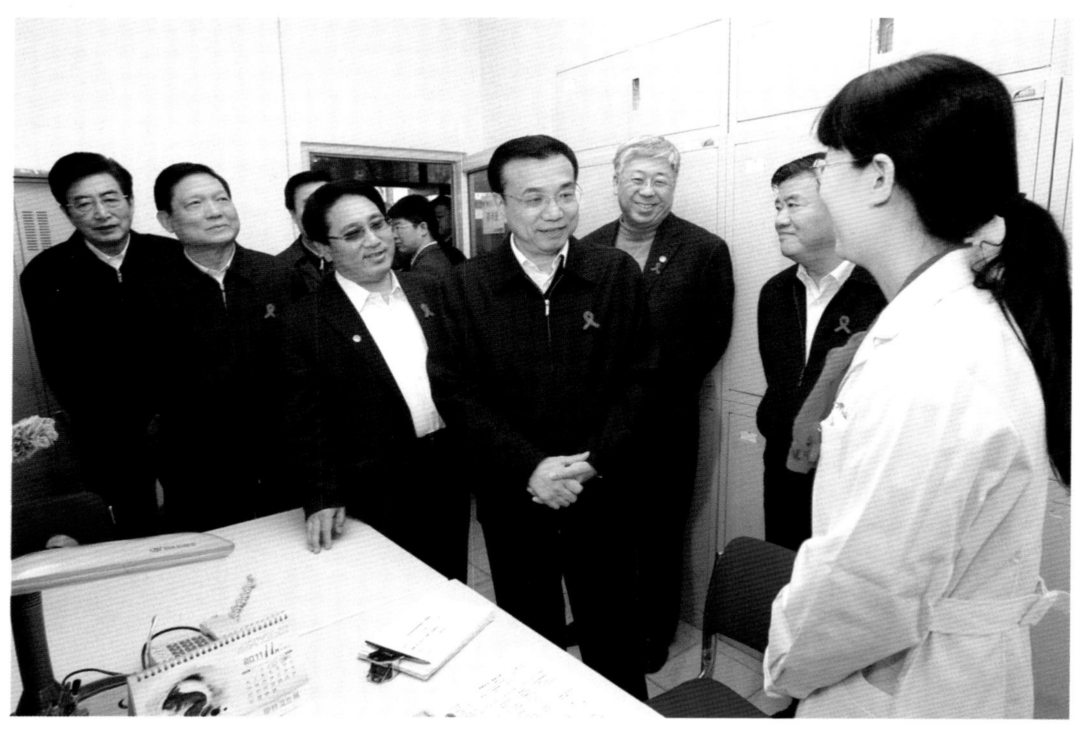

Vice Premier Li Keqiang inspected HIV/AIDS prevention and control in Beijing, November 18, 2011.

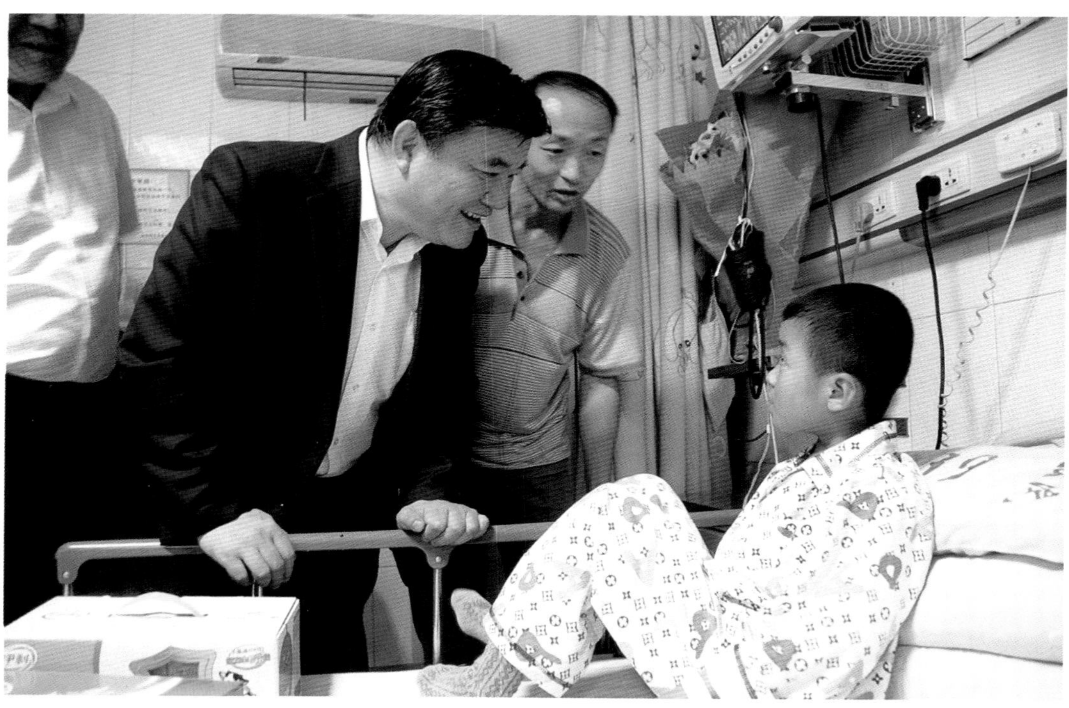

Health Minister Chen Zhu, on his inspection tour in Xinjiang in June 2011, called on a little post-operative patient with congenital heart disease, who benefited from “Spring Seedling Project”.

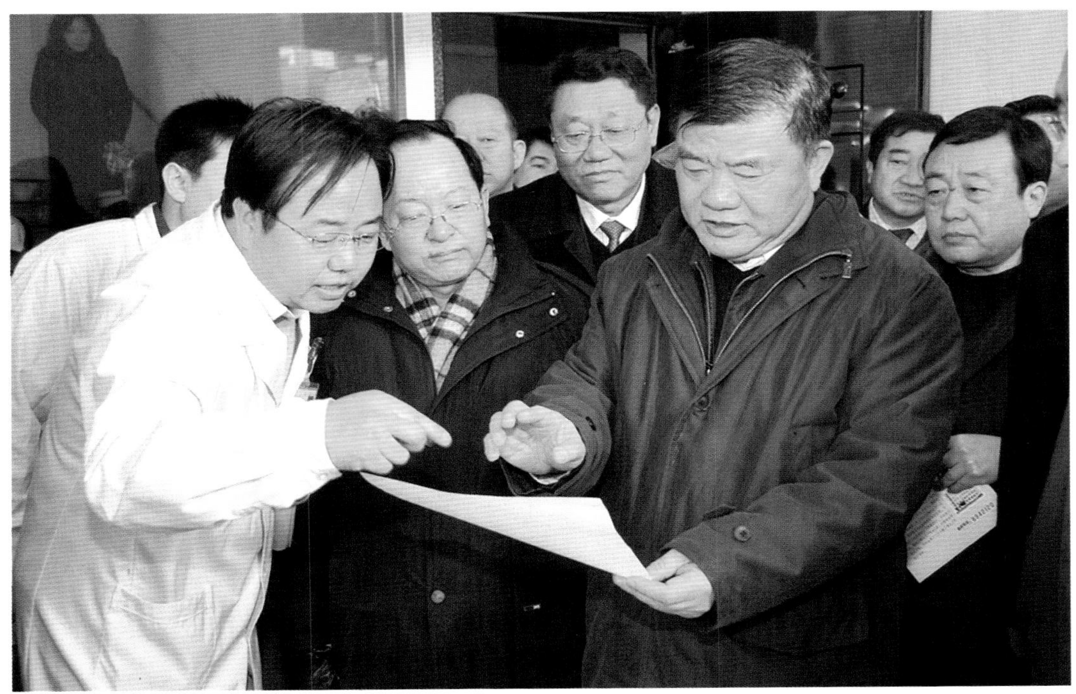

Health Minister Chen Zhu conducted survey and research in the People's Hospital of Fugu County in Shaanxi, January 31, 2011.

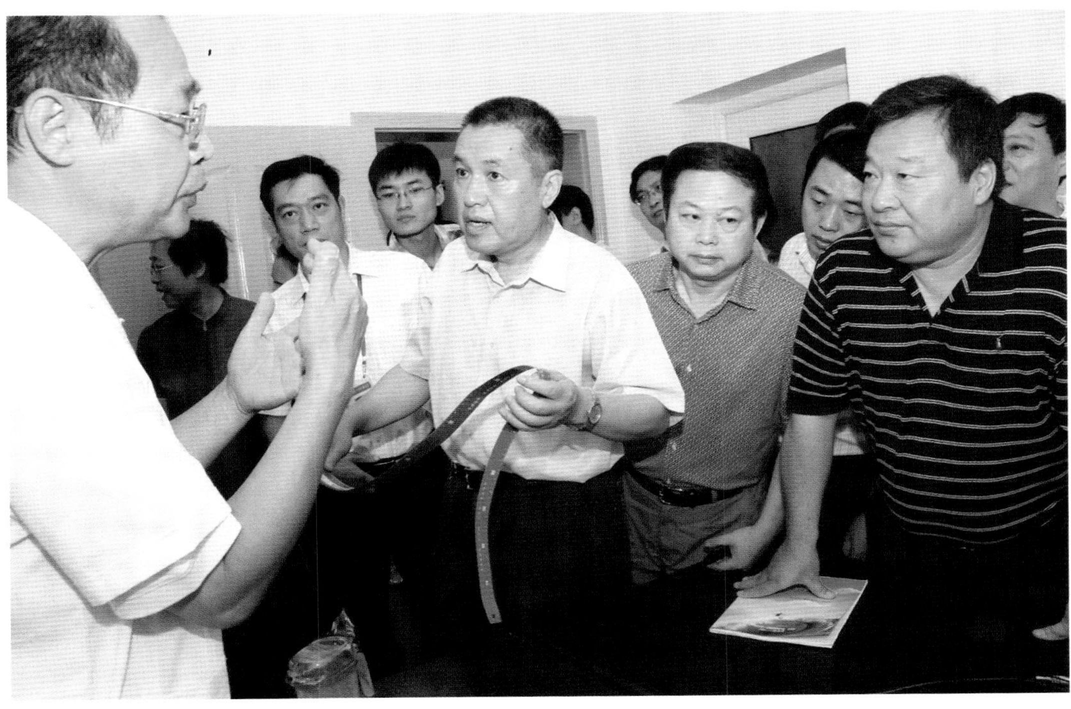

Secretary of the Party Leadership Group and Vice Minister of the Ministry of Health Zhang Mao guided the local medical reform and schistosomiasis prevention during his survey and research in Zhuzhou in Hunan, July 21-23, 2011.

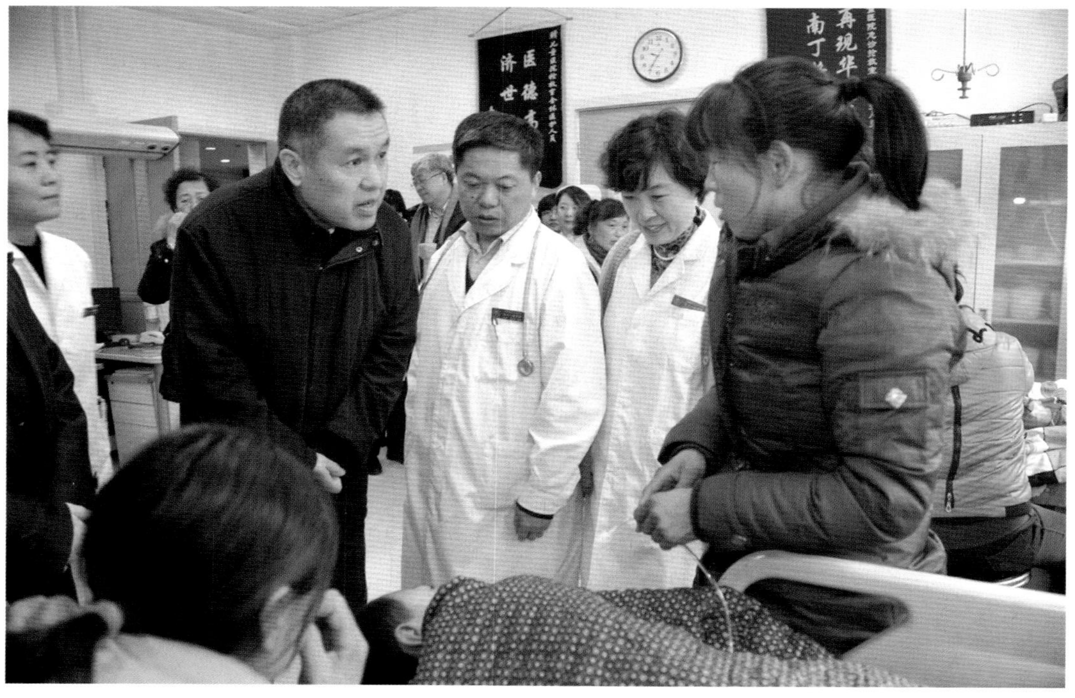

Secretary of the Party Leadership Group and Vice Minister of the Ministry of Health Zhang Mao conducted survey and research in Beijing Children's Hospital, January 28, 2011.

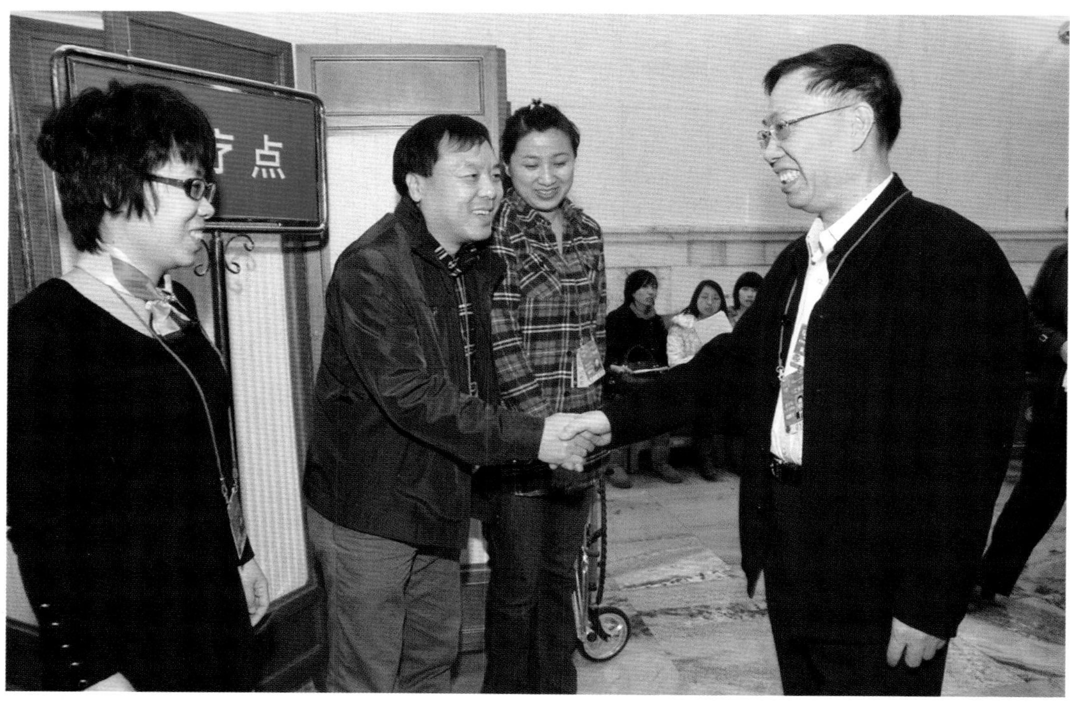

Vice Health Minister Huang Jiefu inspected and guided the work in the clinic for "Two Sessions" held in the Great Hall of the People in March 2011.

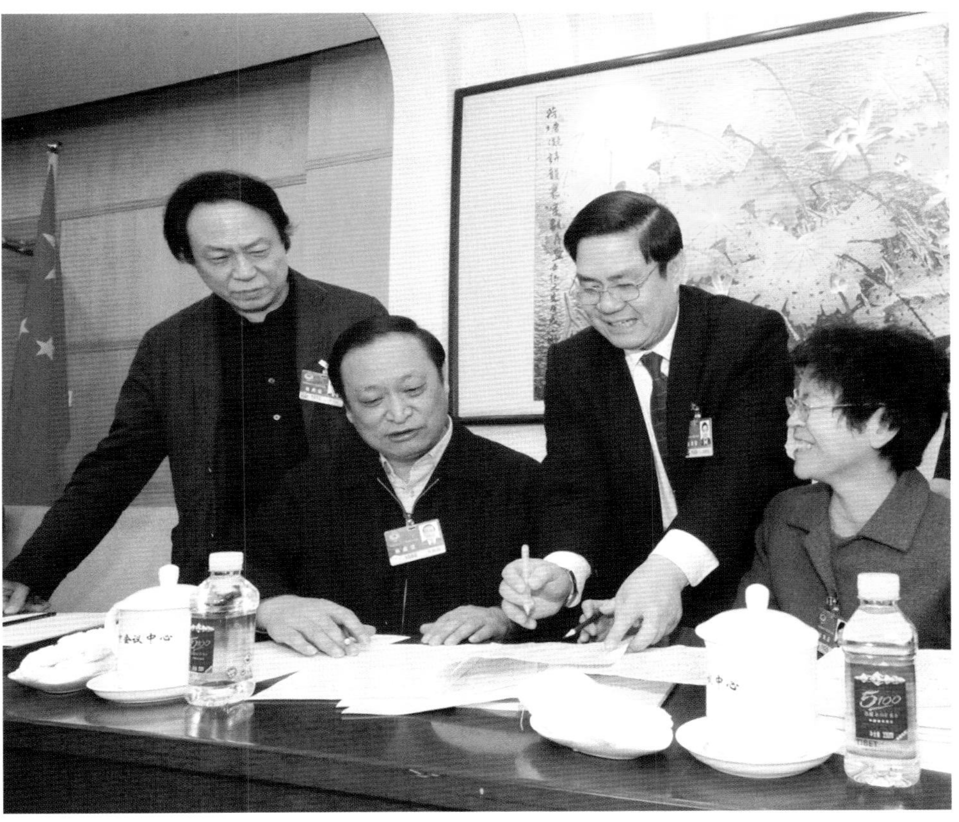

Vice Health Minister and Commissioner of the State Administration of Traditional Chinese Medicine Wang Guoqiang had a heated discussion with the members of medical circles of "Two Sessions" on public hospital reform in March 2011.

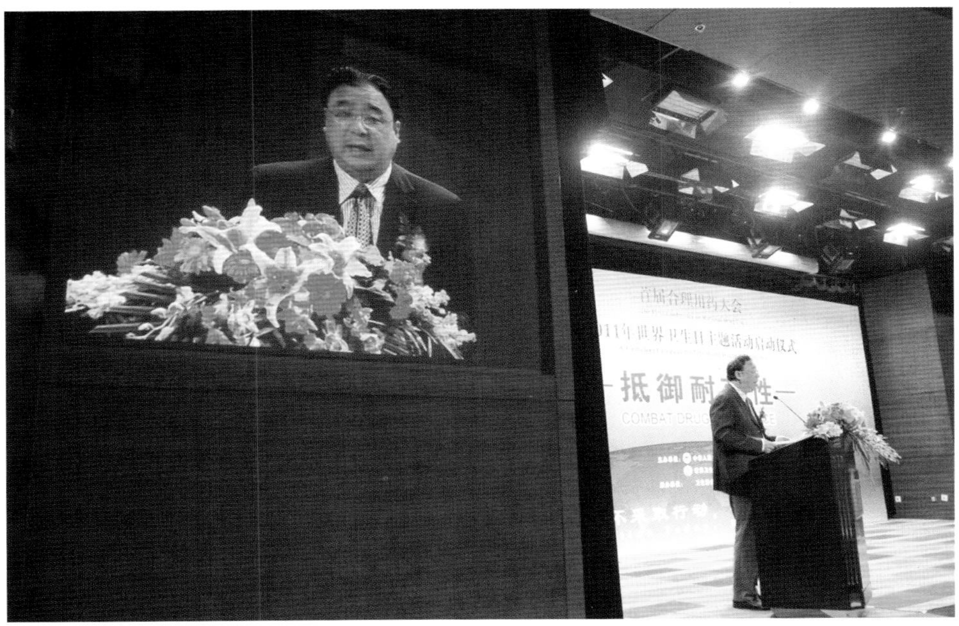

Vice Health Minister Ma Xiaowei addressed the Launching Ceremony for 2011 World Health Day Activities, April 7, 2011.

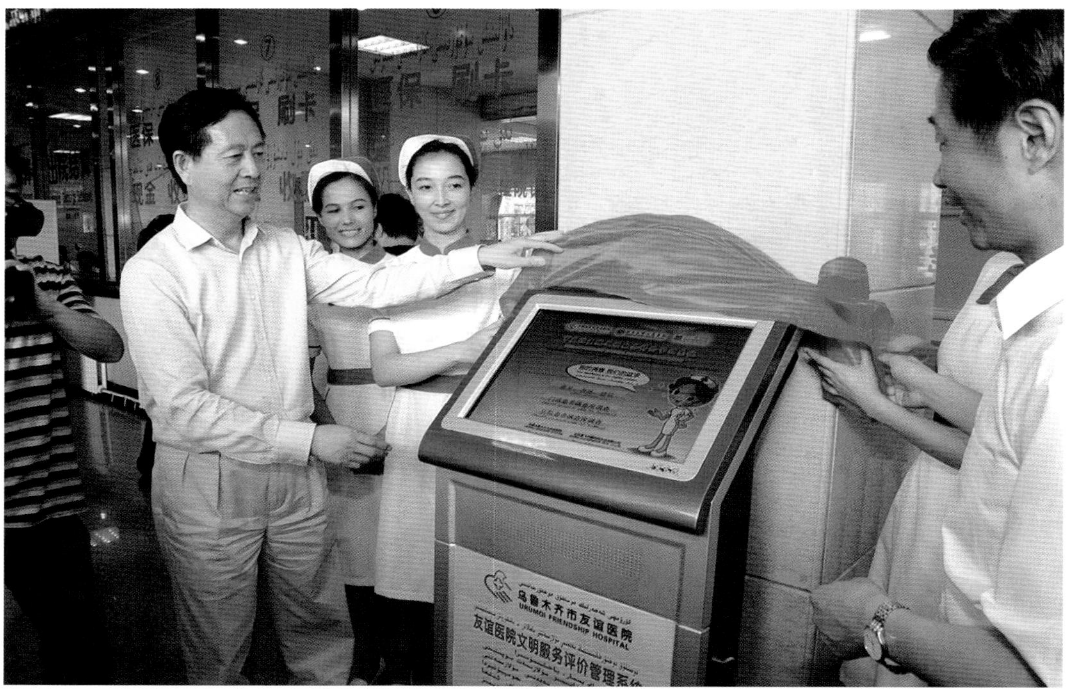

Vice Health Minister Chen Xiaohong inaugurated the touch screen for the evaluation and management of quality service in Urumqi Friendship Hospital, June 14, 2011.

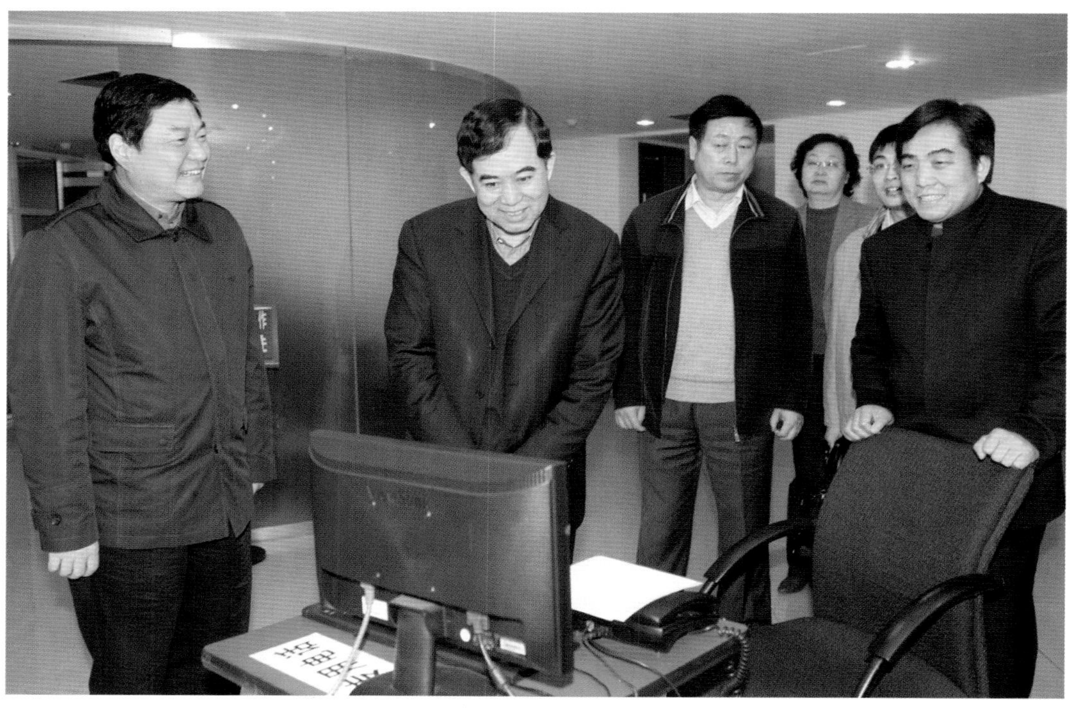

Li Xi, head of the resident discipline inspection group of Central Commission for Discipline Inspection of the CPC in the Ministry of Health, guided the work of medical examinations at the National Medical Examination Center, April 1, 2011.

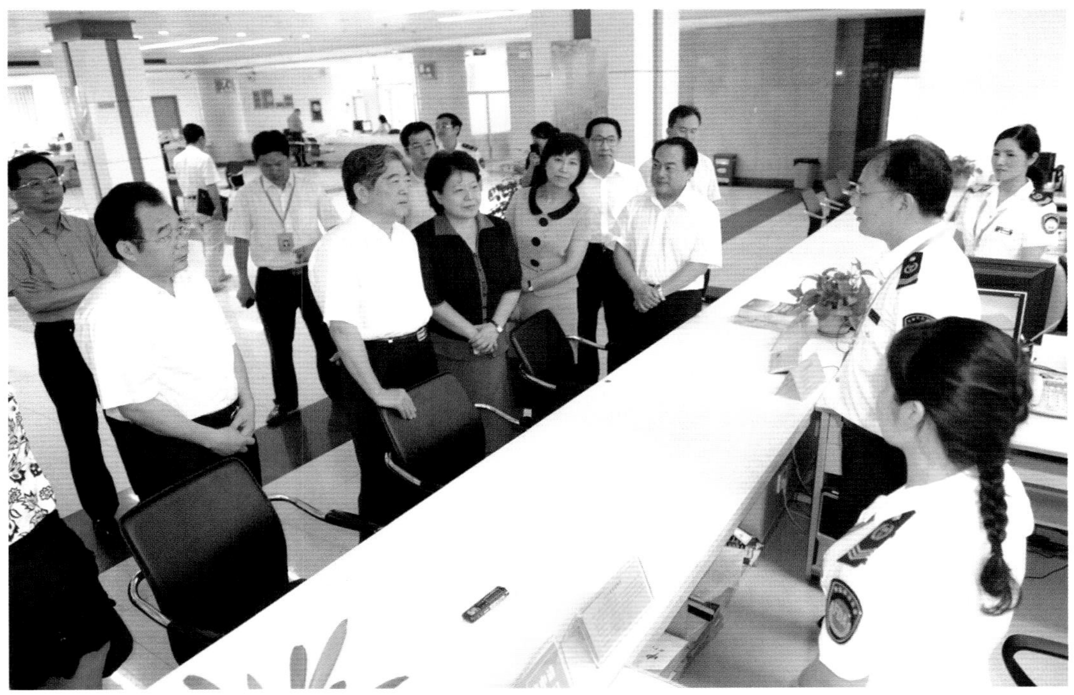

Vice Health Minister and Commissioner of the State Food and Drug Administration Shao Mingli inspected the food and drug regulation at the Administrative Service Center of Guangxi Zhuang Autonomous Region in June 2011.

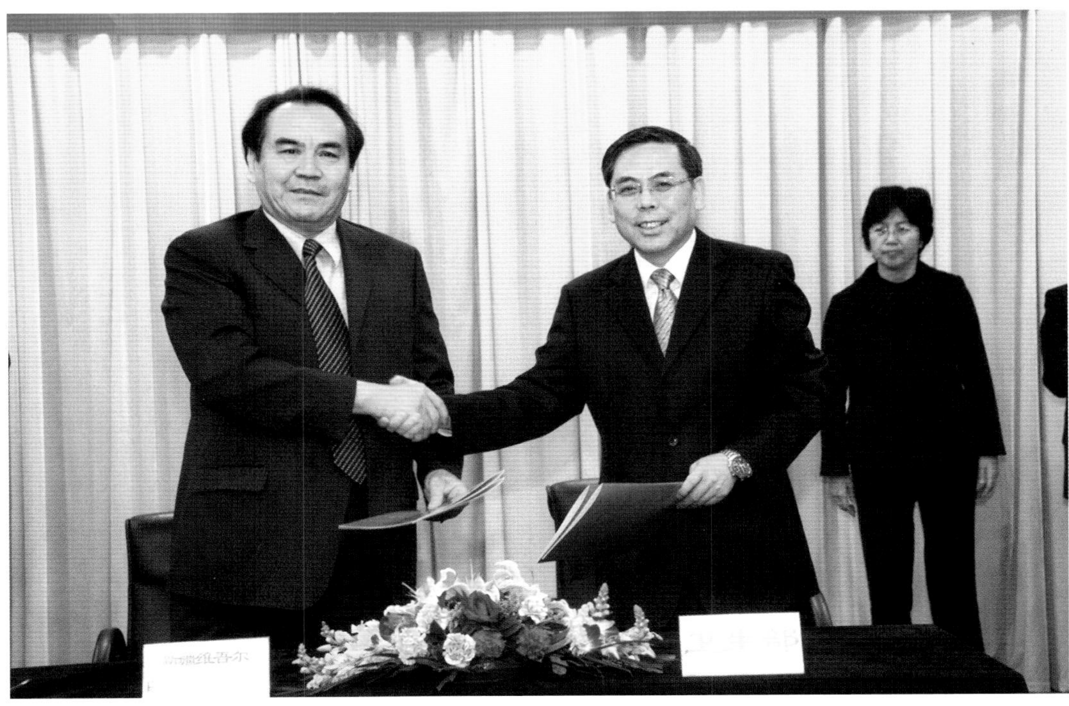

Vice Health Minister Liu Qian and Vice Chairman of Xinjiang Uygur Autonomous Region Tiliwaldi Abdulrixit signed the Collaborative Agreement on Further Deepening the Work of Providing Aid for Xinjiang, January 4, 2011.

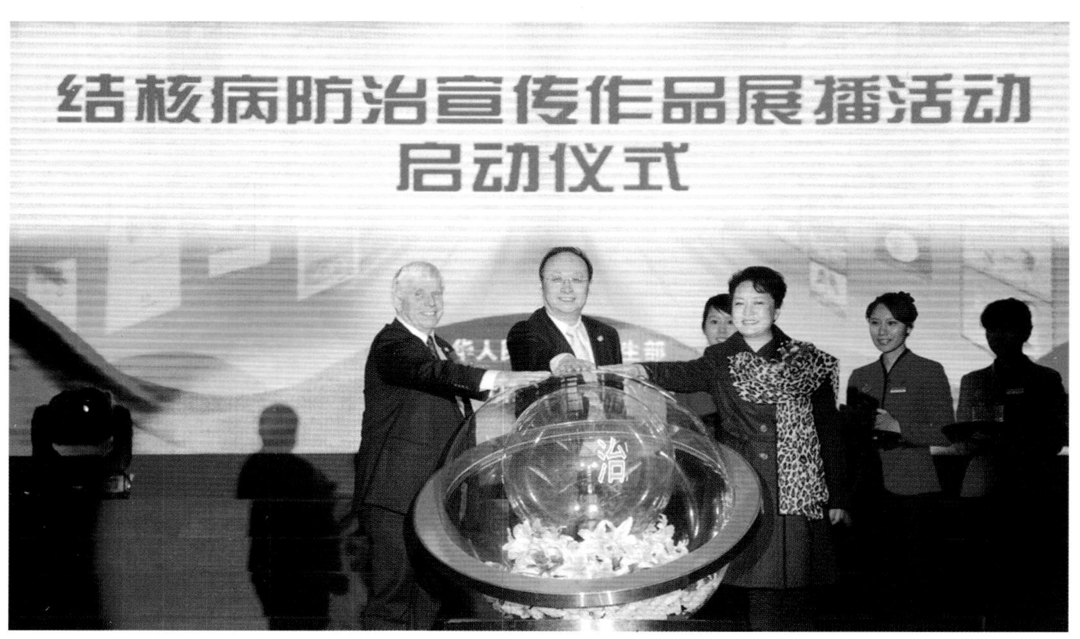

Vice Health Minister Yin Li attended the campaign for 2011 World Tuberculosis (TB) Day, March 22, 2011.

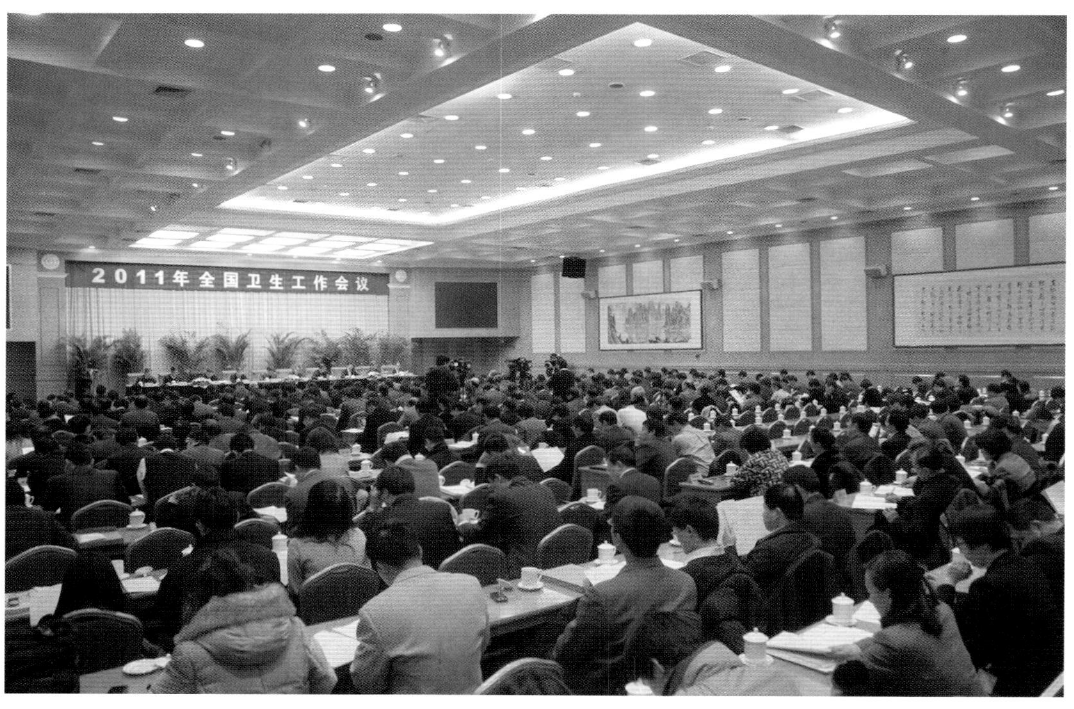

2011 National Conference on Health Work was held in Beijing, January 6, 2011.

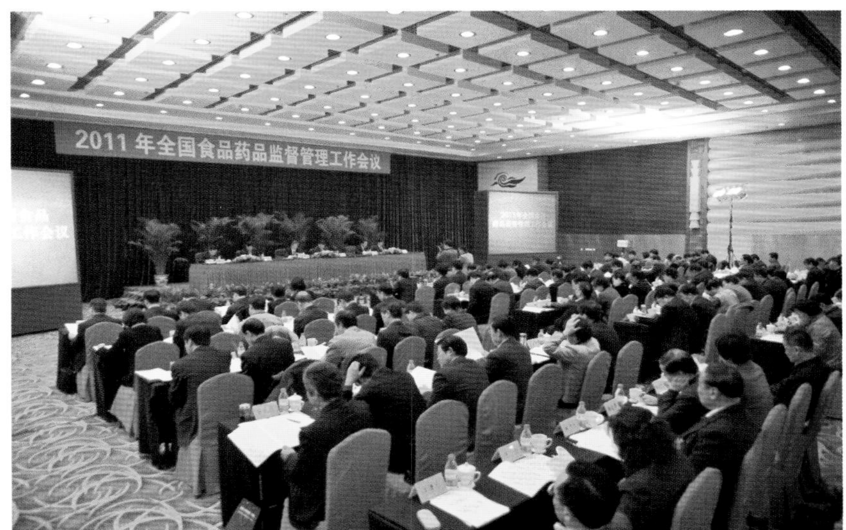

2011 National Conference on the Supervision and Management of Food and Drug was held in Beijing, January 13-14, 2011.

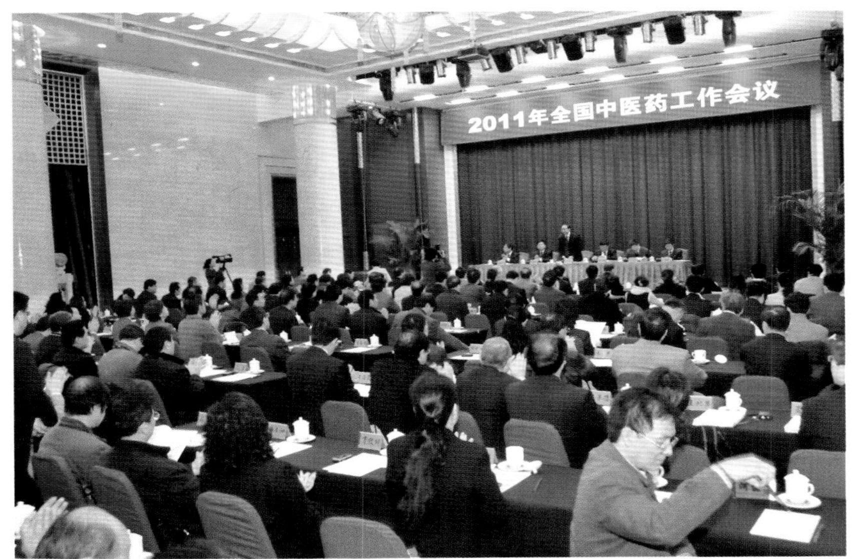

2011 National Conference on Traditional Chinese Medicine was held in Beijing, January 13-14, 2011.

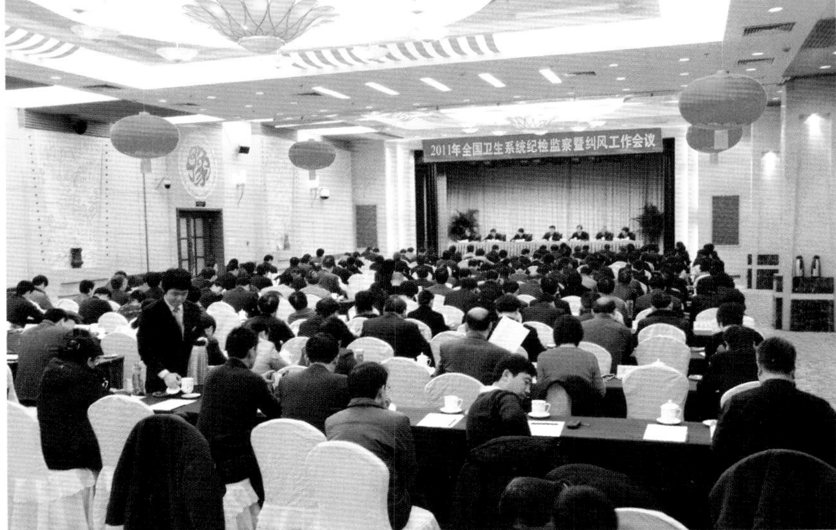

2011 National Conference on Discipline Inspection and Medical Ethics Rectification in Health Circles was held in Beijing, January 13-14, 2011.

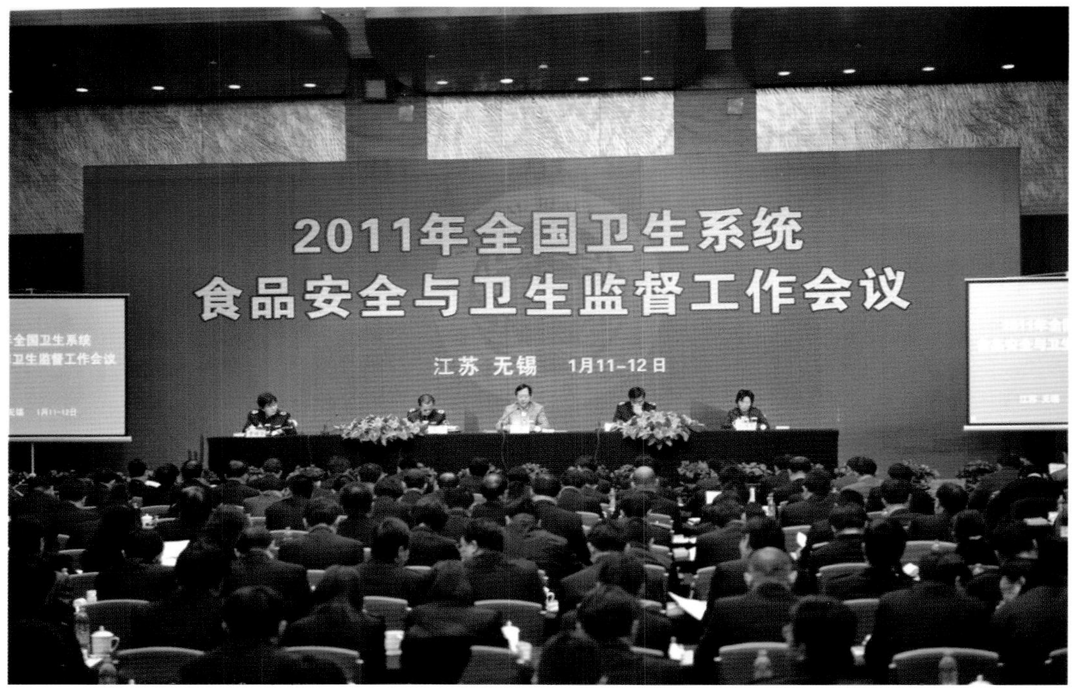

2011 National Conference on Food Safety and Health Supervision of Health Circles was held in Wuxi in Jiangsu, January 11-12, 2011.

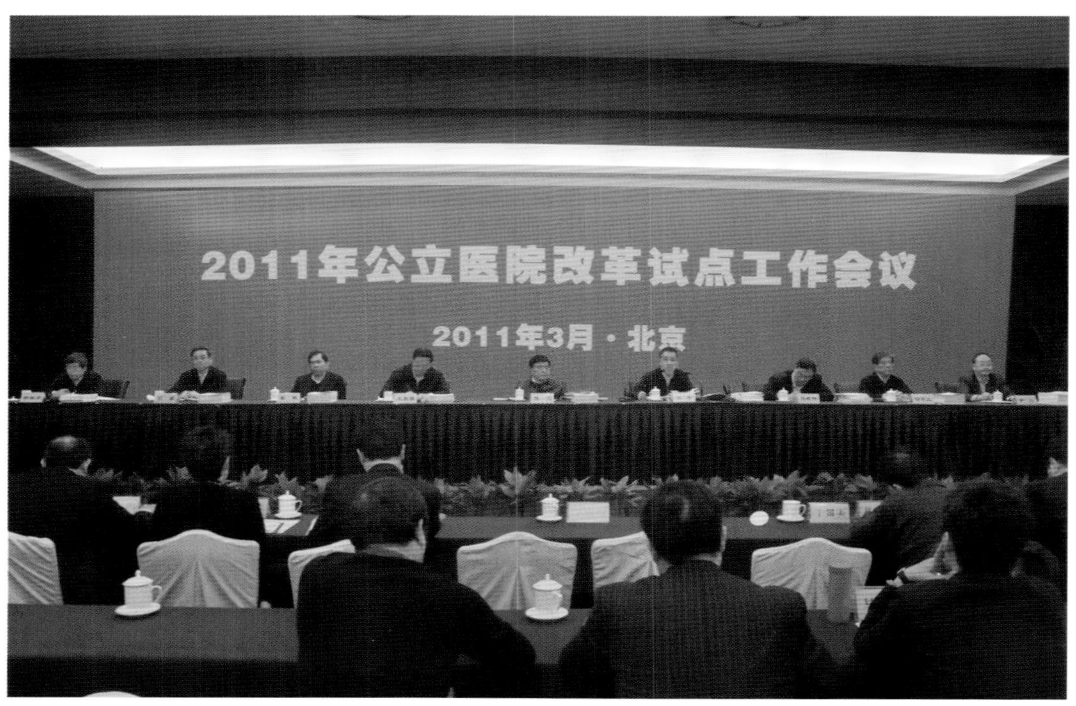

2011 Meeting on Pilot Projects for Reforming Public Hospitals was held in Beijing in March 2011.

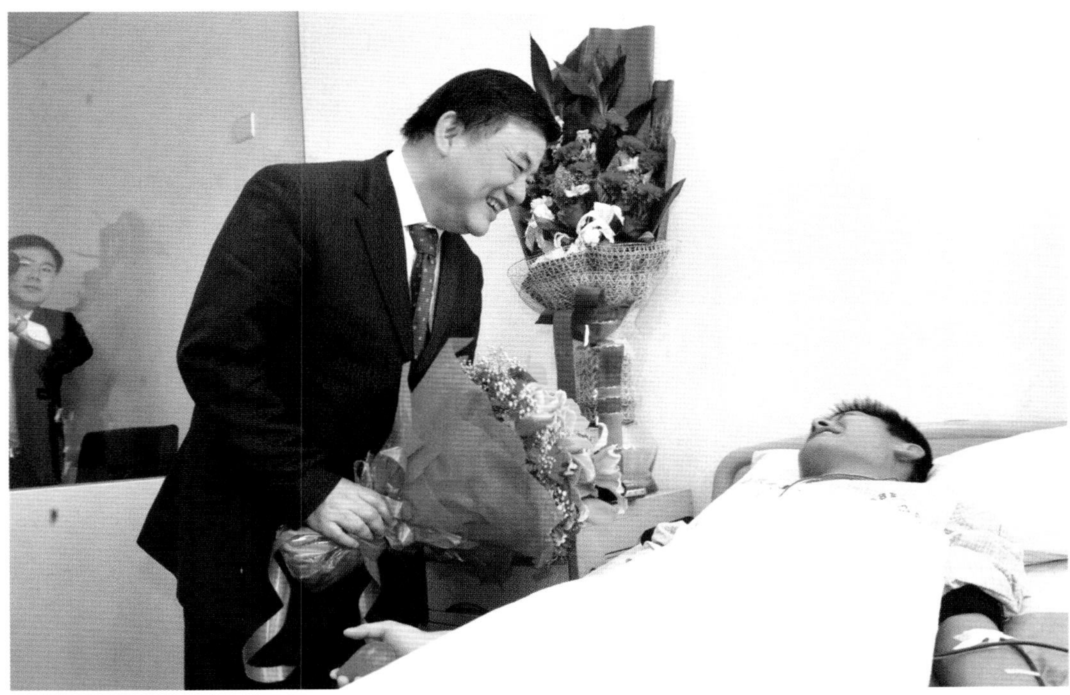

Health Minister Chen Zhu called on Wang Kai, a volunteer donating hematopoietic stem cells for Zhang Guangxiu who was a college-graduate village official from Yantai in Shandong, at 307 Hospital of PLA, March 7, 2011.

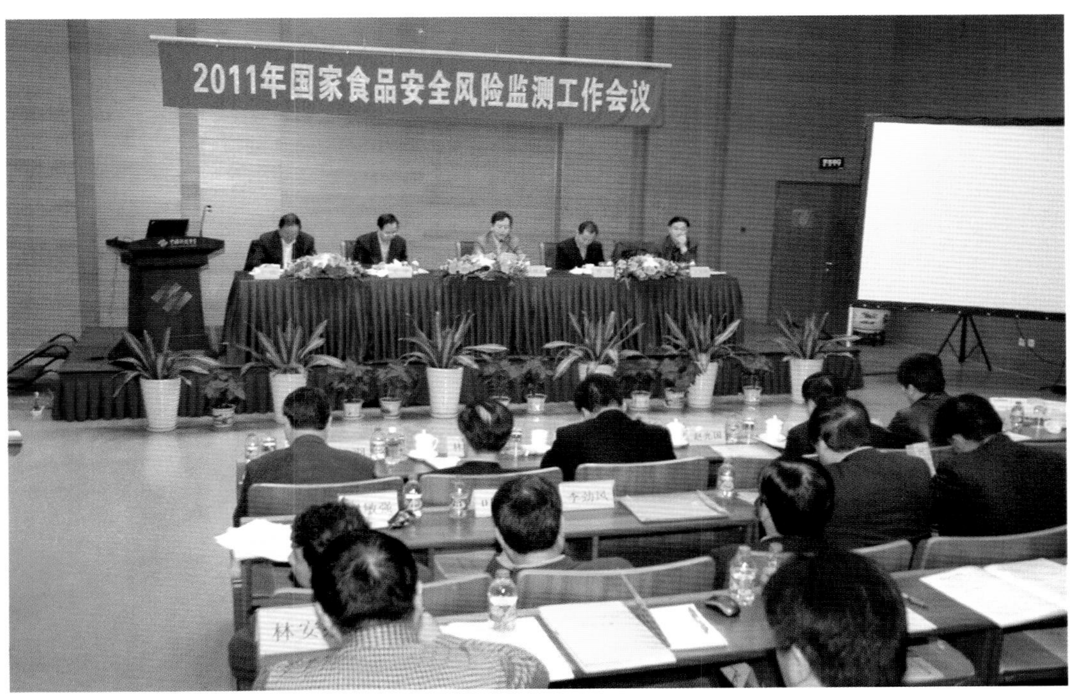

2011 Meeting on National Food Safety Risk Monitoring was held in Beijing, March 17-18, 2011.

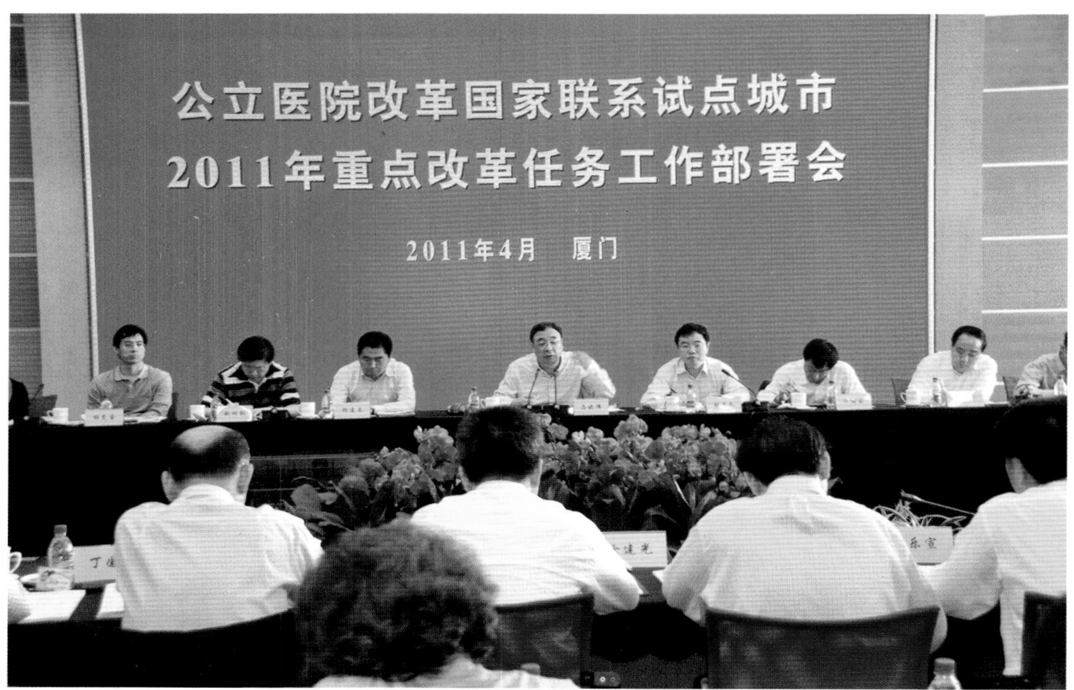

The meeting on 2011 work arrangements for key reform tasks of state liaison pilot cities for public hospital reform was held in Xiamen in April 2011.

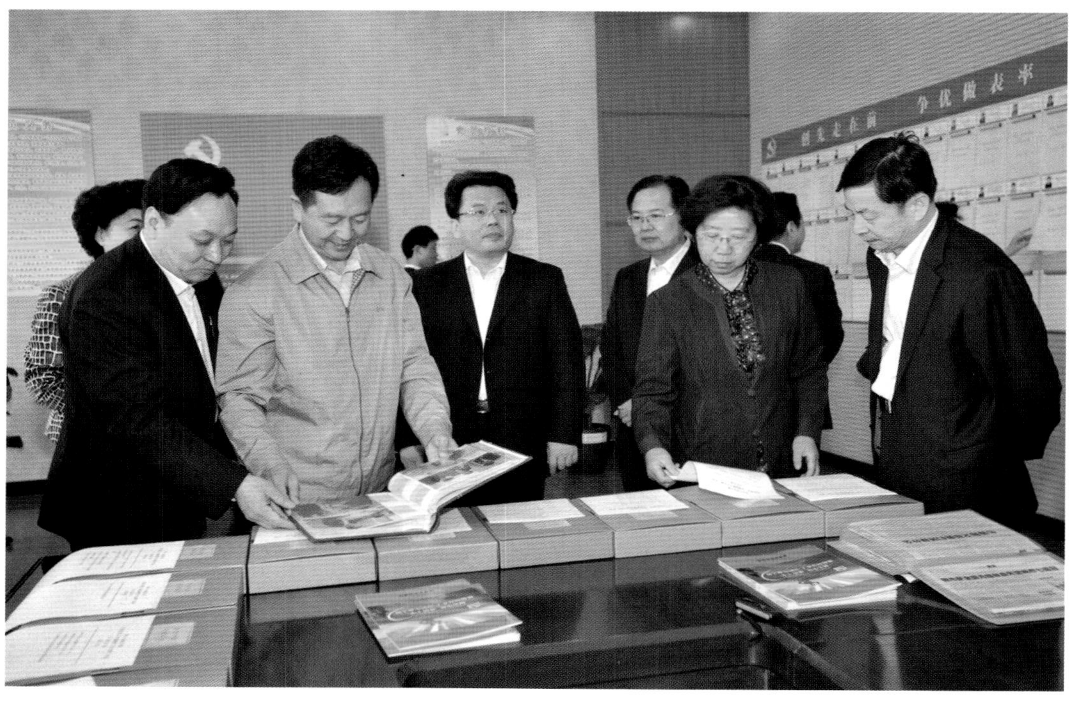

Vice Health Minister Chen Xiaohong and his group conducted survey and research on striving for excellence in performance in medical and health circles in Shandong, April 25-29, 2011.

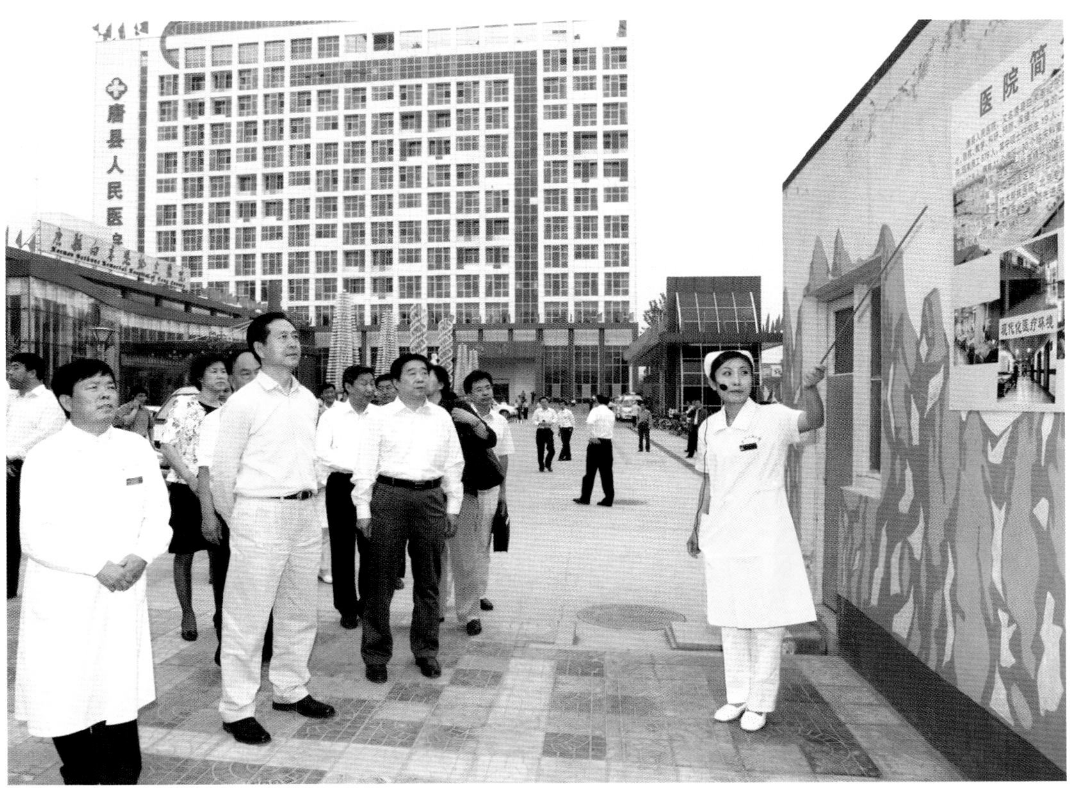

The steering group for striving for excellence in performance in national medical and health circles held the symposium on learning Yang Shanzhou's spirit in Shijiazhuang, May 17, 2011. The picture shows the meeting delegates visiting the People's Hospital of Tang County.

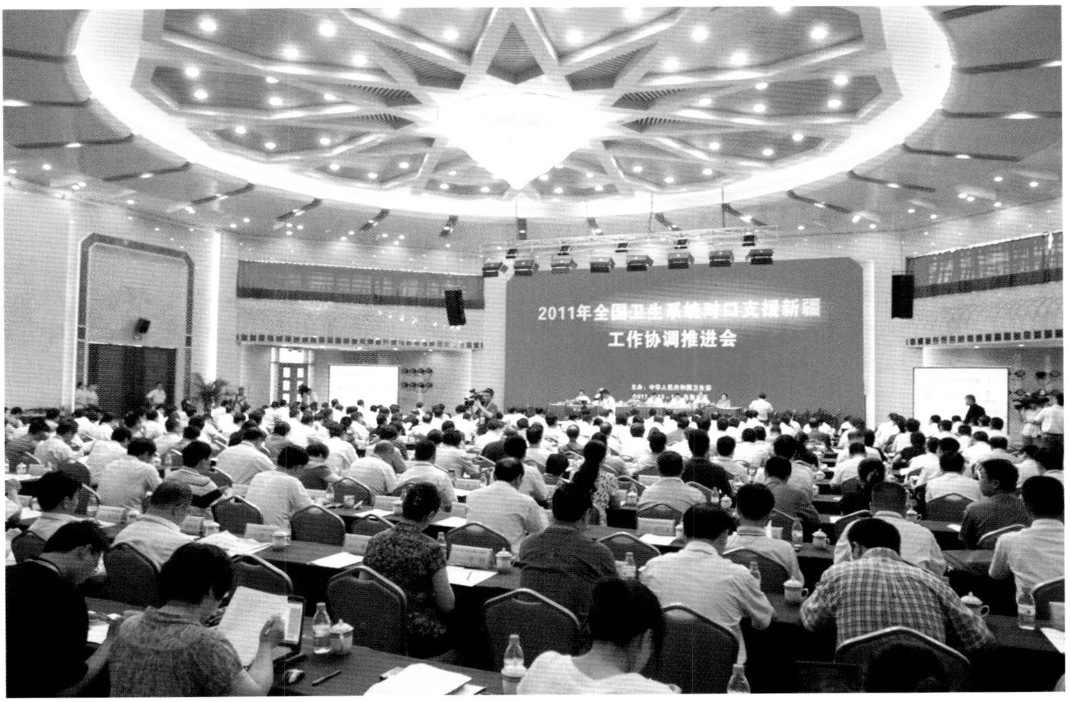

The Ministry of Health held the coordination meeting on counterpart assistance for Xinjiang within national health circles in Urumqi in Xinjiang, June 13-14, 2011.

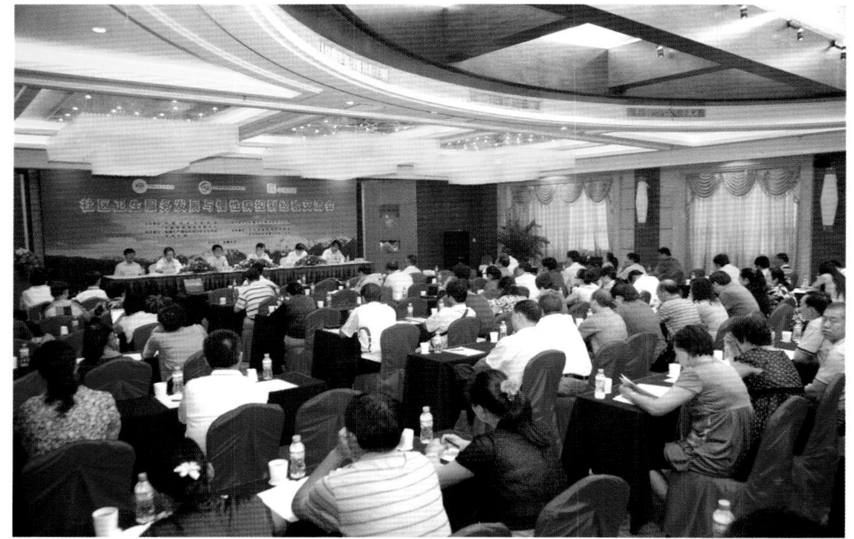

The experience exchange meeting on the national development of community health services and chronic disease control was held in Urumqi, capital city of Xinjiang, June 3, 2011.

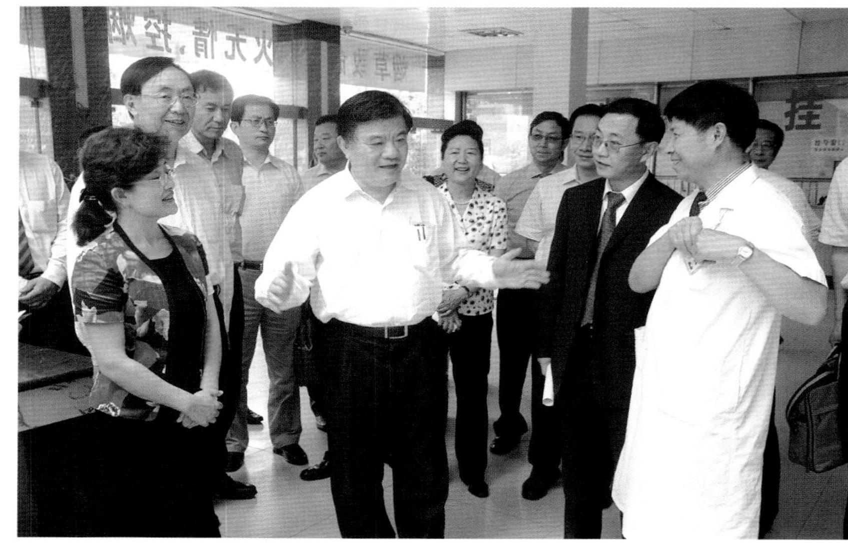

Health Minister Chen Zhu and his group conducted survey and research on public hospital reform and HIV/AIDS prevention and control in Yunnan, June 20, 2011.

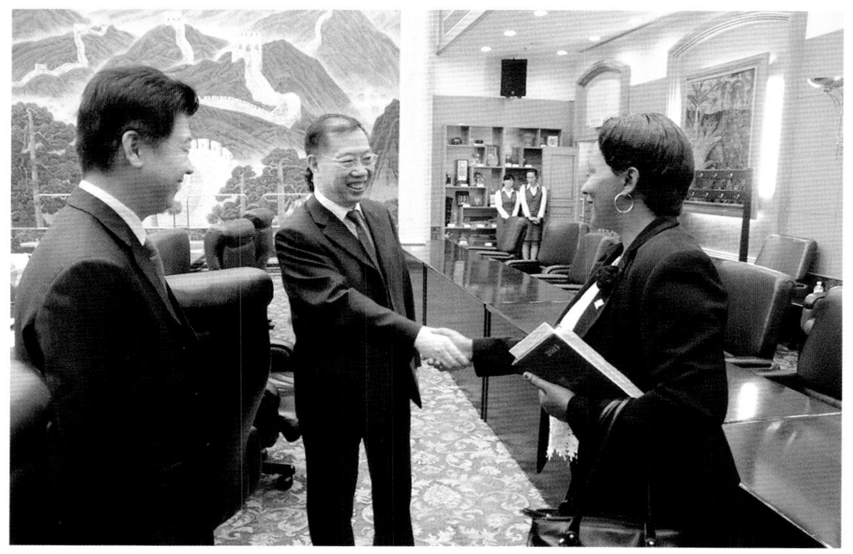

Vice Health Minister Huang Jiefu met with Burundian Minister of Public Health and HIV/AIDS Control Sabine Ntakarutimana, June 28, 2011.

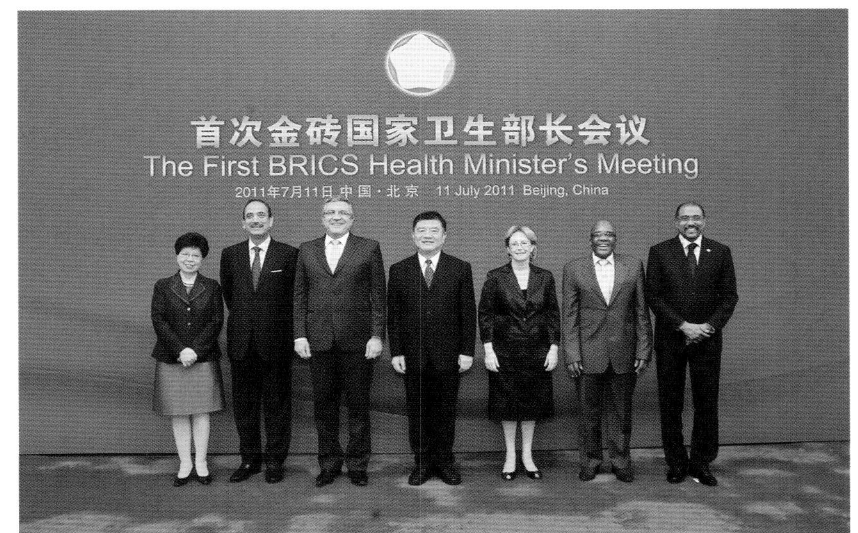

Health ministers from five countries, Director-General of the WHO and Executive Director of UNAIDS, who attended the First BRICS Health Minister's Meeting, had a group photo taken at Diaoyutai State Guesthouse, July 11, 2011.

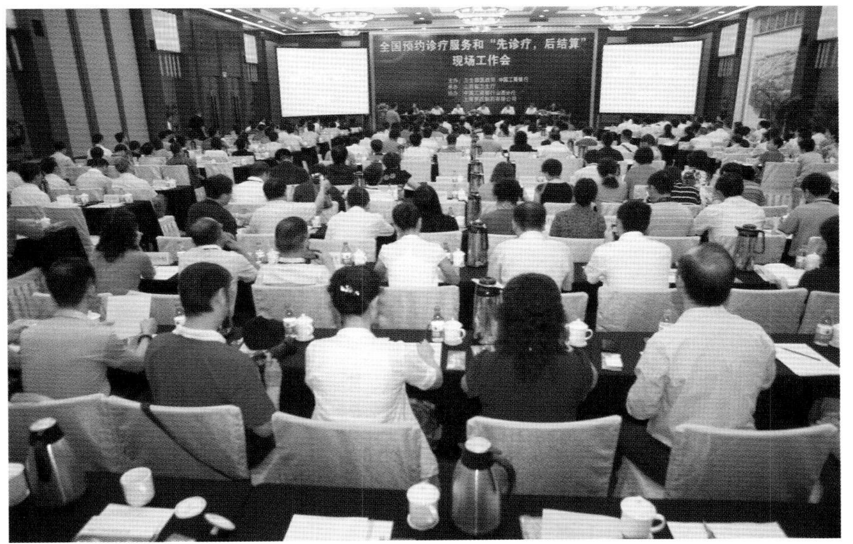

The national on-the-spot meeting on the service of diagnosis and treatment by appointment and "diagnosis and treatment first, accounts settlement second" was held in Taiyuan, capital city of Shanxi, August 18, 2011.

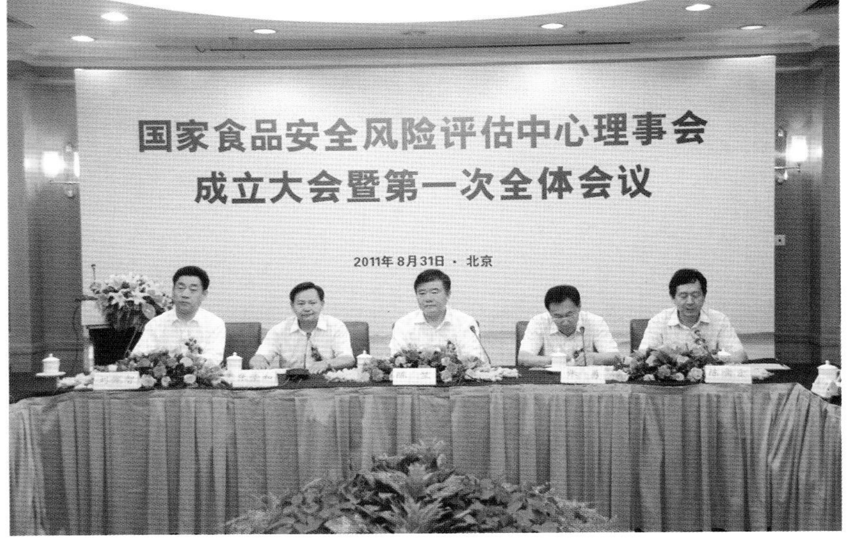

The Inaugurating Meeting for the Council of China National Center for Food Safety Risk Assessment was held in Beijing, August 31, 2011.

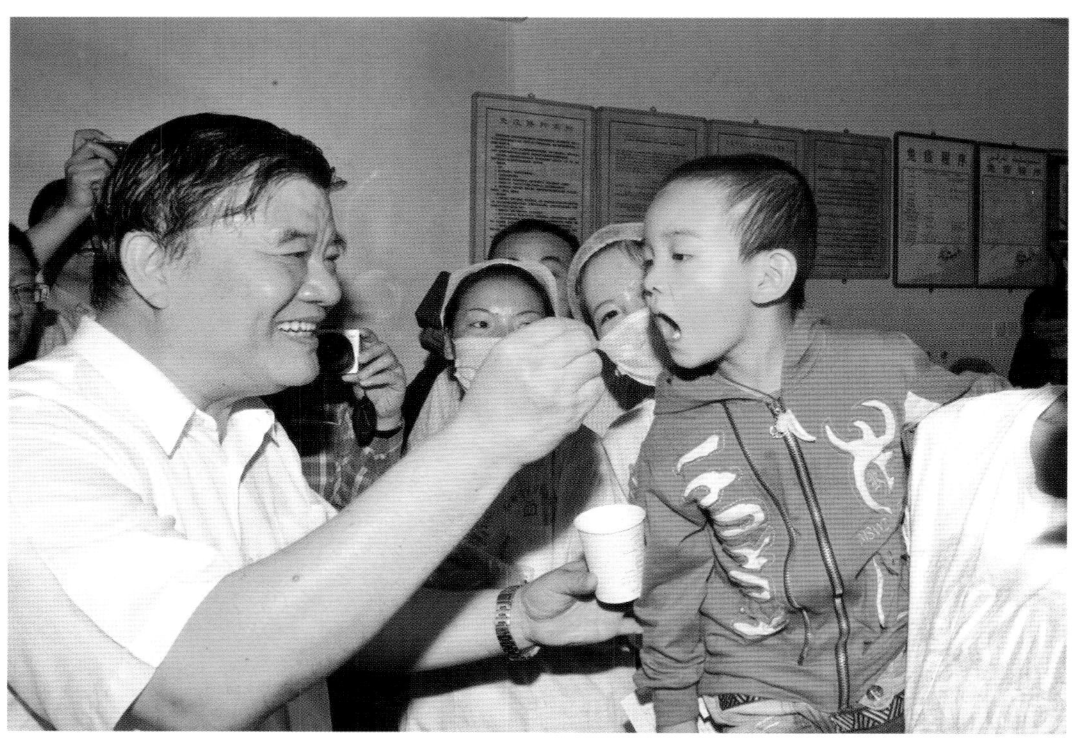

Health Minister Chen Zhu conducted survey and research at Hotan Prefecture in Xinjiang, September 8, 2011. The picture shows Chen Zhu feeding a baby on sugar pills.

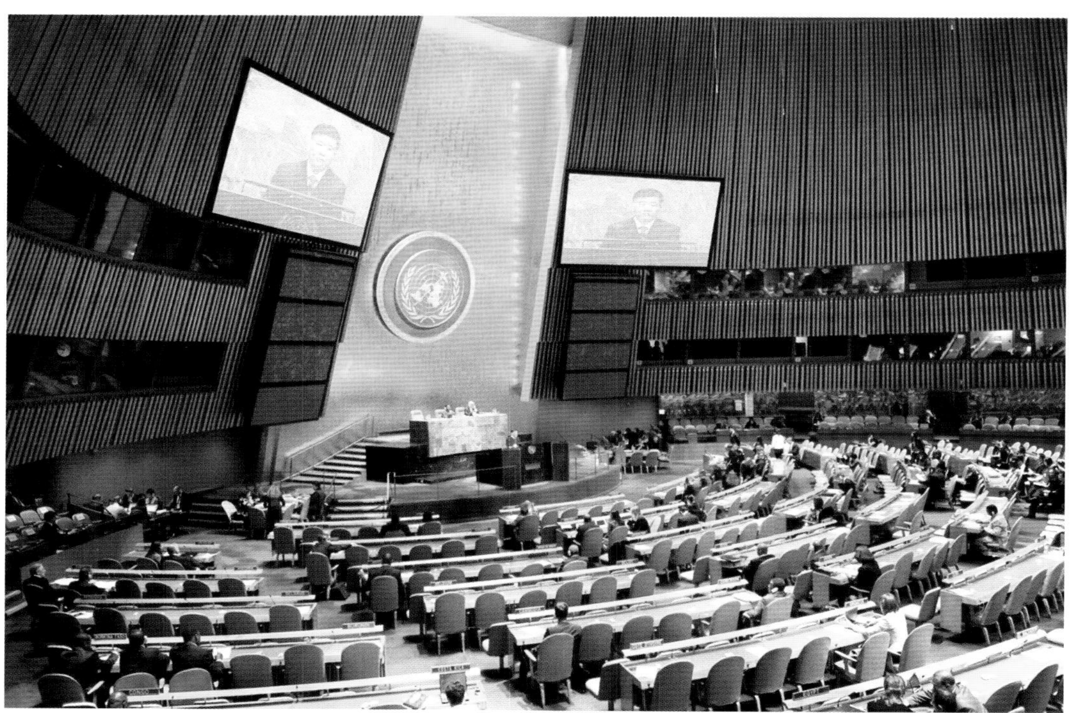

Health Minister Chen Zhu addressed the high-level meeting during the 66th Session of UN General Assembly, September 19, 2011.

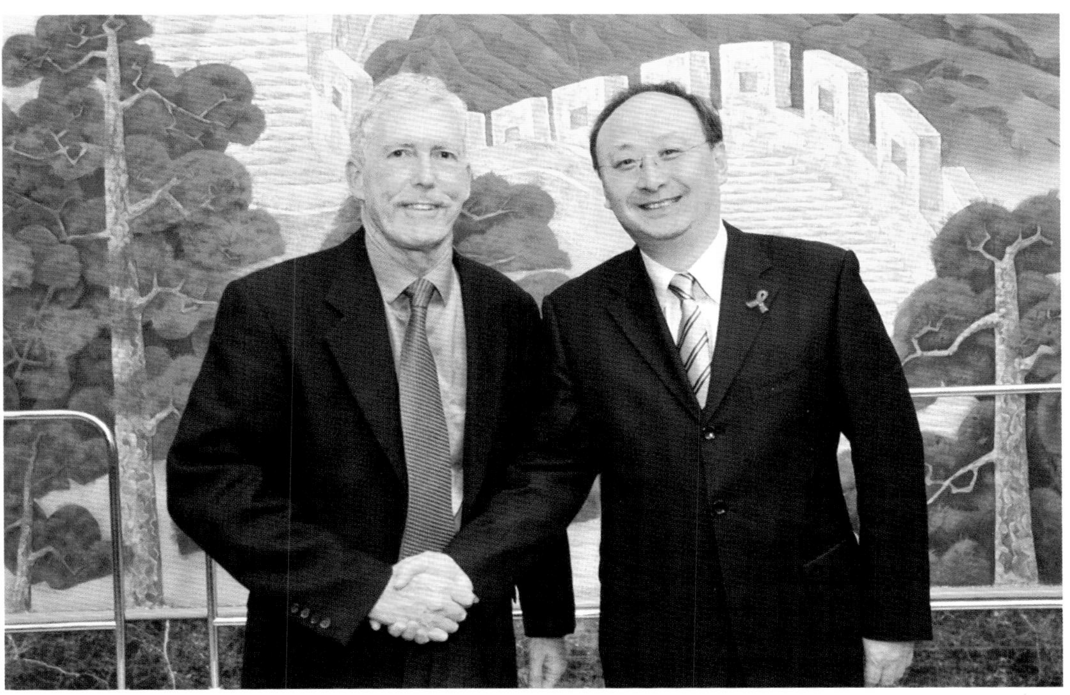

Vice Health Minister Yin Li met with Executive Director of Global Health Program under the Bill & Melinda Gates Foundation Chris Wilson, September 20, 2011.

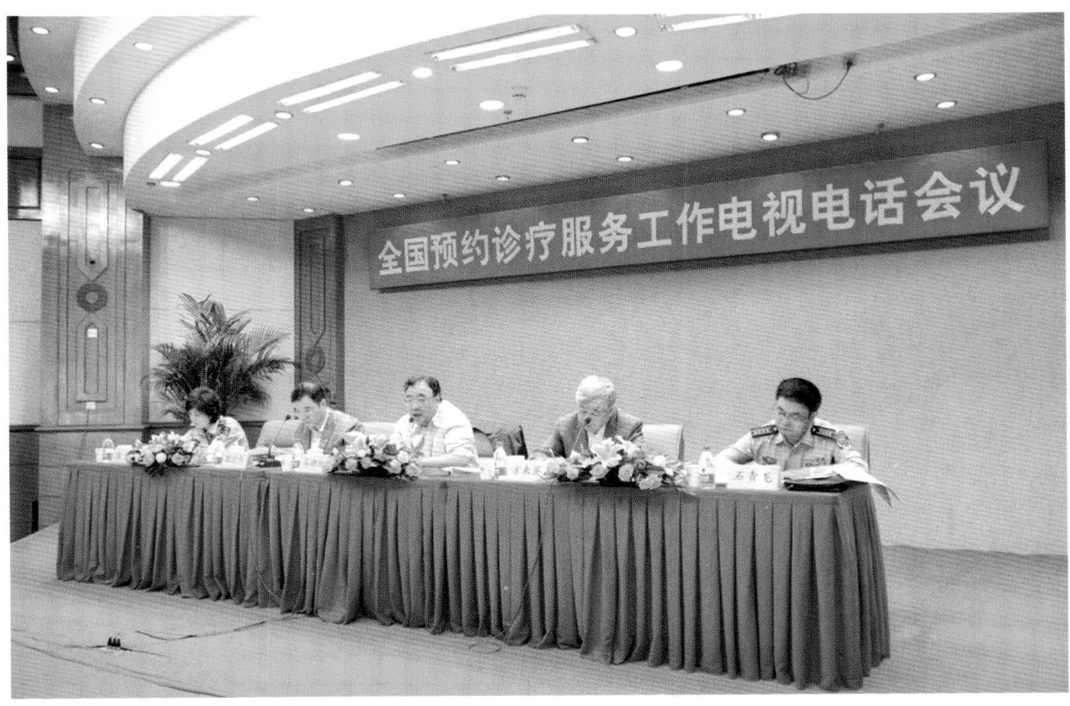

The National Video-and Teleconference on the Service of Diagnosis and Treatment by Appointment was held in Beijing, September 22, 2011.

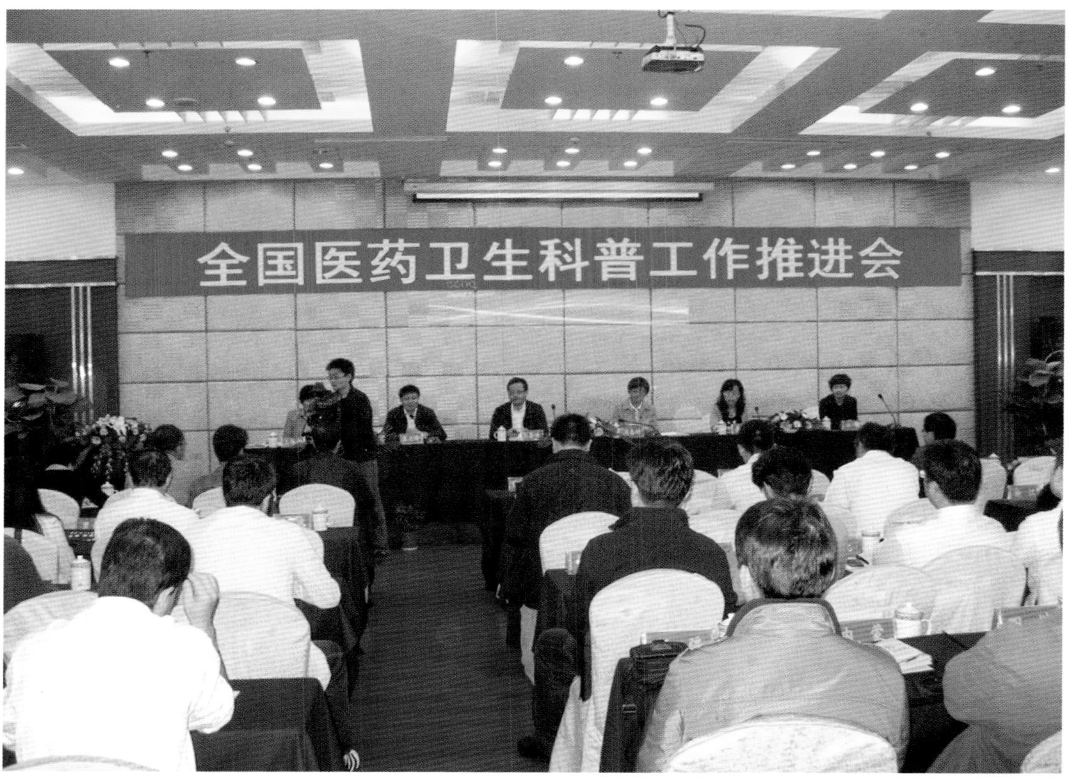

The Ministry of Health held the National Conference on Promoting Medical and Health Popularization in Guizhou, September 29-30, 2011.

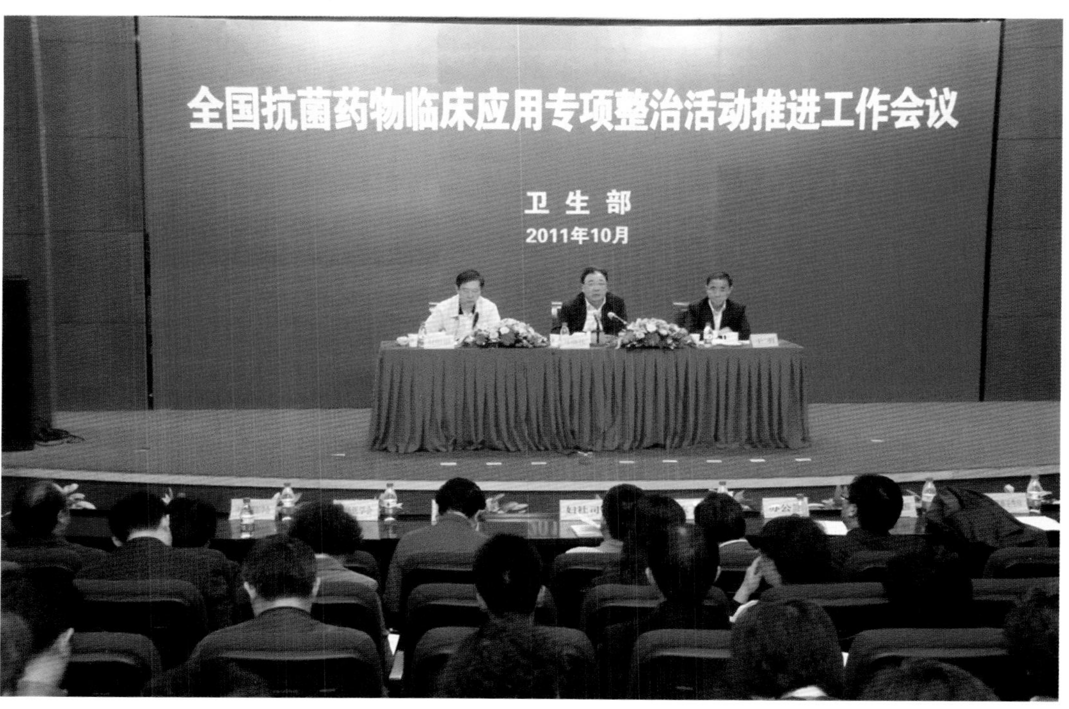

The Ministry of Health held the National Conference on Specific Rectification for Clinical Use of Antibacterial Agents in Beijing in September 2011.

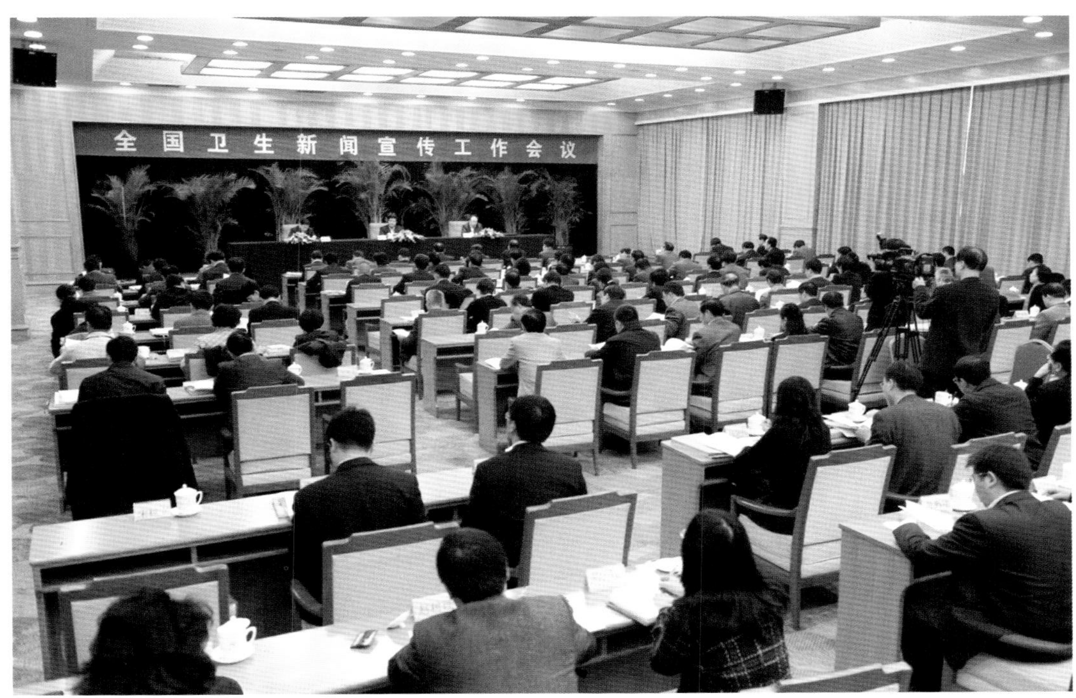

The National Conference on Health News and Propaganda was held in Beijing, November 5, 2011.

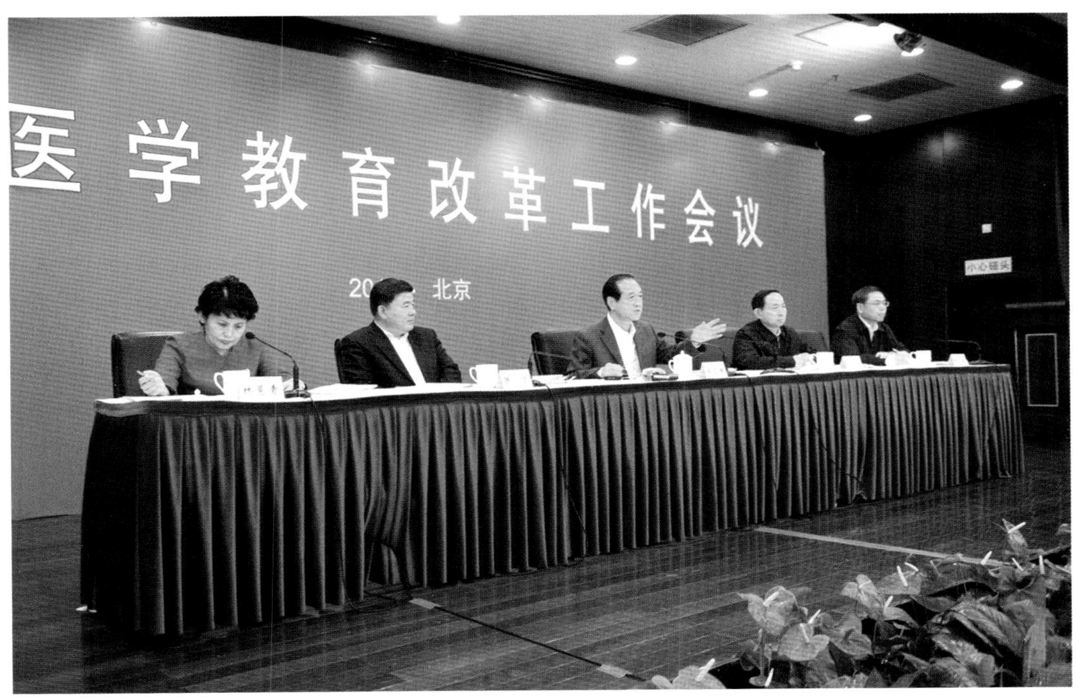

The Ministry of Health and the Ministry of Education jointly held the National Conference on the Reform of Medical Education, November 6, 2011.

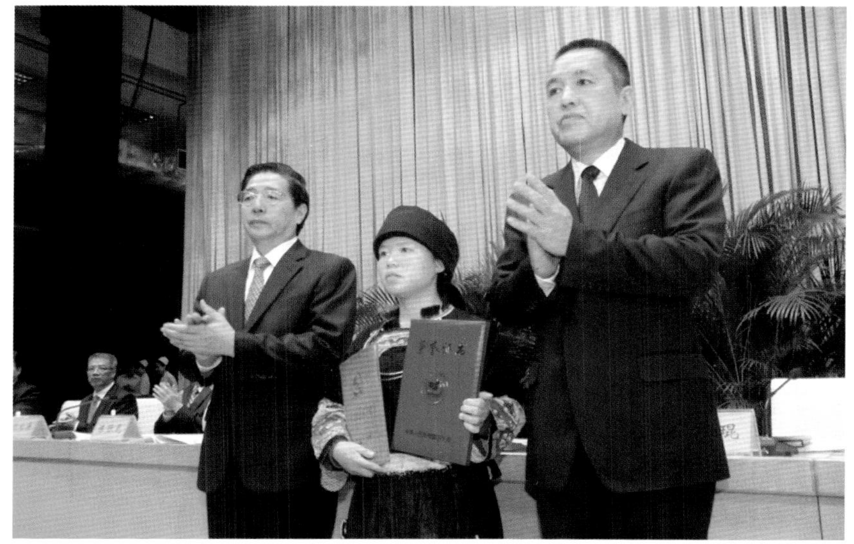

Secretary of the Party Leadership Group and Vice Minister of the Ministry of Health Zhang Mao presented the Certificate of Honor to Meng Chaoying, dependent of village doctor Lan Yun, November 23, 2011.

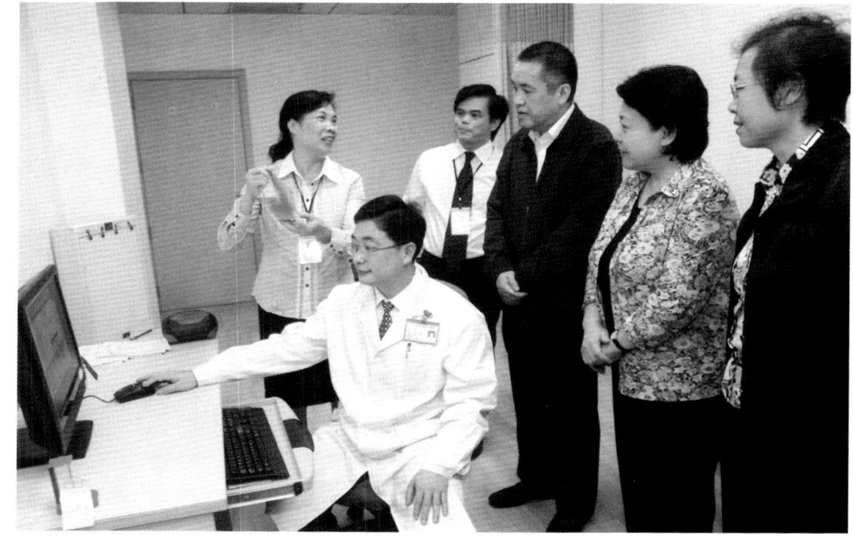

Secretary of the Party Leadership Group and Vice Minister of the Ministry of Health Zhang Mao conducted survey and research on medical reform in Guangxi, November 24, 2011.

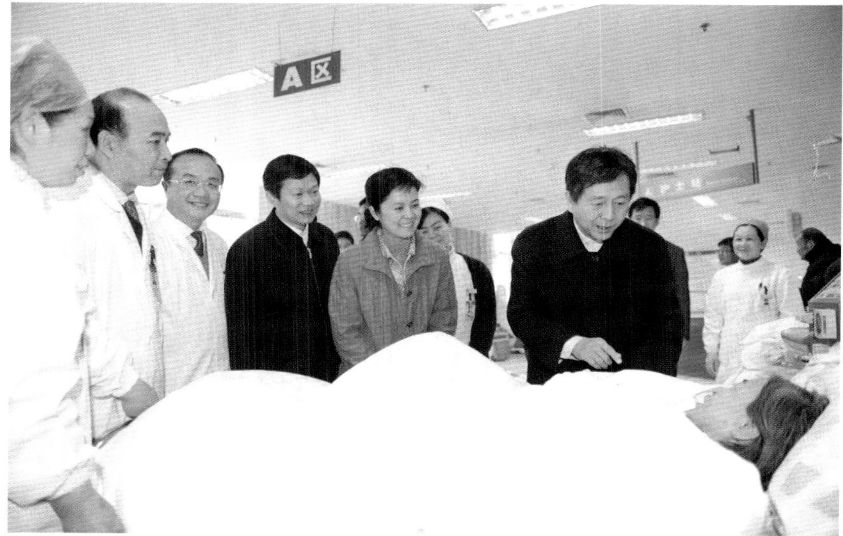

Vice Health Minister Chen Xiaohong inspected the free hemodialysis treatment for uremia in Jiangxi Provincial People's Hospital, December 15, 2011.

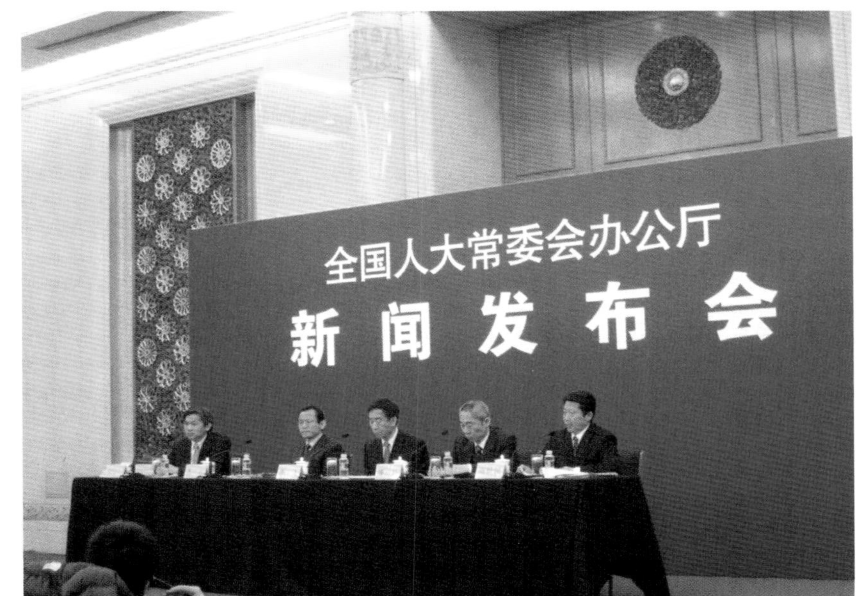

The Ministry of Health attended the Press Conference for the new *Law of the People's Republic of China on the Prevention and Treatment of Occupational Diseases* held by the General Office of the NPC Standing Committee, December 31, 2011.

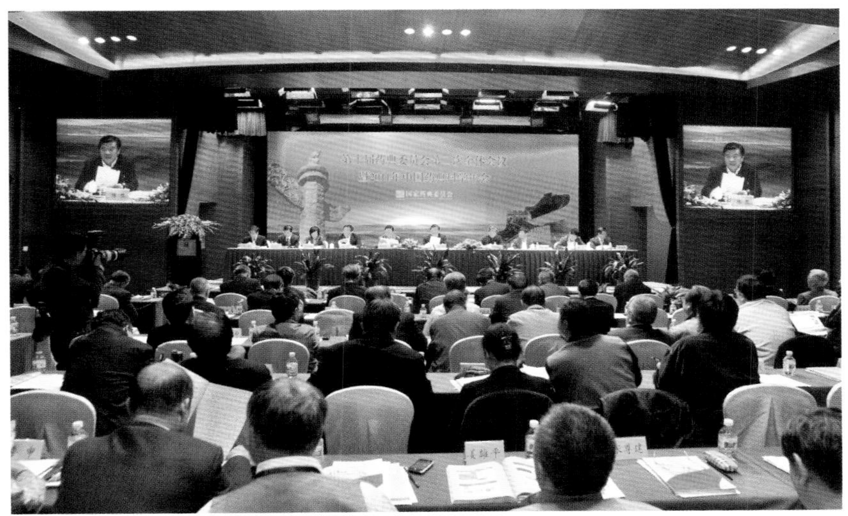

Chinese Pharmacopoeia Commission held the 2nd Plenary Session of the 10th Chinese Pharmacopoeia Commission and 2011 ChP Scientific Annual Meeting in Beijing, November 15-16, 2011.

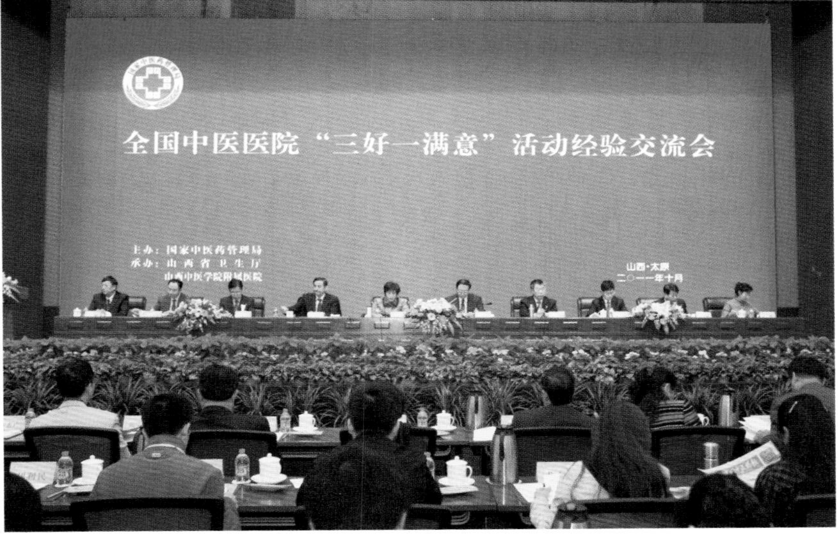

The National Experience Exchange Meeting for Good Service, Good Quality, Good Medical Ethics and Public Satisfaction of Hospitals of Traditional Chinese Medicine was held in Shanxi, October 28, 2011.

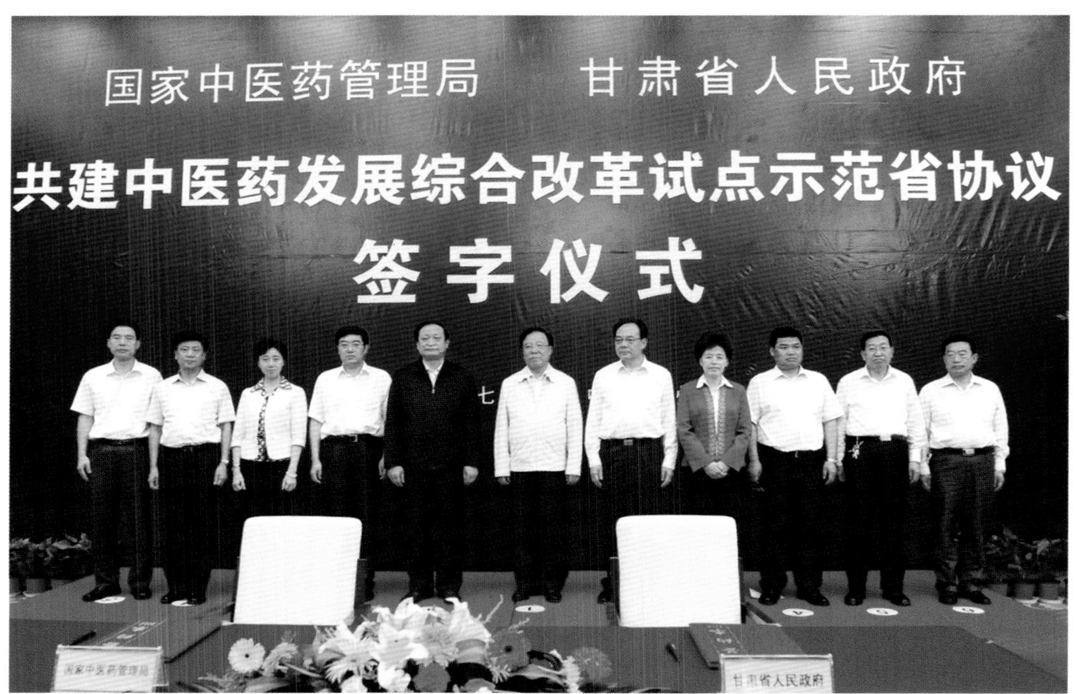

State Administration of Traditional Chinese Medicine and Gansu Provincial People's Government signed the agreement on co-establishing the demonstration province for the comprehensive reform pilot of the development of Traditional Chinese Medicine, July 5, 2011. Gansu became the 1st Chinese demonstration province for the comprehensive reform pilot of the development of TCM.

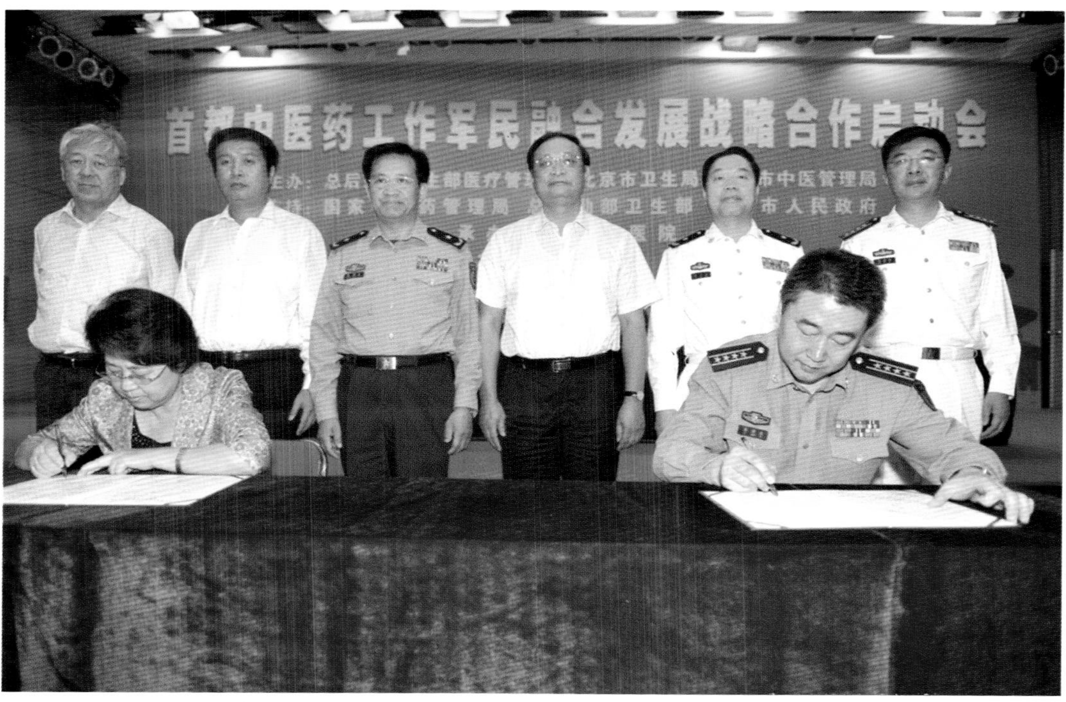

The Medical Administration Bureau of the Health Department of PLA General Logistics and Beijing Municipal Administration of Traditional Chinese Medicine signed the framework agreement on strategic cooperation of civil-military integrative development in the capital's work of TCM, September 28, 2011.

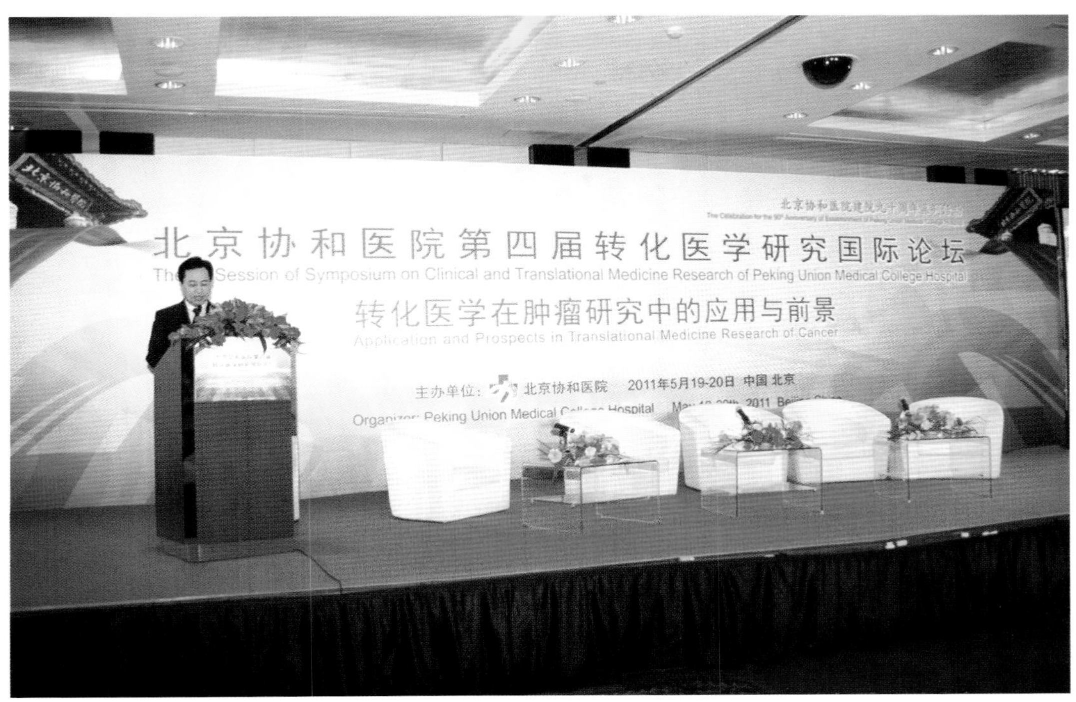

The 4th Session of Symposium on Clinical and Translational Medicine Research of Peking Union Medical College Hospital was held in Beijing, May 19-20, 2011.

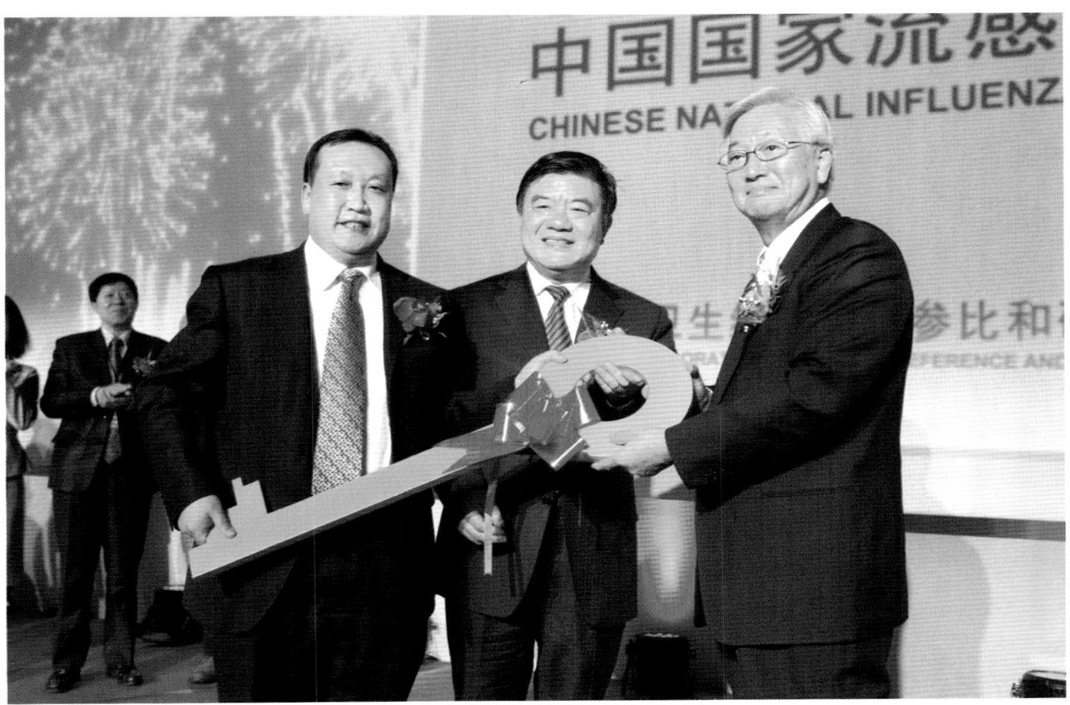

WHO Collaborating Centre for Reference and Research on Influenza under China-CDC was inaugurated in Beijing, March 14-16, 2011.

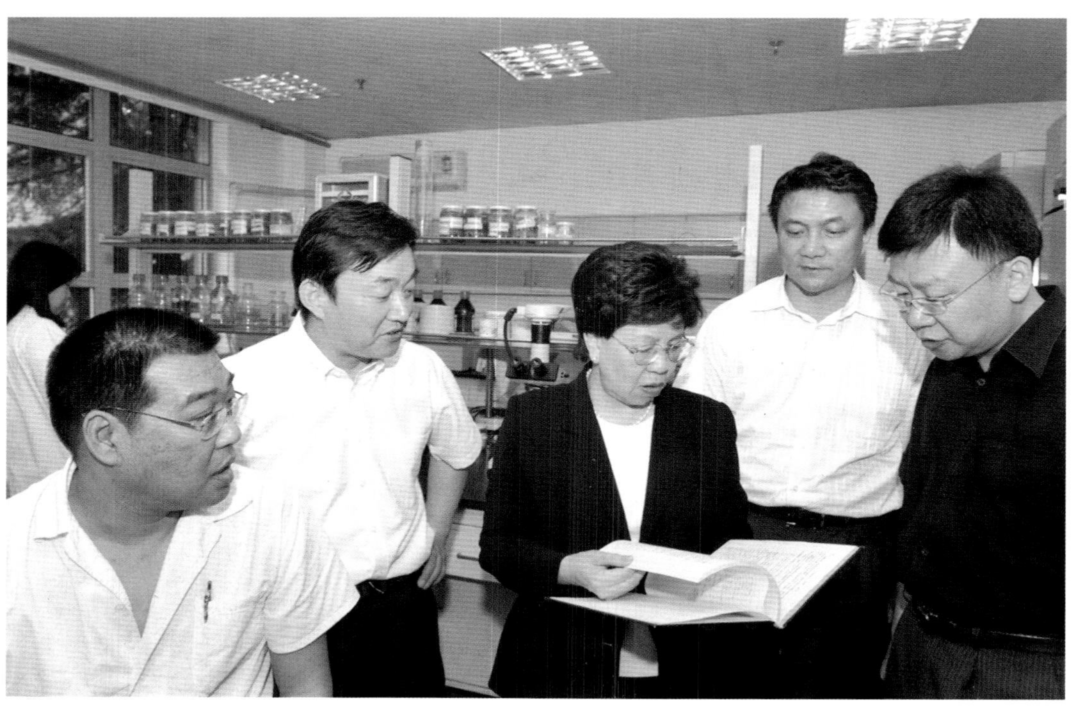

WHO Director-General Dr. Margaret Chan visited China-CDC, July 15, 2011.

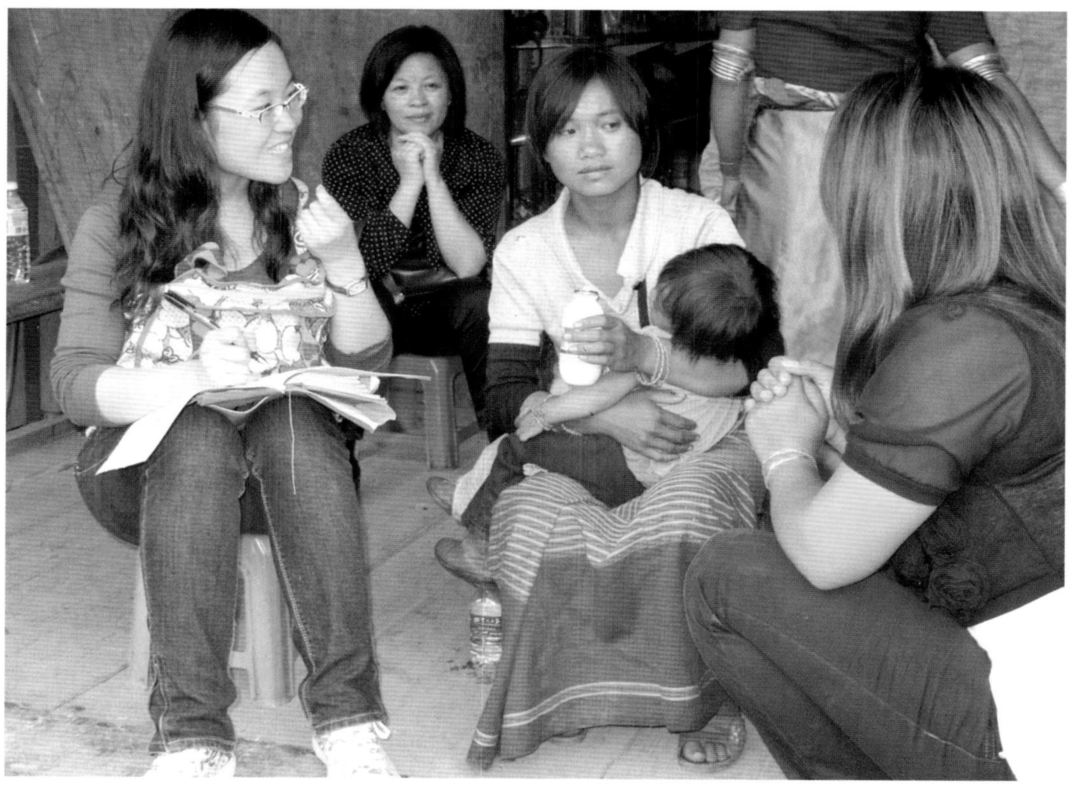

Experts from National Center for Women and Children's Health under China-CDC conducted a questionnaire survey on the causes and influential factors of infant mortality, October 23, 2011.

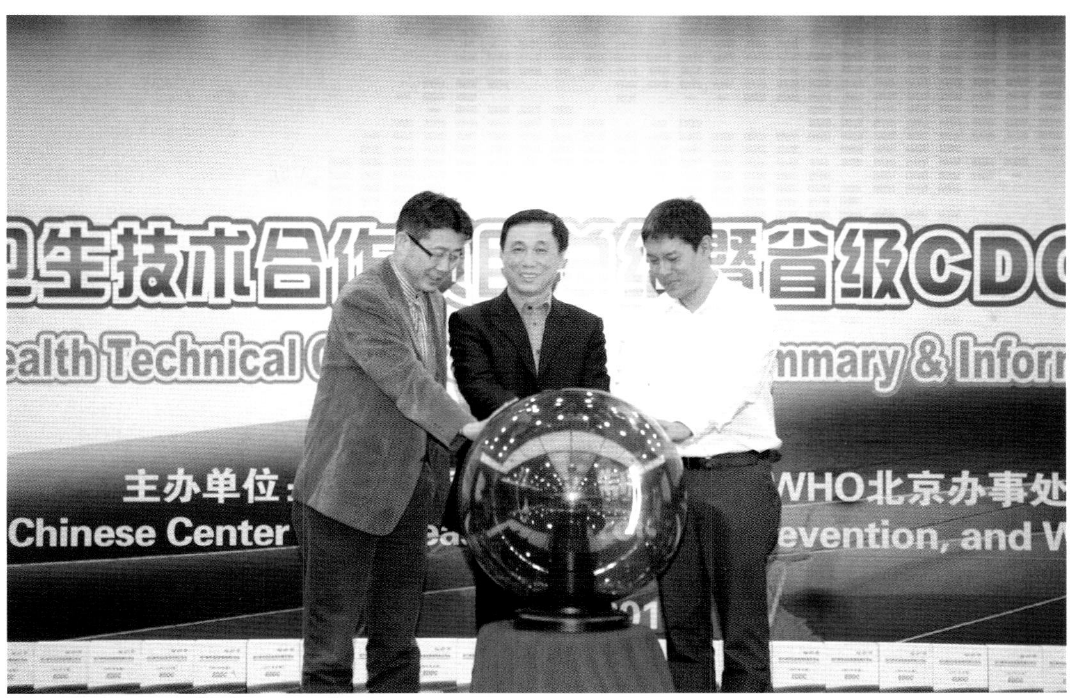

China-CDC issued Chinese-English edition of the cloud platform for dynamic data acquisition of epidemiological survey which was developed independently in December 2011.

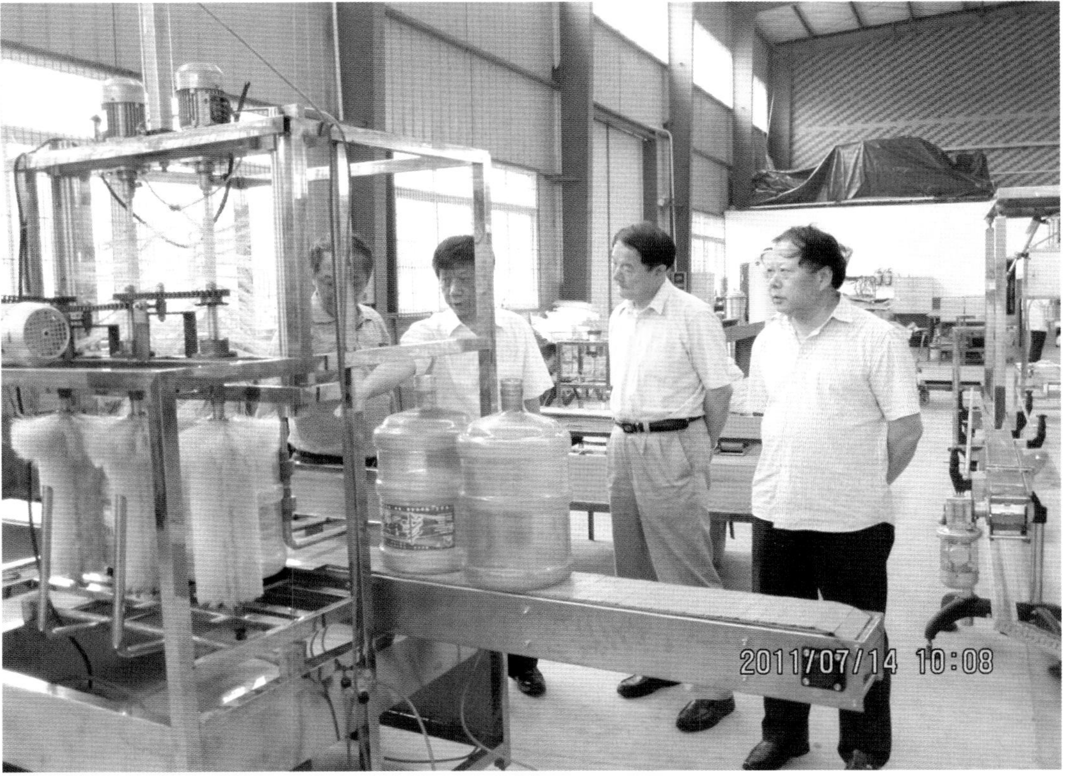

Director of National Center for Health Inspection and Supervision under the Ministry of Health Wang Suyang led his group to conduct a spot check on water-related products nationwide in July 2011.

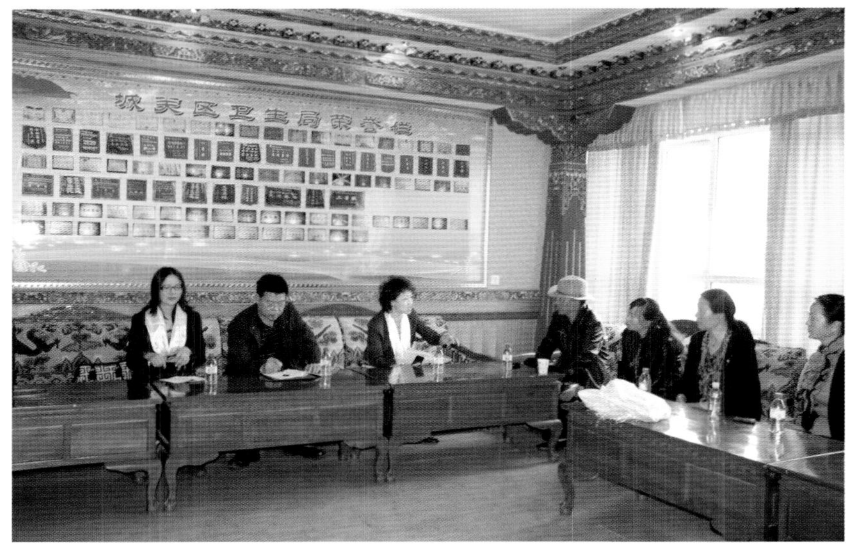

Deputy Director of National Center for Health Inspection and Supervision under the Ministry of Health Lu Jiang led his group to conduct survey and research on assistance to Tibet in September 2011.

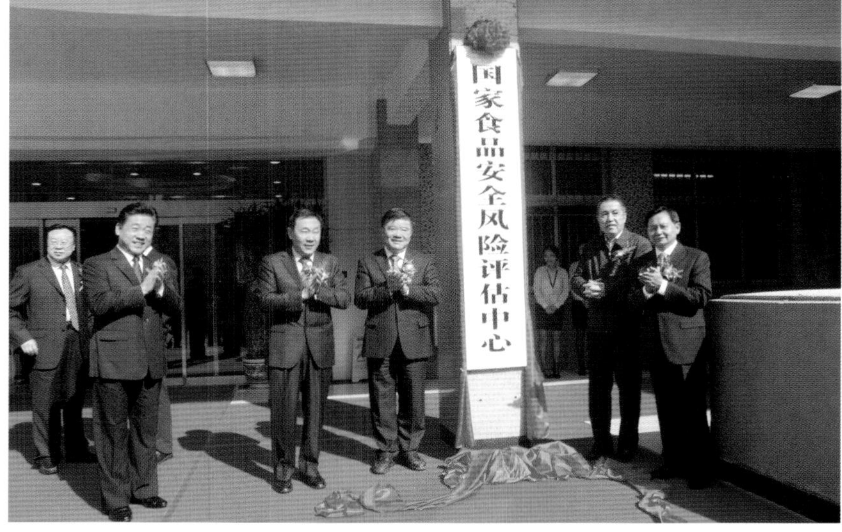

The Food Safety Commission Office of the State Council, the State Commission Office for Public Sector Reform (SCOPSR) and officials of the Ministry of Health inaugurated China National Center for Food Safety Risk Assessment, October 13, 2011.

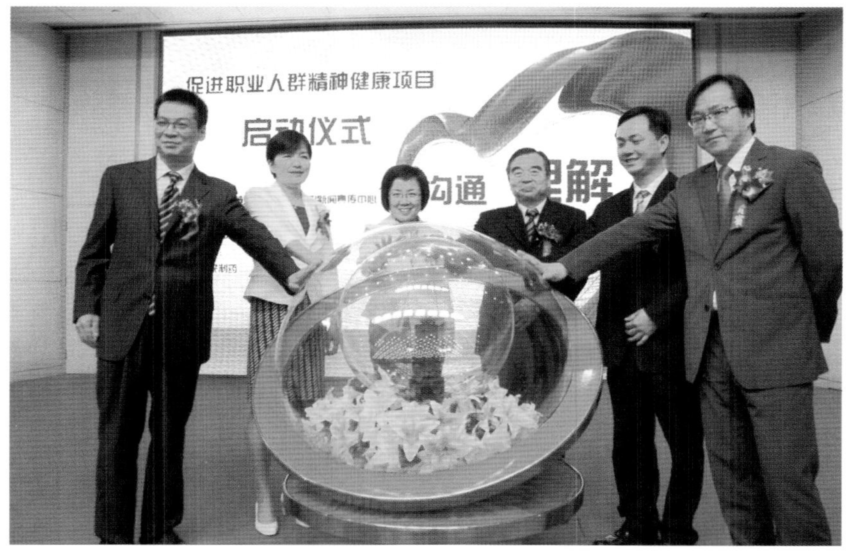

Chinese Center for Health Education (News Center of the Ministry of Health) held the Launching Ceremony of the Program for Promoting the Mental Health of Occupational Population with the Theme of Communication, Understanding and Caring in April 2011.

Chinese Center for Health Education (News Center of the Ministry of Health) held the Launching Ceremony of Balance between Eating and Exercising, Moving toward Health, an incentive plan for Chinese Health Knowledge Dissemination, June 10, 2011.

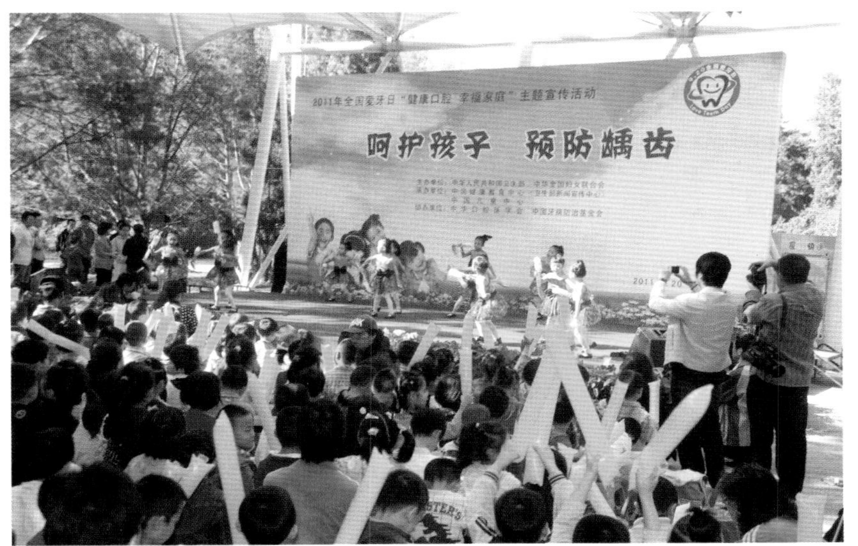

Chinese Center for Health Education (News Center of the Ministry of Health) hosted the campaign for China's Teeth Care Day with the theme of Oral Health, Happy Family, September 20, 2011.

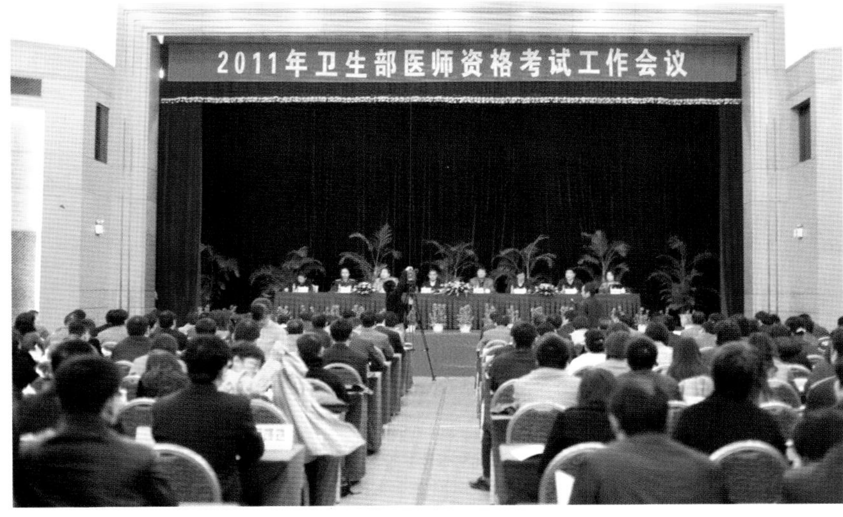

The Meeting of the Ministry of Health on 2011 Examination for Doctors' Qualifications was held in Nanning, capital city of Guangxi Zhuang Autonomous Region, March 3-4, 2011.

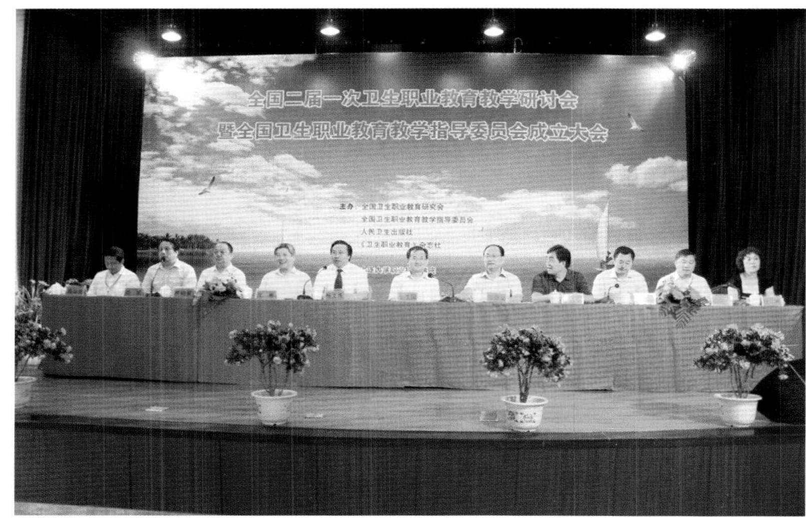

The Inaugurating Meeting for the Teaching Instruction Committee of National Health Vocational Education was held in Dalian, July 2-3, 2011.

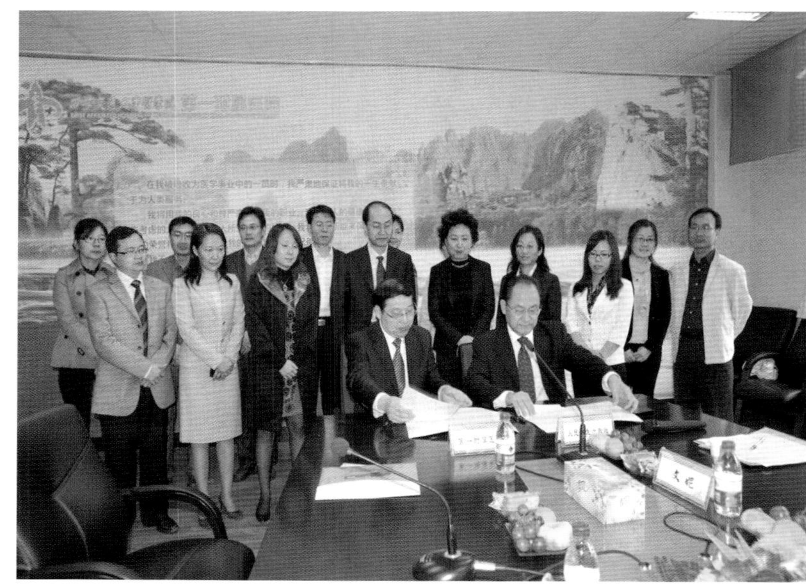

People's Medical Publishing House Co., Ltd held the signing ceremony for the inauguration of Xi'an Translation and Publishing Center under People's Medical Publishing House Co., Ltd, September 28, 2011.

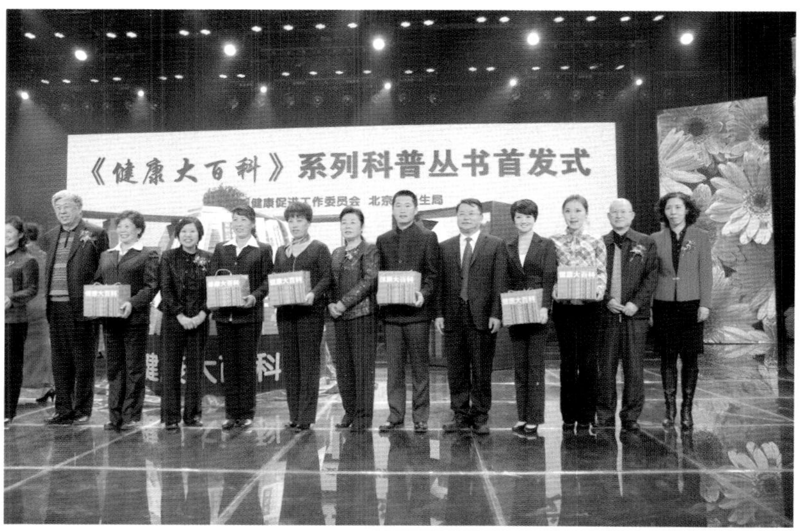

The news conference on a series of popular science books of *Health Encyclopedia* was held in Beijing, December 29, 2011.

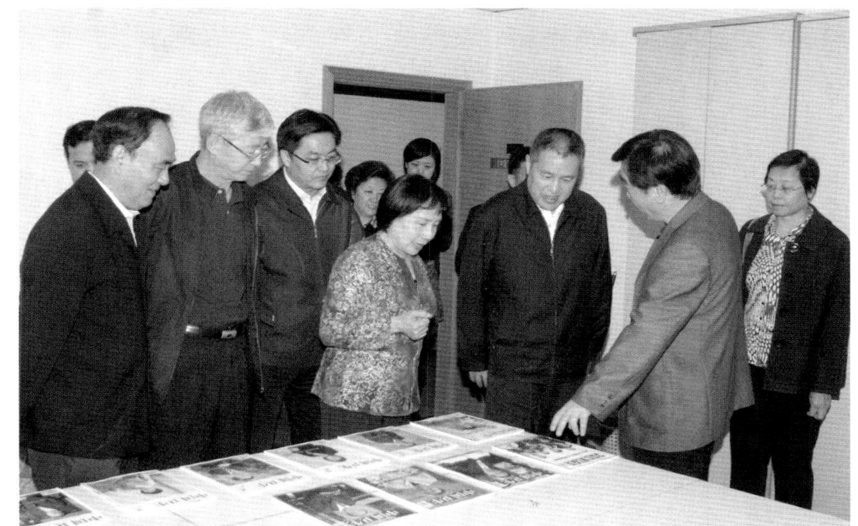

Secretary of the Party Leadership Group and Vice Minister of the Ministry of Health Zhang Mao paid an inspection visit to the editorial department of Chinese Health, April 21, 2011.

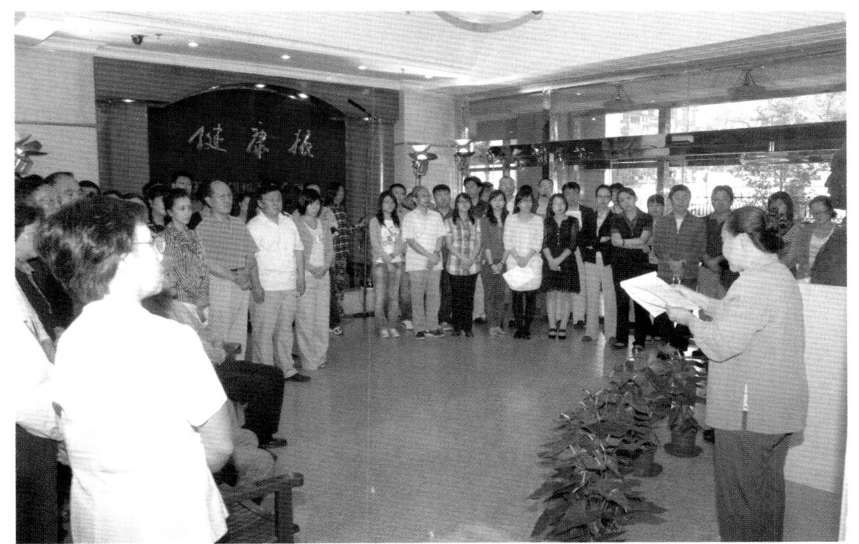

The statue of General He Cheng who was the originator of Health News was inaugurated at the office of Health news, September 9, 2011.

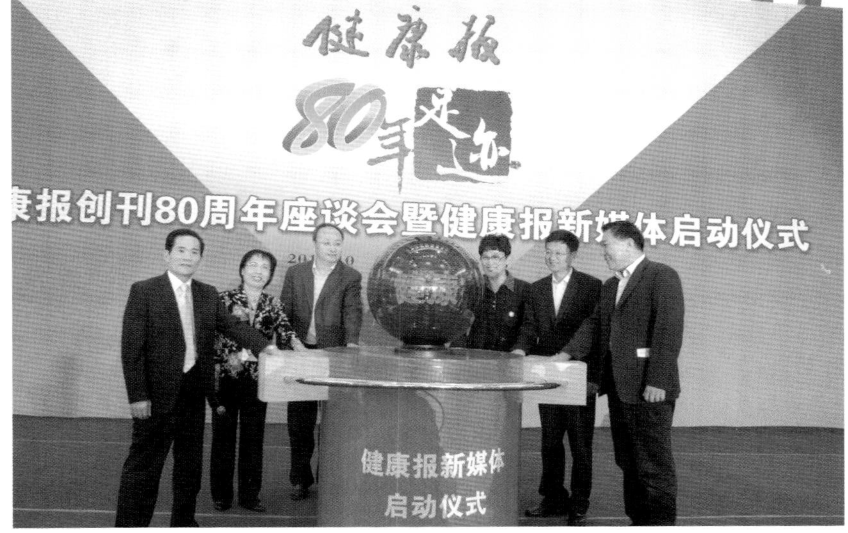

The symposium to mark the 80th anniversary of Health News and the launching ceremony of the new media for Health News was held at Diaoyutai State Guesthouse, October 19, 2011.

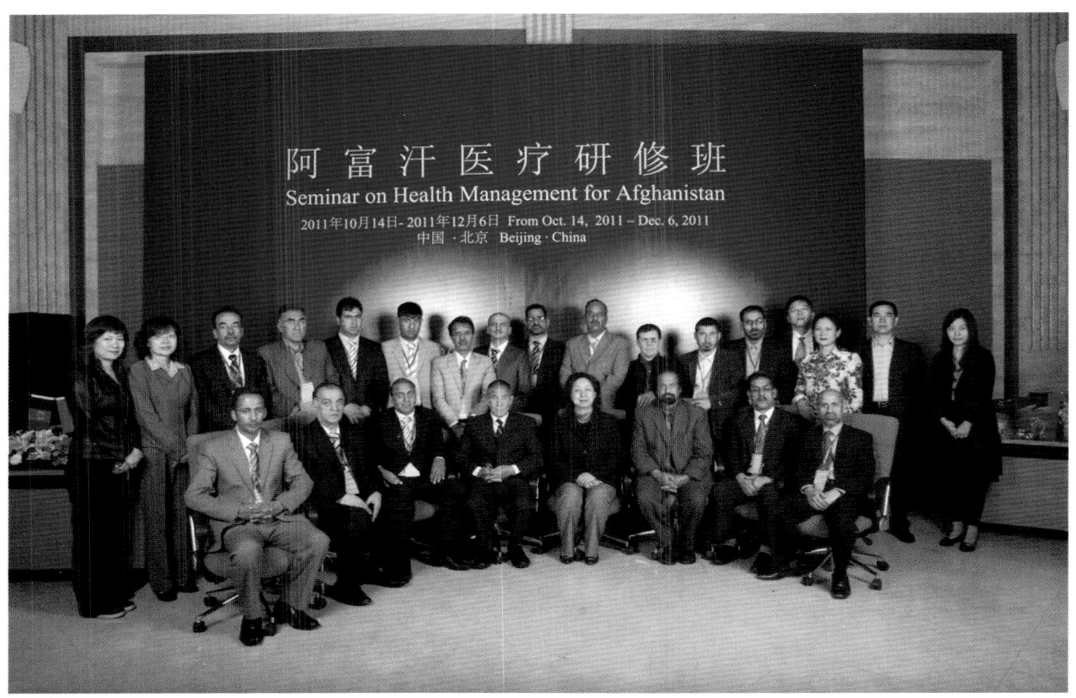

Seminar on Health Management for Afghanistan was held in Beijing, October 14-December 16, 2011.

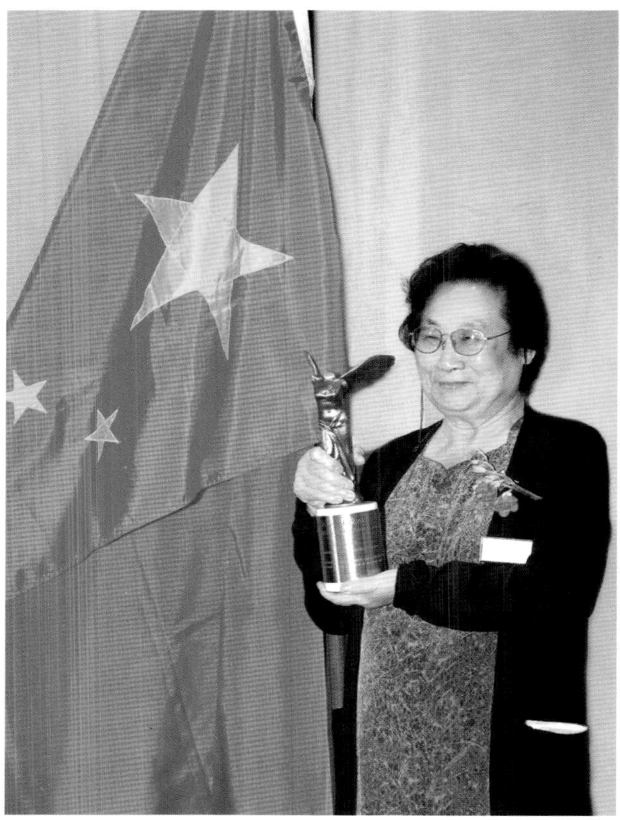

Tenured and lead researcher of China Academy of TCM Tu Youyou won 2011 Lasker Medical Research Awards, September 23, 2011.

The Service Center for Human Talent Exchange of the Ministry of Health held the 1st training class for the national directors of health bureaus at the county level, September 17, 2011.

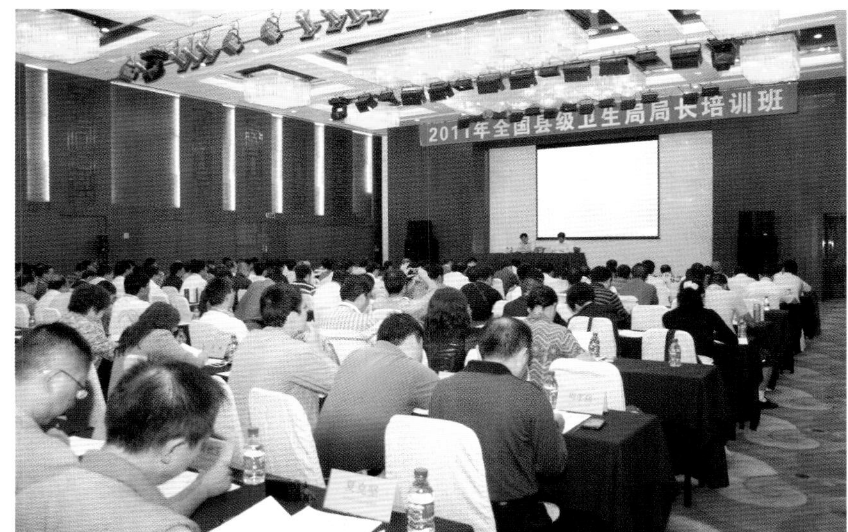

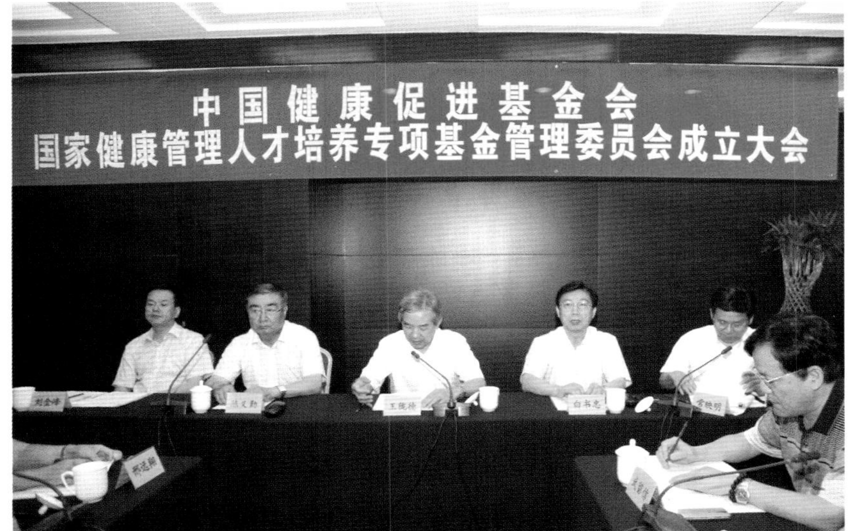

The regulatory commission of special fund for the training of national health management talent was inaugurated in Beijing, June 19, 2011.

International Symposium on Human Resources for Health of Health Emergency Preparedness and Response in Asia-Pacific Region was held in Nanning, capital city of Guangxi, May 21-22, 2011.

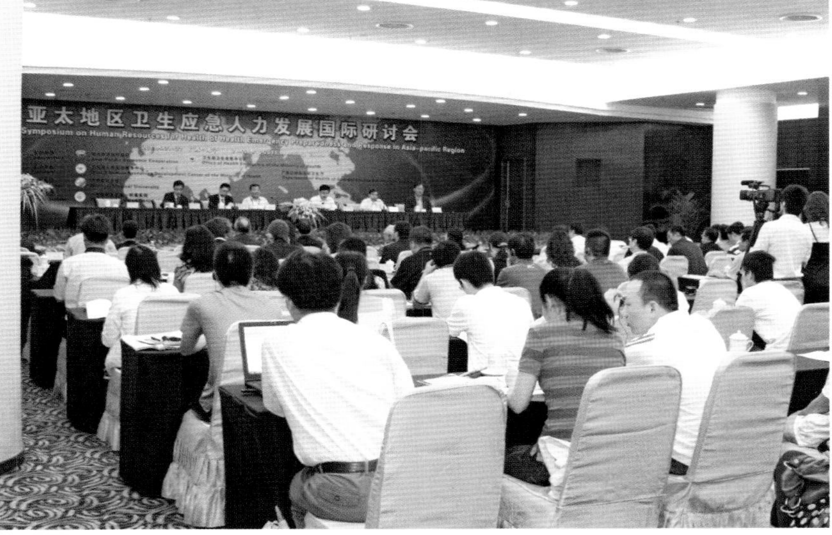

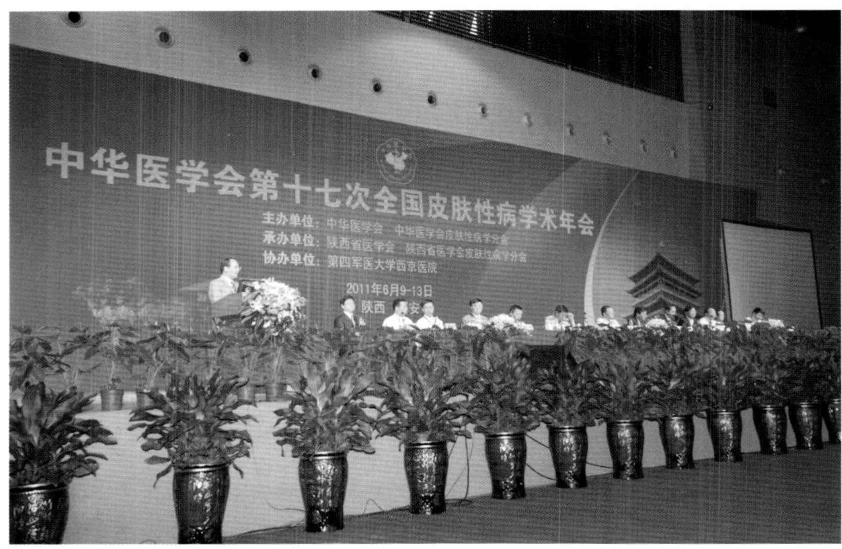

The 17th National Academic Annual Conference of Chinese Medical Association (CMA) for Dermatovenerology was held in Xi'an, capital city of Shaanxi, June 9-13, 2011.

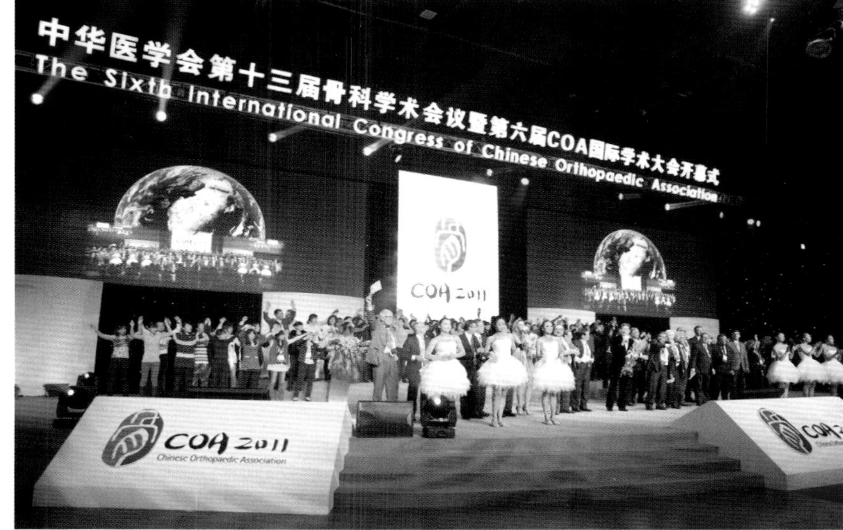

The Thirteenth Orthopedic Academic Conference of Chinese Medical Association (CMA) and the Sixth International Congress of Chinese Orthopedic Association was held in Beijing, December 1, 2011.

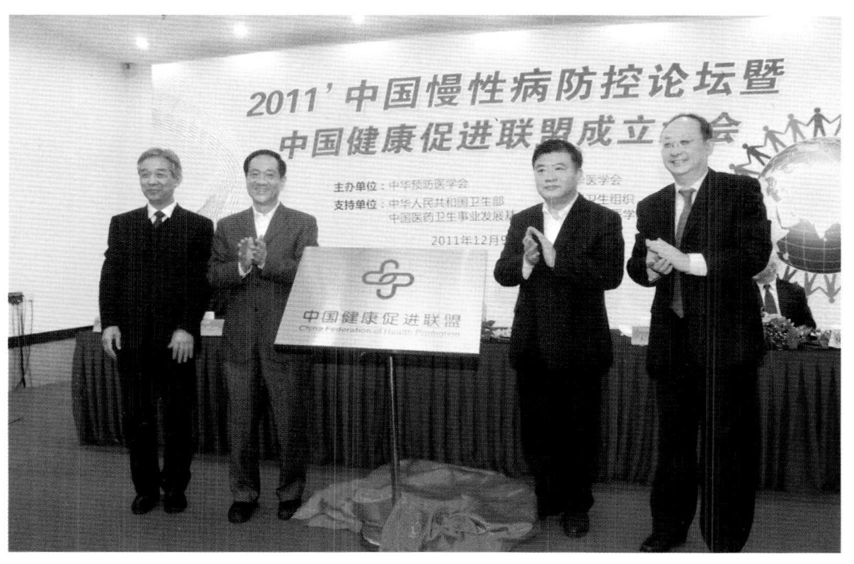

Vice Chairman of the Standing Committee of NPC Han Qide and Health Minister Chen Zhu inaugurated China Federation for Health Promotion, December 9, 2011.

(Wang Dian)

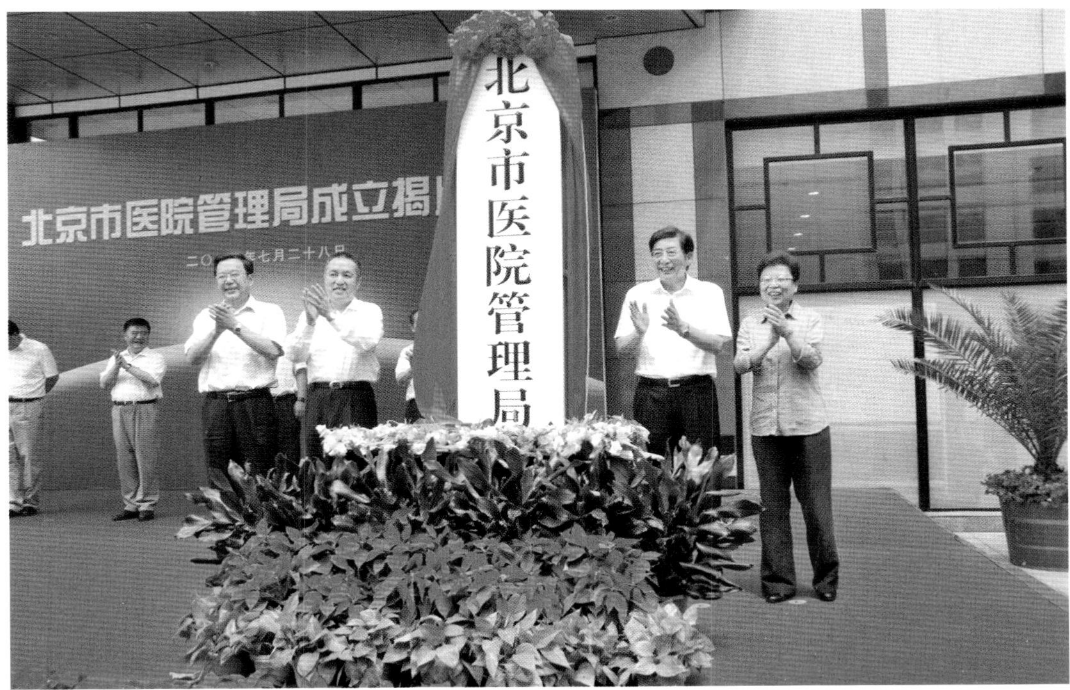

Beijing Municipal Administration of Hospitals was inaugurated, July 28, 2011. Secretary of the Party Leadership Group and Vice Minister of the Ministry of Health Zhang Mao, Beijing Mayor Guo Jinlong, Director of the Health Reform Office of the State Council Sun Zhigang and Director of Organization Department of Beijing Municipal Committee of the CPC Lu Xiwen inaugurated Beijing Municipal Administration of Hospitals.

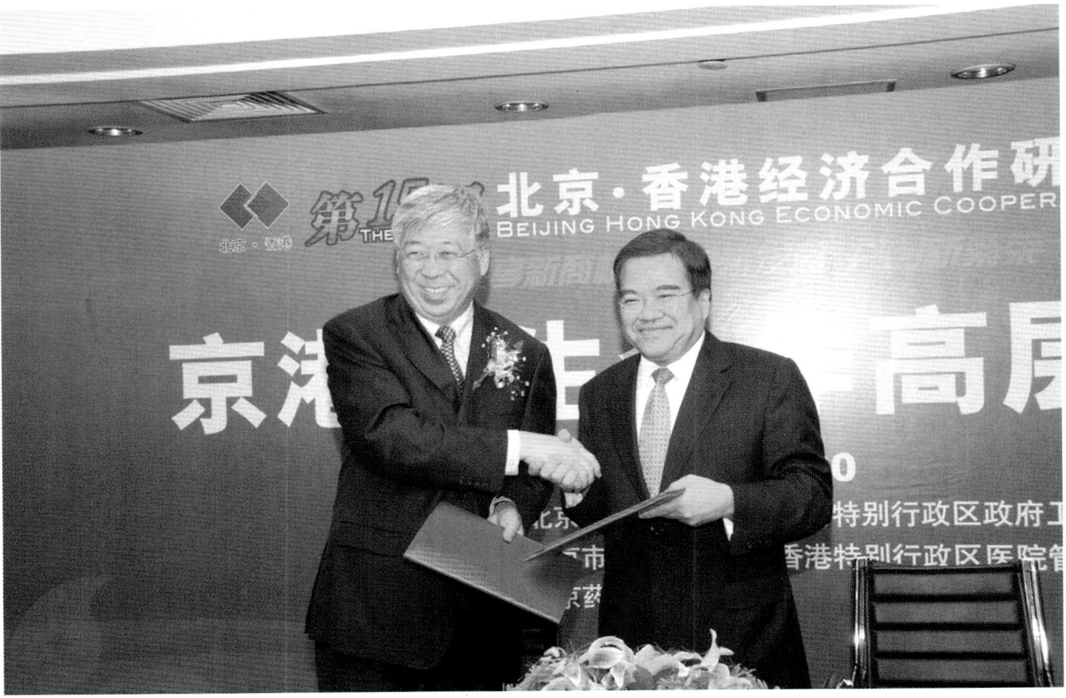

Beijing Municipal Bureau of Health and Hong Kong Department of Health co-organized the special event of health collaboration for the 15th Beijing Hong Kong Economic Cooperation Symposium and signed the Letter of Intent for Cooperation, October 20-21, 2011.

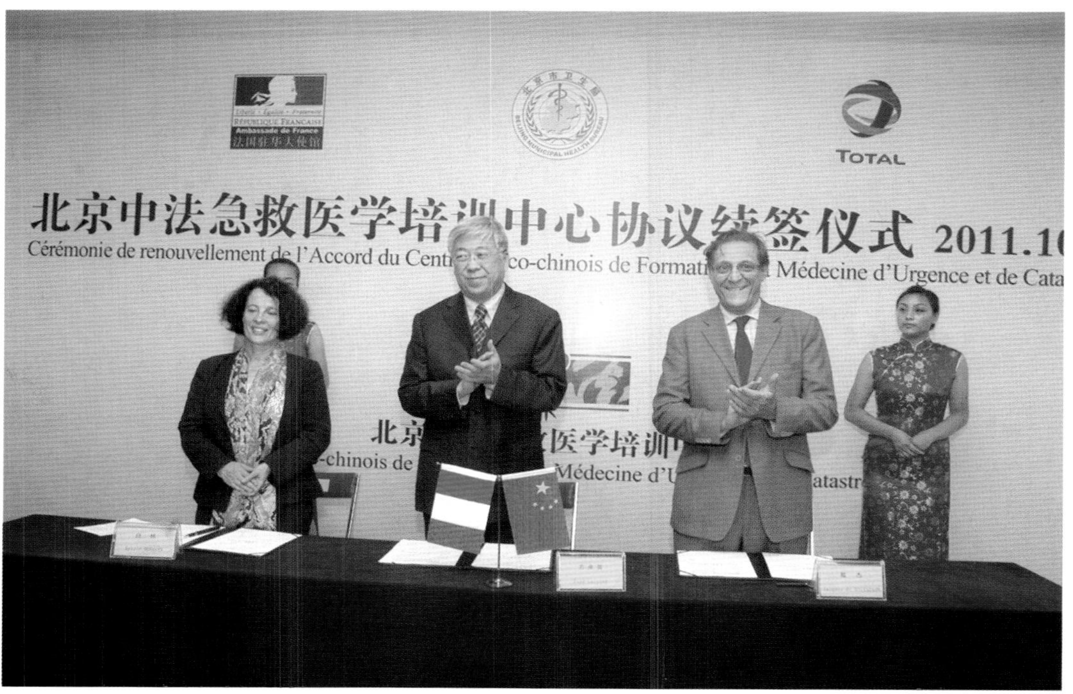

Beijing Municipal Bureau of Health and French Embassy in China and French Total Group renewed the three-year Cooperation Agreement for Beijing China-France Training Center for Emergency Medicine in October 2011.

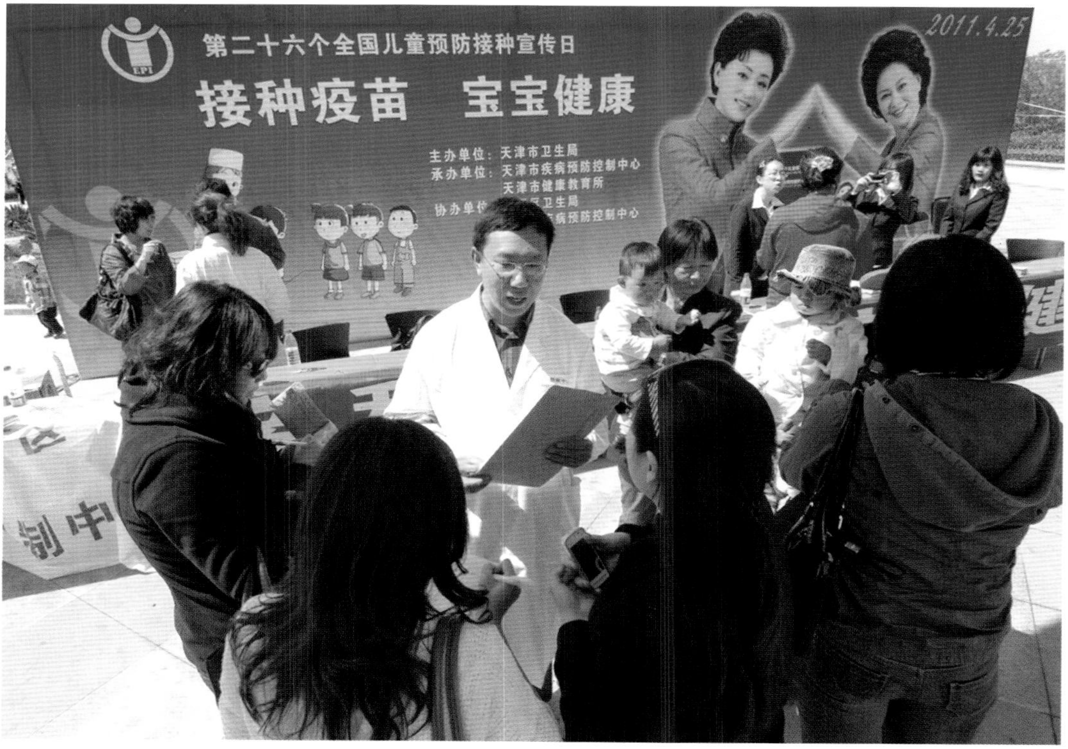

Tianjin Municipal Bureau of Health held the campaign for the 26th China Prophylactic Vaccination Day, April 25, 2011.

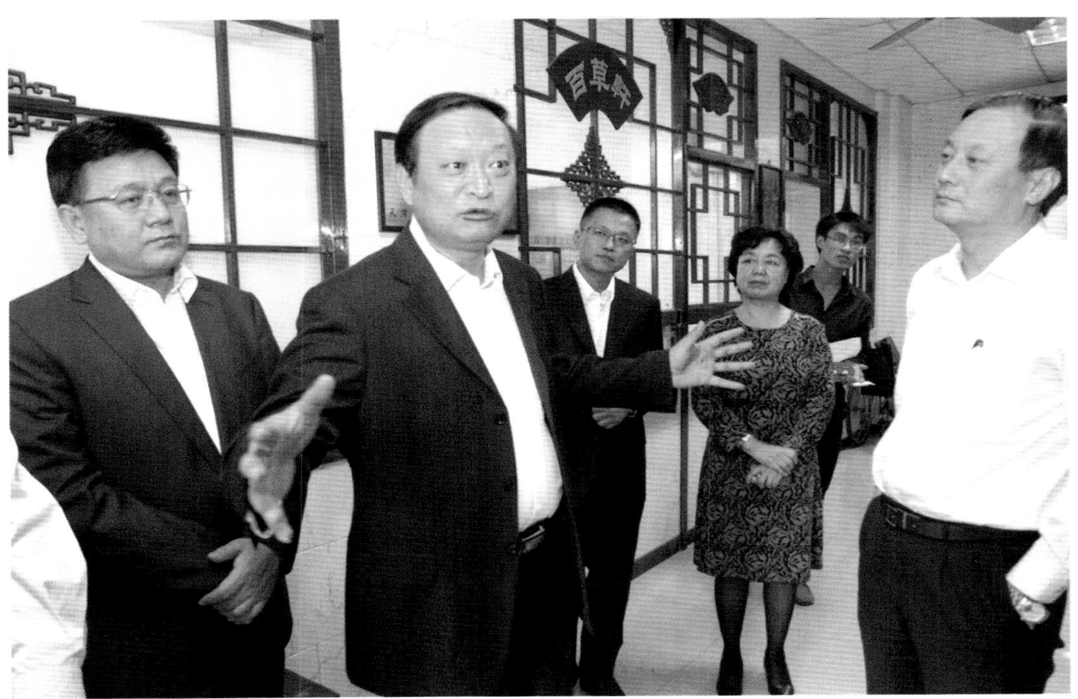

Vice Health Minister and Commissioner of the State Administration of Traditional Chinese Medicine Wang Guoqiang inspected the work of Traditional Chinese Medicine in Tianjin, September 21, 2011.

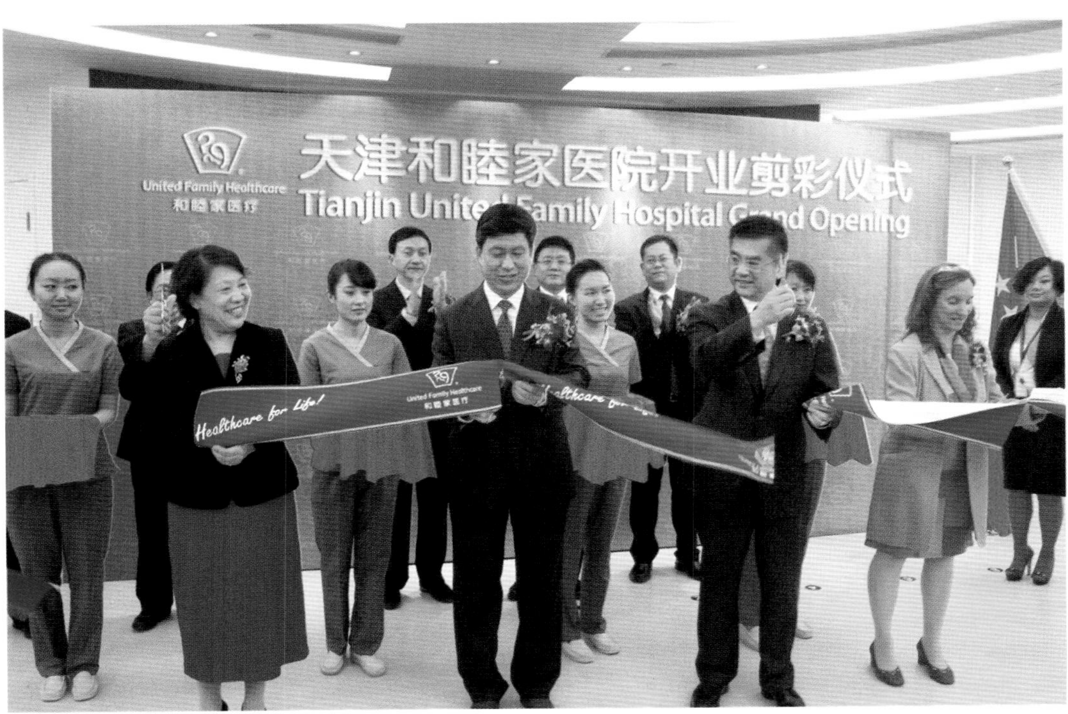

Tianjin's first foreign hospital with international standard went into formal operation, December 16, 2011.

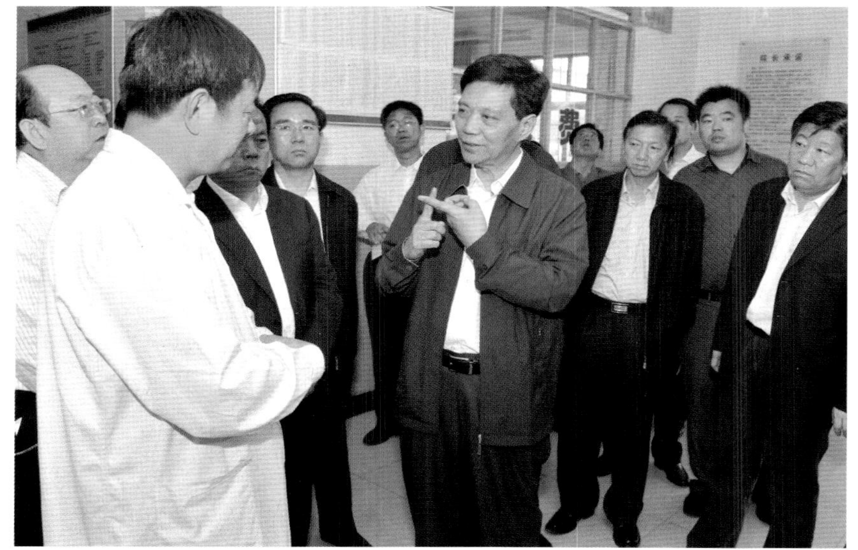

Secretary of Hebei Provincial Committee of the CPC Zhang Yunchuan learned about how the New Rural Cooperative Medical System (NCMS) and medical reform were being pushed on at the township health center of Shangbi in Handan County, May 31, 2011.

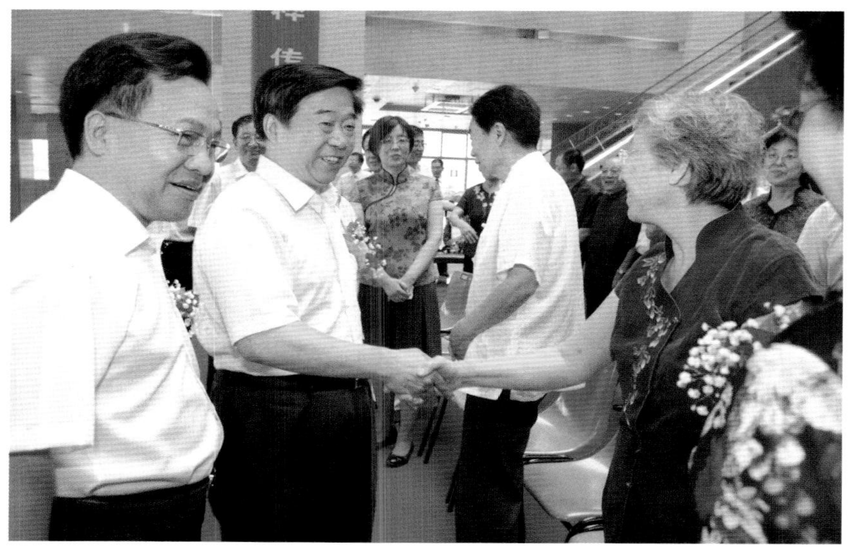

Secretary of the Party Leadership Group and Director-General of Hebei Provincial Department of Health Yang Xinjian attended the formal mentor-apprentice ceremony for prestigious TCM doctors' heritage, August 30, 2011.

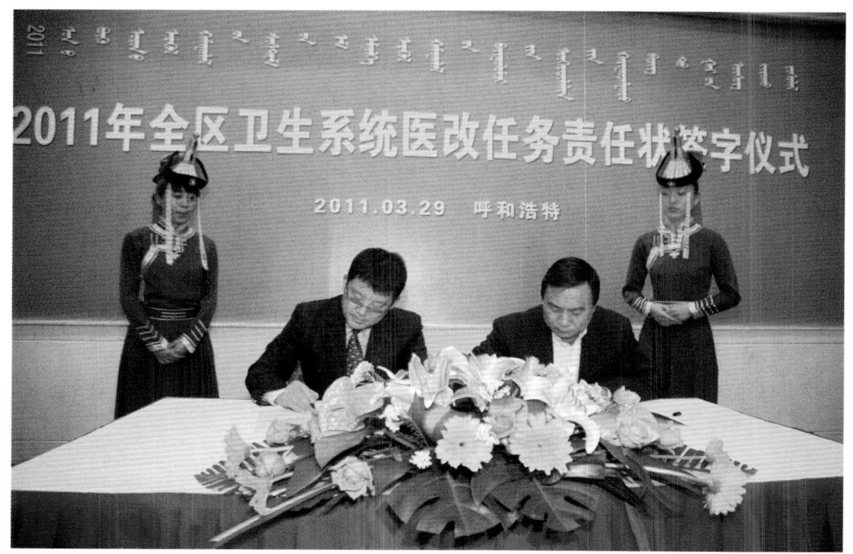

Director-General of the Department of Health of Inner Mongolia Autonomous Region Bi Lifu and various cities of the Region signed the responsibility certificate for medical reform, March 29, 2011.

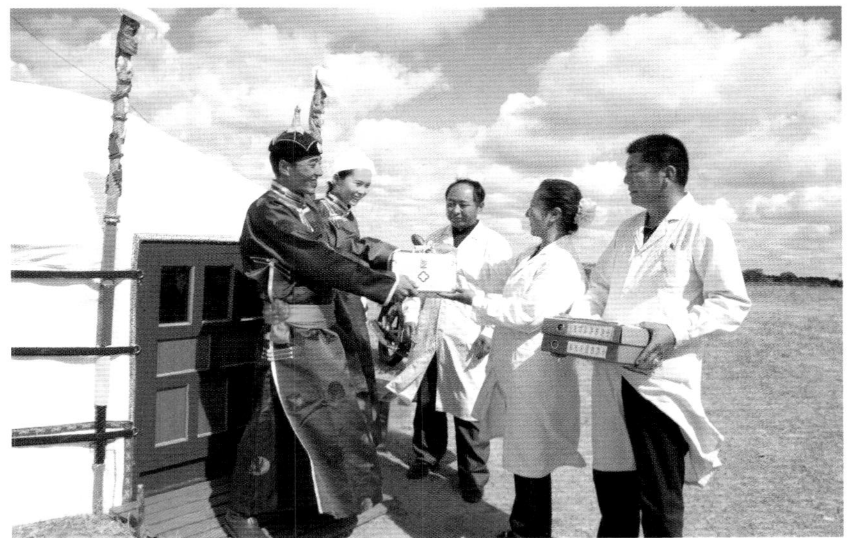

Health workers from Xinzuoqi of Hulun Buir gave out medical kits to the herdsmen, September 16, 2011.

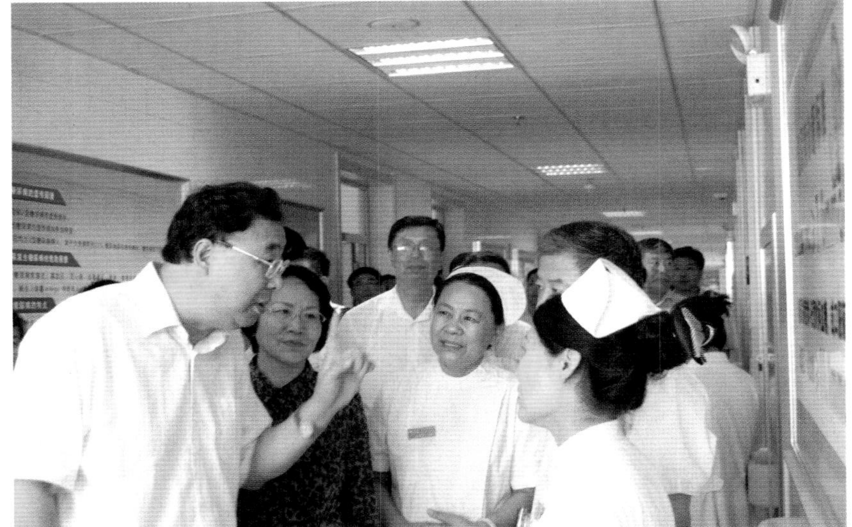

Director-General of Liaoning Provincial Department of Health Jiang Chao and Shenyang Deputy Mayor Wang Ling went along with Vice Health Minister Ma Xiaowei to Xinmin Hospital of Shenyang for the inspection and guidance of the work in July 2011.

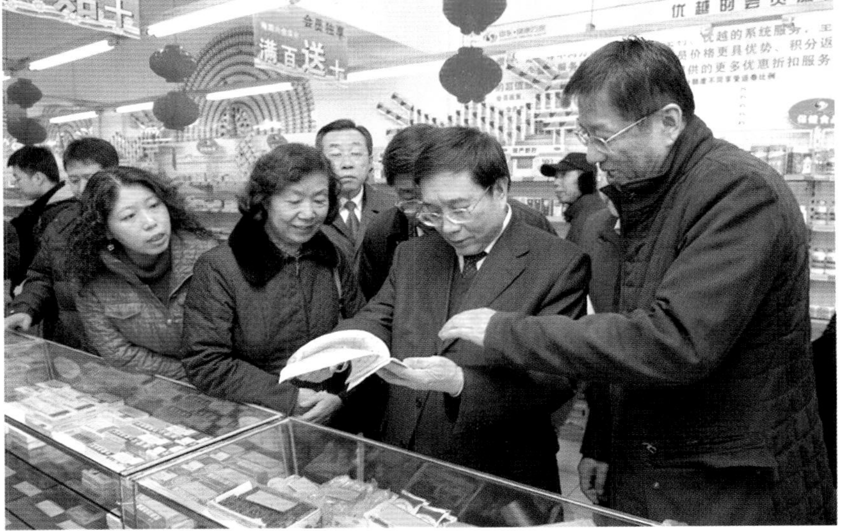

Director-General of Jilin Provincial Department of Health, Deputy Director of Jilin Provincial Food and Drug Administration Qi Youwei and related officials from Changchun Municipal Bureau of Health and Changchun Municipal Food and Drug Bureau paid an inspection visit to the pharmacy in January 2011.

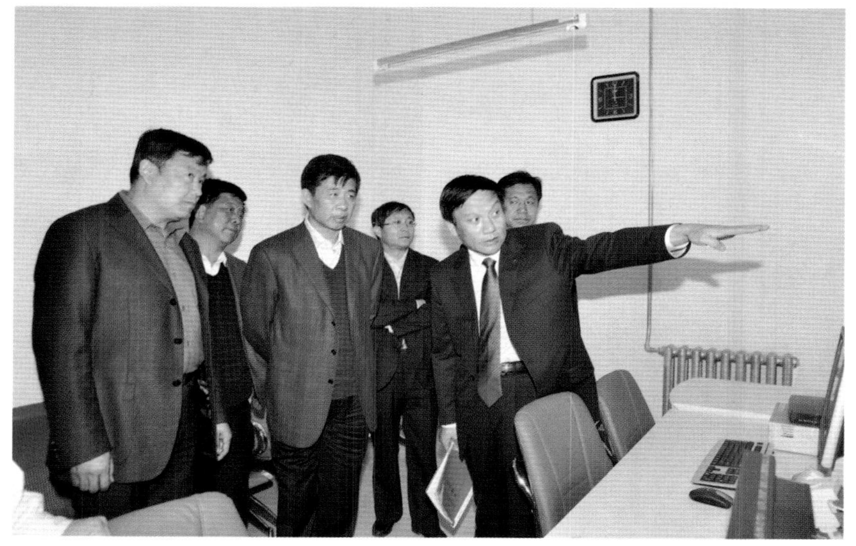

Officials from Heilongjiang Provincial Department of Health inspected the work of the drug distribution center designated by hospitals.

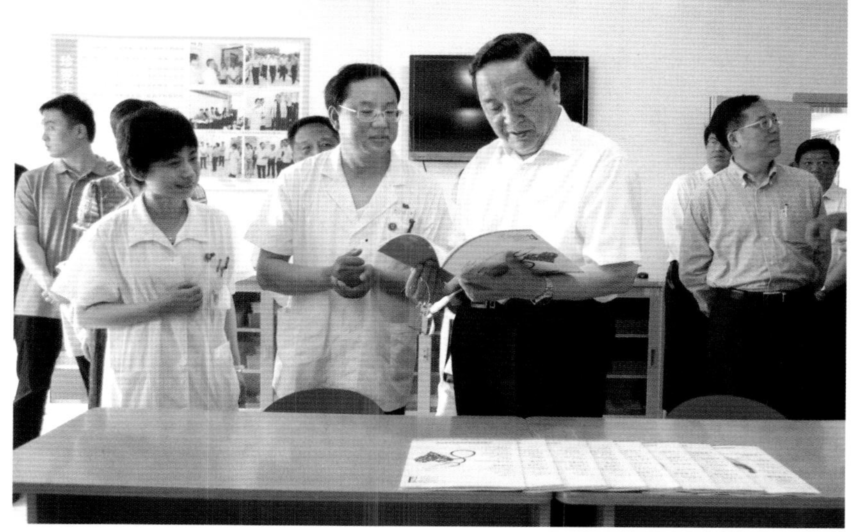

Secretary of Shanghai Municipal Committee of the CPC Yu Zhengsheng inspected the work of mental health at the Branch Center for Mental Health of Changning District, June 23, 2011.

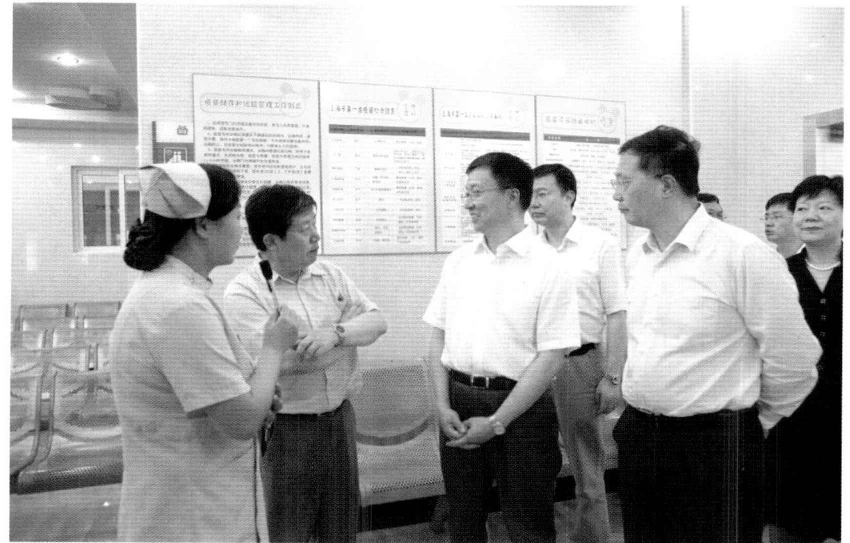

Shanghai Mayor Han Zheng conducted survey and research on the health work of health service center of Gumei Community in Minhang District, June 23, 2011.

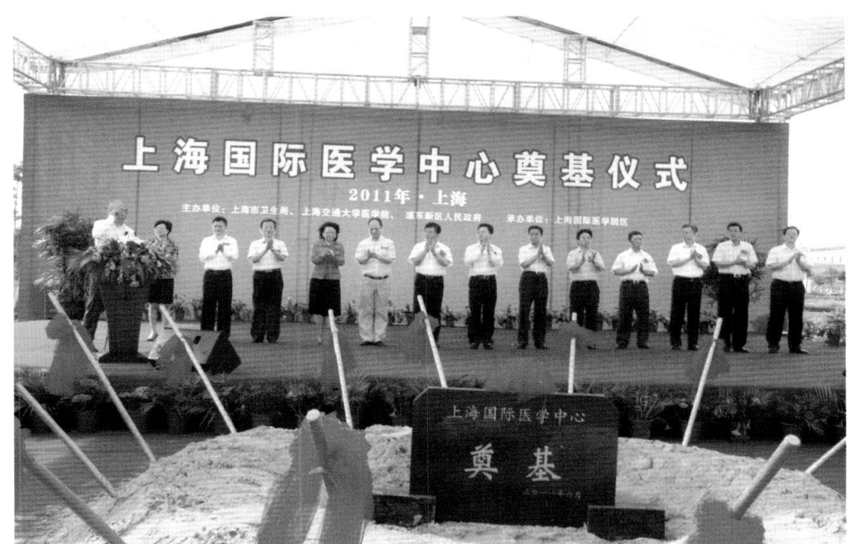

The Foundation-Laying ceremony of Shanghai International Medical Center was held at Shanghai International Medical Zone (SIMZ), June 24, 2011.

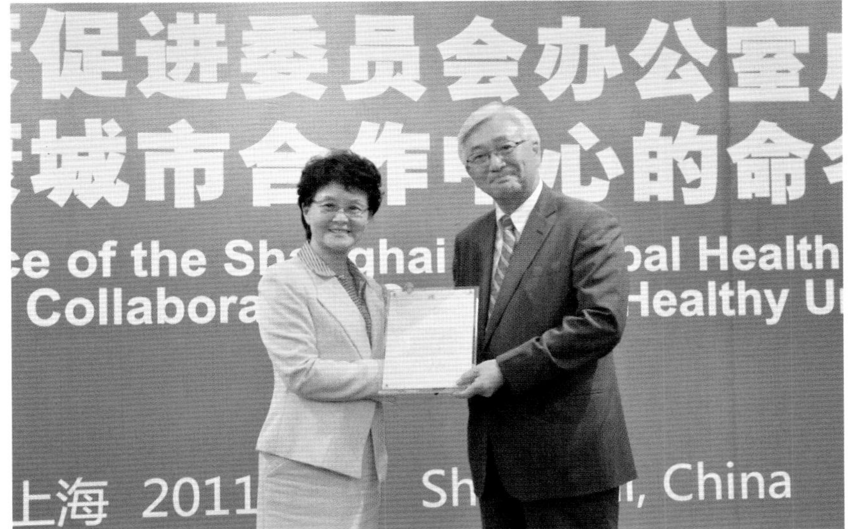

China's first WHO Health City Cooperation Center was set up in Shanghai, August 29, 2011.

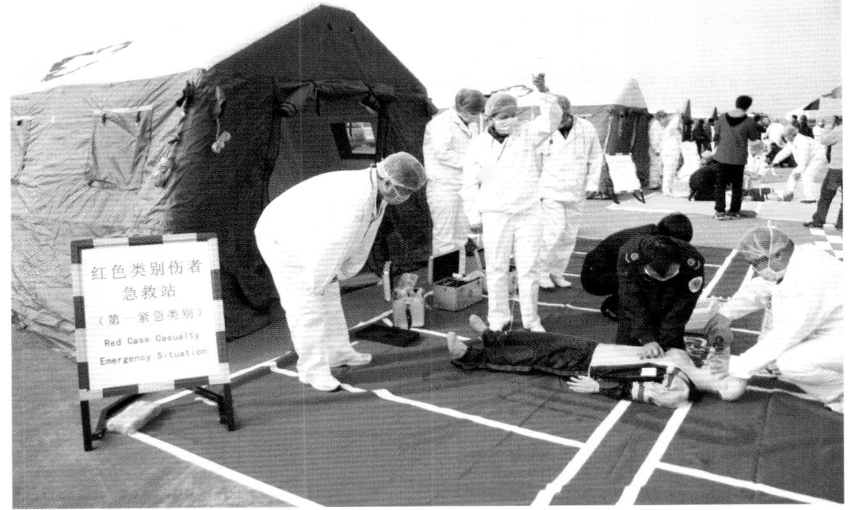

Jiangsu's first emergency exercise of medical rescue for flight accidents of civil aircrafts was held in Xuzhou, November 15, 2011.

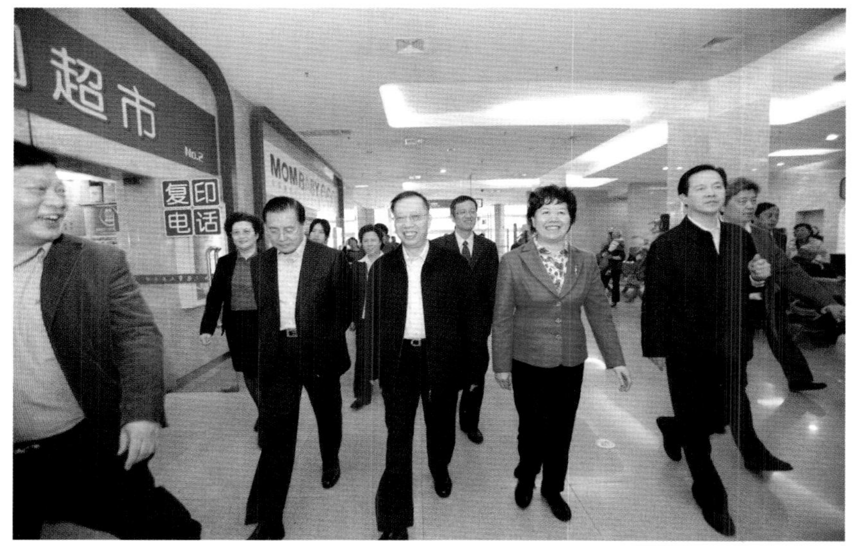

Director-General of Jiangsu Provincial Department of Health Wang Yonghong went along with Vice Health Minister Huang Jiefu to pay an inspection visit to Wuxi Municipal People's Hospital, November 16, 2011.

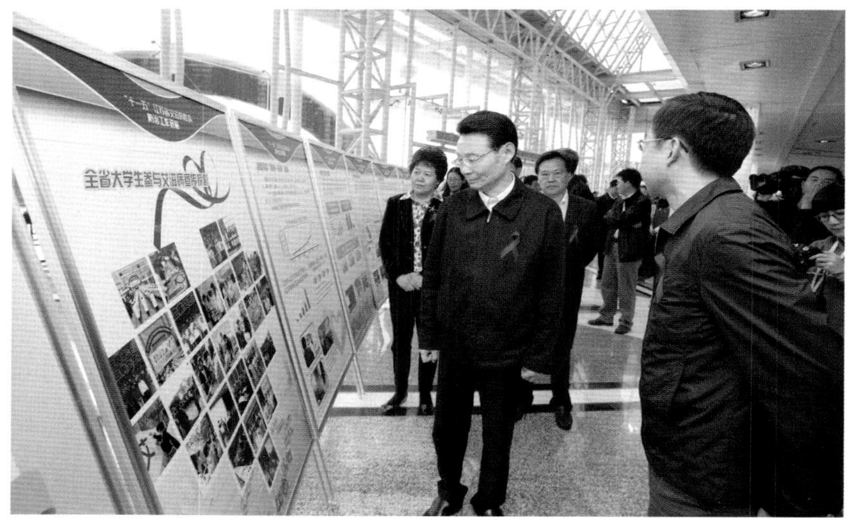

The Campaign for 2011 World AIDS Day was held in Jiangsu, November 30, 2011.

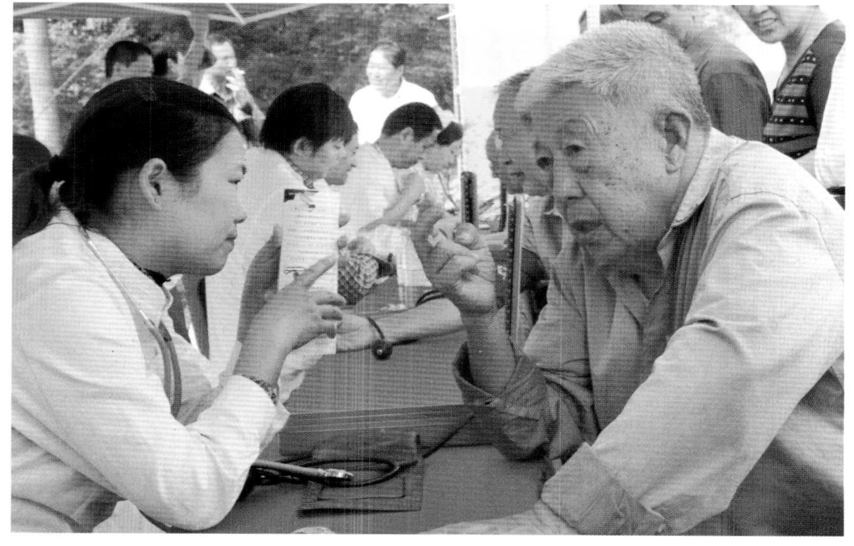

Anhui Provincial Department of Health held the campaign at the square for China Hypertension Day, October 8, 2011.

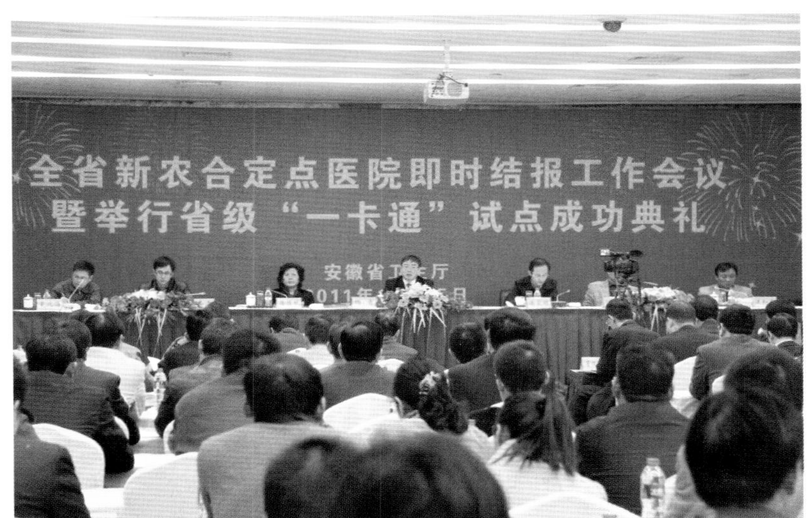
全省新农合定点医院即时结报工作会议
暨举行省级“一卡通”试点成功典礼

Anhui Provincial Department of Health held the ceremony to mark the successful pilot of “all-purpose card” for the New Rural Cooperative Medical System (NCMS), November 14-15, 2011.

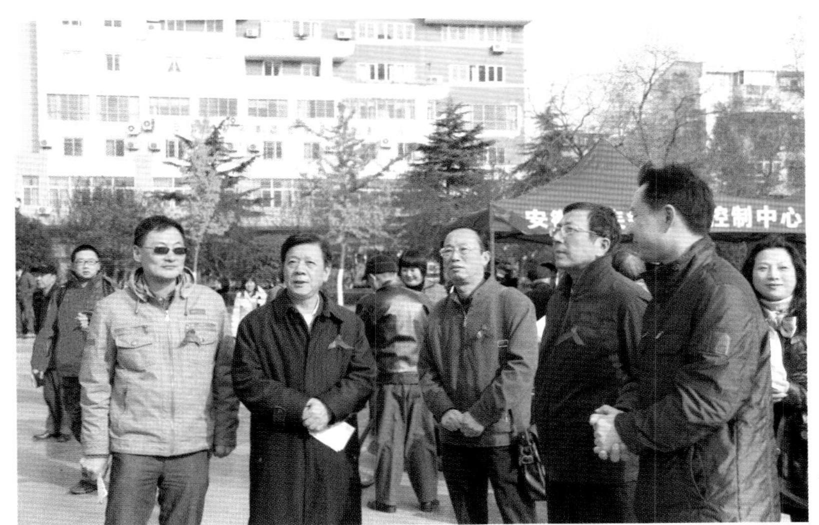

Anhui Provincial Department of Health held the campaign at Peace Square for HIV/AIDS, December 1, 2011.

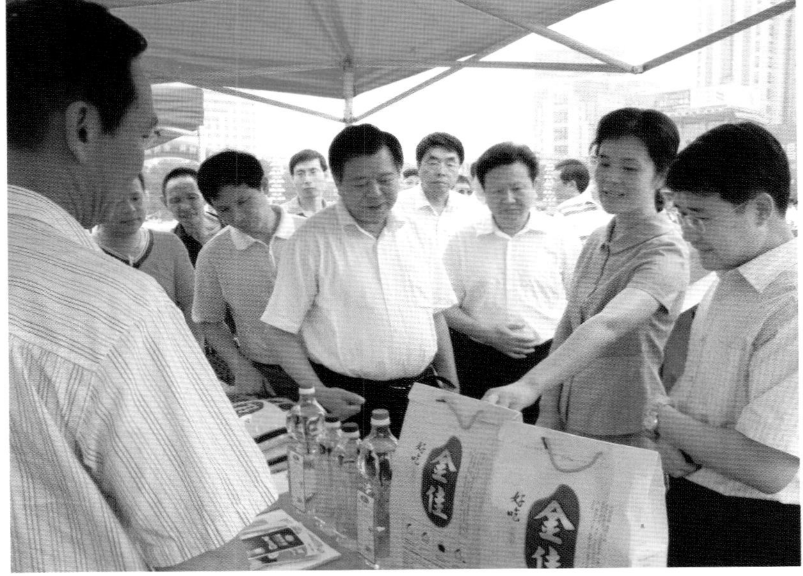
金佳

Deputy Director-General of the Standing Committee of the People’s Congress of Jiangxi Hu Zhenpeng and Jiangxi Vice Governor Xie Ru attended the campaign of awareness week for food safety held by Jiangxi, June 20, 2011.

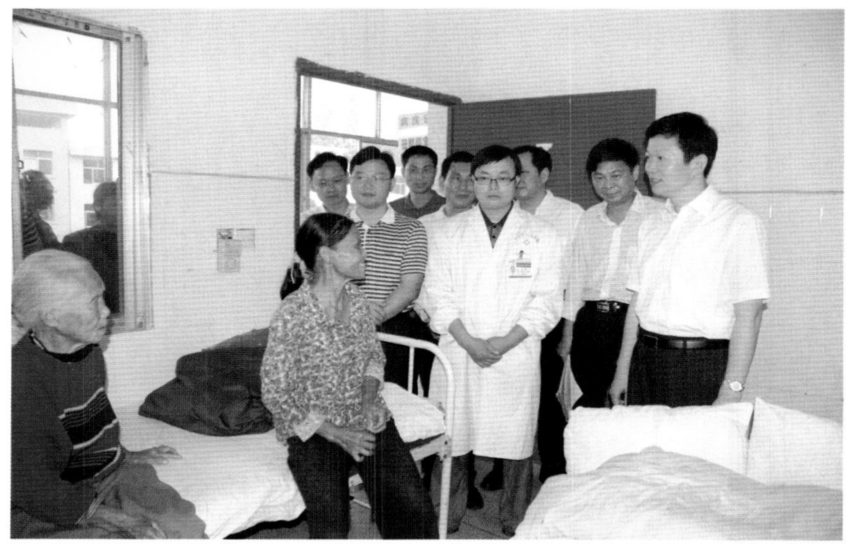

Director-General of Jiangxi Provincial Department of Health Li Li conducted survey and research and guided the work of medical reform at the primary level, October 11, 2011.

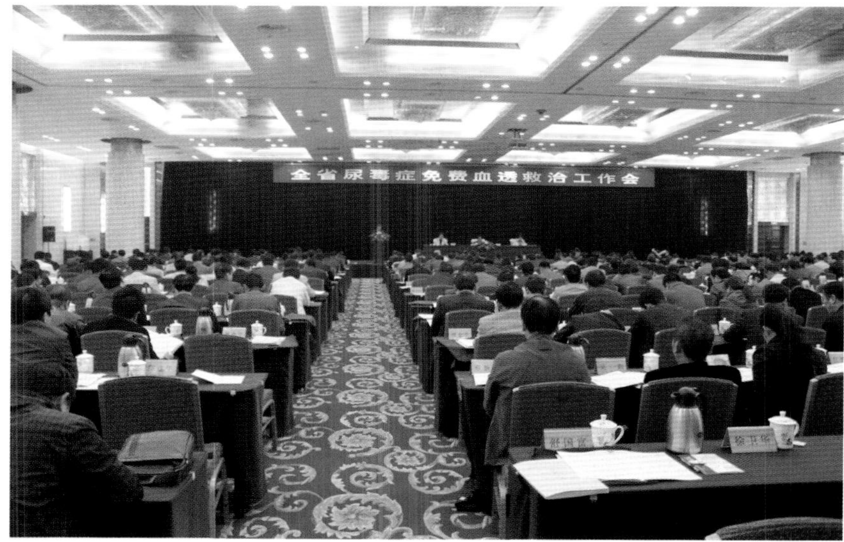

Jiangxi Provincial Department of Health held the provincial meeting on free hemodialysis treatment for uremia, November 23, 2011.

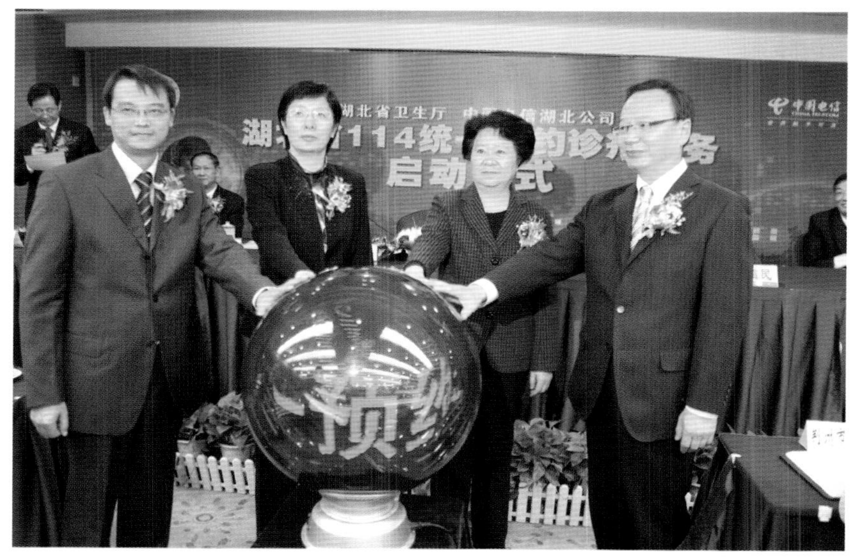

Member of the Standing Committee of the CPC Hubei Provincial Committee and Vice Governor of Hubei Zhang Daili and Director-General of Jiangsu Provincial Department of Health Jiao Hong attended the launching ceremony of medical services by calling 114, October 27, 2011.

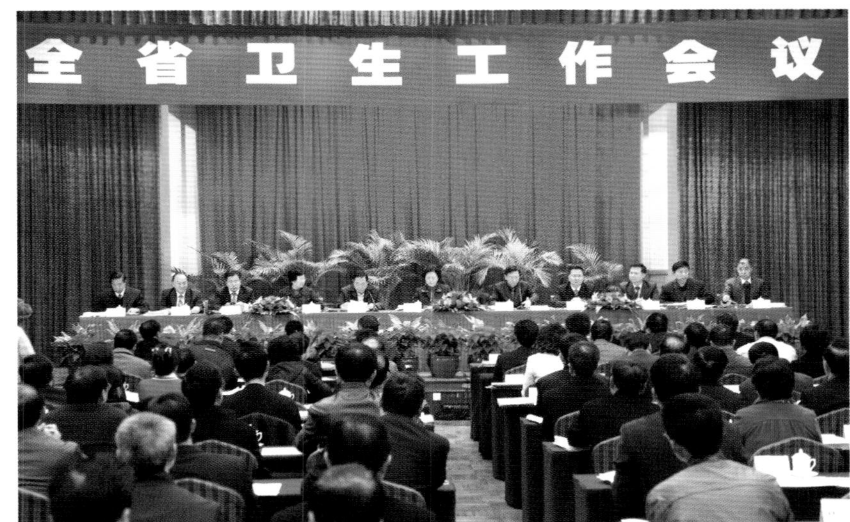

Guangdong Provincial Meeting on Health Work was held in Guangzhou, capital city of Guangdong, January 27, 2011.

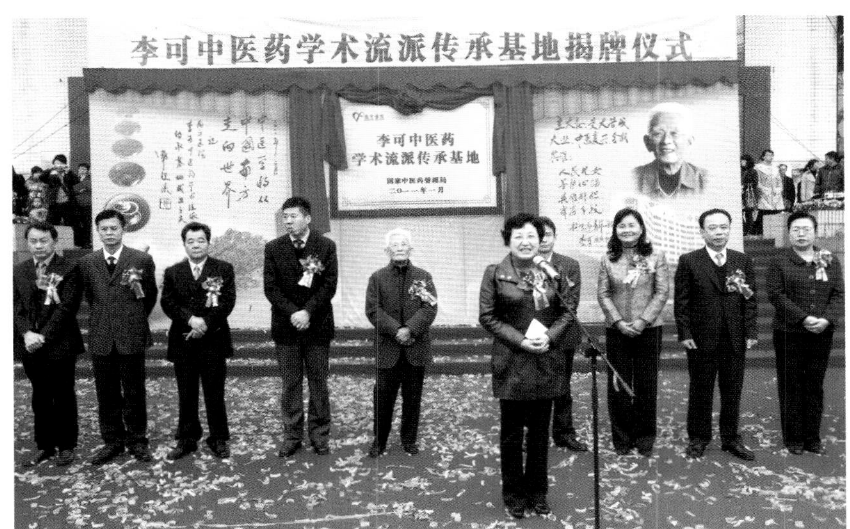

The Base for Inheriting Li Ke Academic School of Traditional Chinese Medicine of Southern Hospital of Southern Medical University was inaugurated, March 9, 2011.

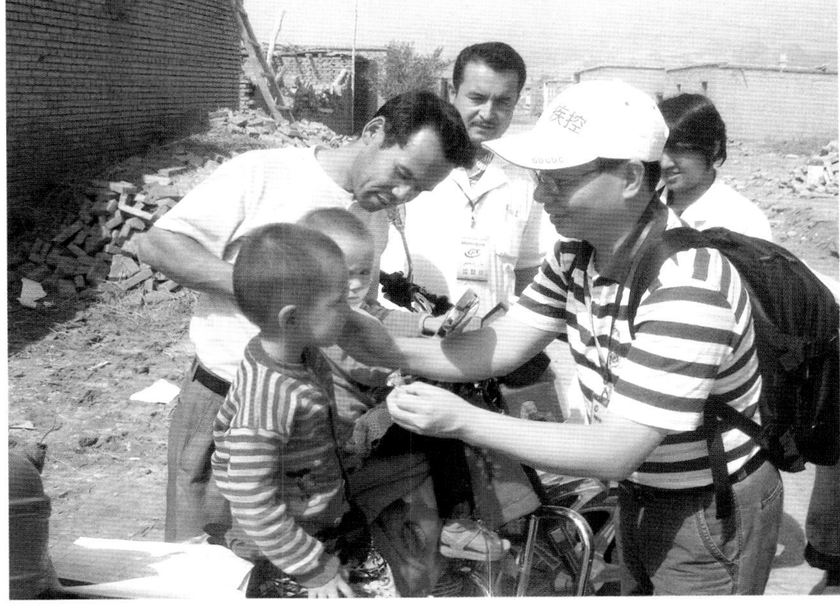

Guangdong-CDC gave aid to the prevention and control of poliomyelitis in Kashgar Prefecture in Xinjiang, September 8, 2011.

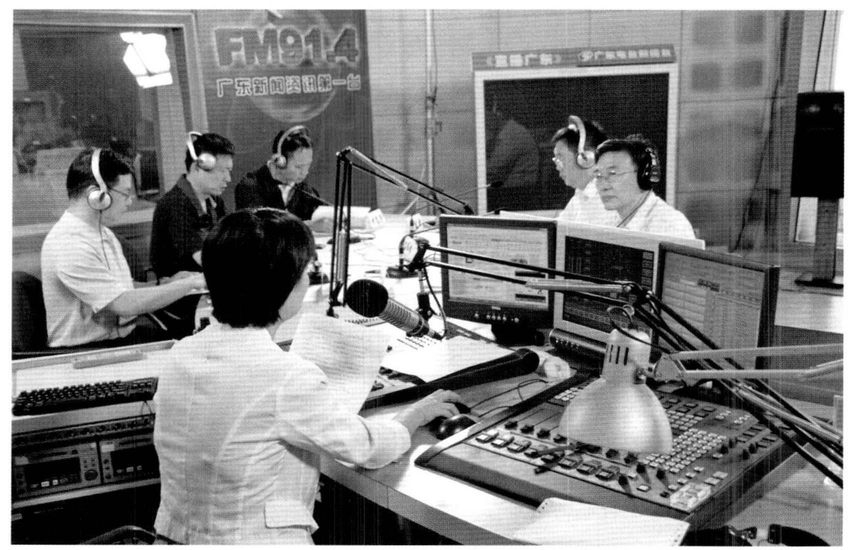

Director-General of Guangdong Provincial Department of Health Yao Zhibin had conversations with the people in answering the phone hotline for people's livelihood, November 8, 2011

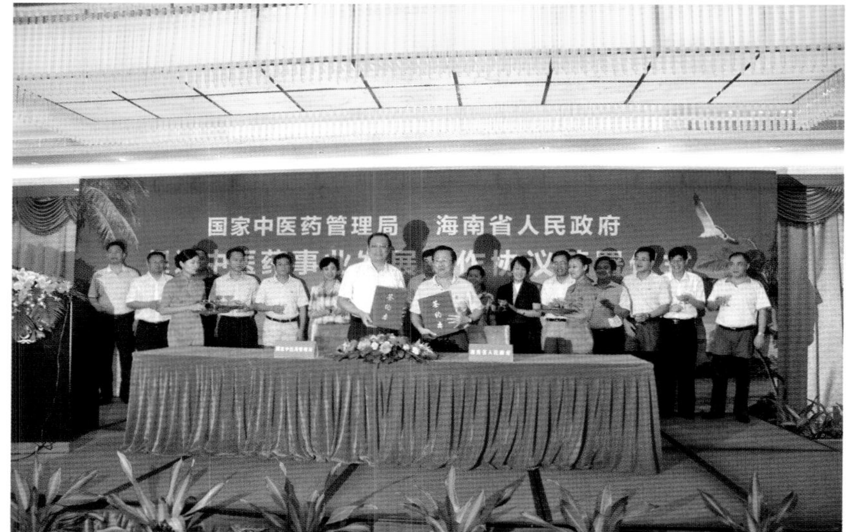

State Administration of Traditional Chinese Medicine and Hainan Provincial People's Government signed the *Cooperation Agreement on Promoting the Development of Traditional Chinese Medicine*, September 19, 2011.

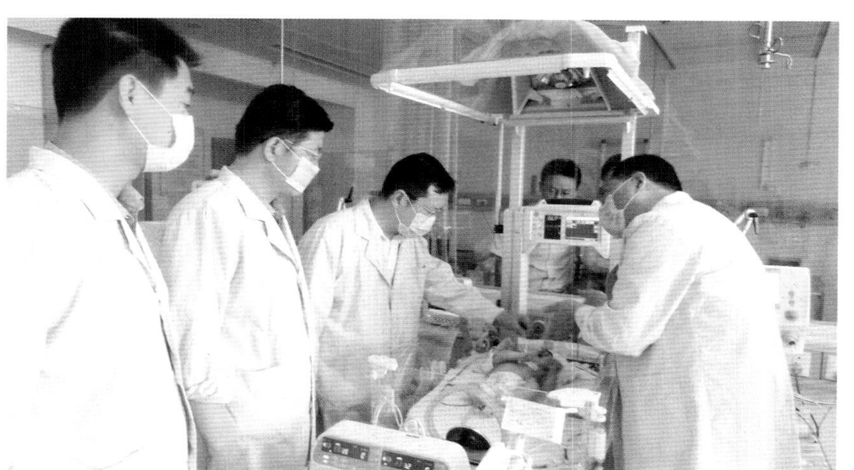

Xinqiao Hospital of the Third Military Medical University received and treated China's first two-headed baby girl twins sharing one trunk and with limb deformities, May 9, 2011. Surviving for 150 days and 17 hours, the conjoined baby was the longest-living two-headed monomer baby in Asia to this day.

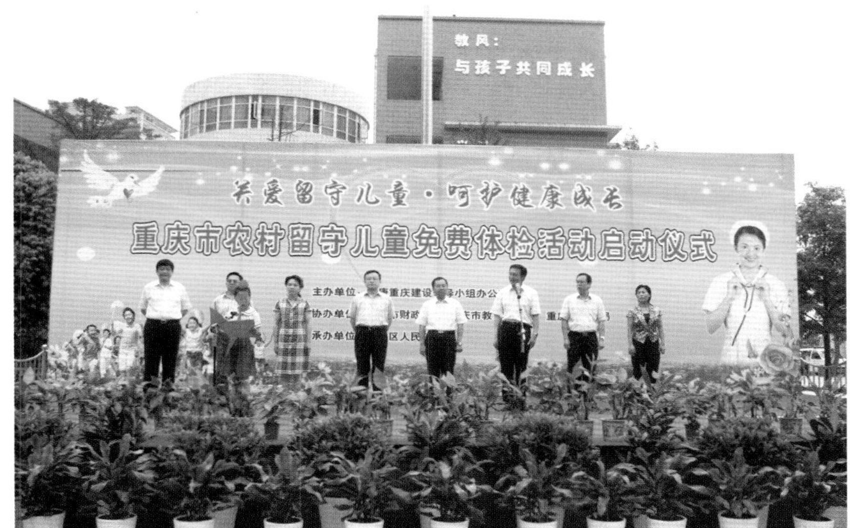

The activity of free physical examinations for left-behind children in rural areas was launched in Chongqing, June 21, 2011.

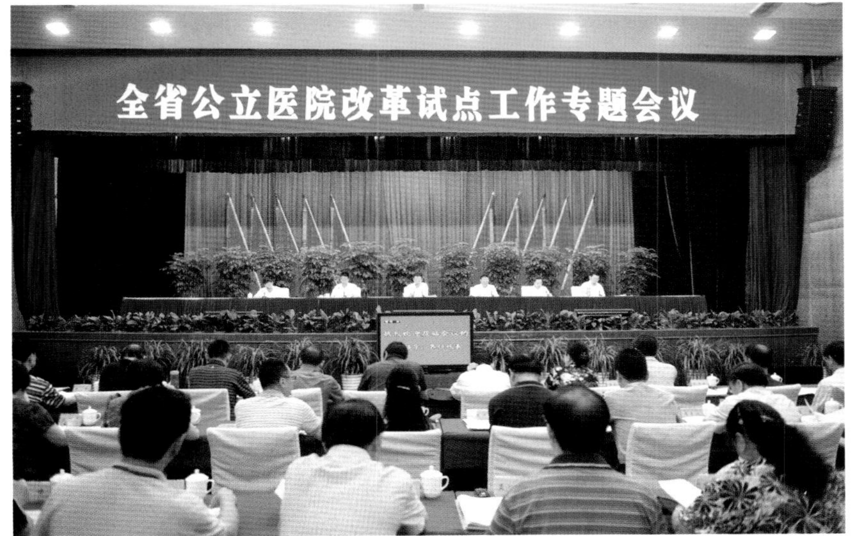

The Special Session on Pilot Reform of Sichuan Provincial Public Hospitals was held in Nanchong, July 28, 2011.

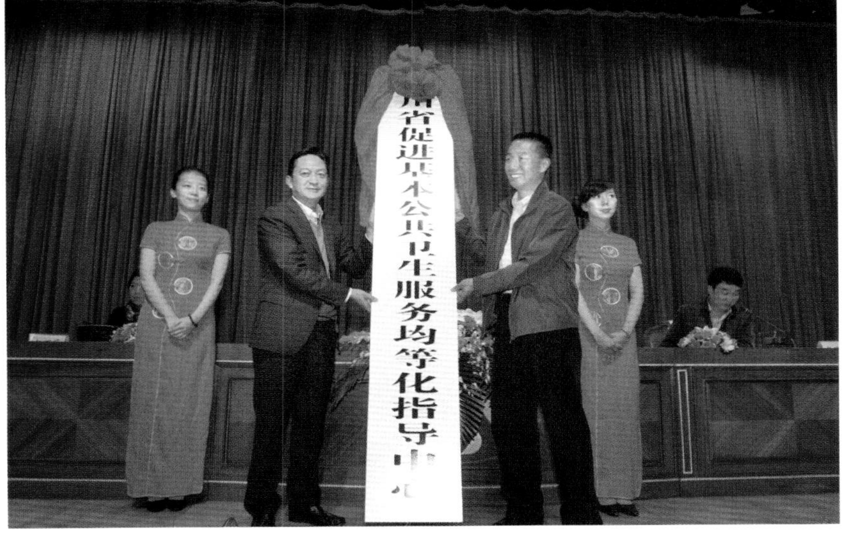

Director-General of Sichuan Provincial Department of Health inaugurated the newly established Guidance Center for Promoting Equal Access to Basic Public Health Services, October 31, 2011.

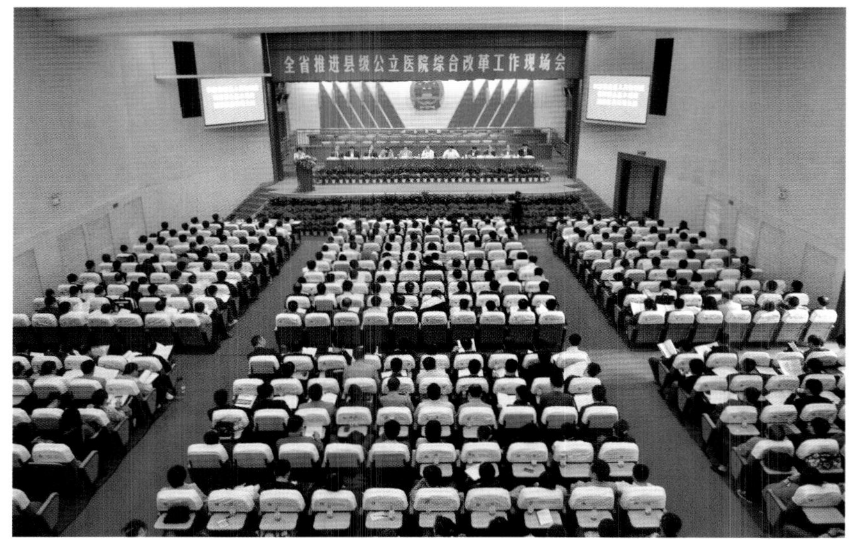

The Provincial On-Site Meeting on Promoting the Comprehensive Reform of Public Hospitals at the County Level was held in Shaanxi, September 29, 2011.

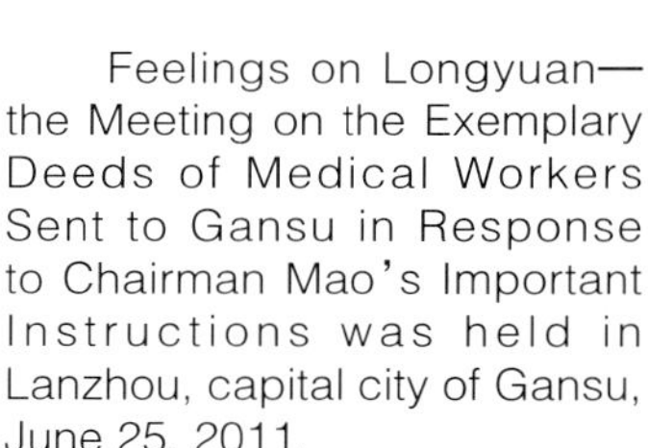

Feelings on Longyuan—the Meeting on the Exemplary Deeds of Medical Workers Sent to Gansu in Response to Chairman Mao's Important Instructions was held in Lanzhou, capital city of Gansu, June 25, 2011.

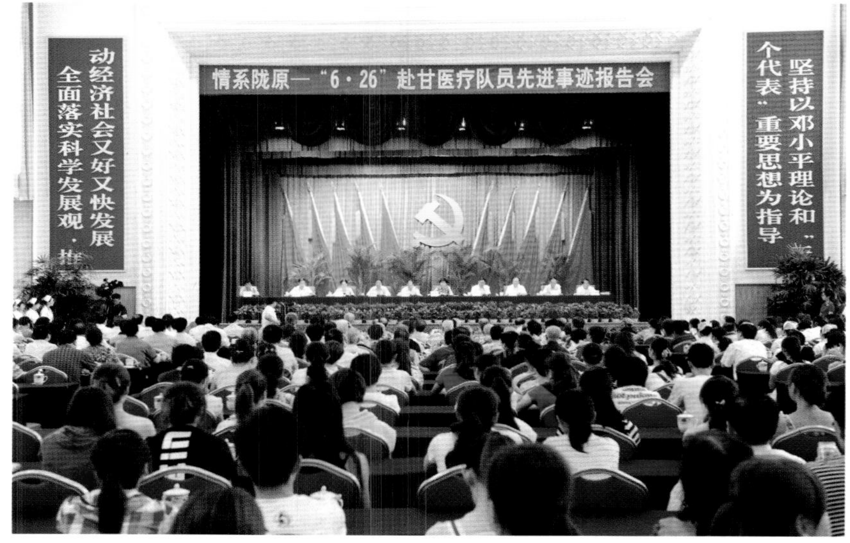

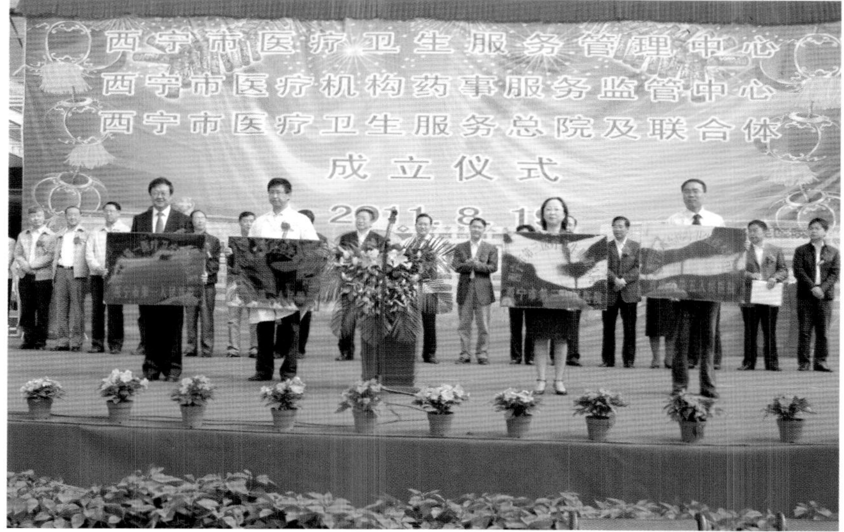

Qinghai's Xining General Hospital of Medical and Health Services and the Associates were established in August 2011. It marked the substantive progress made in the pilot reform of urban public hospitals in Qinghai.

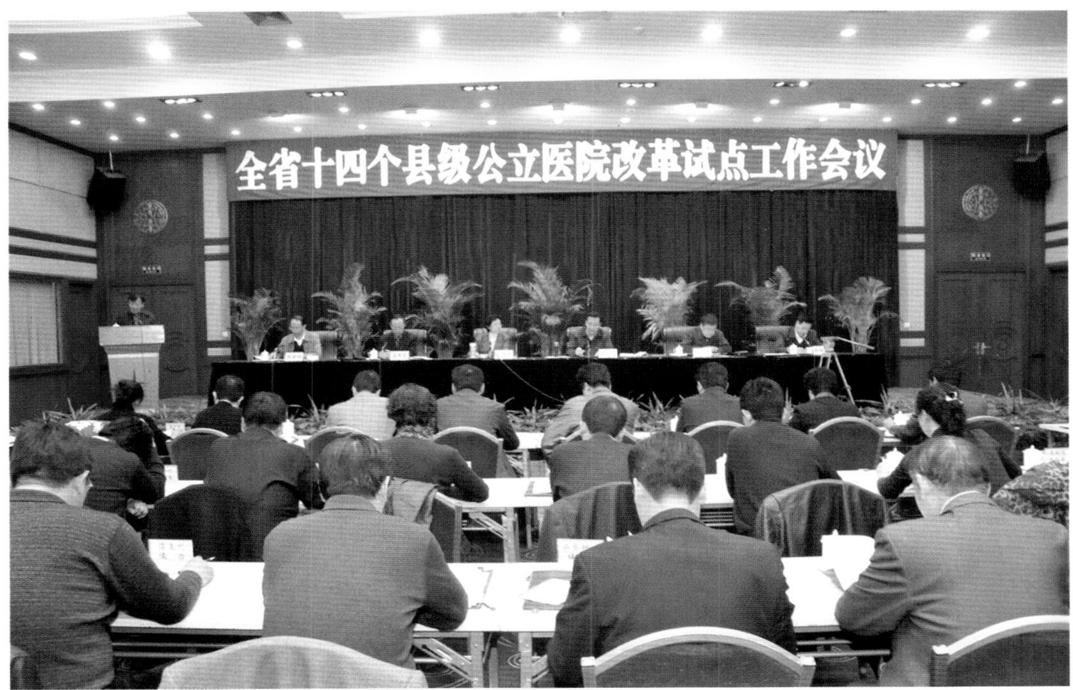

The Provincial Meeting on the Pilot Reform of 14 Public Hospitals at the County Level was held in Qinghai, November 12, 2011.

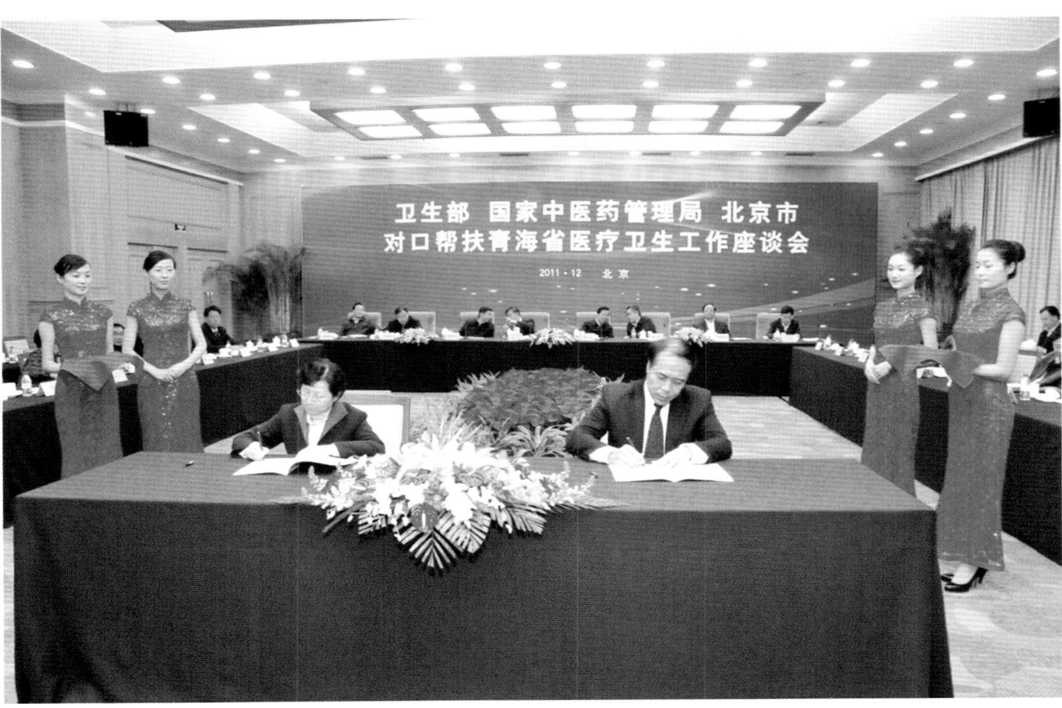

The Symposium on the Counterpart Assistance of the Ministry of Health, State Administration of Traditional Chinese Medicine and Beijing City to Qinghai Provincial Medical and Health Services was held in Beijing in December 2011.

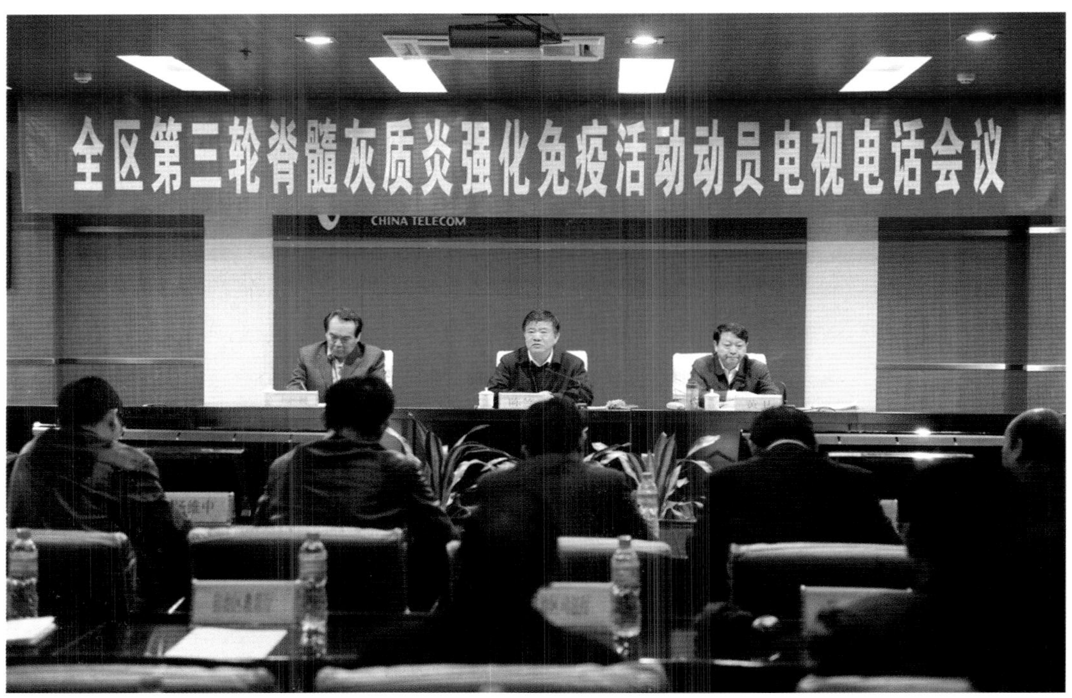

The Region's 3rd Round of Video- and Teleconferences on the Mobilization of Supplementary Immunization of Poliomyelitis was held in Xinjiang Uygur Autonomous Region, November 12, 2011.

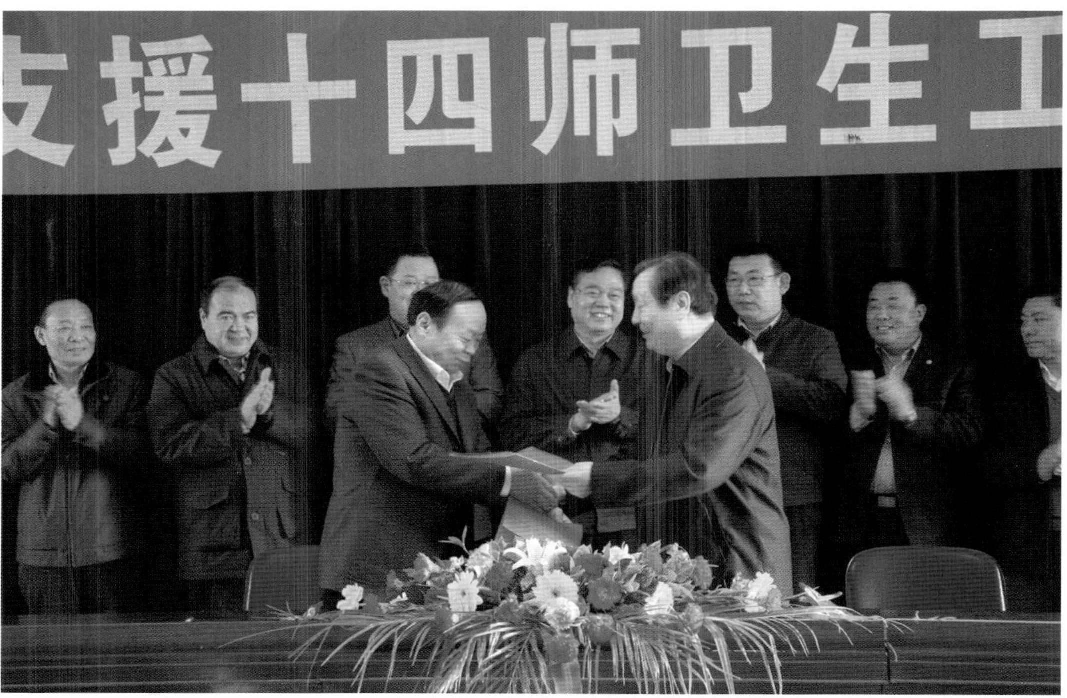

The Health Bureau of Xinjiang Production and Construction Corps signed the ten-year support agreement with Hetian Division 14, January 14, 2011.

(Wang Dian)

2012

YEAR BOOK OF HEALTH IN THE PEOPLE'S REPUBLIC OF CHINA

Editor-in-Chief
Chen Zhu

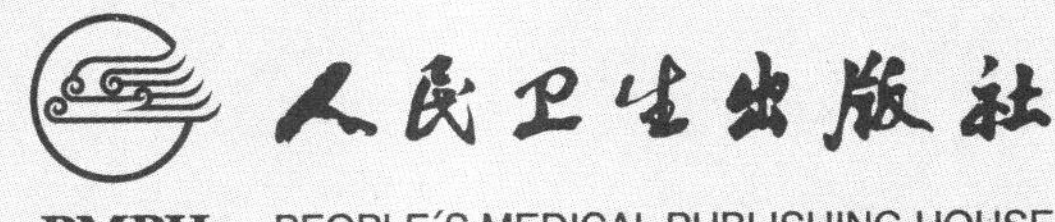

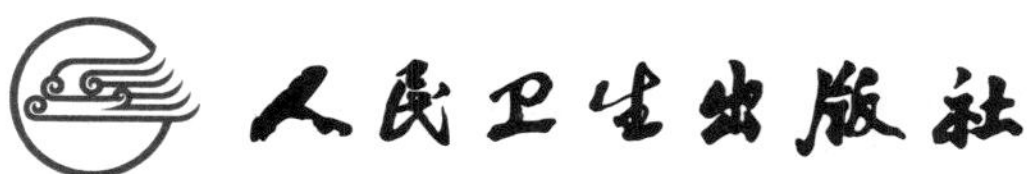

PMPH PEOPLE´S MEDICAL PUBLISHING HOUSE

http:// www.pmph.com

Book Title: 2012 Year Book of Health in the People's Republic of China
2012 中国卫生年鉴

Contact address: No.19 Pan Jia Yuan Nan Li, Chaoyang District, Beijing 100021, P. R. China
phone/fax: 86 10 6761 7315, E-mail: pmph@pmph.com

Disclaimer

This book is for educational and reference purposes only. In view of the possibility of human errors or changes in medical science, neither the author, editor nor the publisher nor any other party who has been involved in the preparation or publication of this work guarantees that the information contained herein is in every respect accurate or complete. The medicinal therapy and treatment techniques presented in this book are provided for the purpose of reference only. If readers wish to attempt any of the techniques or utilize any of the medicinal therapies contained in this book, the publisher assumes no responsibility for any of such actions.

It is the responsibility of the readers to understand and adhere to local laws and regulations concerning the practice of these techniques and methods. The authors, editors and publishers disclaim all responsibility for any liability, loss, injury, or damage incurred as a consequence, directly or indirectly, of the use and application of any of the contents of this book.

First published:
ISBN: 978-7-117-18161-7/R·18162

Cataloguing in Publication Data:
A catalog record for this book is available from the CIP-Database China.

Printed in P. R. China

Contents

Part I Significant Reports in Conference 1

Part I Significant Reports in Conference

1. With Strenuous Efforts to Carry Forward Our Cause into the Future, Create a New Situation in the Development of Health Science

—A Work Presentation Given by Health Minister Chen Zhu at 2011 National Meeting on Health Work (January 6, 2011)

Comrades,

This is an important meeting convened at the crucial stage of deepening the medical system reform. The meeting is also convened at the new development stage of the 12th Five-Year Plan. The State Council attaches great importance to this meeting. Li Keqiang, member of the Standing Committee of the Politburo of the CPC Central Committee, Vice Premier of the State Council, and head of the leading group under the State Council for deepening the medical and health system reform, specially made important written instructions. He gave explicit requirements on the meeting, health work in the year 2011 and fulfillment of every task of deepening the medical system reform. We must seriously study his instructions, get a full understanding and fully implement them.

The theme of this meeting is as follows: Act on the spirit of the 17th CPC National Congress, the spirit of the third, fourth and fifth plenary session of the 17th CPC Central Committee, and the spirit of the Central Economic Work Conference. Under the guidance of Deng Xiaoping Theory and important thought of Three Represents, further study and practice the scientific outlook on development. Summarize the health development achievements in the period of the 11th Five-Year Plan and health work of the year 2010. Analyze the situations and tasks facing health reform and development. Centering on deepening the medical and health system reform, assign tasks for health development in the period of the 12th Five-Year Plan and health work of the year 2010. With the thoughts unified and efforts concerted, lay a foundation for the fulfillment of the three-year key tasks of deepening the medical and health system reform. Therefore, the scientific development for health service in the period of the

12th Five-Year Plan will be achieved.

Now I will talk about things in three parts for your discussion.

I. Health Development in the Period of the 11th Five-Year Plan and 2010 Health Work Review

(1) Health development achievements in the period of the 11th Five-Year Plan. The period of the 11th Five-Year Plan was a truly extraordinary time in the course of the country's health development. It was also a time for the new situation of health work.

In the past five years, a new idea for health reform and development has been firmly established. After the turn of the century, especially after the anti-SARS campaign, the CPC Central Committee put forward the scientific outlook on development. The outlook established the concept of development for people, relying on people and shared by people, which highlighted health development. The 17th CPC National Congress set the goal that everyone would have access to basic medical and health services. In addition, the Congress pointed out a basic direction that public medical and health care services serve the public good. It also made clear the historical task of establishing a basic medical and health care system. Over the five years, the national health system has firmly established aim awareness and a concept of health services for the people wholeheartedly. The maintenance of the people's interests has been taken as the starting point and foothold of health work. Around the most practical health issues of the greatest and most direct concern to the people, all thinking was unified, development thoughts were adjusted, weak links were strengthened, operation mechanism was restructured, and service effectiveness was improved. On the whole, the scientific development concept of being people and health oriented was truly achieved in health work. That is the ideology foundation for the achievements of health work. It is also important spiritual treasure which is worth summarizing and carrying forward.

In the past five years, a new way of thinking for health reform and development has been set. On the basis of years of exploration, the CPC Central Committee and the State Council formulated *Opinions on Deepening the Reform of Medical and Health System*. In the *Opinions*, the general idea, basic framework, policies and measures and recent work focus of reform were clarified. By way of institutional innovation, conflicting issues around system, mechanism and structure would be settled. In addition, the people's health benefits would be maintained by the basic system. According to the principle of providing the people with the basic medical and health care system as public products, "basic medical care should be guaranteed, primary care, strengthened, and medical mechanism, established". Over the past two years, significant progress and remarkable achievements have bee made in all the areas of health reform.

In the past five years, new steps have been taken in the development of health services. Infrastructure construction and talent team building were strengthened in public health and basic health services. And service capability was greatly improved. Health care programs were conducted for such focus groups as women, children and old people. More urban-rural residents were provided with access to standardized service for major health problems, especially chronic non-communicable diseases. The number of people involved in the new rural cooperative medical system increased from 179,000,000 in 2005 to 835,000,000 in 2010, with a coverage rate of 95.9%. Thus, the obligatory target of the country's 11th Five-Year Plan was met ahead of schedule. With a coverage rate of rural-urban medical security system rising from 30% to 90%, the country's equity of health financing was greatly improved and leapfrog development was achieved in the security system. As there was a growing international influence, the role of traditional Chinese medicine in the medical and health service system with Chinese characteristics was becoming all the more prominent. The effectiveness of food and drug surveillance and comprehensive coordination was dramatically enhanced. As a result, the situation of food and drug safety was greatly improved and remarkable progress was made in food safety and every health surveillance task.

The 11th Five-Year Plan period was a time when there was the fastest growing health investment of government. In 2009, health expenditure of governments at all levels amounted to a total of 468.5 billion RMB Yuan, three times that of 2005 (155.2 billion RMB Yuan). A new pattern of government health expenditure was formed, in which priority was given to public health and basic medical services, and consideration was given to both the supply and the demand. The weak links existing in the health system for long was greatly strengthened and unbalanced development got to be improved. From the end of 2005 to the end of 2009, medical and health institutions at all levels and of all sorts increased from 882,000 to 917,000, with an increase of 4%; hospital beds increased from 3,368,000 to 4,417,000, an increase of 31.7%; and the number of health professionals increased from 4,460,000 to 5,535,000, an increase of 24.1%. There was a trend that the regional disparity for health resources per capita was being reduced. In the eastern and mid-western areas, the proportion for hospital beds dropped from 1:0.79:0.79 to 1:0.83:0.84.

In the past five years, the people have obtained more health benefits as a result of the remarkable improvement of national health index. In the period of the 11th Five-Year Plan, the country's average life expectancy was expected to rise to one year. Maternal mortality rate dropped from 47.7/100,000 in 2005 to 31.9/100,000 in 2009, falling by 33.12%. Infant mortality rate dropped from 19.0% in 2005 to 13.8% in 2009, falling by 27.4%. The goal of the 11th Five-Year Plan for both rates was achieved ahead of schedule. In 2009, the country witnessed 5.488 billion outpatient attendances and emergency room visits, 1.391 billion more than 2005, or an increase of 34%. In the same year, there were 130,000,000 hospital admissions, 60,720 more than 2005, or an increase of 84.5%. The people's demand for medical services was greatly satisfied with an easier access to seeking medical advice. Due to the significant change in health cost structure, the share of individual health expenditure in total health expenditure dropped from 52.12% in 2005 to 38.19% in 2009. Therefore the trend of rapid growth of residents' individual medical and health expenditure was further contained.

In the past five years, medical and health workers have made outstanding contributions for the people's health. Over the five years, we have stood the test of Wenchuan earthquake and influenza A (H1N1). At the time when needed most by the people, the medical and health workers braved all dangers and risked their lives in saving lives, rescuing the wounded and stemming the epidemic. They fulfilled their mission of protecting the people's lives and health. We fulfilled the task of health security for Beijing Olympic Games, Shanghai World Expo and the 60th anniversary of the founding of the PRC. We also properly handled public health events like the event of melamine-tainted milk powder. As a result, social security and stability were maintained. Over the five years, the country's 7 million medical and health workers have worked hard for maintaining the people's health at their ordinary posts. They produce an excellent performance with selfless devotion. It has been proved by practice that the country's medical and health workers have stood the test and are trustworthy.

Comrades, after five years of efforts, we have fulfilled the major target and task of the 11th Five-Year Plan. Health work plays an irreplaceable role in maintaining democracy, promoting stability and pushing forward the coordinated development of the economic society. Health achievements in the period of the 11th Five-Year Plan have laid a solid foundation for a new level of health development and the goal of everyone's having access to basic medical and health services.

(2) The 2010 work summary

Over the past year, according to the unified deployment of the CPC Central Committee, the Ministry of Health set up the leading group for excellent performance of the country's medical and health system. Health departments and bureaus in all localities also set up industry guidance groups to arouse medical and health workers' enthusiasm for fulfilling their duties, plunging into the medical reform and professional dedication. As a result, the implementation of pushing forward every task of deepening the medical reform was provided with organization guarantee and internal motivation. And the obvious stage result was fully affirmed by leaders of the CPC Central Committee. In accordance with 2010 work arrangements for medical reform of the State Council, the national health system, centering on the five priority areas of work for medical reform, strengthened responsibilities, made greater efforts, highlighted priorities and steadily carried out the reform. So the five priority areas of reform generally went smoothly. Footy tasks led by health departments are being pushed forward as scheduled. In the meantime, encouraging progress was made in every health task.

1) The new rural cooperative medical system was further improved. The coverage of the new rural cooperative medical system continued to expand solidly with a participation rate up to 90%. The levels of financing and security were further raised with the per capita financing of 155.3 RMB Yuan, of which the government grant per capita amounted to 126.1 RMB Yuan. In over sixty percent of the pooling areas, the pooling of outpatient service was conducted. The inpatient reimbursement ratio within the policy range in the pooling areas rose by five percentage points higher than the previous year. The pay cap was six folds of the average income of rural residents countrywide. The pilot program for improving medical security level of rural children's major diseases was under way. In Anhui, Jiangxi, Hunan and Inner Mongolia, the pilot programs were expanded provincially (regionally). The compensation ratio for rural children's leukemia and congenital heart disease exceeded 70%. Those families qualifying for medical assistance of civil administration could obtain 20% of the subsidy. The management and operation level of the new rural cooperative medical system was constantly improved. In nearly 90% of the pooling areas, the medical expenses of the designated medical institutions within the counties could be reimbursed immediately. In more than half of the pooling areas, the accounts could be settled directly with the designated medical institutions outside the counties. In over one-third of the counties (cities, districts), payment reform was carried out, such as per capita payment, payment by type of disease and global budget. In over half of the pooling areas, the unified service platforms of the new rural cooperative medical care and rural medical assistance were established. In Jiangsu, Henan, Fujian and Guangdong, explorations were being made for the participation of commercial insurance institutions in the operation and management of the new rural cooperative medical system.

2) The national system for basic drugs was steadily pushed forward at the primary level. Over the past year, some policies of basic drugs have been promoted in all localities, such as standardizing procurement, controlling price, organizing distribution, rational use and zero-profit sales. Active explorations were also made in the comprehensive reform at the primary level. According to the latest monitoring

results, the system for basic drugs has been implemented in 57.2% of the government sponsored medical and health institutions at the primary level. In Beijing, Shanghai, Anhui, Tianjin, Ningxia, Jiangxi, Inner Mongolia, Shaanxi, Gansu and Hainan, full coverage of the system for basic drugs was preliminarily achieved. In Anhui, *Duplex Letter* bidding, single source commitment, and unified payment were adopted to reduce basic drug price and ensure quality and supply. In all localities, clinical application guidelines and formulary for basic drugs were positively employed to ensure reasonable clinical use. Where the system for basic drugs was implemented, it was encouraging that, at medical and health institutions at the primary level, outpatient and inpatient expenditures dropped while the number of inpatients and outpatients was on the rise. As a result, the people's burden of medical cost was obviously reduced and the effectiveness of the system implementation preliminarily appeared.

3) The medical and health service system at the primary level was further perfected. In 2010, the central government continued to put an investment of 20 billion RMB Yuan to support the business house constructions of 891 county hospitals, 1,620 township hospitals, 11,200 village clinics and 1,228 community health service centers. On the basis of the general improvement of the hardware of medical and health institutions at the primary level, the construction of medial staff at the primary level focusing on general practitioners was greatly enhanced. The implementation of performance salary policy for public health institutions and medical institutions at the primary level was being accelerated. In those years, there was a directional enrollment of 500 medical students who were from the rural area and received gratis training. 8,938 practicing physicians were recruited for township hospitals. Long partner assistance relationships were established between 2,381 county hospitals and top-level hospitals, and between 15,300 township hospitals and second-class hospitals. The project of tens of thousands of doctors aiding rural health was carried out as always. And 17,500 elite doctors from county hospitals were sent to the top-level hospitals for further study. 475,000 medical workers from the township hospitals, 977,000 from the village clinics and 214,000 from the community health service institutions received on-the-job training. 16,000 general practitioners received job-transfer training. In Shanghai, Tianjin and Shenzhen, the standardized training for resident doctors and general practitioners was explored. In thirty provinces (regions, cities) countrywide, the subsidy policy for rural doctors was further carried out. In Ningxia, Xinjiang, Fujian and thirteen other provinces (regions), the subsidy standard was raised. In some provinces (regions) led by Anhui, the comprehensive reform for the medical and health institutions at the primary level was pushed forward, including the nature determination, post determination, staff allocation, personnel distribution,

performance assessment, multi-channel compensation, medical insurance payment reform and rural integration management. With the task of reform fulfilled, the people's benefits were improved greatly.

4) New progress was made in the equalization of basic public health services. Nine programs for the national basic public health services were conducted in urban-rural areas. Recent surveillance data show that the accumulated rate of record establishment for urban-rural residents' health records was 48.7% and 38.1% respectively. Therefore the annual targets were achieved ahead of schedule. Among the old people of 65 years of age or older, the number of physical checkup amounted to 57,142,000. 35,538,000 hypertension patients, 9,189,000 diabetes patients and 1,706,000 serious mental disorder patients were brought into the standard management of chronic diseases. In Shanghai and Hangzhou, the range of basic public health services was expanded. In 2010, the national per capita funding subsidies for basic public health services amounted to 17.4 RMB Yuan. Major public health projects progressed steadily. 35,100 cases of cataract operations for poverty-stricken people countrywide were performed. 29.629 million children under the age of 15 received vaccination against hepatitis B. The annual task was completed ahead of schedule. 8.847 million rural pregnant women had access to subsidies for hospital childbirths and the rate of rural hospital childbirths was 95.7%. 8.307 million rural childbearing women took folic acid with 85.1% of the annual task completed. 473,000 rural women were examined for breast cancer with 118.2% of the annual task completed. 4.892 million rural women were examined for cervical cancer with 122.3% of the annual task completed. Innocuous toilets were built for 7.833 million rural households and kitchen range transformation against coal-burning fluorosis was carried out for 1.439 million households. The annual task was completed ahead of schedule. New special public health projects were launched in all localities, such as the prevention of mother-to-infant transmission of HIV. In Hubei, Jilin, Sichuan, Henan, Hebei and Chongqing, performance assessment was further perfected, and the management of project funding, work procedures, measures of awards and punishment were all regulated. Service quality and efficiency were improved.

5) Pilot reforms of public hospitals were accelerated. The safety and quality of medical services were further enhanced. In 16 state-level pilot cities and 31 provincial-level pilot cities, pilot work was launched successively. In such pilot cities as Anshan of Liaoning and Weifang of Shandong, full explorations were made in the following areas of public hospitals: layout, management system, compensation mechanism, payment system, internal management, service improvement, support for institutions running hospitals and encouraging hospital running. As a result, preliminary experience was gained. Countrywide, focusing on strengthening service, public

hospitals pushed through some effective and easy-to-operate measures for reform and management. In 1,200 top-level hospitals countrywide, appointment diagnosis and time-phased doctors' visits were under way; in 3,828 hospitals, high-quality nursing care was developed; in over 1,300 hospitals, clinical pathway pilot was launched for 100 types of diseases. In nearly 100 hospitals of 22 provinces (regions, cities), pilot for electronic medical records (EMR) was launched. In 5 provinces (cities), pilot for practicing physicians' multi-sited license was launched, too. In all localities, reform and exploration laid a foundation for accelerating the pace of public hospital reform.

Medical quality and safety control and medical service regulation were further strengthened. Medical Quality Around the World, tour inspection of large hospitals and national key clinical specialty assessment were launched countrywide as always. Medical technology and clinical use of medical devices were standardized. Pharmacy administration was intensified and comments on prescriptions were standardized to promote rational drug use. With voluntary blood donation pushed forward, rational blood use, safety of blood products and regulation of human organ transplantation and donation were constantly strengthened. Mutual accreditation between hospitals of the same level was launched to optimize medical process and make it convenient for patients to seek medical advice. Mediation by the third party for doctor-patient conflicts and medical liability insurance were actively pushed forward. Remarkable achievements were made in the elevation of patients' contentment, medical safety security and the construction of harmonious doctor-patient relationship.

6) New achievements were made in health emergency, control of major diseases and maternal and child health care. In all localities, remarkable progress was made in the core capability construction of emergency system and mechanism, emergency preparation and on-the-site disposal. Disasters were properly dealt with, such as Yushu earthquake in Qinghai and Zhouqu massive landslide in Gansu. Powerful coordination and timely rescue made it possible to prevent major post-disaster epidemics. The task of health security was fulfilled for Shanghai World Expo and the Guangzhou Asian Games. The prevention and control of public health emergencies were further strengthened. Many major epidemics such as plague and human cases of avian influenza were effectively handled to maintain social stability.

The prevention and control of major diseases were effectively strengthened, such as HIV/AIDS, tuberculosis, Schistosomiasis and hepatitis B. The work on national expanded program on immunization was steadily pushed forward. The reported cases of fifteen infectious diseases including diphtheria were remarkably reduced. The supplementary immunization of measles vaccine (MV) for 102 million people was completed countrywide. The morbidity of measles dropped by 25.8% compared with the same period of a year earlier. The prevention and cure of major endemic disease were strengthened. The comprehensive interference and control of chronic diseases, like the prevention and control of major mental disorder and early diagnosis and early treatment of major cancers, were greatly pushed forward. Patriotic public health campaign, health education and health promotion were launched in a positive way. Therefore more and more people developed a healthy lifestyle.

The administration of maternal and child health care was intensified. Neonatal disease screening was further standardized, and the prevention and control of birth defects were also pushed forward. The program of reducing maternal mortality and eliminating neonatal tetanus was carried out thoroughly. And the promotion of knowledge of breast feeding and normal delivery was greatly publicized and popularized.

7) Efforts to regulate food and drug were strengthened constantly. Specific rectifications were launched for the safety of drug and medical devices. The regulation of food service, health food and cosmetics was intensified. The examination and approval of drug and medical devices were strengthened. Besides, the regulation of the whole process of pharmaceutical research was implemented. The quality criteria for the update of drug, food and medical devices were accelerated. *Chinese Pharmacopoeia* of 2010 Edition was promulgated to perfect the management practices of quality control of drug manufacturing. The task of medical reform was carried out to ensure the quality of basic drugs. In addition, with the sampling inspection of the evaluation and supervision of basic drugs, electronic monitoring of all varieties of basic drugs was launched. Moreover, a monitoring system for adverse drug reactions was established. The scientific popularization of Focusing on the Countryside in Safe Medication was launched. To ensure the people's medication safety, the conduct of replacing drugs with non-drugs was contained, and the manufacturing and sales of fake drugs were cracked down on.

The work on food safety was further strengthened. In order to investigate cases of illegal crimes in food safety, the rectification of food safety and check on "tainted milk powder" was launched. Adding non-food substances illegally was cracked down on and special rectification of abuse of food additives was launched. A system of "black list" of illegal food additives was established with preliminary results. With *Food Safety Law* implemented, the reform for the management system of comprehensive coordination of food safety and function adjustment were accelerated. One hundred and sixty-three criteria for national food safety were set and promulgated. The setting and revision of food basic criteria for food additives, food contaminants and mycotoxin were completed. The network for food contaminants detection and risk detection for food-borne food safety took shape initially, covering 31 provinces (regions, cities). As a result, the work on the risk detection of food safety went smoothly. Some food safety incidents were properly handled to maintain social stability, such as "Sheng Yuan Milk Powder", "Crayfish" and "Salt Iodization". Remarkable achievements were made in the food safety rectification of edible farm products, food production and circulation, catering consumption, poultry slaughter and health food.

8) Health supervision/law-enforcement was constantly strengthened. With *Prevention and Control Law of Occupational Diseases of the PRC* implemented, an institution for departmental joint session was established for occupational disease prevention and control. The purpose was to further make clear departmental duties, perfect work mechanism and push forward the implementation of national planning for the prevention and control of occupational diseases. The inspection of occupational health surveillance for employers was intensified. Many major health hazard events such as pneumoconiosis and heavy metal pollution were properly handled. The regulation for the protection of radio diagnosis and radiotherapy was strengthened. And so was drinking water surveillance. A network for drinking water surveillance was initially set up, covering 15 provinces (regions, cities). The quantitative and level-to-level management for the health supervision of such public places as accommodation and swimming complexes was completed. Special random inspection was launched for disinfection products, products of drinking water hygiene and safety, school health and blood plasma stations. The crackdown on illegal medical practice proceeded as always. The supervision and inspection for blood plasma stations were launched. The training program for health supervisors of the central and western regions was conducted as always, with the result of constant improvement of health supervision/law-enforcement.

9) New progress was made in the work on Traditional Chinese Medicine (TCM). In deepening the reform of medical and health system, we positively implemented *Several Opinions of the State Council on Supporting and Promoting Traditional Chinese Medicine* to give full play to the role of Traditional Chinese Medicine. Through the guide of basic medical security system, the service role of Traditional Chinese Medicine was promoted. The network construction of Traditional Chinese Medicine service at the primary level and reform of public hospitals of Traditional Chinese Medicine were accelerated. New progress was made in the health project of "preventive treatment of disease" of Traditional Chinese Medicine. The role of Traditional Chinese Medicine was constantly enhanced in the prevention and control of major infectious diseases and public health emergencies. Some projects were pushed forward quickly, such as clinical research bases for Traditional Chinese Medicine, key laboratories, key clinical specialty construction, talent training for Traditional Chinese Medicine and the maintenance and use of ancient books of Traditional Chinese Medicine. The

Promotion of Traditional Chinese Medicine in China pushed forward "TCM in Villages, Communities and Families". As TCM acupuncture and moxibustion was included in UNESCO's World List of Intangible Cultural Heritage, Traditional Chinese Medicine was gaining wide international acceptance.

10) New Progress was made in other health work. The punishment of health system and the construction of anti-corruption system were solidly pushed forward. The implementation and inspection of policies for promoting economic growth by boosting domestic demand were under way. And so were the protruding issues in the construction of medical projects and special rectification of "hidden coffers". A pilot project was launched for the monitoring mechanism construction of power operation. The accountability of work style rectification and the system of medical ethics assessment for medical workers were carried out. With the centralized drug procurement pushed forward, anti-bribery was intensified to a greater degree to rectify the evil trends in drug procurement and sales and medical services. The work on health care was strengthened to care for the veteran leaders' lives and health and support them in playing a role of reference and consultation.

The supporting role of health science and technology was further enhanced. The smooth overall progress was made in the management system and mechanism of two special innovations of science and technology, namely "the prevention and control of major infectious diseases" and "the development of new drugs". In order to strengthen the management of bio-safety, the interdepartmental coordination mechanism of laboratory bio-safety was established. Some appropriate technologies were spread with primary care strengthened.

Interstate and interregional exchanges and co-operations were widely conducted. Health diplomacy was developed to serve national interests and health reform and development. Experience in the international health system management was widely gained to provide our country's formulation of medical reform policies with reference. Through multiform and multilevel international exchanges, such as multilateral, bilateral, intergovernmental and nongovernmental exchanges, international co-operations and trust were improved. With the management of medical teams aiding foreign countries, more than 400 health workers were trained for Asian and African countries. Deep-level health co-operations with Hong Kong and Macau were strengthened to promote the cross-strait health exchanges. Due to the positive spread of our country's health reform policies and health development achievements, the country's medical reform gained extensive concern and acceptance of the international community.

In 2010, the central government put 126.8 billion RMB Yuan, an increase of 9.1% compared with the previous year. On the basis of deep analysis and study, the formulation of Outline of Health Program in the period of the 12th Five-Year Plan was organized. The management of capital and disposition of major medical equipment was intensified. Meanwhile, drug procurement policies were further perfected. Remarkable achievements were made in post-disaster reconstructions. Consequently, the reconstruction target of "fulfilling three years' task within two years" set by the CPC Central Committee. The spirit of Central Work Conference on Xinjiang and the 5th Central Work Conference on Tibet was seriously carried out and implemented. The 2010 work conference of national health system on the partner assistance to Xinjiang and the 5th work conference on health assistance to Tibet were convened. There were nineteen provincial and municipal health departments giving partner assistance to Xinjiang and seventeen provincial and municipal health departments giving partner assistance to Tibet. Together with the parties receiving the assistance, they worked out plans, signed agreements and organized project dockings. So the work on giving partner assistance to Xinjiang and Tibet was under way in an orderly way.

Hospital information construction, with electronic medical records (EMR) as the core, was positively pushed forward to accelerate health information construction, including residents' electronic health records and health service information platform. A risk evaluation mechanism of health system for maintaining social stability was established. And so were the mediation mechanism for medical disputes and the long-term working mechanism for letters and calls concerning health. As a result, conflicts had been resolved and stability was maintained. Press publicity on deepening medical reform was under way to strengthen typical publicity and public opinion guidance, so that a good public opinion atmosphere could be set up.

Comrades, over the past year, positive results have been achieved in health reform, which had played an important role in maintaining the people's health benefits and promoting the coordinated economic and social development. All those were due to the close attention and strong leadership of the CPC Central Committee and the State Council, the great support of Party committees and governments at all levels as well as the central departments. Moreover, the results were attributed to the concern and participation of various circles of the society and the people. What's more, they were due to the selfless devotion and joint efforts of the cadres and workers of the country's health system. Hereby, on behalf of the Ministry of Health, I would like to express our heartfelt thanks and highest respects to Party committees and governments at all levels and departments concerned which attach great importance and support health service development. Also, our thanks and respects go to various circles of the society, the news media and the people who support health work. Finally, the country's health workers deserve the heartfelt thanks and respects.

II. Study the Spirit of the Fifth Plenary Session of the 17th CPC Central Committee and Guide Health Reform and Development in the Period of the 12th Five-Year Plan with Scientific Outlook on Development

(1) Have a deeper understanding of the new requirements of the Fifth Plenary Session of the 17th CPC Central Committee for health reform and development.

The Fifth Plenary Session of the 17th CPC Central Committee was an important one which summarized the past, planned for the future and made clear the development direction and goals. The Session suggest that the country's development is still in a period of strategic opportunities in which much can be accomplished. In the period of the 12th Five-Year Plan, it must be themed by scientific development to promote the long-term, steady and rapid economic development and social harmony and stability. Also, it must follow the acceleration of the transformation of economic development pattern to do so. *Suggestions of the CPC Central Committee on Formulating the 12th Five-Year Plan for National Economy and Social Development* (hereinafter referred to as *Suggestions*) put forward the guiding ideology, development goals and main tasks of the 12th Five-Year Plan. The *Suggestions* take the safeguard and improvement of the people's livelihood as the basic starting point and foothold of accelerating the transformation of economic development pattern. Also, the *Suggestions* highlight the important role the safeguard and improvement of the people's livelihood in promoting the economic and social development and maintaining social harmony and stability.

Health is a major issue of livelihood. The *Suggestions* give priority to the acceleration of the reform and development of medical services and the improvement of the people's health. In addition, the *Suggestions* explicitly suggest that, in accordance with the requirement of "guarantee the basic medical care, strengthening the primary care and establishing the medical mechanism", fiscal revenue should be increased and the reform of medical and health system be deepened. Besides, medical workers' enthusiasm should be aroused, the people be provided with the basic medical and health care system as public products, and the people's demands for basic medical and health care be a top priority. Finally, the *Suggestions* further designate the focal points and tasks of accelerating the reform and development of medical and health services in the period of the 12th Five-Year Plan.

Seriously studying and understanding the spirit of the Session, we should effectively put together our thinking and the basic situation judgment of the CPC Central Committee. Also, we should unify our thinking and the strategies of the CPC Central Committee about the economic and social development in the period of the 12th Five-Year Plan. And what's more, we should unite our thinking and the specific requirements of the CPC Central Committee for health reform and development. Seizing favorable opportunities, we will strive to improve the people's health and livelihood, push forward the reform of system and mechanism, and transform the mode of health development.

(2) A new situation facing health reform and development in the period of the 12th Five-Year Plan

In analyzing the situation, we must first see the unprecedented favorable conditions and external environment facing health development in recent years. Attaching great importance to health work, the Party and government clarify the direction and way of thinking of health reform and development. Various circles of the society pay considerable attention to and support health work. The continued growth of comprehensive national power has laid a solid foundation for health development. Valuable experience has been gained by health work in the development progress of science. To sum up, no changes will have taken place in the long-term health development toward favorable external environment and conditions in the period of the 12th Five-Year Plan.

Meanwhile, we should also see that, at present and in a period to come, profound changes will take place continuously. And in health work, new situations, new issues and new features have emerged. So we must scientifically judge and accurately grasp the new situation and development trend. Seizing the opportunities, we must settle the health issues of millions of people's concern.

Multiple challenges about health will be brought about at the new stage of economic and social development. Since the new century, the country's economic and social development has entered a new stage. The economic development has just gone past the threshold for high-middle income, yet there remains a wide urban-rural and regional gap. And the processes of industrialization, informatization, urbanization, marketization, globalization and ageing population are accelerating continuously. Therefore health problems facing us remains more complicated. For one thing, the issues of food and drug safety, drinking water safety, occupational safety and environment brought about by eco-environment, production mode, changes of life-style and social factors are increasingly coming out, which affect greatly the people's health and bring great challenge to social health management. For another, the pattern of dual burden of infectious diseases and non-infectious diseases facing our country has not changed, and instead, its threat to the people's health and influence on economic and social development are increasingly getting worse. The situation remains worse in the prevention and control of such major infectious diseases as AIDS, hepatitis and tuberculosis. Some infectious diseases, once eradicated, have resurged. For example, SARS, human avian influenza, influenza A (H1N1) and other newly emerged infectious diseases have emerged constantly. In particular, blowout changes have taken place in the hazards of such chronic noninfectious diseases to health, like cardiovascular and cerebrovascular diseases, malignant tumors and diabetes. To respond the challenges brought about by the above-mentioned changes, corresponding adjustment and changes must be made in our macro-thinking and work strategies of health. Also, long-term strategic arrangements must be made.

A new stage of economic and social development will bring about new changes for residents' health demands and expectations. Our country has entered a new period of building a well-off society in an all-round way. With residents' living standard continually improved and various social security systems perfected step by step, rapid transformation and upgrading are occurring in the consumption concept and consumption structure of urban-rural residents. Their demands for basic material consumption being met, the people pursue life quality, health and safety all the more. And there are higher diversified demands for health care. Also, there are higher and more sensitive demands for health care including seeking medical advice. In response, there must be corresponding adjustment and changes in the service concept, service pattern and service range of health work.

Have a clear understanding of the prominent contradictions in the country's present health development. We must see that there still exist the issues of imbalance, disharmony and unsustainability in the country's health development. Firstly, health equity remains to be further improved. In the allocation of health resources, utility of health services and residents' health level, there remain significant urban-rural, regional and population discrepancy. Secondly, the development of medical and health services, as a whole, lags behind social and economic development. Meanwhile, in the internal structure and development mode of health development, there remain many issues in different degrees. They are as follows: attaching more importance to treatment and less importance to prevention; attaching more importance to scale of development and infrastructure construction and less importance to delicacy management and mechanism transformation; paying more attention to the development of high-end technology and less attention to the spread appropriate technology; and paying more attention to technical service and less attention to humanities construction. Thirdly, the people's individual medical spending remains a heavy burden. The study of WHO shows that only when the share of individual spending drops by 15%~20% of a country's total health expenditure can the issue of "poverty due to illness" be resolved. What needs to be focused on is that per capita medical expenditure is on the rise in recent years, of which the unreasonable rise due to mechanism issues is worthy of attention. Currently, medical expenditures for major diseases remain a heavy burden to urban-rural residents. The above-mentioned issues are the prominent conflicting issues which must be prioritized in the period of the 12th Five-Year Plan.

Have a clear understanding of the deep-seated issues in the country's health development. Over the past 30 years of reform and opening-up, especially in the period of the 11th Five-Year Plan, the weak links and areas restricting the country's health service development were strengthened step by step. With the reform entering a crucial stage, some systems, mechanisms and structural problems restricting health service development have become increasingly prominent. As a unified, efficient health management system and a steady public input mechanism have not taken shape, such key issues of reform as "separation of management and enforcement", "separation of medicine and pharmacy" remain to be further explored. In addition, the constructions for legal system of health and talents, development of health care industry, medical research and construction of health informatization relatively lag behind. Some major issues involving the orientation of health reform and development still need to gather consensus and be embodied in the practice of reform and development. Therefore some specific policies and measures of reform remain to be further improved. And these issues also bring up new requirements for health reform in the period of the 12th Five-Year Plan.

Comrade, from the global height of the country's economic and social development, grasping the favorable conditions of health work and the new situation facing us can boost our confidence, make us strategically situated,put ourselves in an accurate position and assign tasks for the next five years. Meanwhile, it will be of help to enhance our senses of mission and responsibility to do the work specifically and in an down-to-earth way for the next five years to analyze matter-of-factly the principal contradictions and prominent issues facing health development.

(3) Transform the mode of health development to achieve scientific development for health services.

Health work in the period of the 12th Five-Year Plan should be themed by scientific development and follow the transformation of development mode, so that the issues of imbalance, disharmony and unsustainability in health development can be resolved. Through deepening the reform of system and mechanism, we will improve the equity and accessibility of basic medical and health services. An by transforming the mode of health development, we will achieve sound and sustainable development of health services to make sure that the goal of everyone's having access to basic medical and health services will be achieved.

Firstly, we must establish an overall concept and pay more attention to the all-round and coordinated development. Health development must proceed from the overall situation of maintaining residents' health and promoting economic and social development. And the integrity and coordination of health development should be enhanced. Local interest and overall interests should be considered as a whole, and so should immediate interests and long-term interests. Therefore the coordinated development of health services and economic society will be achieved. We should scientifically define the rights and obligations of government, society and individual in the basic medical and health services to take interests of various sides into full consideration and maintain the people's health interests. Also, we will take into full consideration the coordinated development of the systems of public health, medical services, medical security and drug supply, so that a more perfect system of basic medical and health care can be established. In the period of the 12th Five-Year Plan, we will still value highly the health services in the countryside, at the primary level and in the Mid-western region to narrow continually the regional and populations gaps in health services and health levels.

Secondly, based on China's national conditions, we must pay more attentions to the overall benefits of development. In the period of the 12th Five-Year Plan, health development still cannot be separated from the actual situations of the country. Proceeding from the level of economic and social development and the people's affordability, health development must lay a solid foundation for public health and basic medical services. In addition, we will continue to increase government investment in health, optimize the input structure and control medical costs and develop human resources and technology in health. Performing the immediate and most effective intervention in major diseases and major hazards affecting the people's health, we will strive to get the maximum benefits out of the limited resources and really set out on a health path with Chinese characteristics.

Thirdly, we must attach great importance to the transformation of service mode, centering on health improvement. For some time to come, the rapid transformation of the country's disease patterns requires that health development should transform from the emphasis on treatment to health promotion, from the emphasis on individual service objects to families and social groups. And service contents should range from specialties to more emphasis on general practice, so that a continuing service pattern covering everyone's entire life cycle can be established. With the prevention-oriented policy carried out fully, health investment should tilt toward preventive care even more. Moreover, service institutions should adjust, perfect and intensify the function of preventive care. With health education and health promotion enhanced, public health awareness improved, and a healthy lifestyle developed, a new situation of social involvement and everyone's being responsible for health will take shape.

Fourthly, adhering to paying equal attention to both Traditional Chinese Medicine (TCM) and western medicine, we must think highly of giving full play to the advantages of TCM characteristics. As a branch of medical science with original advantages in our country, TCM possesses an extensive and profound basis among the masses. In addition, TCM is an indispensible component of socialist medical and health services with Chinese characteristics. TCM possesses the characteristics of "being simple, convenient, cheap and effective", emphasizes the health care concept of "preventive treatment of disease" and stresses the human spirit of "virtue of great physician" and being people-oriented. All those have promising prospects in the transformation health development pattern. Adhering to the policy of paying equal attention to both Traditional Chinese Medicine and western medicine, and perfecting the system and mechanism which help play a role TCM, we should make TCM play a greater role in improving the people's health quality.

Fifthly, we must adhere to the strategy of talent priority development and think more highly of talent construction. For some time to come, human resources in health remain a key factor restricting health development. In health development, we should attach importance not only to the construction and improvement of facilities and conditions but also to talent cultivation. Both talent scale development and talent quality are to be emphasized. Making the cultivation of top-quality talents in health a priority, we will restructure the system and mechanism of talent building and talent employment to bring up a health talent team with superb techniques and noble medical ethics, which can adapt to the future transformation of medical pattern and the people's demands for health.

(4) The main task concerning the health reform and development for the 12th Five-Year Plan

In accordance to the spirit of the Fifth Plenary Session of the 17th CPC Central Committee and in combination with relevant study results, I will talk about some basic ideas for your discussion and reference on working out plans.

The first idea is the overall target concerning health development for the 12th Five-Year Plan. By 2015, the basic medical and health system covering urban-rural residents will have been established. Moreover, the system of basic medical security will grow more perfect; the system of public health service and the system of medical services will become more complete; and the system of drug supply guarantee will be more standardized. The management system and operation mechanism of medical and health institutions will become more scientific. The accessibility of basic medical and health services will be enhanced significantly. As a result, the residents' burden of individual medical expenses will be reduced significantly and the people's health level will be raised further. In addition, the difference between regional allocation of resources and population health status will be narrowed, and the level of national health will be at a leading position among developing countries. It is proposed that the average life expectancy should be 74.5 years, infant mortality and children under five years old be reduced to 12% and 14% respectively, and maternal mortality, to 22/100,000. With the proportion of government and social health expenditure for total expenditure on health raised, individual health expenditure will be reduced 30%.

The second idea is the basic thinking on health development for the 12th Five-Year Plan. With scientific development governing various health work and the sustainable development of health service driven by the transformation of develop pattern, we will adhere to the nonprofit nature of public medical and health care services. Also, we will adhere to the policy of prevention first, focusing on the countryside and attaching equal importance to TCM and western medicine. With the improvement of public health and urban-rural basic medical services as a highlight focus, we will coordinate and push forward the constructions of public hospitals, security system and drug supply system. And health talent cultivation and the constructions of informatization and health law will be accelerated. Finally, we will carry out government responsibilities, increase health investment, intensify supervision and management and establish the system of basic medical and health care covering urban-rural residents in an all-round way.

The third idea is the main task concerning health development for the 12th Five-Year Plan.

Strengthen the capacity construction of medical and health institutions and improve the level of medical and health services. Intensify the regional health planning and the establishment planning of medical institutions to clarify the functions and responsibilities of all sorts of medical and health institutions. Optimize the scale, structure and layout to establish a system of medical and health services for the combination of prevention and control, paying equal attention to TCM and western medicine, functional complementation, information sharing and interactions between the top and bottom. Strengthen the construction of public health services to improve facilities of professional public health agencies, such as those of disease prevention and control, mental health, maternal and child health, health supervision, health emergency, occupational disease prevention, blood collection and supply and health education. Continue to strengthen the standardization construction of rural emergency system, township hospitals and village clinics. Push forward the standardization construction of hospitals at the county level to reach the level of second grade on the whole. Integrate the medical and health resources of the counties to push forward the comprehensive reform, transform the operation mechanism, perfect the performance pay and achieve the transformation of service function and service pattern. Push forward positively and steadily public hospital reform, improve the service system of public hospitals, and restructure the management system, governance mechanism, operation mechanism and compensation mechanism. Strengthen the medical quality management and control as well as medical safety regulation, and improve the service quality continuously. Promote the management of scientification, refinement and specialization to improve the service and efficiency. Establish initially the system of national medical center and strengthen the construction of regional medical centers and key clinical specialties. Continue to strengthen the construction of community health services and strive to establish a government-run community health service center within each neighborhood office. Establish a new system of urban health service based on community health service, and with rational division of work and close collaboration between community health services and hospitals and professional public health institutions. Inherit and innovate TCM to establish a more complete service system of prevention and healthcare for TCM as well as a system of scientific research innovation. Strengthen the construction of TCM team and play the role of traditional medicine in protecting the national health. Step up the construction of health law, and put into effect the constructions of medical talent training base and medical informationization to provide great support for health reform and development. Encourage and support the social capital in establishing nonprofit and profit medical institutions. Therefore they can get involved in the development of such health services as health management, nursing for the aged, dental care and rehabilitation. And thus a diversified medical structure will take shape to meet the needs of diversified and multi-level medicine, prevention, healthcare, provision for the aged and rehabilitation.

Perfect the medical security system to improve the economic risk sharing of disease. Improve the coverage and security level of the basic medical security system to narrow the medical security gap of urban-rural areas. Per capita financing level of the new rural cooperative medical system aims for 300 RMB Yuan and above. And outpatient service will cover all areas. Raise further the reimbursement of hospitalization expenses within the policy range. Perfect the urban-rural medical aid system to raise the coverage of disadvantaged families. Extend the security scope of major diseases with the reimbursement rate of no less than 90%. Improve the fund management in order to prevent any fund risk.

Prevent and control major disease to control health risk factors. With the improvement of prevention and control system of major diseases, bring under basic control malaria and meet the target of measles elimination. Contain the spread of tuberculosis, venereal disease and HIV/AIDS, and reduce the prevalence of hepatitis B. The main endemic diseases and parasitic diseases will meet the national control standard. Extend significantly the coverage of chronic disease prevention and control. Increase the awareness rate and control rate of diabetes, hypertension and other chronic diseases. Continue to strengthen the capacity construction of disease prevention and control. Improve the prevention and control of mental health and mental disorder. Strengthen the prevention and control of key occupational diseases to reduce genuinely the threat of occupational hazard to people's health.

Improve step by step the equalization of basic public health services. Raise substantially the per capita standard for expenditures on basic public health services. Expand gradually the content of basic public health services and make sure that it can cover all the residents. Implement effective intervention in major diseases and bring the control measures of risk factors into the major public health services of the country. Resolve the issue of public health services among the shifting population, especially the rural migrant workers in cities.

Strengthen genuinely the social management responsibilities of governments at all levels over public health to ensure residents' life and health safety. Establish and improve a security system of drug supply based on national system for basic drugs. Regulate heavily the quality of drug and medical devices. With the improvement of the surveillance rate of drugs, perform random check on the full coverage of basic drugs and perform electronic supervision on wide varieties of drugs. With the establishment and improvement of the management system of standard drug use at second-class and third-class hospitals, strengthen the surveillance and evaluation of reasonable drug use to reduce the occurrence of adverse drug reactions. Establish a responsibility system for drug safety to ensure people's drug safety and safety in medical devices.

Improve and perfect constantly the supervision and management system and mechanism for public finances in disease prevention and control, food safety, drinking water sanitation, occupational health, school health and health emergencies. Establish and improve a monitoring system, perfect regulation agencies and upgrade the regulatory capacity. Perform risk surveillance, evaluation and early-warning. And strengthen the regulation and law-enforcement for catering, health food and cosmetics to reduce greatly the occurrence of unsafe incidents. Improve the risk surveillance coverage for food safety, the surveillance rate for the occupational health of laborers engaged in the occupational-disease-inductive operation, hygienic qualification rate of urban drinking water quality and hygienic qualification rate of rural centralized water supply.

What I said above is a general consideration for the main target and key content of health development planning in the period of the 12th Five-Year Plan. All localities should combine the local actual situations to come up with planning targets, development ideas and work focus in the regions. We should closely integrate the tasks with health reform in the period of the 12th Five-Year Plan, make steady headway and lay a solid foundation for achieving the goal that everyone will have access to basic medical and health services in 2020.

Ⅲ. Spare No Efforts to Do 2011 Health Work

It is the last year in which the recent work focus for medical reform is carried out. It is also the first year of the Twelfth Five-Year Plan. Therefore it is of great significance to do well this year's work.

(1) Complete five tasks for medical reform with focal points highlighted.

Medical reform remains the most important of all the health work for 2011. In accordance with the requirements of Central Economic Work Conference, we should emphasize the construction of basic drug system and pilot reforms in public hospitals for this year's medical system reform.

1) Lay stress on the improvement of national system for basic drugs. The first is to consolidate and expand the implementation scope for basic drug system. Government-run medical institutions at the primary level will put into effect the basic drug system. In localities where conditions permit, it is encouraged that village clinics and non-government medical institutions at the primary level are brought into the implementation range of basic drug system. The second is to study and adjust without delay the list of national basic drugs (at the primary level) to better meet the people's needs for drugs. On that basis, start in due time the formulation of basic drug list in full edition for the use of medical institutions at all levels. The third is to perform the procurement and distribution of basic drugs as required by *Circular of the General Office of the State Council on Printing the Guiding Opinions on Establishing and Standardizing the Procurement Mechanism for Basic Drugs of Government-run Medical Institutions at the Primary Level.* The fourth is to strengthen the management of equipment and use of basic drugs to make sure that all the government-run medical institutions are equipped with basic drugs, use them and conduct zero-profit sales. The fifth is to perfect the reimbursement and disbursement policy for basic drugs to make sure that the rate for reimbursement of basic drugs is significantly higher than non-essential drugs. The sixth is to perform the surveillance and evaluation for the implementation of basic drug system by medical institutions at the primary level to strengthen capacity building for surveillance. The seventh is to encourage medical institutions at the county level and above to make a study of how to carry out the basic drug system. The eighth is to strengthen the guidance of upper-level hospitals over medical institutions at the primary level through assistance to counterparts. In promoting the basic drug system, all localities should learn from the experience of Anhui. By way of comprehensive supplementary reforms and carrying out the policies

of medical institutions at the primary level, such as functional orientation, formation, financial aid, mechanism transformation and performance assessment, all localities should genuinely reduce the burden of medical expenditures. As a result, people can really benefit from the policy of basic drug policy.

2) Step up the pilot reforms in public hospitals. As required by the leading group of the State Council for medical reform, the method of "highlighting the focal points, starting with easy things first" should be adopted. The service measures of benefiting people and for their convenience, which are maturer, more effective and easy to handle, will be popularized throughout the country. Therefore the people can benefit from public hospital reform. The first is to optimize the layout and structure of public hospitals. Strengthen the planning and management, especially the capacity building in the weak areas, in order to promote reasonable allocation of resources. The second is to establish a mechanism of division of responsibilities between public hospitals and urban-rural hospitals at the primary level. Through the upper and lower linkage, give play to overall functionality of medical service system. The third is to give priority to the construction of county hospitals. With the promotion of the comprehensive pilot reforms of county hospitals, there will be a public hospital at level II and above in any county with a population of 300,000 and above by the end of 2011. The fourth is to carry out the service for the convenience of people and strengthen the internal management. With the expansion of the service range of quality service, promote the service measures of benefiting people of appointment outpatient service and inter-accreditation of results. Expand the disease entities and implementation scope of clinical pathway and strengthen the cost control. Proceed with Medical Quality around the World. The fifth is to carry out the reform for the pattern of fee settlement and medical insurance payment. Push forward and carry out the reform of such payment methods as payment by type of disease and global budget. The sixth is to arouse the enthusiasm of medical workers by improving treatment, multi-sited license, establishing standard the training system for resident doctors, perfecting the conditions for career development, improving the professional development and other measures. The seventh is to speed up the promotion of the informatization construction with electronic medical record (EMR) as the core. The eighth is to promote the reform and development of public TCM hospitals. Meanwhile, explore in depth the major issues of system and mechanism concerning public hospital reform in pilot cities and localities according to the principle of separating government administration from medical institutions, management from operation, medical care from pharmaceuticals and for-profit from nonprofit operations. As a result, the experience can be summed up. As for public hospital reform, formulate special document and convene special meeting for deployment. In accordance with the spirit

of speeding up public hospital reform and above focus, all localities can make an early study, early preparation and early deployment for promoting and deepening public hospital reform.

I here would like to lay special stress on controlling the growth of medical expenses. Since 2010, various channels have reported rapid growth of medical expenses. It cannot be denied that, in view of experiences in various countries and with the economic development, technological progress, population ageing and the development of basic medical security system, there will be growth of medical expenses by a certain margin. The growth of CPI will also affect the level of medical expenses. However, the rise in medical expenses must be in harmony with the level of economic development and fit in with the endurance of government finance, basic medical security and individuals. The rapid rise in medical expenses within a short time will affect the people's immediate interests and perception of medical reform. For this reason, it is decided by the Party Committee of the Ministry that it is an important task of this year to control the rapid growth of medical expenses. Therefore, all localities please make a deep analysis and study of the tendency and reason for the rise in medical expenses in the region. From a practical standpoint, set scientifically a control goal and index for per capita outpatient expenses and hospitalization expenses. Adopt the measures of administration, economy, law and information in a comprehensive way to control unreasonable drug use, unreasonable examination and rapid rise in the medical expenses of some key specialties. In addition, make a study of the long-term mechanism of controlling medical expenses. Health administrative department in all localities should publicize regularly the information concerning the change of medical expenses in the affiliated medical institutions for public supervision. The Ministry of Health and all localities should conduct special evaluation and examination for expense control under the surveillance of medical reform.

Strengthen genuinely medical safety and quality control. Push forward the construction of the national center for medical quality management and control and the center for medical quality control of key clinical specialty at the state level. Establish a system of report and warned conversation for any incident of medical quality and safety. Organize and start the review and appraisal of medical institutions and inspection tours of large hospitals. Put into effect the construction project of the country's key clinical specialty. Strengthen the regulation of human organ transplantation and donation. Strengthen the management of blood quality and safety to push forward unpaid blood donation and reasonable clinical use of blood. Strengthen the capacity building of rehabilitation medicine. In combination with the activities of deepening the reform for medical system and excelling in our performance, start the activity of "excellent service, superior quality, excellent medical ethics and people's satisfaction" in the entire medical circle this year. Always upgrade medical service, continuously improve medical quality, carry forward noble medical ethics, put in place the measures of benefiting the people and strive to establish hospitals to the needs of people.

3) Consolidate and perfect the system of new rural cooperative medical care. The first is to improve further the security level of NCMS on the basis of steady rate of participation. Strive to raise the subsidy standard of government again in 2011. Raise the highest pay limitation for hospitalization compensation and steadily expand the scope of overall implementation of outpatient service. Push forward the pilot work on medical security for children's major diseases in the provinces. And launch a pilot program for the security and treatment of major diseases, such as serious mental illness, breast cancer, cervical cancer and uremia. The second is to improve the fine management of the agencies of NCMS to standardize fund management for fund safety. Perfect the agencies of NCMS to improve the capacity of management and service. Speed up the promotion of constructions of NCMS information platform at the state level and information systems in various localities. In the provinces where conditions permit, start the pilot One-Card for rural residents' health. Rural residents participating in NCMS will be able to seek medical advice on their own and obtain immediate settlement for medical expenses. Push forward the work on immediate settlement in provincial and municipal medical institutions. The third is to regularize the service behavior of designated medical institutions and expand the scope of payment reform of NCMS. The fourth is to improve unceasingly NCMS and give an overall consideration to basic medical security and medical services. Promote the pilot work on regulating as a whole the urban-rural basic medical security system. Summarize the useful experience of insurance industry involved in the operation and management of NCMS and spread it gradually. The fifth is to promote the legislation of NCMS to strive to issue as soon as possible *Control Regulations on the New Rural Cooperative Medical Care System.*

4) Promote the gradual equalization of basic public health services. The first is to raise the per capita standard for the expenditures of basic public health services. After the central government set and issued the new standard for subsidy, all localities must ask for full supporting funds. Health departments should work closely with financial departments to guarantee the timely arrival of funds. The second is to add service contents, improve service standards and adjust service standards after the input increase to benefit more people. The third is to improve the management. Seize the opportunity of integrating the township health informatization and equipping village clinics with computers. Improve the management tool of rural basic public health

services to achieve step by step the standardized and refined management. The fourth is to establish a system, divide work explicitly and put into effect the responsibilities. Work out *The State Standards for Basic Public Health Services* (2011 Edition) to conduct surveillance and assessment of how to implement the basic public health services. The fifth is to carry out further the project of major public health. Sum up the two years' experience, seek weak links and improve the project management to promote the implementation of various major public health projects. The sixth is to enhance the capacity building of maternal and child health care system. Continue to carry out the program of reducing maternal mortality and eliminating neonatal tetanus. Strengthen the prevention and control of birth defects; strengthen the management of Baby-Friendly Hospital; promote natural childbirth; and start the pilot work for child nutrition and health surveillance. The seventh is to carry out in an all-round way the construction of prevention and control system for mental health. The eighth is to push forward the establishment of smoke-free medical institutions. Start the activity of national healthy lifestyle and the special operation of health education. Clarify the responsibilities and tasks of health education of various health institutions and professionals. Through unremitting health education and health promotion, improve the health quality of the whole nation. In particular, contain the tendency of rapid rise of chronic, non-infectious diseases.

5) Perfect further the system of medical and health services at the primary level. The first is to accelerate the standardization construction of medical and health services at the primary level. Complete the constructions of county hospitals, township health centers and community health service agencies. Meanwhile, ensure quality and speed up the process in order to complete the constructions as early as possible and produce results. County hospitals should highlight the construction of comprehensive service capacity and key specialties. Use genuinely the funds, issued recently, for equipment and facilities of medical and health institutions at the primary level. Achieve the combination of houses, equipment and personnel through the construction. The second is to promote the comprehensive supplementary reforms of medical and health institutions at the primary level. Carry out *Opinions of the General Office of the State Council on Establishing and Perfecting the Compensation Mechanism of Medical and Health Institutions at the Primary Level* to ensure normal operation of medical and health institutions at the primary level. The third is to deepen the reform of personnel distribution system. Carry out appointment system for entire employees, carry out post responsibilities, carry out performance pay and intensify performance assessment to arouse the enthusiasm of medical workers at the primary level. The fourth is to continue to implement the policy, system and project of talent training for grass-root level organizations. On the basis of raising the subsidy level, standardize

step by step the subsidy policy for village doctors and encourage any region where condition permits to provide retirement pension for village doctors. In particular, we must give full play to the advantage of medical institutions at the primary level with the constant perfection of service facilities of medical and health institutions at the primary level and gradual implementation of financial subsidy policy. The reason is that medical institutions at the primary level are always community-oriented and close to people. Adhere to the functional orientation of "combining prevention with treatment" and restructure the operation mechanism of "subsidizing medical services with drug sales". Transform the service pattern of waiting for patients. Instead, take the initiative to provide public health service and basic medical service, such as disease prevention, health care, chronic illness management and health education. Therefore the policy objective of improving medical and health service system at the primary level can be achieved.

(2) Proceed with the work for health emergencies and major disease prevention.

With effective response to various emergencies as the goal and with the improvement of on-the-spot disposal capacity for health emergencies as the core, push forward the construction of health emergency system. The first is to accelerate the promotion of the construction of command & decision-making system of health emergencies and the construction of health emergency team to ensure timely information, rapid response and smooth command. The second is to start the construction of national base for emergency medicine rescue to lay the groundwork of medical rescue for major accidents or disasters. The third is to strengthen the capacity building of emergency response to various public emergencies. The fourth is to conduct prevention and control of plague, human-infected avian influenza and unknown diseases to be on guard against various public health emergencies.

Positively push forward the prevention and control of major infectious diseases, chronic disease, endemic disease and mental disorder as well as patriotic public health campaign. The first is to perfect the systems of disease prevention and control and patriotic public health. Improve the system of public health physicians in disease prevention and control to fully promote performance assessment. The second is to strengthen the dynamic surveillance over infectious diseases, such as AIDS, venereal disease, hepatitis C, tuberculosis, influenza and hand-foot-mouth disease. Continue to carry out the routine vaccine immunization for national immunization program. Carry out the follow-up revaccination for measles supplementary immunization to achieve the target of eliminating measles as scheduled. The third is to carry out the prevention and control of such key parasitic diseases as schistosomiasis and malaria as well as key endemic disease. The fourth is to work out and implement *Guiding Opinions on Strengthening the Prevention and Control of Chronic Diseases*. Establish national demonstration areas for comprehensive prevention and control of chronic diseases. Intensify the combination of prevention and control of major mental disease with comprehensive management of social order. Extend the content and coverage of comprehensive intervention in children's oral disease of Mid-western Region. The fifth is to continue to strengthen the construction of innocuous toilets in rural areas. Carry out surveillance over the safety of rural drinking water. Promote and standardize the construction of clean cities.

(3) Strengthen the regulation of food and drug.

The first is to carry out the 12th Five-Year Plan to promote the transformation of medical and economic development pattern. The second is to perfect the accountability system for drug safety to improve regulation efficacy. The third is to strengthen the regulation of basic drugs to ensure the safety of basic drugs. The fourth is to improve the work mechanism to enhance the capacity of duty execution. The fifth is to strengthen the construction of laws and regulations. Promote the issue of *Regulations on Supervision and Management of Health Food* to raise the level of supervision according to law. The sixth is to intensify supervision and management to standardize further drug manufacturing and operation order. The seventh is to push forward the reform of cadre and personnel system to strengthen the team building and improve the comprehensive quality of supervision and management team in an all-round way.

(4) Strengthen further the comprehensive coordination of food safety and health supervision/law-enforcement.

In strengthening food safety, the first is to improve further the comprehensive coordination mechanism. Push forward the perfection of food safety regulations and perfect the system of unified announcement for food safety information. The second is to carry out the task of food safety rectification. Continue to carry out special rectification of cracking down on illegal addition of non-food substance and abuse of food additives. Perfect the system of "black list" and investigate illegal and criminal activities for food safety. The third is to clean up and perfect state criteria for food safety to strengthen the publicity, training and follow-up evaluation of food safety criteria. The fourth is to push forward the institution setup of risk evaluation for state food safety. Give priority to five items of risk evaluation including lead in food and trans-fatty acids. Strengthen the constructions of early-warning system for the risk evaluation and risk evaluation capacity of food safety. The fifth is to perfect the investigation system of major accidents of food safety to improve the capacity of emergency investigation and disposal for food safety emergencies.

In the improvement of health supervision/law-enforcement, the first is to attach importance to the self-construction of health supervision/law-enforcement team.

Perform performance assessment for health supervision to raise the level of health supervision and inspection. The third is to carry out and implement *National Program for Occupational Disease Prevention and Control (2009-2015)* to promote the capacity building of institutions for occupational disease prevention and control. Conduct surveillance and investigation over key occupational diseases. Push forward the pilot work for basic occupational health service. Carry out the supervision and management of occupational health examination, and occupational disease diagnosis and appraisal. Strengthen the qualification accreditation and daily supervision for institutions for chemical toxicity identification. The fourth is to intensify the supervision and inspection of radiological health, focusing on the radiation hazard of medical institutions. The fifth is to strengthen health supervision and management of drinking water and disinfection products related to water. Carry out the system of quantified and graded management in bathing and hairdressing establishments. The sixth is to strengthen the supervision and inspection of infectious disease prevention and control as well as the supervision and management of school health. Crack down on such criminal activities as illegal medical practice and illegal blood collection and supply.

(5) Do well the work of TCM

The first is to fully carry out *Several Opinions of the State Council on Supporting and Promoting the Development of Traditional Chinese Medicine*. Establish and improve any system, mechanism and input policy which help give play to the characteristics of TCM. The second is to organize and develop the construction of clinical cooperation center for preponderant illness in TCM. Speed up the promotion of the capacity construction of health emergency response of TCM medical institutions and the construction of emergency system for the prevention and control of emerging infectious diseases by TCM. Improve the capacity of TCM emergency rescue and prevention and control of major diseases. The third is to continue to push forward the health project of "preventive treatment of disease". Make a study of and carry out a menu-driven service for "preventive treatment of chronic disease". Promote the capacity construction of preventive health care of TCM institutions at all levels and of all types. The fourth is to perfect the construction of scientific system for TCM inheritance and innovation. Step up the training of TEM talents and technical elite at the primary level. The fifth is to carry out in a deep-going way the activity of "Promotion of Traditional Chinese Medicine in China—Culture and Science Popularization Week". Encourage the service of TCM to "go into the countryside, community and family". Intensify the base construction of TCM culture, publicity and education as well as the publicity and popularization of TCM knowledge. The sixth is to push forward the process of TCM legislation and construction of TCM criteria. The seventh is to accelerate the promotion of the process of bringing TCM to the world and the development of the trade for TCM service.

(6) Fulfill the task for health talent construction and improve the work capability of health science and education.

Carry out and implement *2010-2020 Development Plan for Medical and Health Talents*. The first is that central and local health departments should continue to strive for funds. They should also set up special funds to intensify talent training at the primary level. In 2011, the central government will give priority to the training of fine doctors, professional and technical talents for county hospitals. The government will recruit practicing physicians for the township health centers of poverty-stricken areas. And the government will also start the program of training medical students gratis for the countryside. The second is to summarize experience and finish the on-job training for urban-rural health workers at the primary level as required by the task of three-year medical reform. The third is to establish initially a system for the standardized training of general practitioners to intensify the job-transfer training for general practitioners. The fourth is to perfect relevant policies, strengthen the construction of nursing team and increase the number of nursing staff. Start the pilot training for the standardization of public health workers. Push forward the training for clinical pharmacists, especially those at the primary level. In 2011, 10,000 pharmacists from urban-rural medical institutions at the primary level will be trained. Make a study of establishing a pharmacist system.

Depending on science and technology, promote the implementation of medical reform and the development of health services. The first is to intensify the popularization of appropriate technology based on the requirements of strengthened primary. Establish a long-term mechanism of selection, development, popularization and evaluation of appropriate technology. The second is to organize the implementation of various major scientific plans and intensify the process supervision. The third is to work out health science and technology plan for the 12th Five-Year Plan to explore the construction of medical science and technology innovation system. Give full play to the supporting role of science and technology to promote the cultivation and development of strategic emerging industries. The fourth is to intensify the management of laboratory biosafety. And strengthen the construction of the key laboratories of the Ministry of Health and other scientific-research bases. The fifth is to perfect the management system of medical science and technology research. Push forward the construction of the systems for ethical review, management of intellectual property and research integrity of biomedical research.

(7) Speed up the promotion of the construction for health information system.

The first is to plan the health information development in the period of the

12th Five-Year Plan. On the basis of strengthening information standardization and platform of public service information, intensify the construction of national health information strategy with the promotion of electronic health record (HER), electronic medical record (EMR) and telemedicine as the breakthrough points. The construction focuses on public health, medical service, medical security, basic drug system and comprehensive management. Work out and issue guiding opinions on health information construction and launch comprehensive pilot projects. The second is to accelerate the information construction of medical and health institutions at the primary level. With some provinces (regions, cities) chosen as the pilot areas, strengthen the training of information knowledge and skills for village health workers while unifying the information equipment. Unify and standardize the information management and technical criteria at the rural grassroots. Improve as soon as possible the levels of rural public health, medical security and administrative management of health, depending on information technology. The third is to accelerate the construction of tele-consultation system. Launch the pilot project of the construction for tele-consultation system between top-level hospitals affiliated the Ministry of Health and provinces and municipal general hospitals in the remote areas, and between provincial hospitals and county hospitals in the remote areas. The fourth is that health administrative departments at all levels should look closely at interconnection and information sharing. They should also integrate the needs of health information and existing resources. In addition, they should strive for financial support, lead research institutions and social forces to get involved in and promote health information construction.

(8) Launch deeply and solidly an activity of excelling in performance.

It is the political impetus and organization guarantee of deepening medical reform to strengthen the Party construction and excel in performance. Centering on health work, we should launch an activity of excelling in performance. The first is to start such activities as public commitment, leadership comments and mass appraisal, combining the tasks of medical reform. Stimulate and arouse the enthusiasm of a large number of Party members, cadres and workers to perform their duties and responsibilities and fully complete every task of medical reform. The second is to launch an activity of selecting and rewarding exemplary primary-level Party organizations, outstanding Communist Party members and outstanding Party workers within the medical and health circles of the country. In addition, launch an activity of learning from the exemplary organizations or individuals and achieving success to promote the construction of Party organizations at the primary level and play the role of combat fortress of Party organizations and the vanguard and exemplary role of Party members. The third is to publicize and carry forward the exemplary models and exemplary deeds with medical and health circles. And also create a sound atmosphere of learning from the exemplary individuals or organizations, catching up with them and promoting the reform. The fourth is to perfect and establish an assessment criterion for civilization units, intensify the assessment and push forward the creation activity for civilization units within the industry.

(9) Make overall arrangements to do well other health work.

With the planning guidance strengthened, work out the health development plan and special health plan for the 12th Five-Year Plan. Play the guiding role of regional health planning in the reasonable allocation of health resources to optimize the allocation of large medical devices. Strengthen the management of health funds and projects. Fulfill genuinely the tasks of restoration and reconstruction in disaster areas and assisting Xinjiang and Tibet in health.

Strengthen the construction of legal system of health. Push forward the legislations of health care of basic medical care, mental health and TCM. And push forward the formulation of standards for health rules and regulations. Strengthen the promotion of knowledge of the laws and administrative reviews of health. Centering on the issues concerning theory and practice in the course of reform and development, conduct a research into health policies.

Perfect unceasingly the systems of punishment and corruption prevention within health system to ensure the implementation of the central decisions and arrangements about anti-corruption and advocating integrity. In combination with health matters, strictly carry out the construction of CPC Party work style and clean government and accountability for rectification. Do a solid work for medical ethics appraisal, centralized drug procurement and making hospital affairs public. Strive to achieve new results of rectification in health and bribery control.

Give play to the advantages of health to serve state diplomacy. Strive for technical support from international organizations to conduct medical evaluation. Take the initiative to start multilateral diplomacy in health and deepen bilateral and regional health cooperation. Expand our way of thinking and bring about a new situation of medical care. The mainland should keep in close contact with Hong Kong, Macau and Taiwan to put into effect the signed agreements.

Step up the establishment of mechanism of risk evaluation of the social stability for major events within health circles. Strengthening the work of health complaints, summarize and spread the experience of the adjustment and handling of the third party in doctor-patient disputes to effectively guard against and reduce doctor-patient conflicts. Establish peace hospitals. Take the initiative to carry out publicity on health and further strengthen the publicity of major decisions about health, medical reform results and exemplary models. Do well the work of publishing hot issues of health and emergencies and opinion orientation. Push forward openness in government affairs and take the initiative to accept social supervision.

Attach importance to the work of health care and improve work level. Care for the lives and health of veteran cadres and veteran workers, and give play to the role of veteran cadres.

Comrades, for achieving the stage goal of medical reform, it is of great significance to do well this year' health work to open a world for health development in the period of the 12th Five-Year Plan. Under the strong leadership of the Party Central Committee with Comrade Hu Jintao as the General Secretary, let us forge ahead with determination with strong confidence and one hear and one mind to do solid work. And let's strive to open a new world for the scientific development of health services to commemorate the 90th anniversary of the CPC with excellent results.

(Shan Yongxiang)

2. Taking Advantage of the Opportunities, Building Consensus and Effectively Strengthening Food Safety and Health Supervision

—An Address Delivered by Chen Zhu, Minister of Health, at the 2011 National Work Conference of Food Safety and Health Supervision (January 12, 2011)

Soon after the conclusion of 2011 National Health Work Conference, we hold this National Work Conference of Food Safety and Health Supervision to study and implement the essence of the national work conference and deploy the work of food safety and health supervision this year, which means the conference is of great importance. A short time ago, Comrade Li Keqiang, member of Standing Committee of the Political Bureau of the Central Committee and the Vice-premier of State Council, made special instructions at the National Health Work Conference, in which he fully recognized the remarkable achievements made by the national health system last year, expressed his sincere greetings and gratitude to all the health workers and meanwhile proposed clear demands for the work this year. As for the important instructions of Vice Premier Li's, we must carefully study it, deeply understand it and fully implement it.

The CPC Central Committee and the State Council attach great importance to promoting the reform and development of health care undertaking, regarding it as an important part of ensuring and improving the livelihood of the people and an important measure of promoting social harmony. The reform and development of health supervision system has always been an important part of the reform of health care undertaking. In the past ten years, under the leadership of the party committees and governments at different levels and with the care and support of relevant departments, all walks of the society and the people, the comrades in the field of health supervision have made great progress with their persistent efforts and exploration. The health supervision systems at the provincial level, municipal level and county level have gradually taken shape, which are being extended to the township level, with nearly 100,000 health supervisors nationwide. Consequently, the law enforcement has been intensified and management of the team is more normative. Health supervision has become an indispensable force to secure people's health and interest and safeguard the order of public health service and the harmony and stability of the society, which has also obtained the attention and recognition of the governments at different levels and the people. Here, on behalf of the Ministry of Health, I would like to express our cordial greetings and honorable respect to all the staff members working diligently in the field of health supervision and all the comrades working in relevant fields of food safety and public health. Meanwhile, I would like to express our sincere gratitude to the leaders and comrades of party committees, governments, people's congress committees, political consultation committees at different levels and various departments who care for and support the development of health supervision.

The year 2011 is one in which the most difficult key work of recent medical reform will be solved, and it is also the first year of the Twelfth-Five-Year-Plan, which means that we must spare no effort to determinedly push forward the reform of health supervision system and the construction of health supervision system in accordance with the deployments of the Central Committee and the State Council and earnestly fulfill our duty for food safety and health supervision in accordance with the requirements of the laws and regulations. In the following parts, I will present my opinions on four aspects.

I. Intensifying the sense of mission and fully understanding the importance of food safety and health supervision

Health is a major aspect for people's livelihood. At the fifth plenary session of the 17th CPC National Congress, it was clearly required that more importance should be attached to ensuring and improving people's livelihood and ensuring and improving people's livelihood should be regarded as the starting point and fundamental goal of accelerating transforming the mode of economic development. In the proposals for the Twelfth- Five-Year-Plan by the Central Committee, it was clearly required that food safety should be strengthened and prevention and pre-warning of food safety and the emergency handling mechanism of food safety should be improved. At the Central Economic Work Conference, special requirements were made on food safety.

Food safety and health supervision is a major problem concerning the livelihood and the stability of the society. Therefore, our thoughts must conform to the requirements of the CPC Central Committee on the reform and development of health care and we must center on ensuring people's health interest and safeguarding social equality and justice to promote food safety and health supervision effectively.

With the acceleration of industrialization and urbanization in our country and the rapid development of economic globalization, food safety and health supervision are faced with even more severe tasks and challenges. In the aspect of food safety, there have been successive incidents of food safety in recent years, and there have been local risks of serious food safety incidents. In the aspect of occupational disease control, the occurrences of some occupational diseases that would seriously harm the health of the workers, such as pneumoconiosis and occupational poisoning etc., have been on the rise year by year, and there have been occasional occurrences of severe and mass occupational diseases. In the aspect of drinking water safety, there were some water containment incidents in some places. Besides, the illegal medical practice has reoccurred in some places and the potential hazards for the safety of blood plasma collection and supply still exist. All these problems are the concern of the leaders at all the levels, of the people and of the media, for they are the sensitive problems closely associated with the health and interest of the people. It must be realized that our abilities and methods to cope with these problems are far from satisfactory. Meanwhile, if not handled properly, these problems will have impacts on the health of the people, the stability of the society and the credibility of the government. Therefore, we must intensify our sense of mission and sense of responsibility to strengthen food safety and health supervision, give priority to ensuring people's health, effectively establish the awareness of giving priority to people's health and safety, improve our initiative for working, take effective measures, crack down on all the crimes that harm the safety of people's health and lives, push the safety of food, occupational diseases and drinking water safety for the better and effectively protect people's health interest.

II. Converting our ideas and fulfilling the duties of food safety and health supervision by law

Firstly, we must have a correct understanding of the adjustments of our duties of health supervision. In recent years, the CPC Central Committee and the State Council have made successive adjustments of the duties of food safety and the supervision of occupational disease control. Some of our staff members hold different views on these adjustments, for they think the specific duties of supervision of the health departments have been weakened after the adjustments, which influences the stability of the team. Besides, in the regions where financial input was not sufficient, they may worry that such adjustments will influence the development of health supervision and their own benefits. I can understand such views. But how can we correctly understand the adjustments of the duties? Now, I will share my personal views. The adjustments of food safety and occupational health supervision are the important decisions the CPC Central Committee and the State Council have made to better fulfill the duties of the government and protect the health interest of the people more effectively. Therefore, the health department must implement and enforce the adjustments effectively. In accordance with the regulations of *Food Safety Law* and its implementation regulations as well as the programs of "Three Organizational Rules", the food safety duties of health administrative department mainly include comprehensive coordination, risk surveillance and assessment of food safety, formulation of food safety codes, organizing investigation and handling of food safety incidents and mutual reporting and releasing food safety information etc. The duties taken by the local health departments are of vital importance, especially duties such as incident reporting, emergency handling and incident investigating etc. The duties taken by the institutions for disease control and prevention at various levels are also of vital importance for their highly professional techniques such as hygiene disposal of scenes for food safety incidents, epidemiological survey, risk surveillance and tests etc. The decision of the State Commission Office for Public Sector Reform on the division of duties of occupational health supervisory departments clearly regulates that the health departments take lead in drafting laws and regulations, formulate codes for occupational health, propose programs for occupational disease control, focus on the occupational health examination, diagnosis, appraisal of the occupational diseases and their supervision and management, and do the technical and basic work of surveillance on occupational disease and special investigations etc. From all these, it can be seen that the adjustments of the duties require the health departments to give full play to their professional and technical advantages and make full use of the limited supervisory resources and professional technology to provide better professional services to the people and laborers, to analyze and asses the hazards scientifically and to fulfill the duties of supervision regulated by laws and regulations. With the duties adjusted, we are faced with higher and more specific requirements and greater responsibilities. But at present, our resources and capabilities are insufficient to fulfill these tasks. Therefore, we must convert our ideas, convert our functions, establish firmly the awareness of fulfilling duties by law, seize the opportunity of deepening health care reform, further strengthen the construction of capability and try to do all the work more effectively, more carefully and more fruitfully. As for the insufficient financial input for supervision, the central finance will increase the input. All the localities should also coordinate with the development and reform departments and financial departments initially to obtain their support for food safety and heath supervision so as to effectively safeguard people's interest.

Secondly, we must administrate strictly by law. Last October, the State Council clearly required in the opinions on strengthening the construction of the government of laws that: "The administrative organizations at all levels should exercise their powers in accordance with statutory jurisdiction and procedures. We should fulfill the duties of the government, pay more attention to social management and public services, focus on ensuring and improving people's livelihood and effectively solve the problems of medical health care and other concerns of the people. We should intensify administration and law enforcement and investigate and severely punish all the criminal cases concerning food safety to safeguard public interest and economic and social orders." The health administrative departments at all levels must, in accordance with the laws and regulations and the programs of "Three Organizational Rules" by the local governments, fulfill the duties of supervision on food safety, occupational disease control, radiation protection, drinking water safety, school health, public place health as well as the supervision on contagious disease control, cracking down on illegal medical practice and illegal blood collection and provision etc. The health departments at all levels must further sort out the duties and put in place all the duties, which means both the promotion for the cause and the responsibility for people's health. If we can't strictly fulfill statutory duties, the health departments will be blamed and relevant people will also be held accountable. All our staff members must be fully aware of this.

Thirdly, we must convert our methods of work. The duties of food safety and health supervision, by the nature of the duties, can be divided into three categories: first, the duty of comprehensive coordination, including the duties of food safety, occupational disease control and environment and health related duties; second, the duty of supervision and law enforcement, including administrative permits, daily supervision and inspection, administrative punishment, administrative coercion and law enforcement inspection etc. third, the duty of administration on public health, including the construction of professional capability related to health such as laws, regulations and codes of health supervision, the construction of health supervisory system and health surveillance and assessment etc. Due to the different natures, the working modes and methods are bound to be different. Therefore, the traditional supervision modes can no longer meet or cater for the needs of fulfilling our duties, which means we must innovate our thoughts, dare to explore, take effective measures and means to push forward our work, pay more attention to the effects and improve the efficiency. In the aspect of comprehensive coordination, efforts will be made to coordinate with relevant departments, establish and improve inter-departmental coordinative mechanism, strengthen information communication and collaborate closely to build up synergy. In the aspect of supervision modes, some methods have proved effective in recent years such as the system of quantitative management of health supervision at different levels implemented by the Ministry of Health and the publicity system of health supervision information as required by opening government affairs etc. All the localities must effectively convert the working methods so as to improve the capability and levels of health supervision and law enforcement to satisfy the people.

III. Focusing on the key work and effectively pushing forward food safety and health supervision

Efforts will be made to closely connect food safety and health supervision with the requirements of improving people's livelihood by the Central Committee and the State Council as well as the task of deepening medical reform, firmly establish the awareness of people's livelihood and effectively work well on food safety and heath supervision. I will stress on several work:

(1) Working well on food safety effectively

We have learned from our working experiences on food safety that food safety, especially cracking down on violations of law concerning food safety, will be a long, arduous and complicated process, which not only requires all the relevant departments to administrate strictly by law and strengthen supervision on every link of food safety but also requires governments at all levels to strengthen comprehensive coordination to build up synergy and endeavor to solve the prominent problems of food safety. In February 2010, the State Council established Food Safety Commission and set the independent Commission Office for Food Safety, which was an important measure to strengthen food safety by the government. The Commission Office for Food Safety of the State Council is responsible for the task of comprehensive coordination entrusted by the Food Safety Commission and supervising and inspecting the implementation of food safety law and regulations as well as the policies and deployments of the Food Safety Commission. The duties of the Commission Office for Food Safety of the State Council does not take the place of the duties of relevant departments for the management of food safety and the relevant departments will work in accordance with the division of their duties. At present, twenty-four provinces (regions, municipalities) are known to have set the comprehensive coordination organs for food safety in the health administrative departments. Acting on the regulations of *Food Safety Law*, all the localities will further clarify the responsibilities and effectively fulfill the duties of comprehensive coordination taken by the health departments. Efforts will be made to rely on the local party committees and governments, clarify functions as soon as possible, promote reform forcefully and divide the duties soon. In 2011, in accordance with the unified deployments of the State Council, the health administrative departments at various levels must work earnestly to rectify food safety, proceed with cracking down on illegal adding of non-edible substances and the special rectification of abusing food additives with the focus on the rectification of illegal additives included in the "Black List", and join hands with relevant departments to severely investigate and punish the violations of laws concerning food safety. All the localities must formulate the 2011 programs for the surveillance on food safety risks in time by law and organize the implementation. Potential hazards or risks of food safety, once found, must be notified to relevant supervisory departments and reported in time. All the health administrative departments must further sort out the duties regulated by food safety laws, put in place of the duties of comprehensive coordination of food safety, reporting of incidents, handling of emergencies, investigation of responsibilities and releasing of information etc, improve our abilities to handle food safety incidents, release timely pre-warning of risks and guide public opinions correctly.

(2) Pushing forward occupational disease control initially

Occupational disease control is of great significance for the physical health and lives of the laborers and the harmonious and stable development of our economic society. Since the State Commission Office for Public Sector Reform has adjusted and clarified the duties of the Ministry of Health, State Administration of Work Safety, the Ministry of Human Resource and Social Security and All-China Federation of Trade Unions, I hope all our staff members can keep the overall interests of occupational disease control in mind, give priority to protecting the health of the laborers, further sort out our thoughts in accordance with the new division of duties, convert our working modes, stress on the key work and join hands with relevant departments initially to effectively promote the implementation of *Law of the People's Republic of China on Prevention and Control of Occupational Diseases and National Occupational Disease Control Program (2009-2015).* Herein, I will especially stress that the health departments at all levels must seize the opportunity of deepening the reform of medical and health care system, effectively strengthen the capability construction of the prevention and control institutions for occupational diseases, the examination institutions for occupational health and the diagnosis institutions for occupational diseases, improve rules continuously, strengthen management and work well on the examination of occupational heath and the diagnosis and appraisal of occupational diseases. Pilot on basic occupational health service will be carried on. Surveillance on the key occupational diseases such as pneumoconiosis, occupational poisoning and occupational radioactive diseases etc. will be organized, assessment on the risks of occupational health will be carried out and the publicity and education on the prevention and control of occupational diseases and promotion of occupational health will be strengthened. The prevention and control of occupational diseases for the migrant workers will be attached special attention to. The heath supervisory institutions at all levels must strengthen the supervision on the prevention and control of occupational diseases with the focus on supervision and management on the examination of occupational health, and the diagnosis and appraisal of occupational diseases, and strengthen the supervision and management on the control of radioactive hazards in medical institutions.

(3) Working well on health supervision and management

The health administrative departments at all levels must strengthen the leadership on food safety and health supervision, clarify the keys of supervision and put in place of all the duties on the basis of their local reality. The health supervisory institutions must be given full play to so as to intensify health supervision and law enforcement. Supervision and inspection must be strengthened to ensure the complete implementation of all the supervisory duties by law.

Under the leadership of the health administrative departments, the health supervisory institutions at all levels must intensify routine supervision and inspection. Efforts must be made to improve and innovate the ways of supervision and law enforcement to achieve scientific supervision and management, normative supervision and management and effective supervision and management so as to make the best of the limited financial and human resources of health supervision.

The disease control and prevention institutions and occupational disease control and prevention institutions at all levels take on the responsibility empowered by law for food safety and risk surveillance, assessment and appraisal related to health supervision as well as the investigation and handling of health hazards like poisoning and contaminant etc. Such great responsibility requires that we should further strengthen the instruction of the institutions and regulate management system and working procedures; we should strengthen education and training for the staff to improve their policy level, legal awareness and professional quality; we should regulate inspection and certification to ensure that the inspection is legal, scientific, just and timely. The implementation of all work must be associated with performance evaluation. Chinese Center for Disease Control and Prevention must, in accordance with the new functions and work requirements, organize as soon as possible the formulation of work norms for the disease control and prevention institutions and occupational disease control and prevention institutions at all levels and further clarify the duties and tasks. The disease control and prevention institutions and occupational disease control and prevention institutions must, in accordance with the requirements of the duties, effectively improve the technical capability, establish and complete the surveillance network for food contaminant and foodborne diseases, the quality of drinking water and waterborne diseases, occupational diseases and medical radiation protection etc., formulate and implement programs for surveillance, and make full use of the surveillance information to provide scientific basis for policy making.

The health administrative departments at all levels must strengthen the leadership, and the health supervisory institutions and relevant public health institutions like disease control and prevention institutions must strengthen collaboration, establish and complete the mechanism of institutionalized collaboration and give better play to the overall efficiency of the health departments.

IV. Seizing the opportunity and effectively strengthening the construction of health supervisory system and capability

In the suggestions of the Central Committee on the Twelfth-Five-Year-Plan, it is proposed that efforts should be made to actively prevent and control five types of catastrophic diseases including occupational diseases and strengthen pre-warning for public health emergencies and food safety incidents and the construction of emergency handling system. Now, the Ministry of Health is assisting National Commission of Reform and Development to formulate health programs during the Twelfth-Five-Year-Plan period and assisting the Commission Office for Food Safety of the State Council to formulate the national Twelfth-Five-Year program of supervisory system for food safety. The next five years will be an important period of strategic opportunity for the development of food safety and health supervision. So we must seize and make the best of the opportunity to make greater achievement during the Twelfth-Five-Year-Plan period.

(1) Constructing the health supervisory system that covers both the urban and rural areas

The Ministry of Health has listed the construction of the health supervisory system that covers both the urban and rural areas as the key work during the Twelfth-Five-Year-Plan period. The main contents are to complete the health supervisory system especially the health supervisory system at the grassroots. Efforts will be made to establish and complete the system of risk surveillance, assessment and pre-warning for food safety and the emergency handling of incidents. Efforts will be made to strengthen the construction of capability of supervision and surveillance on drinking water. Efforts will be made to make the best of resources available, establish a complete system of occupational disease prevention and control, improve the system of surveillance for occupational disease and risk assessment for occupational health to improve the prevention and control of occupational diseases. Efforts will be made to strengthen the construction of capability of health supervision such as radioactive health, school health and medical law enforcement etc. and their technical support institutions. The Ministry of Health has included surveillance on food contaminant and occupational disease prevention and control in the items of medical reform, which will be funded by the central finance. We plan to include food safety, occupational disease prevention and control and drinking water safety into the items of the equalization of basic public health services, meanwhile we are discussing the feasibility of including into the items of national major public health services some major public health issues in fields such as food safety, occupational disease prevention and control and drinking water safety during the Twelfth-Five-Year-Plan period. In 2011, the programs of strengthening the office building for the health supervisory institutions at the county level will be gradually started and then we will coordinate to gradually include the health supervisory institutions at the provincial and municipal levels into the construction programs. Besides, during the Twelfth-Five-Year-Plan period, the national overall program for the construction of health informationization will be implemented, of which the construction of health supervision informationization is an important part. Efforts will be made to fully better the informationization levels for food safety and health supervision, and improve the efficiency of health supervision and law enforcement and the capability of service.

(2) Fully strengthening health supervision and the construction of capability of relevant public health

In recent years, while handling the public health incidents of food safety, occupational diseases and health hazards caused by environment pollution, we have fully realized that our capabilities of risk surveillance, assessment, norm formulation and incident investigation and handling are far from adequate to meet the needs of food safety and health supervision. In the aspect of food safety, at present, only one third of the provincial institutions of disease control and prevention are able to undertake all the surveillance projects of the national risk surveillance program for food safety. In the aspect of occupational disease prevention and control, at present, there are only twelve independent provincial institutions of occupational disease prevention and control, which suffer from severe drain of professionals. In the aspect of drinking water surveillance, only nine provincial institutions of disease control and prevention are capable of inspections for 106 indexes of water quality. Hence, it is of vital importance for the institutions of disease control and prevention and the institutions of occupational disease prevention and control to improve the professional skills on public health, for the work undertaken by this system on risk surveillance, evaluation, norm formulation and epidemiology surveys determines the capability of the health departments. During the Twelfth-Five-Year-Plan period, we will focus our attention on the construction of risk surveillance and assessment system for food safety and try to solve the serious problems of insufficient capability and levels of risk surveillance and assessment for food safety etc. Efforts will be made to strengthen occupational health examination, diagnosis and treatment of occupational disease and the capability construction of the institutions of occupational disease prevention and control, and try to set up the network for occupational disease prevention and control that corresponds to fulfilling the duties and tasks and to the development of local economy. Efforts will be made to further expand the scope of health surveillance on drinking water, complete the national surveillance network for urban and rural drinking water and improve the capability of examining water quality of the institutions for disease control and prevention.

Meanwhile, we will apply scientific methods, endeavor to promote the modernization of supervisory method, improve the equipment for the supervision and law enforcement and the ability to use the equipment and improve administration by law.

(3) Effectively strengthening the construction and management of health supervisory team

Firstly, efforts will be made to lay a solid foundation for the team. At present, we have only 0.7 health supervisor per 10,000 regular residents in China, which is far from adequate. While formulating the Twelfth-Five-Year development program for health talents, we put forth endeavoring to significantly improve the equipment for the health supervisory staff. In *Opinions of the Ministry of Health on Effectively Fulfilling Supervisory Duties and Further Strengthening Food Safety and Health Supervision* issued recently, we put forth the reference standards for calculating the supervisor staffing and all the localities must make applications to the department of public sector reform actively to speed up the staffing of supervisors. Meanwhile, we will better the equipment and device for law enforcement in line with the equipping standards for the supervisory institutions at different levels. Secondly, efforts will be made to strengthen talent cultivation. More top experts and a large number of compound talents who are adequate for comprehensive law enforcement will be needed to meet the needs of food safety and health supervision. All these require that we complete the system for talent cultivation, innovate forms of training and improve the mechanism for motivating talents so that we can attract, retain and give full play to the excellent talents who are committed to health supervision. Thirdly, law enforcement must be strictly regulated. The health administrative department at all levels must further strengthen the campaign of combating corruption and upholding integrity for the heath supervisory team and relevant public health teams, rectify the malpractice in the industry and regulate the management of the team. All the staff members of the health supervisory system must be vigorously committed to the campaign of Excellent Service, carry forth the fine working style and try to cultivate more excellent workers and models for law enforcement to add more glory to the cause of health supervision.

In the new year, I hope that in accordance with the requirements of the party committee of the Ministry of Health and the working deployments made by Comrade Chen Xiaohong in his speech, all of us will unify our thoughts, activate the spirit, unite as one, make joint efforts, work well on health supervision this year and make our contribution to a peaceful and harmonious environment for the people, safeguarding people's health and promoting the sound and fast development of economy and the society.

(Zhao Xuemei)

3. Strengthen the Responsibility and Guarantee the Implementation to Ensure the Completion of 2011 Medical Reform

—An Address Delivered by Health Minister Chen Zhu to the Meeting of Health System on the Arrangements of 2011 Medical Reform (February 15, 2011)

The main task of this meeting is to study and carry out the spirit of the national meeting on deepening the medical system reform, especially Vice-Premier Li Keqiang's important address to the meeting. It is also to arrange and fulfill the 2011 main work of health circles under the five key tasks of medical reform of the State Council with an analysis of the current situation facing the medical reform. In addition, it is to strengthen further the accountability of medical reform within the medical system to ensure that every reform task of this year will be completed as scheduled.

Now I will talk about things in three parts.

I. Accurately Grasp the Current Situation Facing the Medical Reform

The year 2011 is the first year of the "Twelfth Five-year Plan" period and a crucial year for the recent tasks of three years' medical reform as well. This year will witness opportunity and challenge existing side by side, but on the whole, the situation facing the medical reform remains pressing.

(1) Last year's work provided a sound basis for the completion of this year's work. In the past year, with the earnest implementation of the requirements of the Party Central Committee and the State Council, the focus highlighted and steady progress

made, the national health circles completed the yearly task for five key focuses of the medical system reform undertaken by the health system. The first was that the coverage of the new rural cooperative medical system (NCMS) remained expanded. The maximum pay limitation was further improved and the pilot program of medical security for major diseases of rural children was carried out orderly. The second was that the essential drug system was fully implemented in 57.2% of government-run medical institutions at the primary level. Through comprehensive reform, new operating mechanism is taking shape. As a result, where the essential drug system was implemented, the medical costs of inpatient and outpatient service dropped while both outpatient visits and inpatient visits were on the rise. The third was that, with the further improvement of medical service system at the primary level, the primary-level medical team with general practitioners as the focus was strengthened and the service capacity was further enhanced. The fourth was that new progress was made in equal access to basic public health services. Nine programs of national basic public health services were carried out extensively in both urban and rural areas. And the major public health services were promoted steadily. The fifth was that the pilot project of public hospital reform went smoothly. In some pilot areas, initial experience was gained in the layout planning, management system and service improvement of public hospitals. Nationwide, with a focus on strengthening services, public hospitals implemented a number of measures with quick effectiveness and easy operability, which were praised by the people.

(2) There remains a considerable gap between medical reform and the people's expectations and requirements. The people are direct beneficiaries of medical reform and appraisers for the results of medical reform. With the economic and social development, there have been growing expectations and demands of the people for the health and health services. Besides, they pay more attention to the improvement of security system and services. All those make newer and higher demands for the distribution adjustment of resources, the improvement of public health services and regulatory functions, the elevation of medical and health service capacities, the transformation of service mode and the construction of health security system. In the mean time, there remain disequilibrium, disharmony and unsustainability in health development of our country. Also there remain significant urban-rural difference, regional difference and population difference in the allocation of health resources, availability of health services and residents' health status. With the advancement of the reform, some issues of system and mechanism and structure which restrict health development are getting more and more prominent. A unified and efficient health management system has not yet taken shape. Some major issues involving the direction of health reform have yet to build consensus and be reflected constantly

in the practice of reform and development. In addition, some specific policies and measures of reform remain to be further perfected. Now "making up for the weaknesses and paying back the old debts" account for much work in medical reform. For example, in recent years, the government has given priority to the grass-units, public health system and healthcare system in health investment. However, it requires greater investment and deeper reform to really establish steady health investment mechanism. After the investment is increased, it is an important task to establish the operating mechanism through comprehensive reform. Therefore there remains a long uphill journey to satisfy the people's growing and increasingly diverse demands for medical and health services, and maintain all-round and sustainable development of health services. Withal, the chief responsible comrades of health administrative departments at all levels must have a clear understanding and must not take it lightly.

(3) This year's medical reform is faced with a more arduous task. Medical reform is a step-by-step process, from the bottom up, from shallow to deep and from the easier to the more advanced. With the deepening of the reform, the biggest headaches of the recent key tasks have been revealed gradually. The Party Central Committee has made it clear to take the following as the priority of this year's medical reform: the implementation of national system for essential drugs, pilot reform of public hospitals and improvement of medical security system. In the implementation process, we will encounter difficulties and problems. Therefore it is the "required course" of this year's medical reform to solve these problems. It is also a big test of organizing capacity and management and executive ability of leaders of health administrative departments at all levels. Once these problems are not settled, we will fail in our year-end performance. We should sort out these problems into categories and acts appropriately to the situation. The first is that we should concentrate our efforts in the improvement of quality and level for the new rural cooperative medical system (NCMS) and equal access to basic public health services, which have been institutionalized and standardized. With the focus on the strengthening of system construction and refined management, we should also improve further the operating level of fund regulation. And we will do relevant work after the subsidy standard improvement of the new rural cooperative medical system (NCMS) and public health services. The second is that, for the establishment of national system for essential drugs with a clear policy, we should give priority to the standardization of bidding procurement, the implementation of the policy of zero margin drug profit, and the establishment and perfection of compensation and operating mechanisms of medical institutions at the primary level. Besides we should try every means and overcome difficulties to carry out the implementation out and out. And special attention should be paid to the guarantee of village doctors' treatment in order to maintain the stability

of village doctors. The third is that, for such work as pilot reform of public hospitals with whole experience not yet formed, all localities are encouraged to make bold explorations and with continual innovation. With the focus on county-level hospital, positive and steady progress should be made as required by the pilot reform. We should also combine the implementation of measures for the convenience and benefits of the people with the promotion of comprehensive reform and the exploration into the settlement of problems concerning system and mechanism. Therefore both will support each other and promote each other to form sustainable, intrinsic power and establish step by step a long-term mechanism.

(4) In health circles there is something incompatible with medical reform. In the new situation and new requirements, the understanding level, mental state and working methods of some people cannot adapt to work requirements, and they still lack enterprising spirit. Very few take a negative wait-and-see attitude and fail to be active thinkers, throw themselves into timely investigations and researches, tackle problems boldly, or spare no efforts to push forward the reform. With the management level of health departments remaining to be further improved, improvements are to be made in target setting, task decomposition, accountability, supervision and assessment, and information communication. In some localities, falsification and fraudulently obtaining funds are related to the above-mentioned. Without a full departmental cooperation, health departments still lack initiative and strength in departmental coordination. Some departments even go it alone, which is more prominent in health departments at the primary level.

II. Clarify the Targets and Highlight the Focal Points to Make the Results of Medical Reform Better Benefit the People

Centering on the three-year target of five key reforms, *The 2011 Main Work Arrangements for Five Key Reforms of Medical System Reform* issued by the General Office of the State Council set 17 tasks and 67 specific targets for the year 2011. The Ministry of Health is supposed to lead the completion of 46 targets and cooperate with the completion of 18 targets. After the leading group of deepening the medical reform under the Ministry of Health did an in-depth study and repeatedly solicited opinions, those tasks have been, in the form of responsibility certificates, broken down into the health departments (bureaus) of various provinces (regions, cities) and various departments and bureaus of the Ministry of Health. Comparing with the task targets of the responsibility certificates of medical reform, all the health departments (bureaus) of various provinces (regions, cities) and various departments and bureaus of the Ministry of Health should carry out the tasks effectively. Centering on the key and tough issues, I will highlight three areas:

(1) Adhere to consolidation and enhancement and do well the work of basic medical security and perfection of health service system at the primary level and basic public health service. Further consolidate the coverage of the new rural cooperative medical system (NCMS) to ensure the continual steady participation rate of 90% and above. Carry out extensively the out-patient coordination of the new rural cooperative medical system (NCMS) to further benefit the rural residents participating in NCMS. Carry out the pilot project of security for such major diseases as children's leukemia and congenital heart disease at the provincial scale. Go ahead with the improvement of reimbursement standard and expand the range of pilot project. Further reform the payment system of NCMS and cooperate with the promotion of all-purpose card for seeking medical advice to realize immediate settlement.

Perfect the medical and health service system at the primary level. Continue to strengthen the construction of medical and health institutions at the primary level to improve the capacity of service at the primary level. Do a solid job for recruiting free medical students, general practitioners' training for job transfer and training of health personnel of community health service institutions. Encourage and guide medical talents to work at the primary level. Encourage initiative service and door-to-door service. Push forward the establishment of general practitioners' team and team of doctors signed with families to provide convenient and consecutive service of health management for jurisdiction inhabitants.

Promote gradual equal access to basic public health services. With government expenditures on basic public health services increased to an average of 25 RMB Yuan per person this year, innovation will focus on service philosophy, service model and service depth. We should put this money to good use in order to give full play to the role of disease prevention and health care of basic public health services. In premise of ensuring the completion of task, we will expand and deepen greatly the contents of basic public health services, expand service population and improve service quality. We will also do well in basic public health services for rural migrant workers to protect their health rights and interests.

(2) Fully implement the system for basic drugs to shift the operating mechanism of medical institutions at the primary level. Fully implementing the system for basic drugs within medical institutions at the primary level and establishing the internal operating system are related to the overall situation of medical reform, so-called a slight move in one part may affect the whole situation. To effectively implement the system for basic drugs, we should pay special attention to two core links: procurement and distribution and establishment of compensating mechanism. Seizing the favorable opportunities of establishing the compensating mechanism, we should advance in

an all-round way the comprehensive reforms in the staffing management, personnel system, income distribution and performance assessment of institutions at the primary level. In addition, we should establish a new mechanism of maintaining public welfare, arousing enthusiasm and protecting sustainability.

Now it is time in the main for fully implementing the system for basic drugs and pushing forward the comprehensive reform in institutions at the primary level. This year we will achieve a full coverage for government-run medical and health institutions at the primary level. Village clinics and village doctors have done a considerable proportion of work for clinics and basic public health services, which plays a very important role. We should work hard to bring village clinics into the implementation of national essential drugs. With the implementation of multi-channel compensating policies that have been issued as the key grasp, we will give aid to the survival and development of village clinics and give play to their bottom role of medical and preventive health care. We will also explore the possibilities of bringing non-government run medical institutions at the primary level into the implementation of basic drug system, and of giving reasonable compensations in the form of buying services. Give full play to the role of Traditional Chinese Medicine in medical reform and encourage medical institutions at the primary level to offer appropriate technique and services of Traditional Chinese Medicine. During the implementation, pay attention to various influences possibly brought by the adjustment of interest pattern. Finally something should be done in an in-depth and careful way to ensure smooth operation of mechanism and smooth operation of institutions.

(3) Highlight the comprehensive reform of county level hospitals and positively push forward the pilot project of public hospitals. Comrade Keqiang pointed out in his address that deepening medical reform adhered to the top-down train of thought, starting from institutions in urban-rural areas to county level hospitals and further to large hospitals in big cities. In accordance with this train of thought, another battlefield for this year's tough battles is where we will accelerate the pilot project for the reform of public hospitals. Make greater efforts for the pilot project for the reform of public hospitals. Encourage and direct pilot cities to carry out pilot projects for the comprehensive reform of system and mechanism, which are centered on "four divisions". With bold exploration, take the lead in breakthrough and sum up experiences in time to try to explore a basic way as quickly as possible for the reform of public hospitals. Adhere to two-sided tactics. The first is to highlight the pilot work of pilot cities, encourage our minds to be freed and call for bold exploration. The second is to make public in public hospitals nationwide some reform measures with quick effectiveness.

County hospital is a key link in solving poor accessibility and affordability of health care services. It is also a bridge and bond linking large hospitals and medical institutions at the primary level. This year we will put on the important agenda the comprehensive reform of county hospitals and highlight the development of county hospitals, regarding them as the hub of upper and lower linkage and the central link of relieving poor accessibility and affordability of health care services. The goal will be achieved that a county hospital can reach grade A of level 2. A focal point of county hospital reform is to eliminate "supporting medicine with drugs" step by step through improving compensating mechanism and establishing the mechanism of reasonable price formation mechanism of drugs.

As required by upper and lower linkage, internal vitality and external thrust, we will establish the mechanism of improving the labor division and collaboration between public hospitals and institutions at the primary level. We will also consolidate the long-term mechanism of partner assistance. Push forward convenience-and-benefit-for-people measures to promote the scientific and sophisticated management of hospitals. Besides we will accelerate the diversified medical pattern to promote the development of non-public medical institutions.

Ⅲ. Strengthen Responsibility and Tackle the Tough Problems to Finish the Recent Key Tasks of Medical Reform Set by the State Council

At present, the three-year key tasks for deepening medical reform has entering the crucial stage with urgent situation, arduous task and great responsibility. Compared with the goals and requirements of the three-year task, we will carry out every task with better mental status, higher standards, more effective measures and greater strength.

(1) Take the implementation of accountability as the powerful grasp of pushing forward medical reform. Last year, we came up with the new approach to the implementation of medical reform task, that is, to sign responsibility certificates while strengthening the surveillance of the progress of medical reform, which was reported to all the provinces in time. This approach proved very effective. At today's meeting, the Ministry of Health will sign responsibility certificates with the directors of health departments of all the provinces (regions, cities), production & construction corps and relevant bureaus of the Ministry of Health. It is a specific measure for further deepening the "accountability" and gathering the strength of the whole medical system in promoting the reform on the basis of last year's experience summary. Here I will stress that the principal responsible persons of health departments of all the provinces (regions, cities), production & construction corps and relevant bureaus of the Ministry of Health are the first heads for your respective medical reform. You are

supposed to be responsible for medical reform while performing your duties. Health departments at all levels should pay attention to refined decomposition of medical reform items and responsibility implementation. After the signing of responsibility certificates, various localities should hurry up and organize the formulation of specific project implementation plan. For each item of responsibility certificates, there should be specific target index, specific reform steps, specific responsibility subject, specific assessment methods and specific rewards-punishment measures. All the responsibility subjects should promote the target implementation in comparison with task targets and make up work schedules.

Strengthen the surveillance and supervision of medical reform. This year, the Ministry of Health will go ahead with the work on the basis of the adjustment and improvement of index system, standardization and organization of management and improvement of data quality. All the provinces (regions, cities) and production & construction corps are also supposed to establish surveillance platforms with available statistical information systems and carry out and improve constantly the surveillance & supervision of medical reform over cities and counties. The Ministry of Health will strengthen the scheduling for the project progress with quarterly reporting. Departments concerned will supervise the implementation of the projects with slow progress. All the provinces (regions, cities) and production & construction corps will also strengthen the supervision of medical reform with reference to this practice. In addition, mid-term evaluation will be performed by the state for the implementation of medical reform, which is an important measure for promoting effectively medical reform. Health departments at all levels should fully understand the significance of this work and cooperate with related departments to perform the evaluation for deepening medical reform.

Powerful organization and leadership is the guarantee for finishing the task of medical reform. All localities should continue to stick to the work method of "four changes and four concentrations": change of work idea, change of way of thinking, change of work pattern and change of work style; concentration of manpower, concentration of time, concentration of energy and concentration of wisdom. They must push forward medical reform with effective and powerful organization and leadership. Strengthen further the construction of medical reform office and choose key personnel with sound knowledge structure and strong business ability to enrich the team of medical reform. Strengthen study, training and researches to improve the quality and level of related personnel. Allot necessary funds in financial budget of institutions based on medical reform task to ensure smooth start of work.

(2) Strengthen overall coordination to form resultant force of pushing forward reform. The wider area health work and reform task involve, the more we need

to strengthen communication and coordination. The practice in recent two years show that it is the important guarantee of performing the task of medical reform to strengthen departmental cooperation and form resultant force under the leadership of government. The leadership system for medical reform involving multiple central and local departments has also created good conditions for departmental communication and coordination. Within such a coordinating work mechanism, health departments, proceeding from the whole situation, should take the initiative to work. Analyzing the progress of tasks in time, they should also find prominent problems and listen to the opinions of relevant departments. Moreover they should put forward suggestions to the leaders' group of medical reform and build consensus to work on policy and measures for solving problems and pushing forward work. A good work atmosphere should be created for departmental mutual respect, mutual support, timely communication and working together. A work mechanism should be established and perfected for conforming to local situations, giving full play to the advantages of various departments and arousing the enthusiasm of all the departments.

Horizontally we should strengthen coordination and cooperation. In cooperation with other departments, we should establish global consciousness and overall consciousness without any shuffle.

Vertically upper and lower linkage should be formed for transition. Medical reform in all localities is the important part of the whole situation of medical reform nationwide with characteristics of their own. All local authorities should strengthen work transition from department to department to ensure the full advancement of all the tasks for medical reform without weaknesses.

Attach importance to mobilizing all social forces to get involved in reform and mobilize all positive factors in favor of advancing reform. We should make the people aware that it is the duty of both the government and everyone in the whole society to ensure health. In the improvement of medical service environment, it takes the efforts of not only medical workers, but the support and coordination of patients and all social forces.

(3) Strengthen publicity and guidance to create an atmosphere beneficial to reform. The first is to strengthen the publicity for health policy and health knowledge. We should strengthen the publicity of medical reform policy to increase the people's awareness rate of policy. Closely follow public opinions, study in time the key and hot issues concerning medical reform, improve the pertinence and effectiveness of health publicity and education, and strive for the understanding and support from all sectors of society. Health policy concerns mostly daily preventive health care and habits of seeking medical advice and medication. It also concerns medical workers' daily behavior of medical and health services. We should take the process of publicity

to the people as the form of policy popularization and the means of health promotion. Publicity should be in the form that is popular and easy to understand and loved by the people, which let the people understand and remember. The second is to positively publicize the progress and results achieved by medical reform. The people's feelings about the reform are derived mostly from their own experiences and media interpretations and reports. There is a gradual manifestation process of health reform results, which is invisible in the short run. Strengthen positive publicity and boost confidence of all social sectors in the reform. Through giving publicity to the progress of reform, we will establish models for reform and publicize exemplary people to make the people feel the results of reform. The third is to guide social rational expectations. Medical reform is a lengthy, arduous and complicated process that is impossibly a one-time effort. So we should make the people aware of the chronicity, arduousness and gradualness of medical reform, so that the reform can advance steadily in a comfortable favorable environment.

Comrades, hardship gives birth to great causes and arduous struggle results in glorious achievements. For 2011 work of deepening medical reform in medical system, time is pressing, tasks, arduous, responsibility, heavy, and opportunity, rare. Health system nationwide should further unify thinking, boost spirits, forge ahead in a pioneering spirit and guarantee the implementation. We believe that, under the strong leadership of the CPC Central Committee and the State Council, and with the involvement of medical and health care workers and their joint efforts, we will surely be able to complete the 2011 task of medical reform in health system. We will also push forward the deepening of medical system reform to benefit the people and encourage medical workers.

(Shan Yongxiang)

4. Consolidate the Foundation, Improve the Local Condition and Make Efforts to Open up a New Prospect in the Work of the Medical and Health Aid to Xinjiang

—A Speech Delivered by Health Minister Chen Zhu at the Coordination and Promotion Meeting on the Counterpart Aid to Xinjiang of the National Health System

Today, the 2011 Coordination and Promotion Meeting on the Counterpart Aid to Xinjiang of the National Health System is convened by the Ministry of Health in Urumqi. It is an important meeting which will implement the decisions and arrangements made by the Second Meeting of Central Government on the Counter Aid to Xinjiang and which will greatly promote the leap-forward development of the health work in Xinjiang. The main task of the meeting is: to put into practice the principles set up in the Second Meeting of Central Government on the Counter Aid to Xinjiang, to exchange the development of the medical aid to Xinjiang after the Conference on the counter aid to Xinjiang by the National Health System in 2010 and to coordinate the two sides to make plans, create new projects, raise funds and usher in a new era in the medical aid to Xinjiang.

Here, I will assert several opinions of mine.

I. Affirm our achievements. The National Healthcare System's counterpart aid to Xinjiang region started with great success.

According to the CPC Central Committee's plan for the counterpart aid to Xinjiang and the work requirements of the Health Ministry, the health executive departments from 19 provinces and municipalities have devotedly carried out their aiding work with the help of the party committees, the provincial and municipal governments and the mass people. Thus, the successful beginning of the whole project is achieved.

Firstly, building a comprehensive organization. The health administrative departments from 19 provinces and municipalities have put into practice the principles established at the Central Work Conference of Xinjiang and the National Work Conference on Counterpart Aid to Xinjiang and the Conference of National Health System on the Medical Aid to Xinjiang in 2010. Moreover, being in charge personally, the major leaders established the organizations, formulated the working mechanisms and raised funds. Thus, the development of the medical aid to Xinjiang was organizationally and systemically safeguarded. For instance, chiefs of health administrative departments from 18 provinces including Jilin, Anhui, Hubei, Hunan, Guangdong acted personally as group leaders of the medical aid to Xinjiang. They coordinated the local governments and the related departments, made great efforts for the investment to Xinjiang and supervised the whole process. This has safeguarded the development of the medical aid to Xinjiang.

Secondly, working out special plans scientifically. The health departments of provinces and municipalities which are engaged in the counterpart aid to Xinjiang, should carry out investigations there, which should cover the current situation, hindering factors and needs of the health undertaking in Xinjiang. This will take full advantage of all the resources and lay a solid foundation for the special plans of medical aid to Xinjiang. By far, the plans of 19 aid-providing provinces and municipalities have been basically achieved and 265 programs supported. The total input amounts to 4.28 billion RMB Yuan, among which 3.71 billion RMB Yuan is from special financial fund, making up 7% of the total. The plans cover various areas, mainly including construction of infrastructures, purchase of medical equipment, talent cultivation and informationization of the health sectors. In Fujian Province, the input for special plans of the medical aid to Xinjiang is 420 million RMB Yuan, including financial capital 260 million RMB Yuan, accounting for 17.2% of the total from Fujian Province, and the ratio is the highest among all the provinces included. The investment of Zhejiang Province is 810 million RMB Yuan, ranking first for the total amount among all the aiding provinces and municipalities.

Thirdly, carrying out the pilot programs actively. In accordance with the central government's requirement and actual needs of the recipients, the aiding provinces and municipalities have accurately pinpointed the direction and taken immediate actions to push forward the development of the pilot programs. As a result, outstanding achievements have been made and a solid foundation laid for the implementation of the special plans for the medical aid to Xinjiang. By far, 104 pilot programs have been developed with an input of 1.01 billion RMB Yuan. Funded by Beijing, the outpatient and emergency buildings of the People's Hospital in Moyu County and the comprehensive hospital building of the People's Hospital in Luopu County are under construction. Five mobile vans and other medical equipment worth 74.8 million RMB Yuan provided by Shanghai for Kashi Prefecture have been put into use. Built by Shenzhen, the new People's Hospital in Taxkorgan covers an area of 9,000 square meters. Now with its main structure completed, the building will be put into use in this August. Funded by Hebei Province, the construction of Hebei Hospital in Korla has also been basically completed and the outpatient building of the People's Hospital in Hejing Prefecture and the emergency comprehensive building of the People's Hospital in Ruoqiang Prefecture are both under construction. Aided by Shandong, the remote medical consultation center is being built and the bid for the remote line equipment has been initiated. Later, at this conference, 56 ambulances will be provided on spot.

Fourthly, pushing forward the intellectual support steadily in the medical aid. To counter the lack of medical staff in the recipient regions, the aid-providing provinces (municipalities) vigorously strengthened health personnel training in recipient regions and meanwhile, in order to increase the ability of the recipients, the aid was combined with the self-reliance of the aided areas. Up to now, a total of over 700 cadres and health technicians have been sent to Xinjiang province, more than 500 health workers of Xinjiang have been accepted by the supporting regions and over 7,000 people from Xinjiang have received specialized training. Professional and technical health personnel in Heilongjiang province carried out a variety of training in the Altay region for 72 times and 1,880 medical staff were trained. In addition, 77 health workers in recipient regions went to the Heilongjiang provincial medical institutions for follow-up training. Shanxi province has built a long-term mechanism which would help the recipients to train health talents. 17 provincial, prefecture-level medical institutions of Shanxi have been identified as pilot institutions to help the 19 counterpart medical institutions in Xinjiang and the medical service and management of the recipient organizations have been greatly enhanced.

Fifthly, protecting the health of the mass people. The aid-providing provinces (municipalities) sent high-level medical teams to recipient regions, promoted the advanced technology, and actively carried out medical practice and surgery. As a result, the mass people of the recipient regions enjoyed real benefits brought by the health aid to Xinjiang province. All these efforts protected the health of people from all ethnic groups. Up to now, 52 batches of medical teams, a total of 596 people, have been sent to Xinjiang. They examined 205,000 people and carried our surgery for nearly 9,000 people. Fujian province sent 16 batches of medical teams, all together 122 people, to Xinjiang. They examined 27,000 people and carried out operations for 1531 people. Henan medical teams focused on improving medical technology in the assisted areas and helped carry out eight new technologies. Tianjin medical teams participated actively in mobile medical service, carried out diagnosis and treatment for nearly 400 people, and distributed medicine worth nearly 4 million RMB Yuan. Jiangsu medical teams actively carried out clinic tour, popularized health knowledge and directly brought medical resources to the public.

5 subordinates of the Health Ministry and the aid-providing Health Bureaus attached great importance to the medical aid to Xinjiang province. Chief leaders went for field research to keep track of the statue quo so that the work could be done according to the needs of the recipient regions and the advantages of the aided regions can also be brought to full play. The medical aid to Xinjiang focused on scientific research, talent training, technical guidance and intellectual support, which greatly improved the service capability in Xinjiang medical and health institutions and laid the foundation for high-quality health service for the local people. People's Hospital of Peking University, Xinjiang Urumqi Friendship Hospital and First Affiliated Hospital of Xinjiang Shihezi University of Medicine established medical and health service community. Via a variety of ways including video conferences and video lectures, advanced medical technology was adopted and medical teleconsultation system connecting experts in Beijing was established .By carrying out special technical training, giving operational guidance and adopting other means to help the recipient regions, China's Disease Prevention and Control Center helped improve capacity of the recipient regions in the control and emergency response to AIDS, leprosy and other major infectious diseases and endemic diseases in Xinjiang.

Institute of Pharmacology and Institute of Medicinal Plant Development of Chinese Academy of Medical Sciences exchanged researchers with the recipient hospitals. And they cooperated in the application of research projects, and actively carried out academic exchange. As a result, the scientific research ability and technical level of assistance- receiving hospitals were effectively improved. Tongji Hospital, the affiliated hospital to Tongji Medical College of Huazhong University of Science and Technology, selected a number of resident experts with clinical experience and scientific research ability to instruct the medical staff of assistance- receiving hospitals in advanced diagnostic techniques and methods. Meanwhile, 11 key technical personnel from assistance- receiving hospitals were received by Tongji Hospital for further study and famous experts were designated as their tutors, which effectively improved the level of medical technology in assistance-receiving hospitals. China Academy of Chinese Medical Sciences opened traditional Chinese medicine (ethnic medicine) postgraduate courses in 14 hospitals and a Medical College in Xinjiang to train senior Uygur medical staff. In addition, together with the recipient hospitals, China Academy of Chinese Medical Sciences set up a Joint Research Lab of Scientific Data Application in traditional Chinese medicine and Uygur medicine in order to share information and provide a scientific basis for clinical studies.

The Health Ministry and the State Administration of Traditional Chinese Medicine attached great importance to the medical counterpart aid to Xinjiang. The chief leaders took the command personally. They formulated the overall plan, mobilized all the available forces and spared no efforts in supporting the leap-forward development of the health undertaking in Xinjiang region. Firstly, in terms of capital input, 2.8 billion RMB Yuan of special central government financial investment was arranged by coordinating the relevant departments in 2010, which was 39% than that of 2009. In 2011, the input would be further increased. Only in the first quarter 1.4 billion RMB Yuan was invested to support the key health work like the deepening of the medical reform in Xinjiang region.

Secondly, as for the infrastructure construction, they supported the infrastructure construction and the purchase of basic equipment for 485 county (regiment) level hospitals, center township health centers, community health service centers, village clinics and mental health prevention institutions. The emphasis was laid on improving primary hardware facilities and conditions of service in the grassroots medical and health institutions.

Thirdly, when it comes to the public health service, Xinjiang was included in the major science and technology programs as the pilot area of the comprehensive prevention and treatment of AIDS, viral hepatitis and other major infectious diseases and was given key support. The prevention and control efforts of endemics like iodine deficiency disease, endemic fluorosis and endemic drinking water arsenic poisoning were intensified. And the phase goal of elimination of iodine deficiency was achieved.

The central government gave the highest proportion of 80% to the basic public health service grants, implemented a number of major public health programs like the national immunization project and made great efforts to improve the life quality and health of the people in Xinjiang. Xinjiang is recognized as a project province of national health emergency team-building and support was given to the construction of the command and decision-making system for public health emergency .

Fourthly, in the matter of the cultivation the professional talents, the program of sending tens of thousands of doctors to the rural area was supported, and the training of backbone doctors for the county hospitals and the health workers for the rural areas was carried out. By this way, the medical technique and hospital management ability in Xinjiang was improved and a batch of permanent and available medical talents were cultivated.

Fifthly, in the information construction, Xinjiang was chosen as a pilot region for the national health information construction. Support was focused on the pilot work of the construction of the primary medical and health information system at grassroots level. A horizontal network connecting the medical service, disease prevention, health supervision, woman and child healthcare, health knowledge popularization and a vertical network connecting the provinces, prefectures, towns and villages would be established in the pilot region. What's more,priority was given to the pilot work of remote consultation system, making the high-quality medical and health recourses available to the local hospitals in Xinjiang. As the entire Xinjiang region was covered with the remote medical service system, the ability to treat the difficult and critical cases and the medical service capacity were greatly improved.

Sixthly, in the aspect of the development of TCM (traditional Chinese medicine), support was given to the following projects: the construction of clinical research base of TCM, the construction of pharmacies of TCM in county-level TCM hospitals, the training of general practitioner of TCM, the construction of specialized acupuncture rehabilitation clinics in rural areas, the construction of key clinical disciplines of TCM , the workshops for inheriting the experience of national famous TCM doctors' and etc.. Finally, efforts were made to build new partnership of counterpart aid. According to the principle of full coverage, 15 assistance-providing hospitals like the First Affiliated Hospital of Beijing University were organized to support the relevant medical and health institutions of the Xinjiang region and the Xinjiang Production and Construction Corps. They strengthened the efforts to cultivate related personnel in the recipient institutions and effectively improved their technical and service ability. Up till now, 20 hospitals at the national level have been organized to form counterpart aiding partnership with the relevant institutions in Xinjiang region.

With the joint efforts of the national health system and the recipients in Xinjiang region, the counterpart aid was successful initiated and the achievement was remarkable. There are four points standing out during last year's work: Firstly, the chiefs were required to shoulder the task personally. The aid-providing health administrative departments at all level and the aiding institutions stuck to the new needs for the leapfrog development of Xinjiang. Their leaders conscientiously carried out their responsibility in the aiding work and the work was well organized and completed. Secondly, we should steadfastly uphold the Scientific Outlook of Development. After comprehensive and thorough survey, the needs of the recipients were identified. All the supporting organizations made arrangements of programs according to the actual needs so as to ensure the formulation and implementation of the special plans would meet the targets. Thirdly, the recipients' capability of self-development was consistently elevated. In order to realize recipients' development potential, when programming and implementing the projects, the characteristics of the recipients were taken into consideration and the assistance was combined with self-reliance. Fourthly, the construction of both the software and the hardware in the pilot region was pushed forward. The basic facilities and medical service ability of the medical institutions in Xinjiang needed improving urgently. Therefore, when formulating and implementing the specialized programs, the construction of the hardware like the housing, medical and research equipment as well as the construction of the software, such as training of health workers, scientific research cooperation and technical guidance were both enhanced.

Over the last year, in order to accelerate the leapfoward development of Xinjiang's health undertaking, much work was dong and a great amount of capital was invested,which was unprecedented in the history. As a number of health-pilot programs were started and many urgent difficulties were solved, the upbeat changes were taking place in the region:

The overall health resources enjoyed a sustained growth. The maternal and infant mortality decreased steadily. The physical quality of the whole area was significantly improved. Great progress was made in building the medical health service system. A comprehensive medical, preventive and supervisory system was formed. The infrastructure facilities and service capacity were further improved.

The full coverage of the new rural cooperative medical system was realized and the basic medical security was constantly improved. The essential medicine system was steadily implemented and the reform of the public hospitals was further pushed forward. The incidence of statutory infectious diseases decreased steadily. Serious infectious diseases and endemics were effectively controlled.

All of these achievements were made with the broad vision and the wise leadership of the Party Central Committee and the State Council, the arduous work of all the workers and cadres of Xinjiang and XPCC (Xinjiang Production and Construction Corps) and the selfless assistance from all the aid-providing provinces/ municipalities.

Hereby, on behalf of the Ministry of Health, I extend my sincere gratitude and high tribute to all the people who gave support to and participated in the medical aid to Xinjiang.

II. Raise awareness and clarify the profound meaning and needs for the medical aid to Xinjiang.

According to the CPC Central Committee's unified deployment, this year is the first year when the new round of projects of counterpart aid to Xinjiang will be fully carried out. Meanwhile, it is also an important year when the foundation of counterpart medical aid to Xinjiang will be laid. We must assess the situation with greater sense of urgency and responsibility, deepen the medical reform, solidify the fundamentals, plan and implement the projects and manage the aiding work scientifically. The enthusiasm for the construction and development should be well protected, guided and tapped.

(1) The new resolutions of the Central Work Conference of Xinjiang pointed out the direction for the counterpart aid to Xinjiang. During 27-29 May, the Second National Work Conference on Counterpart Aid to Xinjiang was held. Hu Jintao, General Secretary of CCP, made Important instructions. Li Keqiang and Zhou Yongkang attended the conference and delivered important speeches. They clarified the working direction, contents and requirements for the future work.

The achievement of the counterpart aid was Fully affirmed at the meeting. It was made clear that the aid to Xinjiang is an important part of our party's general plan and that it was an inevitable requirement for implementing the 12th Five-Year Plan, accelerating economic transformation and boosting domestic demand. Moreover, it's also a major initiative to promoting new growth pole for west development, lift the living standard of the people from all ethnic groups accelerate Xinjiang's leap-forward development and maintain our nation's long-term stability.

The conference stressed that this year is the beginning year for the 12th Five-Year Plan as well as the first year of the new round of counterpart aid to Xinjiang. We should seize these opportunities to push forward the development and stability in Xinjiang and to a new prospect will be created. Firstly, we should give top priority to protect and improve the people's livelihood. The project concerning the people's livelihood should be steadily pushed forward. We should concentrate our efforts on major issues and real work and try to solve urgencies and important matters to facilitate the equality of the basic public service. Secondly,we should boost the self-developing capability of Xinjiang. The construction of key infrastructures and competitive industries should be pushed forward. Thus, the advantages of Xinjiang in resources and geography will be turned into the advantage in economy. Thirdly, we should push forward the implementation of the differential economic policies. More flexible policies should be adopted for tackle special cases with special methods, which will greatly boost Xinjiang's development. Fourth, We should deepen the counterpart aid to Xinjiang in an all-round way. We should combine all the resources in economy, education, technology, cadres and talents and carry out the construction in both hardware and software to speed up Xinjiang's development. The Conference's required that the leadership should be strengthened in all localities, departments and enterprises. The working conception and system should be constantly innovated and the work should be done in a practical, scientific and efficient way. The projects and funds should be strictly managed and the constructions should be accomplished with quantity and quality. Thus, the aid to Xinjiang can be really fruitful.

The conference also emphasized that all cadres and talents in this counterpart aid project are the nucleus strength and they should be supported in work, life and politics. Thus, they can cooperate together with the people in Xinjiang to turn the grand blueprint of the counterpart aid work into reality.

With the aim to carry out the important instructions of the state leaders and the spirit the Central Conference, we must look from the overall perspective to unify our thoughts, raise our awareness and further enhance our sense of mission and responsibility.

(2) The working direction should be determined by the existing problems.

In the Guiding Opinions of Ministry of Health on Supporting the Leap-forward Development of the Medical and Health Undertaking in Xinjiang, the medical and health aid to Xinjiang will be carried out in 3 phases: The preliminary phase will last form 2011 to 2012. The improvement phase will last from 2013 to 2015. And the rapidly-developing phase will last from 2016 to 2020.

We should fully recognize that good preparations are the objective requirement for the long-term goals and the scientific development of the counterpart aid to Xinjiang. They are also the fundamental guarantee for the realization of Xinjiang's leapforward development. In addition, they are the important prop for solving the problems and promoting the sound and fast development of the health undertaking in Xinjiang. Thus, we must earnestly sort out the problems and gaps in our work and figure out practical solutions.

Firstly, there was an imbalance of the counterpart aid to different regions. In terms of the aiding plans provided by all aiding provinces/municipalities, there is a huge gap in the total capital investment in the medical aid to Xinjiang. It swings from the most 770 million to the least 20 million and ranges from 17.2 percent to only 2 percent of the total aiding investment. Though there is difference among the aiding regions in economic level, economic aggregate and quota of aiding missions, the attention given to the counterpart aid work and the implementation of the project differs among the aiding provinces/municipalities. According the strategic arrangements of the central government, in the new round of medical and health counterpart aid to Xinjiang, the top priority should be unwaveringly given to the people's livelihood. As the medical and health work is an important part of people's livelihood project, the medical aid investment shouldn't be less than 5%.

Secondly, the problem of laying more emphasis on hardware rather than software still exists. In the project planning and pilot programs, it is prevalent that more efforts are made in building houses and purchasing equipment than in the training of talented people and technical support. Once ample funds are invested, the hardware can be significantly upgraded in a short period, but the soft power, including talents, technology and management, requires a long-term accumulation.

Thirdly, the planning for the aiding projects is not closely integrated with the planning for the development of local medical undertaking and the medical reform. Some partners of the counterpart aid failed to make overall and long-term plans and their special counterpart aiding projects couldn't be well integrated with the comprehensive plan of the nation and Xinjiang Autonomous Region.

Fourthly, the aiding funds should be further integrated with other capitals. For example, a large sum of money has already been invested by the central government into the construction and renovation of country-level hospital buildings as well as the medical equipment. However, for most aiding provinces/municipalities, they also put a certain amount of funds into the hospital construction. This part of money should be used together so as to improve Xinjiang medical service quality in an all-round way.

In view of the above problems, all the participants in the counterpart aid should carry out the work jointly from an overall perspective. They should take joint action and give support to one another in project planning, project implementation fund raising and intellectual support to guarantee the success of the counterpart medical aid to Xinjiang and the medical reform in Xinjiang.

(3) The present working thoughts for the medical and health aid to Xinjiang should be directed by the new missions. Taking the central government's requirements and the actual working situation into consideration, we have formed the working plans for the preliminary phase of the medical and health aid to Xinjiang. The work should be guided by the outlook of scientific development and focused on the medical reform. Under the requirements for meeting basic needs,developing grassroots

institutions and establishing new mechanisms, we should intensify our efforts, practically carry out the aiding projects and strive to accomplish the three major tasks —laying a solid foundation, ,improving the local conditions and lifting our ability. Importance should be attached to the construction of a talent contingent and the self-developing ability. Thus, basic health care system can be initially set up and a new prospect in the medical and health aid to Xinjiang can be opened up.

1) We should stick to the core mission and set up the basic health care system.

Taking deepening medical reform as our central task, we should follow the comprehensive arrangements of the aiding and aided regions, actively participate in the medical reform, continuously improve the funding and insurance level of NCMS and make sure that the basic medical insurance covers all the urban and rural residents. We should effectively implement the compensation policy in medical organizations and preliminarily establish the essential medicine system. Meanwhile, the service ability should be enhanced to ensure the completion of constructing the basic medical and health service system at grassroots level. In addition, we should further develop the major projects of public health service and ensure the equality and availability of the public health service. Finally, we should lend full support to the pilot reform of the public hospitals to ensure the effectiveness of the reform and lay a solid foundation for the preliminary establishment of the basic healthcare system.

2) We should follow the following two paths and spare no efforts to strengthen the foundation in the health and medical aid to Xinjiang.

The first path is to focus on the requirements of meeting basic needs,developing grassroots institutions and establishing new mechanisms. This is the basic path to guarantee that the basic medical and health service can be provided as public product for all the people. Meeting basic needs means that we should do well in the basic medical security and comprehensively improve our basic medical and health service. We should reasonably establish the medical security standards with all of our efforts but not out of our ability. And the standards should be gradually elevated with the development of the society and economy, and thus, the overall coverage of the basic medical service can be realized. Developing grassroots institutions means that we should gradually improve the service ability of the grassroots medical and health institutions and set up medical service platform and network for effective disease prevention and treatment as well as hospitalization costs control. In order to improve the grassroots institutions, we should pour more human, physical and financial resources into them. Establishing new mechanisms means that We should establish scientific working mechanisms to guarantee an efficient operation of the medical and pharmaceutical system. In order to set up new mechanisms, we should closely integrate the establishment of mechanisms with the increase of investment in the process of medical reform. We should effectively strengthen the establishment of mechanisms and turn the increased investment into a driving force and make all the participants work more actively.

The second path is to make overall arrangements, highlight the key points and proceed in proper sequence. It is fundamental to promote the sustainable development of the health undertakings in Xinjiang. We should coordinate the development in urban and rural areas; give consideration to both suppliers' and demanders' interests, and focus on integration of the prevention, treatment and rehabilitation. Meanwhile, we should balance the relationship among government, medical institutions, pharmaceutical enterprises, medical workers and the people. In addition, we should also highlight the key points and solve the main problems. By focusing on the priorities, the efficacy of medical reform and development can be promoted tremendously. The current economic and social development status of Xinjiang determines that it's impossible to achieve the leapforward development overnight, so the work should be done step by step. The medical and health undertaking in Xinjiang involves all the aspects that are closely linked with one another. By consolidating the foundation of health care at the grass-roots level, the prominent problem, the relatively backward situation in the construction of the medical and health system at the grassroots level in Xinjiang, can be improved. The medical reform that begins from the grassroots level to the hospitals at the county or city level will greatly facilitate sustainable development of the medical and health undertaking in Xinjiang.

3) The following three tasks should be completed to lay a solid foundation for the medical and health aid to Xinjiang.

To lay a solid foundation. The work should be done in all aspects so as to carry out the overall counterpart aid to Xinjiang and push forward the transformation of the mechanisms. We should lay down the material foundation for health supporting Xinjiang by effectively planning and implementation through the implementation of the projects and the infrastructure construction. In the meaning time, attention should be paid to the integration of capital, talent, technology, management and other resources and the function of the comprehensive aid to Xinjiang should be brought to full play.

To improve the local conditions. The allocation of resources should be optimized and the priority should be given to the grassroots institutions in order to improve the service network at the grassroots level. We should take the work at the grassroots level as the priorities and breakthrough point and invest in more efforts and money. And we should guide the flows of the essential elements of funds, technology, talented people and management into the grassroots level and promote rational distribution and circulation of health resources. Thus, the growth potential of the grassroots institutions can be elevated.

To improve the abilities. To complete this task, we should intensify the intellectual support and the construction of the talent contingent. And priority should be given to the aid in cadres, technology, management and the popularization of appropriate medical techniques. Meanwhile, the technical level of disease prevention and medical serviced quality in the grassroots medical and health institutions should also be elevated. Thus, a group of academic leaders mastering modern medical science and technology and skills will emerge in Xinjiang. In addition, the training in management should be strengthened, new management methods and concepts should be adopted and the management ability in the medical and health institutions should be improved.

4) We should grasp the following 4 key points to realize the fine management in the counterpart aid to Xinjiang.

Firstly, the work progress should be fast yet steady and the working procedures should be lined out in detail. Under the guidance of progressing as-quickly-as-possible, we should refine the work plans and carry them out effectively and timely in order to achieve significant results within a short period of time. The medical and health aid to Xinjiang should be regarded as a long-term and systematic project, so we shouldn't reach for what is beyond our grasp. Besides, we should carry out the work gradually, systematically and in a down-to-earth way. We should do our best within our capability and spare no efforts on practical matters in light of people's requirements. We should do the solid work and avoid the image projects and vanity projects.

Secondly, the aiding work should be done with both quality and quantity and the project implementation should be standardized. On the basis of quality coming first, equal importance should be attached to quantity and quality. And we shouldn't be eager for quick success and blindly seek for high starting point and high speed. All the projects must be implemented under relevant regulations, standards and quality supervision. Thus, no jerry-built projects will appear and the people's long-term benefits can be ensured.

Thirdly, the regulation should be strengthened and the supervision and inspection should be institutionalized. We should strengthen the regulation from the source, innovate the supervisory mechanism, carry out on-site supervision in all dimensions and regularly supervise the projects. Thus, the quality control can be enhanced, the operational regulations can be strengthened. And as a result, the quality of the projects can be effectively controlled. The examining and assessment system should be reinforced to ensure the practical effect. For the work that has been done we should evaluate the result. For the work being undertaken we should pay great attention to the progress. For the work that has not been done we should find out the reasons. For the work that has not been done responsibly and effectively we should demand accountability.

Fourthly, the mass people should benefit from the counterpart aid and the unification of service management should be realized. We should listen to the people's voices and try our best to obtain the firsthand information, and gather all the resources to serve the people. Besides, we should change our thoughts, strengthen the construction of professional ethics, elevate the quality and level of our service, meet the rational needs of the people and construct harmonious relationship between the patients and doctors.

Ⅲ. We should focus on the priorities and make efforts to promote the leap-forward development of the medical and health undertaking in Xinjiang

In order to lay a solid foundation and primarily set up the basic medical and health service system, the aiding and aided parties should effectively integrate the counterpart aid work with the medical reform and get their work well linked with the demands of the leapforward development of the health undertaking in Xinjiang. Meanwhile, all the parties should concentrate their strength on the solutions to the difficult problems and achieve remarkable results.

(1) We should deepen the reform of the systems and mechanisms, especially the reform of the medical system. Nowadays, we have entered "the deep water zone" of the medical reform, where lots of contradictions in the systems and mechanisms have emerged. On May 31, the Ninth Plenary Meeting, held by the Leading Group of the State Council on Deepening the Reform of the Medical and Pharmaceutical Systems,, proposed that we should speed up our reforming and innovating pace and give priority to the establishment of mechanisms in the medical reform.

In order to carry out the Central Government's general deployments, the Xinjiang region should push forward the comprehensive reform of the grassroots medical and health institutions and promote the overall coverage of the essential medicine system. In addition, the efforts should be made to set up the new operating mechanism in the grassroots medical and health institutions and the proper methods and paths of reform should be explored. The following mechanisms should be established and they are the non-profit management mechanism, the competitive personnel mechanism, the incentive distribution mechanism, the standardized medicine-purchasing mechanism and the long-lasting multi-channel compensatory mechanism. What's more, great impetus should be given to the pilot work of the reform of the public hospitals. We should sum up the experience, active explore and pay special attention to comprehensively reform of the country-level hospital so as to explore new models for the reform and development of the public hospitals.

We should further advance the security standard, increase the ratio of reimburse, adopt various measures and carry out bold practice to build a sound medical insurance framework for all the residents. Finally, every aiding province/municipality should do well the support in terms of money and projects. And at the same time, they should take the reality of the recipients into consideration and focus on the exchange of the reform concepts, working thoughts, policies and measures with the recipients so as to inspire and learn from each other and create a win-win situation.

(2) We should strengthen the personnel training and the construction of the talent contingent.

Xinjiang's current condition in medical human resources and its goal for the leapforward development require a scientific and practical medical talent training plan. We should launch the contingent construction of grass-roots health professionals, further carry out the training base construction for the general practitioners and organize and implement the training projects for medical personnel. The aiding provinces/municipalities should take the actual needs of the recipients into consideration and focus on the support to the cooperation in scientific research, discipline construction, technological assistance, vocational training, academic education and other aspects. Thus, the service ability and level of the professional medical technicians in Xinjiang can be actually elevated. At the same time, the interaction between the cadres in charge of the management of medical and health care work in the aid-giving and aided areas should be furthered and both sides should send cadres to get tempered through titular position. They should also study and exchange with each other.

(3) We should put emphasis on the health emergency management and increase the emergency response ability.

Xinjiang, with its social, historic and cultural specificities and complexities and its harsh natural conditions, is sometimes disturbed by natural disasters and public security incidents, which urgently requires a sound management and decision-making system for the health and public emergencies. We also should upgrade the four-tier emergency management system and the information report network and gradually realize the overall commandment and management over the public health emergencies. The monitoring and warning of public health emergencies and the lab testing ability should be enhanced and the ability in early identification, storage of supplies for emergency response and so on should be increased. The construction of a three-dimensional medical rescue system that involves the land and air aid should be strengthened based on the present medical and health resources. All the aiding provinces/municipalities should exert their further assistance in terms of emergency response supplies, first-aid vehicles and the construction of the information system, so as to enhance the recipients' capacity of emergency management. Once an emergency occurs, the aiding parties should actively cooperate, take proactive action and give their full support.

(4) We should continue to boost the construction of telemedicine and raise the level of health information system. Full coverage of telemedicine, which makes the advanced treatment technology available to the whole Xinjiang region, has brought tangible benefits to the mass people of all ethnic groups in Xinjiang, and effectively alleviated their needs of high-quality medical resources.

Xinjiang should further strengthen the construction of the regional information system that focuses on the health file of the residents and fully implement the infrastructure construction of the grassroots medical information network. The information platform for the *New Rural Cooperative Medical System* (NCMS), the health emergency commandment and decision-making system, the health supervision information system and the medical treatment information system should be optimized to improve the level of the construction of Xinjiang's health information system.

We should make full use of the overall coverage of telemedicine in Xinjiang and further increase cooperation between major hospitals in Xinjiang and the ones in the aiding provinces/municipalities, between grassroots medical and health institutions and major hospitals in respects of technical guidance, medical service and resource sharing and so on. We should actively take steps to pursue a development path which will make use of telemedicine to elevate the overall medical and health service ability and bring benefits to the mass people in Xinjiang as a whole. And we will strive to foster a distinctive pattern telemedicine and the common diseases as well as the complicated and serious cases can be cured within Xinjiang.

The aiding provinces/municipalities and hospitals should fully understand the importance of telemedicine to solve the difficulty in getting medical service for the mass people in Xinjiang. The highly qualified experts should be arranged in the telemedicine service to meet the Xinjiang people's demand for medical service and elevate the service ability and level of all the medical and health institutions in Xinjiang. With the advantages of medical education, research and treatment of the aiding hospitals, we should vigorously carry out remote technical consultation and medical education to bring the latest and advanced medical information and technology to Xinjiang and give fully play to the radiation function of telemedicine.

(5) We should make full use of our advantages and improve the service capability of traditional Chinese/ethnic medicine. Traditional Chinese/ethnic medicine is an

important part of the China's health undertaking. Since it's efficient, inexpensive and effective, it is widely accepted and used by people of all nationalities in China.

Efforts should be made by Xinjiang government to establish and improve the systems, mechanisms and investment policies which are beneficial for the development and perfection of Traditional Chinese/ethnic medicine. The guidance to the clinical application of essential medicines of traditional Chinese/ethnic medicine should also be strengthened and the preferential policies that encourage the application and use of traditional Chinese/ethnic medicine should be made. Besides, the service ability of traditional Chinese/ethnic medicine, the construction of the service network and the establishment of specialty disciplines should be enhanced. Furthermore, the ability of specialized medical service should be increased and the selection, research and popularization of the appropriate techniques in the traditional Chinese/ethnic medicine for the common diseases in the local regions should be conscientiously carried out. With these measures, the mass people can be well served and get more benefits.

The aiding organizations should vigorously support the traditional Chinese/ethnic medicine industry in Xinjiang province and give guidance and impetus to the construction of clinical research bases. Moreover, they should strengthen the training of grassroots professionals and backbone technicians of traditional Chinese/ethnic medicine in order to comprehensively boost the inheritance and innovation of traditional Chinese/ethnic medicine industry in Xinjiang.

IV. We should cooperate closely and try our best to maintain the scientific development of the medical and health aid to Xinjiang.

(1) The organization and leadership should be strengthened and the aiding mechanisms should be optimized. Every health department of the aiding provinces/municipality and the subordinates of the Health Ministry and health should regard the counterpart aid to Xinjiang as a long-term task and make unremitting efforts to improve the guarding system of the medical and health aid to Xinjiang.

The chiefs should shoulder the aiding work personally and the leading groups should study careful over the tasks. And the counterpart aid to Xinjiang should always be included in their agendas and plans.

The aiding and aided sides should increase their exchanges and communication, and further improve their connection and communication. By ways of exchange, cooperation and consultation, they should optimize the consultative mechanisms in the counterpart aid and establish a regular reporting and communication system. We should further complete the funding mechanism, the supervision and management mechanisms of projects and funds and the management and appointment mechanisms of cadres to promote the smooth process of counterpart aiding work.

(2) We should focus on the overall plan and effectively guarantee that the work can be persistently carried out. We should adhere to the plan-oriented principle, take projects as the starting point, pay attention to the overall situation and consider both the short-term and long-term benefits. Besides, we should give full consideration to the actual needs of the recipients and the economic and social development level of the aiding provinces/municipalities, act according toour ability and try our best to implement the counterpart aiding tasks. The policies and work arrangements should be firmly carried out and special support should be given to the aspects of policies, capital investment, and project arrangements to ensure the completion of the aiding tasks and the success of the medical and health aid to Xinjiang. We should further carry out the refinement and quantization of the aiding tasks, fix the responsible departments and persons and the deadline should be set. For every task, the responsible person/persons, the deadline, the standards and the specific missions should be clarified to ensure the tasks can be orderly conducted. During the implementation of the project, the plan should be carried out according to the real situation of the project and an inverted schedule should be made. We should overcome the difficulties and spare no efforts to ensure the quality and the timely completion of construction tasks so that the projects can benefit the mass people as soon as possible.

(3) We should strengthen the financial supervision and safeguard the security and benefits of funds. By actively adopting the comprehensive measures, we should further strengthen the supervision and control of the funds to enhance the capital efficiency. As for the media of inspection, the external forces such as the specialized auditing agencies and the social intermediaries can be hired to intensify the inspection and supervision so as to ensure the supervisory transparency. In terms of methods and devices, the modern information tools can be employed to ensure the thoroughness, normalization and timeliness of the supervision. In the matter of the form of supervision, not only should the single lateral horizontal inspection be carried out, but also the all-dimensional inspection of a certain area should be conducted. And thus, the progress and effect of the project can be found out.

(4) We should focus on the publicity of typical models and create a positive social atmosphere. The deeds of the outstanding groups and individuals in the medical and health aid to Xinjiang should be widely promoted and the exemplary methods and experience should be introduced by the media in order to create a sound public opinion and a positive social atmosphere. At the same time, the aiding provinces/municipalities and the aiding organizations should do well the implementation of the

policies and the publicity of the aiding cadres and medical technicians. Their work and life should be care about and the selection, management and appointment of the cadres should be considered as the key linkage of the counterpart aid. By earnestly strengthening the contingent construction and giving full play to the talents, the counterpart aid work can be well guaranteed. We should trust the aiding cadres on a political basis, give them support in their work, care for them in their daily life and feel assured to employ them. Meanwhile, we should help them to solve the difficulty they meet and let them feel the warmth from the organizations and the care from the colleagues. Thus, they can be worry-free, go forward with their burdens discarded and throw themselves wholeheartedly into the work.

As the development goals and working thoughts of the medical and health to Xinjiang has been clarified for the years to come, we should take the Scientific Outlook of Development as the guidance, thoroughly carry the spirits of the Central Conference, unite together, stick to our goals, cooperate closely, implement the plans , lay a solid foundation, try our best to improve the medical and health service ability and the health level for the people in Xinjiang and make great efforts to ensure the leapforward economic and social development in Xinjiang.

(Qu Yang)

5. Summarize Experience, Deepen the Understanding and Make Solid Progress in the Pilot Work of Medical Security for Major Serious Diseases

—A Speech Made by Chen Zhu, Minister of the Ministry of Health (June 28, 2011)

On the occasion of the 90th anniversary of the founding of the Communist Party of China, we hold the conference on the promotion of the pilot work of medical security for major serious diseases, the purpose of which is to carry through and implement the key working tasks for the medical and health reform of 2011, summarize the working experience achieved in the pilot work of medical security for childhood leukemia and congenital heart disease in all the localities in the past year, conduct research on the perfection of policies, carry out the work of the improvement of the level of medical security for these two diseases in an all-round way, expand the range of diseases covered in the pilot and promote the pilot work in a down-to-earth manner so as to celebrate the 90th anniversary of our Party through our concrete actions.

First of all, I should extend thanks to Jiangsu Provincial Government for the strong support offered to the conference. After I heard the introduction made by several provinces, regions and Nanjing Children's hospital just now, I feel encouraged. Their methods and experience are of significance for us to do well the future work.

Next, I'll talk about three points of my opinions.

I. Fully affirm the achievements gained in the pilot work of improving the level of medical security for rural childhood leukemia and congenital heart disease

(1) The pilot work was initiated quickly and carried out smoothly and remarkable results were achieved in the treatment of childhood leukemia and congenital heart disease.

In June 2010, the Ministry of Health and the Ministry of Civil Affairs jointly issued the *Opinions on Improving the Level of medical security for Rural Childhood Leukemia and Congenital Heart Disease* and held meetings in Changsha City of Hunan Province and Chengdu City of Sichuan Province, at which mobilization and deployment for the pilot work were conducted. All the localities immediately took actions after the meeting and within two months, more than half provinces of the whole country issued provincial implementation plans, in which pilot regions, compensatory schemes and designated hospitals for the treatment of childhood leukemia and congenital heart disease were defined. By the end of 2010, 4,329 children participating in the new rural cooperative medical care were treated, of whom 3844 suffered from congenital heart disease and 485 suffered from leukemia. From January to April this year, 4730 children were treated, 4254 suffering from congenital heart disease and 476 suffering from leukemia. Relevant work was further accelerated in recent few months and many children who hadn't got access to medical treatment due to lack of money were rescued and treated effectively. Great achievements were made in the pilot work of medical security for these two diseases, which gained broad recognition and acclaim from all sectors of the society and transformed the concerns the Party Central Committee and the State Council showed to people's livelihood to concrete health benefits they could feel.

(2) Operating mechanisms for the pilot work were formed initially and a critical step towards the exploration of making good use of limited funds to solve the issues on medical security for some major serious diseases was made.

Departments of health, civil affairs, finance and administrative organizations responsible for the new rural cooperative medical care at all levels, especially those in pilot areas, closely cooperated with designated hospitals and for the supreme goal of jointly protecting patients' health right, on the basis of full communication and consultation, in the light of our country's unified policy framework and actual conditions in all localities, established a set of operating mechanisms for the pilot work which provided that the pilot work was mainly funded by the new rural cooperative medical system and the medical assistance and paid appropriately by patients, managed by administrative organizations of the new rural cooperative medical care and designated hospitals rendered medical services. As a result, the management was intensified and the level of medical security for a great number of children with leukemia and congenital heart disease was improved with comparatively less money paid so that children patients' economic burden was relieved remarkably and the prospective policy effectiveness was gained. By the end of April 30, 2011, the new rural cooperative medical system compensated up to 111 million RMB Yuan for major childhood serious diseases and the medical assistance subsidized about 18.355 million RMB Yuan, the two kinds of funds amounting to 129 million RMB Yuan. 9,059 children with leukemia and congenital heart disease got effective rescue and treatment with paying only 20% of the whole medical expenses, so the funds were used with a significant efficiency. In comparison with the situation before the pilot work, payment of children patients' family decreased by 60 percent, so people's medical load was relieved substantially and they just reaped the tangible benefits of the pilot work.

(3) The pilot work made good use of the advantages of the overall-planning management of medical service and medical security, which played an exemplary role in the solid promotion of the comprehensive reform of medical and health system.

Despite the limited coverage of diseases, the pilot work gave full play to health departments' systemic advantages in the overall-planning management of medical security and medical service. By intensification of comprehensive management, the industrial supervisory management, the professional guidance and the reform in the payment of the new rural cooperative medical care were closely integrated. Designated hospitals were also required to carry out management on clinical pathways and standardized diagnosis and treatment for pilot diseases so that medical service conducts were regulated. Particularly, the mode of quota payment for specific diseases compelled medical institutions to maintain the balance of financial revenue and expenditure by increasing service efficiency and decreasing medical cost, which changed the operating mechanisms of medical institutions, helped them get rid of irrational incentive mechanisms and interest chains and effectively controlled the unreasonable increase of medical expenses. Medical institutions maintained the balance of financial revenue and expenditure as well as produced social benefits and led to a virtuous circle of the decrease in cost and the improvement in development.

From 2004 to 2010 in Caidian District of Wuhan City, children patients' average expanses for the treatment of congenital heart disease were 39,000 RMB Yuan, of which 11,800 RMB Yuan were compensated by the new rural cooperative medical systém and individual payment was 27,000 RMB Yuan. After the implementation of the pilot work, the average medical expanses for the children patients with congenital heart disease decreased to 22,300 RMB Yuan, of which 16,100 RMB Yuan were compensated by the new rural cooperative medical system; 4,600 RMB Yuan were offered by the medical assistance and individual payment was only 1,600 RMB Yuan, so that medical expanses and personal load were substantially decreased and the masses spoke highly of the services of medical institutions; many doctors felt that the pilot work of the treatment of childhood leukemia and congenital heart disease enabled them to regain the high sense of responsibility and pride on the job.

(4) The pilot work promoted the construction of related disciplines and the improvement of service capacity of designated hospitals and improved the cooperation between medical institutions.

The pilot work of the treatment of childhood leukemia and congenital heart disease remarkably reduced the burden of medical cost on children patients' families, improved the accessibility to the medical service and particularly satisfied the need of such patients who failed to be treated due to lack of money. Some designated hospitals reported that the number of patients in three months after the pilot work was much more than that of the whole year before the pilot work. To deal with the sharp rise in work load and ensure medical quality, designated medical institutions standardized medical conducts, intensified internal management, with the help of the technical coordination and guidance from regional cooperative centers and expert panels, effectively promoted the construction of related disciplines, accelerated the talent cultivation and improved the comprehensive managerial capacity of designated hospitals as well.

Most of the designated hospitals for the pilot work of the treatment of two diseases were provincial tertiary hospitals, while the first choice for farmers participating in the new rural cooperative medical care was township health center or county hospital, so the improvement of timely and accurate diagnosis of first-visit medical institutions would increase the working efficiency of provincial designated hospitals and decrease the disputes brought about by the disagreement on the first diagnosis and follow-up diagnoses. Therefore, numerous designated hospitals took the initiative in the improvement of the diagnostic level of grassroots medical and health institutions by offering technical assistance, personnel training and guidance on management, while county-level hospitals and township health centers were also active in conducting propaganda and transferring patients and all-level medical institutions closely cooperated and coordinated so that the level of the treatment of major childhood diseases was heightened comprehensively, which laid a sound foundation for the future spread of mature techniques to county-level hospitals with service capacity.

All these accomplishments are attributed to the great attention and energetic support of all-level Party committees and governments, the active cooperation and unified promotion of departments of health, civil affairs, finance and other departments concerned and the hard work of the staff of administrative departments and medical workers. Here, on behalf of the Ministry of Health, I express my heartfelt thanks to all the comrades.

In the one year's pilot work, all the localities worked creatively in accordance with the requirements of the Party Central Party and the actual local conditions and effective methods were formed. These valuable experience and successful methods are of vital importance for the full development of medical security for the two childhood diseases and further fulfillment of the pilot work. Viewed from a more macro perspective, these experience and methods are significantly important to the future work of medical security for our country's broad masses' major diseases and the exploration of the health road with comparative low input, good health benefits and Chinese characteristics. The important points of experience in the pilot work are as follows.

Firstly, high attention of all-level Party committees and governments, close cooperation and unified promotion of relevant departments guaranteed the smooth development of the pilot work. Many provinces (autonomous regions and cities) regarded the improvement of the work of medical security for childhood major serious diseases as a vital issue of people's livelihood and pushed forward it energetically and the establishment of accountability system, the intensification of departmental cooperation and especially the close coordination and concerted promotion of the departments of health, civil affairs, finance and other departments concerned effectively guaranteed the smooth development of the pilot work. Secondly, scientifically-made plans and subtle management laid a foundation for the successful implementation of the pilot work. With limited time and high demands, all the localities adopted the scientific attitude when working out implantation plans and organized experts to carry out thorough investigations. On the basis of the baseline survey on the incidence of diseases and the medical cost and according to the actual local conditions, all the localities adjusted assistance range, compensatory level and payment forms. The new rural cooperative medical system, departments of medical administration, supervision and management of medical services, planning and finance, medical institutions and other departments had clear division of work and responsibilities so that smooth implementation of the pilot work was ensured. Thirdly, standard medical services with focus on the management of clinical pathway and standardized diagnosis and treatment and effective control on medical cost with limited or quota payment for specific diseases were the key to the success of the pilot work. Management of clinical pathway and standardized diagnosis and treatment conducted in the pilot work guaranteed the standard service of medical institutions, which avoided excessive treatment and unreasonable medical conducts. Limited or quota payment for specific diseases made medical institutions change their ideology, improve the quality as well as reduce the cost, so that such medical institutions with high skills, qualified services and low cost attracted more patients and achieved economies of scale. Since there were both full cooperation and mechanism restriction in medical treatment and medical security, hospital-patient relationship transformed from the opposite to mutual trust and a win-win situation emerged and developed soundly.

While fully appreciating the achievements in the treatment of childhood leukemia and congenital heart disease, we should also realize the pilot work is at the very beginning and there exist a number of difficulties and problems, for instance, some leaders of health departments in some localities haven't fully realized the importance of the pilot work of medical security for major serious diseases and didn't work effectively; different localities didn't have balanced development and some localities were obviously fallen behind; grassroots medical institutions had difficulties in the diagnosis, classification and treatment of childhood leukemia and congenital heart disease and phenomena of delayed diagnosis and treatment still existed, so on the basis of the summary of experience, we should further explore laws, perfect policies, make greater efforts and continue to promote the pilot work in an all-round way.

II. Fully realize the importance of the pilot work of medical security for rural residents' major serious diseases

Perfection of the medical security system and improvement of the level of the security for major serious diseases is a big event that improves people's livelihood and promotes the harmony and stability of the society and also is what the in-depth medical and health reform aims at. On the basis of gradual improvement of the general level of all the medical security systems, it is of vital importance to explore ways for the establishment of the system of medical security for rural residents' major serious diseases.

(1) The pilot work of medical security for rural residents' major serious diseases is an engineering of people's livelihood that draws the concern of the Party, governments, and the whole society.

In recent years, with fast development of our country's economy and society and gradual establishment of various social security and welfare systems, people's living standard improves obviously. But with the limits of the basic medical security level, the problem of patients' becoming poor or returning to poverty due to major serious diseases is still unsolved, which is especially prominent among rural residents. Once a family member comes down with a major serious disease, the family will be caught in poverty soon, which not only brings a huge psychological and economic burden to patients' families, but also has a serious impact on work and life and constitutes a hidden danger for social harmony and stability. Media expose some families leading a poor live because of treatment of disease, which creates immense stir in the society and such phenomenon is one of the most prominent problems concerning people's livelihood at present. The Party Central Committee and the State Council attach great importance to the problem and require health departments and relevant departments to do well the work concerned. The call for the solution to the problem of medical security for rural residents' major serious diseases is increasing year by year in the recent two years' suggestions and proposals put forward by the deputies to the National People's Congress and the remembers of the Chinese People's Political Consultative Conference. Doing well the pilot work of medical security for rural residents' major serious diseases and exploring ways to solve the problems concerned is a historical task the Party assigns us, is the broad masses' expectation and desire and also an important engineering of people's livelihood with high expectations of the whole society.

(2) The pilot work of medical security for rural residents' major serious diseases is a major measure to perfect and develop the new rural cooperative medical system.

With several years' rapid development of the new rural cooperative medical system, the capacity for medical security has been improving unceasingly. In 2011, we shall strive to reach the goal of about 70 percent compensation and the highest payment limit of no less than 50,000 RMB Yuan for policy-allowed hospitalization in overall-planning areas. Although these measures can initially solve the problem of rural residents' basic medical security, for some major serious diseases, farmers participating in the new rural cooperative medical care still have a heavy load of medical expenditure. So how to solve the problem of rural residents' medical security for major serious diseases constitutes a major issue that concerns the further development and perfection of the new rural cooperative medical system and also an inescapable one for us to promote the medical and healthcare reform, particularly, the reform of public hospitals.

The present security level of the new rural cooperative medical care is at such a level that a slight increase in the percentage of compensation can't be perceived by farmers. If we can heighten the comprehensive level of medical security as well as allocate a small part of newly-supplied funds to relieving the broad masses' heavy burden caused by major serious diseases, then remarkable social benefits can be created and the masses will increase their sense of identity for the new rural cooperative medical care, which is of positive significance for the development of the new rural cooperative medical system as well as for the establishment and perfection of the system of quota payment for specific diseases; as a matter of fact, this is an work that affects the overall situation. The pilot work of medical security for childhood leukemia and congenital heart disease has already explored a practicable way for us and we shall accelerate the pilot work on the basis of the summary of the experience, which can not only benefit the masses who are plagued by major serious diseases, but also do good to promoting the fund-raising for the new rural cooperative medical care, improving the comprehensive security level and arousing masses' enthusiasm for participating in the new rural cooperative medical care and lay a solid foundation for the sustainable, stable and healthy development of the new rural cooperative medical system.

(3) The pilot work of medical security for rural residents' major serious diseases is an important method to push forward the reform of public hospitals.

Remarkable achievements and substantial progress have been made in medical security, medical service, public health service, reform of public hospitals and drug supply and security in the two years after the medical and healthcare reform and the broad masses have reaped the benefits of the reform, but there remain some deep-rooted problems to be solved in systems and mechanisms. The pilot work of two childhood diseases offers us great amount of experience that we could use for reference. Particularly in the reform of public hospitals, simultaneous promotion of various measures, such as reform in payment systems and management of clinical pathway, has effectively controlled the increase in medical expenses, at the same time, guaranteed the medical quality and led public medical institutions to transform the operation mechanisms so that service efficiency increased whereas service cost decreased, but the income of hospitals and medical staff was not reduced and the purpose of the reform was realized that "the broad masses reaped benefits; medical staff were in high spirits and medical institutions developed". Therefore, acceleration of the pilot work of medical security for rural residents' major serious diseases and active increase of diseases and areas covered by the pilot are beneficial for the promotion of the reform of public hospitals and can enable more masses to get benefits and more public hospitals to develop soundly.

Solution to the problem of medical security for rural residents' major serious diseases is a necessity for economic and social development and also an urgent need for the broad rural residents' health security. In 2011, governments' annual subsidies for the new rural cooperative medical care was increased from last year's 120 RMB Yuan per person to 200 RMB Yuan per person this year and the standard of individual payment also rises. We shall make full use of this favorable opportunity, unify our ideology, improve cognition and on the basis of further improvement of the hospitalization compensation level and full implementation of outpatient overall planning, accelerate the promotion of the pilot work and do well the pilot work of medical security for rural residents' major serious diseases with all our strength.

III. Make greater efforts, accelerate the speed and do well the pilot work of medical security for rural residents' major serious diseases

(1) Fully improve the level of medical security for rural childhood leukemia and congenital heart disease.

The Healthcare Reform Office of the State Council required explicitly in the arrangement for the major work of the medical and health reform that each province (autonomous region, city) carry out the pilot of the full improvement of the level of medical security for childhood leukemia and congenital heart disease and on the basis of the summary and evaluation, increase diseases and areas covered by the pilot. According to the requirement, each province (autonomous region, city) has already initiated the pilot successively. Although there is an imbalanced development in different areas, unexpected better results have been gained on the whole. So far, 15 provinces (autonomous regions, cities) have carried out the pilot work in the whole province and 12 provinces (autonomous regions, cities) are preparing for the start of the pilot work.

With overall implementation of the pilot work, administrative organizations of the new rural cooperative medical care, designated medical institutions, technical cooperative centers and technical guidance experts will undertake more tasks and greater pressure, therefore, in the light of actual increase of children patients, administrative organizations shall properly increase the number of designated medical institutions in order to match the increase in the number of children patients and ensure the capacity for treatment. But since childhood leukemia is a special major serious disease with comparatively lower incidence, fewer cases and difficult and complicated standardized diagnosis and treatment, it is better for tertiary hospitals that have the capacity and conditions for the diagnosis and treatment of childhood leukemia to take on the work.

Designated medical institutions shall strictly carry out the management of clinical pathway and standardized diagnosis and treatment for pilot diseases, ensure high-quality medical treatment and control medical expenses. Health departments and departments concerned shall strengthen the guidance, do a good job in linking up the work of designated medical institutions and grassroots medical institutions, guarantee children patients' smooth first visit and referral and for children patients with leukemia that is difficult for grassroots medical institutions to diagnose and classify, we shall try particularly to avoid waste of a great amount of time, money and delay of timely treatment due to misdiagnosis.

Technical cooperative centers and technical guidance experts shall further enhance technical cooperation with designated medical institutions and render more technical assistance to them. For designated medical institutions in the middle and western regions and those with comparatively low technical level, technical cooperative centers and technical guidance experts must make full use of their technical advantages, offer targeted assistance and set up fixed channels of technical cooperation and assistance so that these regions and medical institutions can rapidly improve their capacity and level that can meet children patients' medical need and ensure the smooth implementation of the work.

Provinces that have already carried out the work comprehensively shall make persistent efforts, further perfect policy measures, improve the implementation of the policies and conscientiously put them into effect. Provinces that haven't initiated the work shall make greater efforts to ensure the overall implementation of medical security for two childhood diseases by the end of September. Regions with suitable conditions may consider taking complex childhood congenital heart disease and acute childhood leukemia into the range of the improvement of security level, in that case, all the rural children with leukemia and congenital heart disease throughout the country, including those in the towns where the work was promoted by urban and rural joint efforts, can reap the benefits of the policy.

(2) Accelerate the pilot work of medical security for newly-added diseases

At present, there are many diseases that affect rural residents' health, but due to low fund-raising level of the new rural cooperative medical care and insufficient service capacity of grassroots medical institutions, these problems can't be solve together, so we have to, in accordance with the actual conditions, first tackle those major serious diseases that seriously endanger rural residents' health, severely affect their production and lives, bring heavy burden to their families and cause extensive social attention and at the same time, the diseases that we tackle first must have sure curative efficacy and comparatively controllable expenses. Last year, we initiated the pilot work of two childhood diseases and remarkable achievements have been gained. This year, we shall give priority to following diseases.

The first is two female cancers, namely, breast cancer and cervical cancer. Protection of maternal and child health is one of the symbols to show the level of a country's civilization. The Party and government pay much attention to it and Premier Wen has listed it in this year's *Report on the Work of the Government*. In the five key tasks for the medical and health reform in 2009-2011, we regarded the provision of health protection for rural pregnant and puerperal women as a basic public health service item and screening of cervical cancer and breast cancer for childbearing-aged women as a major public health item and it is only the first step. The second step is to consider how to solve the problem of medical security for rural women's two cancers, earnestly put the Party Central Committee's policies into effect and make rural women deeply feel the care of the Party and government and enjoy the benefits.

The second is rural serious psychosis. Serious psychosis is a disease with a long therapeutic course and frequent relapses. If not properly treated, patients with serious psychosis are more likely to become the disabled, which is a heavy burden for patients themselves and their families. Also because of patients' serious cognitive impairments and loss of ability to control their behaviors, at the time of stroke onset, they can even bring harmfulness to the society. In recent years, malignant cases brought about by serious psychotic patients have occurred in some places and cause not only casualties and economic losses, but also masses' panic, which affects the harmony and stability of the society. According to current statistics, there are no less than 1.8 million serious psychotic patients in rural areas, many of whom don't get timely and standard treatment because of lack of money. This year, we shall make good use of the opportunity of the increase in the pilot diseases and in the light of the state's management of serious psychosis and special fund allocation for the treatment, tremendously improve the security level for rural serious psychotic patients' outpatient and in-patient treatment, help the families that are plagued by serious psychosis overcome difficulties, share the care and burden of the Party and government and fully play the role of the new rural cooperative medical care in the promotion of harmony and stability of the society.

The third is end-stage renal disease. It is estimated that there are 500 thousand cases of end-stage renal disease in our country's rural areas and this is a large number. If there is such a patient in an ordinary family, the whole family will be stripped bare and lead a hard life because of the long therapeutic course and high expenses of the disease. The event of patients' purchase of dialyzers published by media fully illustrates what I have mentioned above and I am deeply disturbed by the event. At present, many countries take offering of effective medical security for dialysis of patients with end-stage renal disease as a major index to measure the level of medical security. If we can't solve the problem that plagues nearly hundreds of thousands of rural families, what's the point of talking about social development and improvement of livelihood,Then, the medical achievements gained will be discounted. Therefore, we shall focus on considering how to heighten the security level of the dialytic treatment and improve service patterns and the departments of the new rural cooperative medical care, medical administration, supervision and management of medical services and so on shall also enhance cooperation, actively create conditions, popularize peritoneal dialysis which is cheaper and safer and do well the work of medical security for rural residents' dialytic treatment.

The fourth is multidrug-resistant pulmonary tuberculosis. There are about 120 thousand new cases of multidrug-resistant pulmonary tuberculosis each year throughout the country. Compared with patients with common tuberculosis, it takes longer time to diagnose and treat patients with multidrug-resistant pulmonary tuberculosis so that they have longer infective period, more serious harmfulness and need more expenses to cure the disease. We are confronted with a serious situation of the prevention and treatment of multidrug-resistant pulmonary tuberculosis. The World Health Organization has listed our country in one of 27 countries with the heavy load of multidrug-resistant pulmonary tuberculosis. Numerous patients haven't been treated timely due to lack of special funds for the prevention and treatment of multidrug-resistant pulmonary tuberculosis, so in accordance with the actual conditions, the new rural cooperative medical care shall improve the level of subsidiary for the medical expenses that are beyond payment range of the public health program for the prevention and treatment of multidrug-resistant pulmonary tuberculosis and make due contribution for our country's prevention and treatment of tuberculosis.

Furthermore, opportunistic infection with AIDS shall also be considered to be taken into the treatment range in the regions with suitable conditions and beneficial coverage shall be further expanded.

In the light of the methods of the pilot of medical security for two childhood diseases, all the localities shall bring the diseases mentioned above into the pilot of medical security for major serious diseases and conduct management by the way of quota payment for specific disease; the new rural cooperative medical care compensates 70% of medical expenses and all the localities shall make active efforts to get the support of the medical assistance and cooperatively heighten the security level. The Ministry of Health is working out clinical pathways suitable for county-level and above medical institutions to treat the above-mentioned diseases and according to local actual conditions, on the basis of the clinical pathways issued by the Ministry of Health and on the premise of guarantee of quality and being helpful to the reduce of expenses, health departments and bureaus of each province (autonomous region, city) can also formulate standardized schemes of diagnosis and treatment that are more suitable for local patients' actual conditions.

At present, 11 provinces (autonomous regions, cities) nationwide initiate the work that covers more major serious diseases in the pilot and good results have been achieved in some provinces. For example, the Second People's Hospital of Wujiang City, Jiangsu Province establishes a dialysis center where 95% of the expenses was reduced by the new rural cooperative medical care and individual payment is only 20 RMB Yuan; meanwhile the hospital offers patients free lunch and shuttle service. In Jiangyin City, patients' expenses for dialysis are compensated every three month according the standard of once hospitalization treatment and 50% of self-payment within the range of reimbursement is also subsidized, as a result, the actual compensation amounts to 80%, which greatly lightens patients' economic load. On the basis of the overall implementation of the pilot work that improves the level of medical security for two childhood diseases and according to the principle of classified diagnosis and treatment, Anhui Province carries out the pilot work for 65 kinds of major serious diseases respectively in province-level, city-level and county-level medical institutions this year; greater efforts are made to make the work done solidly and meticulously and farmers are expected to get further benefits generally. Shandong Province carries out the pilot of major disease security for hemophilia and all the other provinces that haven't launched the work shall accelerate the speed and see to it that the pilot of medical security for newly-added diseases shall be implemented formally before the end of September. With quickening promotion of the work, rural residents' economic burden of major serious diseases will be gradually alleviated.

(3) Attach importance to the several key links of the pilot work

The first is to rationally designate medical institutions for newly-added major diseases. With the overall implementation of the pilot work of medical security for two childhood diseases and the addition of diseases to the pilot, it will be difficult for tertiary hospitals to fulfill the treatment of all the patients with major serious diseases. In order to ensure designated medical hospitals to rationally undertake the task, we shall designate different hospitals for the treatment of different diseases and this is what "classified treatment" means. In principle, end-stage renal disease, two female cancers and some other major diseases shall be treated mainly by county-level medical institutions and promotion of the pilot work of medical security for major serious diseases and comprehensive reform of county-level public hospitals shall be integrated. By deepening the partner medical assistance of urban tertiary hospitals and county-level hospitals, carrying out the system that tertiary hospitals take turns to dispatch doctors to county-level hospitals and county-level hospitals send backbone doctors to tertiary hospitals for further study, strengthening the cultivation of backbone professional staff, improving medical facilities, equipment and conditions, we can improve medical techniques and management capacity and level of county-level medical institutions and difficult and complicated diseases can be diagnosed and treated in county-level hospitals so as to guarantee the smooth implementation of the work that adds more diseases to the pilot. In accordance with the needs and possibilities, the diagnosis and treatment of major serious diseases shall be gradually delegated to county-level hospitals from tertiary hospitals, which is not only an effective way to reduce the medical cost for the treatment of major serious diseases, but also beneficial to the promotion of the construction of disciplines and comprehensive service capacity and the formation of a rational layout of classified diagnosis and treatment.

The second is to intensify cooperation and do well the work of the control on medical expenses. Health administrations, administrative organizations of the new rural cooperative medical care and designated medical institutions must establish sound mechanisms of communication and consultation and on the basis of baseline survey on medical expenses for different diseases, overall consideration of fund-raising level, regional difference and actual performances of designated medical institutions, rationally set expense standards for newly-added diseases; in the light of fixed expense standards, conduct quota payment for specific diseases and keep medical expenditure for the pilot diseases under reasonable control by adopting comprehensive measures such as management of clinical pathways and standardized diagnosis and treatment; fully consider abnormal conditions that may occur in the process of rescue and treatment, jointly consult and work out countermeasures, build up mechanisms for sharing relevant fees such as money paid for identification of responsibility for surgical accidents and quit of clinical pathways so as to avoid doctor-patient disputes and patients' misunderstanding of policies on the new rural cooperative medical care. When the pilot expands to a certain scale, in purchasing and distributing important medicines and medical consumables, we shall stick to the principle that quality shall be put in the first place; both quality and price shall be taken into consideration; centralized tender and unified distribution shall be adopted.

The third is to improve the capacity of administrative organizations of the new rural cooperative medical care. The administrative organizations of the new rural cooperative medical care shall further perfect working systems, optimize working procedures, strengthen service awareness and particularly, improve service capacity and level by means of accelerating informationized construction and improving service methods. Efforts shall be made to link up the work of different parts so as to ensure patients' timely referral, rescue and treatment and immediate reimbursement of their medical expenses. According to the actual conditions, certain amount of working capital shall be allocated to county-level medical institutions that undertake main task of the new rural cooperative medical care and their advance payment shall be timely settled so that they can function well. Meanwhile, we shall fully do well the work of the connection between the new rural cooperative medical system and the medical assistance system, for those patients who are in conformity with the conditions of the medical assistance, strive to realize "one-stop" reimbursement from the new rural cooperative medical system or provide necessary conditions beneficial to convenient reimbursement from the medical assistance system.

IV. Do well the work of the organization and implementation of the pilot work of medical security for major serious diseases

Leading comrades of health departments and bureaus in each province (autonomous region, city) shall be the first persons responsible for the promotion of the pilot work of medical security for rural residents' major serious diseases, meticulously arrange and deploy the pilot work in person, enhance the organization and leadership, actively do well the work of communication and cooperation with departments of civil affairs, finance, linking up of systems and strive to fully play the role of joint security.

Each relevant department of the health system shall have a clear division of responsibilities, make concerted efforts to cooperate actively and do well the pilot work. Rural health departments (departments of the new rural cooperative medical care) shall take the lead in the enhancement of overall planning and coordination for the pilot work, fulfill the design of schemes for the pilot work and perfection of settlement service for the new rural cooperative medical care and strengthen the agreement management of designated hospitals. Departments of medical administration shall formulate and issue clinical pathways suitable for county-level medical institutions in the treatment of pilot diseases and organize regional technical cooperation and assistance. Departments of supervision and management of medical services shall well supervise and manage medical services and effectively integrate the comprehensive reform of public county-level hospitals with the pilot work of medical security for major serious diseases. Departments of planning and finance shall take part in the control on medical expenses earnestly and jointly fulfill the reform in methods of payment. Departments of drug administration shall make efforts to do well the work relevant to the essential drug system.

Promotion of the pilot work of medical security for rural residents' major serious diseases is a critical arrangement for the medical and health reform and also a requirement for the development of the new rural cooperative medical system, which involves numerous links and departments. We have arduous tasks and great responsibilities. I hope that every comrade shall have the spirit of being highly responsible for the Party and people, proceed with confidence, spare no effort, seize opportunities, forge ahead and innovate and do greater contribution to the promotion of the reform of medical and health system, the maintenance of the broad masses' health rights and the construction of a socialist harmonious society.

(Zhao Yinghong)

6. Deepen the Understanding and Vigorously Carry out the Implementation, Promote the Basic Public Health Service into Deep Development

—A Speech Given by Chen Zhu, Minister of Ministry of Health, at Project Implementation Conference of the State's Basic Public Health Service (September 15, 2011)

Today, we hold a project implementation conference of the state's basic public health service and the purpose of it is to summarize the experience and the achievements obtained in project implementation of the state's basic public health service in the past two years, make deep analysis on the problems, perfect policies and measures, promote the implementation of the basic public health service and let the masses enjoy the benefits brought by medical reform. Next, I'll speak out three points of opinions.

I. Have a Clear Picture of the Situation and Fully Understand the Significance of Project Implementation of the State's Basic Public Health Service

(1) Profoundly Understand Severe Challenge Facing China's Public Health

During the period of the "Eleventh Five-year Plan", considerable progress has been made in China's economic and social development, gross national product has jumped to be the second in the world, people's living standards has been constantly improved, public health undertaking has been developing fast, and health status of the urban and rural residents has been further improved. With the sustainable growth of China's population and the accelerating ageing process, problems of public health are increasingly prominent, such as disease patterns change, population mobility, environmental pollution, food safety, occupational health, mental health, and people's lifestyle. China's public health is facing a very serious situation.

Major infectious diseases are still more serious. In 2010, there were 3,180,000 case reports of grave infectious diseases of Class I and Class II, currently there are 4,990,000 new patients of tuberculosis above the age of 15, which ranks right after India and there are 1,300,000 new patients each year; the situation of prevention and treatment of viral hepatitis is still severe; the numbers of the persons with AIDS virus infection and relapse cases are still rising, which means the diffusion starts from high-risk groups to general population; and other newly-discovered infectious disease and imported infectious diseases appear constantly, which poses a serious threat to people's health and social stability. The situation of chronic disease is becoming more severe. Chronic disease has already overtaken infectious diseases and become the main cause of death of the residents in China, accounting for 85% of the causes of death, which has become the main health problems in our country. Currently, the number of the patients with high blood pressure exceeds 200,000,000, the number of the patients with diabetes mellitus is 90,000,000 and the disease burden brought by direct and indirect chronic diseases is shocking. The report on the number of the patients with heavy mental diseases continuously increases. Due to the absence of management, troubles and accidents caused by patients with mental diseases increase year by year, which has become the hidden danger to residents' health. The unfair health care is still outstanding in our country. Average life expectancy, mortality rate of the pregnant and puerperal women, and child mortality reflect that the gap between comprehensive indexes of health condition in east and mid-west areas, between urban and rural areas, between permanent and transient population are still large. Health status of the residents in some poverty-stricken areas, remote and mountainous areas and regions inhabited by ethnic groups is worrisome. Public health emergencies caused by food safety and drinking water pollution happen occasionally. Occupational hazards increase year by year, and mass disturbances happen occasionally. In addition, health literacy of China's residents is low, unhealthy lifestyle is universal, overweight and obesity rates are rising and smoking rate is high. These outstanding health problems pose new challenges and higher requirements in the construction of public health service system and public health system, which should be replied seriously with comprehensive measures and solved gradually.

(2) Project Implementation of the State's Basic Public Health Service is a Long-range Institutional Arrangement of China's Public Health Undertaking.

The core objective of deepening medical health system reform is to provide all the residents with the basic medical health system as a public product. The affordable basic medical service, especially the free basic public health service is the core content of the basic medical health service and the reform achievement is enjoyed directly by residents. Project implementation of the state's basic public health service means prevention first and the core connotation of health policies. Project implementation of the state's basic public health service bases on the improvement in fairness and accessibility of the basic public health service for all the residents, on the solutions to the present main problems of public health, the improvement in health of all the residents, the changes of operating mechanism for medical health institutions at grassroots, and the promotion of the sustainable development in institutions. Abiding by the basic principle of "safeguarding the basic, strengthening the grassroots and establishing the mechanism" is a new system design in the field of public health.

Projects of the basic public health service are determined based on the current problems of public health and health risk factors in China, including specific service objects, contents, and standards, which directly benefits the masses of people, fully reflects the idea of equalization and equally benefits different groups of people in different areas. Service contents cover not only traditional prevention and treatment of infectious diseases, preventive vaccination, health education, health for the pregnant and puerperal women, and children but also the establishment of health archive of residents, elderly care, chronic disease management, management of heavy mental disease and the assistant health supervision. Service objects expands from women and children in the past to key groups of people and the general population, like the aged, sufferers of chronic diseases, and transient population. Project implementation of the state's basic public health service is a public health intervention strategy with the maximum coverage and benefits people in the broadest areas in the 60 years since the founding of PRC. The funds covering projects of the basic public health service are mainly arranged by the government with clear subsidy standards, and constantly increased with social and economic development, which clarifies the financing responsibility of the government for the basic public health service and provides security conditions for project implementation. The projects of the basic public health service are mainly undertaken by medical health institutions at grassroots, like rural township health centers, village clinics and urban community health service centers (stations). Professional public health institutions provide personnel training, technical guidance and so on, which improves the accessibility of public health service to the hilt for residents.

II. Summarize Experiences and Fully Affirm the Progress and Effectiveness of the Projects of the Basic Public Health Service

Since the launching of the basic public health service projects in July, 2009, Ministry of Health, together with the relevant departments, has taken a series of measures to prefect the system, put the funds in place, carefully deployed, and made overall arrangements so that the projects have been extensively promoted in urban and rural areas nationwide and the remarkable progress has been made in just two years.

The first one was to establish a rather prefect system for project organization and management. A series of systems and documents of standards for the state's basic public health service, guiding opinions for performance assessment, managerial methods for project subsidy funds were issued successively at the national level. Project coordination group and expert group were formed, and the working systems for monitoring, supervising and evaluating the progress of the projects were set up preliminarily. Mechanisms for project organization and leadership were universally established by local governments and so were the health administrative departments at all levels. Many prefectures made the project implementation the important indicators for performance appraisal of the governments, and target letters of responsibility were signed level by level, which provided powerful organic safeguards for project implementation. Based on the requirements of the relevant documents by the Central Government, the prefectures, combining with the realities, further refined the schemes for project implementation, clarified the duties of all departments and all institutions, reasonably determined project targets, refined the appraisal indicators and provided all-round institutional guarantee for project promotion.

The second one was to establish long-term fund safeguard mechanism. In recent two years, the governments at all levels have invested more in medical health institutions at grassroots, which basically guaranteed housing construction, facility equipment and personnel, and provided the basic conditions for the project implementation of the basic public health service. Fund subsidy for projects of the basic public health service was budgeted and arranged mainly by the government. From 2009 to 2011, 39,600,000,000 RMB Yuan of subsidy fund was arranged by the Central Finance and more than 30,000,000 RMB Yuan was invested by local financial departments at all levels. Since 2011, the standard for financial subsidies has been increased from 15 RMB Yuan to 25 RMB Yuan, and the fund appropriation system of "appropriation at the beginning of a year and settlement at the end of a year" was established by the Central Government, and the subsidies at different proportions were given to mid-west areas. Since 2010, in order to strengthen the support in poverty-stricken areas in the west, the Central Government has given the subsidies to 243 counties in 6 provinces according to the standards in the west. All prefectures established the project funds safeguard mechanism of "financial budget, undertaking by different levels, appropriation at the beginning of a year and settlement at the end of a year". The project funds safeguard mechanisms of budgeting and financing by the government, undertaking at different levels, advance appropriation of fund, assessment settlement were basically established from the Central Government to prefectures. Subsidy fund standard for the basic public health service per capita nationwide reached 25.6 RMB Yuan, of which 13.7 RMB Yuan per capita was subsidized by the Central Finance. On the basis of the state's regulation, the fund subsidy standards were upgraded in Shanghai, Tianjin, Zhejiang, Beijing, Jiangsu, Qinghai and other regions.

The third one was to explore the effective methods for project implementation. In the project management, some prefectures explored package management and package purchase in accordance with project management and contract management mode while others practiced two-line management of income and expense in health institutions at grassroots, examined the performance of the basic public health and increased score proportion of public health performance.

In the project organization and implementation, many prefectures determined the responsibilities in project implementation and the tasks of the basic public health undertaken by health institutions at all levels, and established cooperation mechanism of labor division for the guidance of special public health institutions and duty implementation of medical health institutions at grassroots. In the project supervision and management, most prefectures constantly strengthened project supervision and performance appraisal, refined project contents and subsidy standards, improved assessment schemes, introduced assessment methods of the third party, improved the fairness and scientificalness and brought the promoting functions of the assessment into full play, basing on the principle of "apanage management and classification assessment".

The fourth one was to standardize the contents of public health service and enrich service modes. Ministry of Health printed and distributed *Standards of the State's Basic Public Health Service*, which clarified the objects, contents, processes, requirements, and indicators for performance appraisal covered in all projects of public health service. All prefectures further refined service contents combining with local realities. The medical health institutions undertaking projects of the basic public health service positively adjusted staff positions and structures, and enriched the contingent of public health service. Some prefectures established the contingent of general practitioners to visit the households, divide up the work and assign a part to each individual and actively carry out service. Other prefectures fully mobilized the community residents to participate in, fostered a large number of family health workers and let more people enjoy the public health service.

The fifth one was to strengthen the public health functions of medical health institutions at grassroots. For quite some time, there has been the ubiquity of "focusing on treatment while ignoring prevention" in medical health institutions at grassroots. Public health work has been relatively weak in both staff allocation and service provision. After the project implementation of the state's public health service, the governments guaranteed the fund investment for it, and the input of human and material resources by medical health institutions at grassroots has been increased remarkably, which turned the passive service into active service, mobilized the enthusiasm of medical health institutions at grassroots to provide the basic public health service, strengthened the functions of prevention and health care at grassroots and enriched service contents of medical health institutions at grassroots.

The sixth one was to promote the reform of operating mechanism in medical health institutions at grassroots. The funds of the public health service were one of the important channels of subsidy in medical health institutions at grassroots. In the project implementation, all the prefectures took a series of incentive and restraint measures, including publicizing assessment result, linking assessment results with capital, employing fixed subsidies and performance subsidies, outsourcing procurement basing on projects or services, and issuing service vouchers. Some prefectures linked performance evaluation results with presidents' (directors') positions and remunerations, qualification of cooperative medical points, the payment of village doctors and practicing qualification. These measures promoted the changes in service concept and service mode in medical health institutions at grassroots and the reforms on employment mechanism, distribution system, and internal management.

Preliminary achievements in the state's basic public health service have been obtained since the implementation two years ago. The sustainable quantity growth of all tasks of the basic public health service has been increased, the quality been constantly improved and people are experiencing more and more benefits. According to medical monitoring, by the end of June, 2011, the filing rate of national health archives had reached 50.2%, the filing rate of standardized electronic health records reached 27.2%, of which 37.6% were urban residents', and 21.8% were rural residents'. The filing rate of electronic health records in more than 20% counties (districts and prefectures) were above 50%. More than 81,000,000 old people above 65 were given health examination, 44,000,000 patients of high blood pressure, 11,000,000 patients of diabetes mellitus and 2,200,000 patients of heavy mental diseases were supervised. The rate of the counties (districts and prefectures) launching health supervision and assistant service in institutions at grassroots by the governments was over 70%.

Social benefits and economic benefits of project implementation of the basic public health service appear gradually. Recently, Community Health Association of China has made three-year tracking survey on health service agencies in 8 municipal districts community of 6 cities, which shows that with the project implementation of public health service, the rate of follow-up visits to the residents with high blood pressure increased from 69.2% to 87.0%, the control rate of fasting blood sugar of the patients with diabetes mellitus increased from 53.2% to 92.8%; the number of the old people undergoing health examination increased nearly ten times, the number of the children included in health management increased 48%, children's morbidity of anemia, rickets and malnutrition declined to varying degrees and medication compliance of the patients with heavy mental diseases improved significantly. According to the research made by state cardiovascular disease center, 21,000,000,000 RMB Yuan per year and per capita for direct medical costs of high blood pressure has been saved with the project implementation.

Since the project implementation of the state's basic public health service two years ago, we've summed up some basic experience. First, to stick to making the improvement in resident health the fundamental the starting point and the foothold of the project implementation. The ultimate goal of the project implementation of the basic public health service is to improve and enhance resident health status. In project implementation, service mode, cooperation mechanism of labor division, the way of fund subsidies, the indicator of performance assessment and the way of training must center around the theme of improving resident health level, which is the important standard for judging the achievements in the project implementation of the basic public health service. Second, to stick to making the fulfillment of the government responsibility the premise condition of the work. The basic public health service is offered freely to all the residents by the government, who must bear responsibility for fund guarantee, establish perfect system of organization and leadership and the system of supervision and management, organize and mobilize all resources of all departments and institutions of all kinds to form the joint effort for the work. Third, to stick to making medical health institutions at grassroots the implementing subject to provide services. At present, the medical health institutions at grassroots in 700,000 cities and countryside have built double net-bottom basic health care and basic public health service. These institutions distributed in vast rural areas and urban streets, which were close to the residents and maximized the fairness and accessibility of the service. Fourth, to stick to "prevention first, and prevention and treatment combined" of project implementation as the basic policy. Disease treatment and prevention are two different aspects and different stages for maintaining resident health and the inseparable organic integrity.

The working policy of "prevention first, and prevention and treatment combined" corresponds to the basic laws of health maintenance, which has been the basic experience of health work for decades since the founding of PRC. All the institutions and all the personnel can be mobilized to participate in public health service with the service mode combined with prevention and treatment: to make "early detection, early diagnosis and early intervention" and improve the efficiency of health service. Fifth, to stick to making service quality the basic part of the work. The service levels in medical health institutions are generally not high, the residents' trust degrees are low so they must constantly improve service conditions, change service modes, strengthen contingent construction, enhance coordination of labor division among special institutions of public health service, public hospitals and the medical health institutions at grassroots, continue to improve service ability and ensure the effectiveness of the project implementation.

III. Guarantee the Implementation and Further Promote the Launch of the Basic Public Health Service Project

The project of the state's basic public health service is a long-term job. Since the implementation two years ago, it has been generally going smoothly for it has a good start. With the deepening of the implementation, some problems appeared gradually in the practice, which should be focused on.

In management, the management systems in some prefectures were not perfect. The project management lacked unified coordination, the responsibility was not clear, work schemes were not meticulous, the operability was bad, and the assessment became a mere formality. All these impacted quality and progress of the work. In the capital, fund supporting failed to reach the designated positions in some prefectures, cycle of fund appropriation was long and there was occupation and misappropriation of fund in some prefectures. The unreasonable spending of project fund was relatively common, which influenced the efficiency in the use of funds. In the task implementation, the service in some prefectures lacked standardization, and there was shortage of service quantity and the fraud practice, which put the service effect into a great discount. In other prefectures, the propaganda and mobilization failed to reach the designated position, which caused low rates of awareness and unobvious experience from the masses. The reasons for the problems were both subjective and objective. The subjective ones were that the relevant people didn't pay enough attention to, and their understanding did not reach the designated while the object ones were that there was the shortage in health workers at grassroots and their qualities were not high. In the early period of the project implementation, we must attach great importance to these problems, timely research the solutions to the problems, otherwise, they would impact the long-term development of the project.

Starting from 2011, the basic public health service has covered more people, enriched service contents, increased the service items, and provided 41 items out of 10 categories of free basic public health service. All prefectures should combine with their own realities, make the key work outstanding, seize the weak link and fully promote the implementation of all service projects. The first one was to further standardize the establishment of health archives, the process of utilization and management, and improve the utilization rate of health archives. According to the objectives of medical reform tasks, the filing rate of standardized health archives should reach 50%, which, from the current progress in all prefectures, meant a great distance from the goal. Therefore, all prefectures should make great efforts to accelerate informatization construction of health archives, speed up the progress and ensure the timely completion of the objectives of medical reform tasks. The second one was to strengthen mainly the management of the patients with high blood pressure and diabetes, screen and troubleshoot the patients by means of measuring blood pressure in the first diagnosis, routine diagnosis and treatment, and health examination for people above 35, and involve more patients into the management, enlarge the coverage, and improve patients' awareness rate, management rate and control rate. The third one was to implement the management of the patients with heave mental diseases. All prefectures should establish contact mechanism between special institutions of mental health and medical health institutions at grassroots, intensify the training and technical guidance for health workers at grassroots, timely involve the patients with heavy mental diseases found by troubleshooting into management, provide the follow-up visit, evaluation and instructions on drug use and rehabilitation and improve the rate of drug use and the rate of stable diseases. The fourth one was to continue to deepen health management for the aged, children, pregnant and puerperal women. These groups of people are the frequent utilizers of medical health institutions at grassroots. Therefore, we should do solid and good work in health examination, constantly enrich service contents, and make an effort to improve the experience degree and acceptance degree of the service objects. The fifth one was to strengthen health education. All people in medical health institutions at grassroots were required to participate in health education and health promotion, popularize and propagandize health knowledge with popular forms and make people set up good and healthy way of life. The sixth one was to do well in preventive vaccination, and the prevention and treatment of infectious diseases. Immunization is the most effective way to prevent infectious diseases, the priority among key work of the basic public health service, which must not have the least bit slack. We should actively carry out the service, and the key emphasis in work should be tilted to remote rural areas and urban transient population. We should make great efforts to deal with miss vaccination and revaccination, improve vaccination rate, and reduce immune blank. The seventh was to organize as soon as possible the implementation of health supervision and assistant service of information report on food safety, occupational health consultation, drinking water safety patrol, school health, establish working system of health supervision and assistant service, reasonably arrange human resources, strengthen the training for service ability and bring the functions of health supervision and sentinel point of medical health institutions at grassroots into full play.

This year is the year of assaulting fortified positions in all tasks of medical reform. Half of the time has passed and the tasks of the basic public health service are very heavy.

Next, in strict accordance with the requirements of *The Circulation on Doing a Good*

Job in 2011 Basic Public Health Service by Ministry of Health and Ministry of Finance, we should focus on the following several aspects of work.

The first one is to strengthen leadership and further improve project management system. All prefectures should enhance the coordination planned as a whole, organization and leadership of the project, establish coordination mechanism for project management of the basic public health service, determine the leading divisions and the offices of the project, intensify the coordination planned as a whole, establish and perfect the management systems for performance evaluation and capital management of the basic public health service project, formulate the implementation plans scientifically, set up reasonable targets of the project and tasks, clarify the quantity, content and subsidy standards of service projects according to the principle of easy to service, easy to assessment, and easy to supervision, mobilize the enthusiasm of medical staff and medical health institutions at grassroots, establish regular report system and reporting system of the project implementation progress and carry out target responsibility system and accountability system.

The second one is to implement supporting funds and strengthen the project funds management. According to the requirements of the relevant policy reform, all prefectures should implement the subsidy policy to medical health institutions at grassroots. And basing on it, all prefectures should coordinate with financial and other related departments to arrange local matching funds of public health in accordance with the requirements, ensure the standard of $25 per person, strengthen the project funds management and supervision, and ensure the reasonable use of the project funds, combining with the newly issued and implemented accounting system and financial management system and by means of meeting the related requirements of project subsidy fund management measures. The subsidies of the basic public health service are used by medical health institutions at grassroots to provide free basic public health service for urban and rural residents in accordance with the provisions. And other units who do not undertake the tasks of public health service are not allowed to retain, misappropriate and embezzle the subsidies. The supervision and inspection on the progress of fund use should be strengthened and the related departments must be supervised and urged to shorten the cycle of fund appropriation, take the methods of fund of "pre-appropriation at beginning of a year , and assessment and settlement" to ensure timely fund appropriation to the grassroots for service implementation.

The third one is to clarify objectives and the main body of responsibility. The main responsibility of the governments at county level should be brought into a good play. The health administrative departments should strengthen the implementation of the project organization, clarify objectives and time schedule, accomplish the tasks with quality and quantity, reasonably determine areas of responsibility, service crowd, and labor division of each medical health institution, divide up the work and assign a part to each individual, fully bring functions of rural doctors in the implementation of the basic public health service into good play, assign rural doctors to assume a certain percentage of the public health service and give the corresponding subsidies.

The fourth one is to strengthen training and improve service ability at grassroots. Scarce capacity of medical health institutions at grassroots is one of the main restricting factors in project implementation, and personnel shortage and undergrade quality coexist. The pressing matter of the moment is to enrich personnel in medical health institutions at grassroots, enhance training, involve the related contents with the basic medical health service into all kinds of current personnel training projects in the local places supported by the Central Government so as to make the personnel at grassroots proficiently master service skills of the basic public health and standardize service implementation. In the long run, the improvement of service capacity asks for further perfection of service network of the basic public health, a breakthrough in personnel cultivation, training, attraction, and the overall improvement in health contingent at grassroots.

The fifth one is to enhance coordination and distribution of responsibilities and feasibly bring special public health institutions into play. All prefectures should explore to establish working mechanisms for cooperation of labor division. Medical health institutions at grassroots are main implementation bodies. The special public health institutions of disease prevention and control, women and children health care, health supervision should play the roles of organizers, managers and coordinators responsible for technical guidance, examination, evaluation, and professional training. Daily assessment results of special institutions are made the important examining contents of the project implementation of the basic public health service. The related personnel in special public health institutions should be given the intensified training so that they will guide the launching of work at grassroots better. All prefectures should coordinate well and put the required funds for special public health institutions into good place, fully mobilize enthusiasm and initiative, and jointly promote the implementation of tasks.

The sixth one is to progress steadily and attach great importance to the obtainment of actual effect. The ultimate goal of the project implementation of the basic public health service is to improve residents' health and the key lies in the service implementation in accordance with standardization. From the monitoring results of medical reform, the service volume of the basic public health is in the continuing growth, and next, service quality should be paid more attention to. For example, both patient number under management should be increased and the controlling rate of the patients with high blood pressure and diabetes mellitus be improved in the management of the patients with high blood pressure and diabetes mellitus. As for health archives, the filing rate should be increased and the utilization rate be emphasized. Medical health institutions at grassroots should launch service according to standardizations and requirements, change service mode, go to households of the residents, provide active service, and truly benefit people. Fraud practice, halfhearted coping with a check and going in for formalism must be strictly prohibited.

The seventh one is to strengthen supervision and launch performance evaluation of the project. In the first half of this year, Ministry of Health required all prefectures to launch the activities of project supervision and inspection on the basic public health service for once. Those who haven't launched supervision and inspection should take action immediately. The key contents of inspection cover project organization and management, system construction, fund management, service quantity and service quality provided and the satisfaction degree of the residents. The problems found in the supervision must be timely rectified. All prefectures should establish and perfect the performance evaluation mechanism in accordance with the requirements of project performance evaluation guidelines of the basic public health service, perfect the ways and methods of examination, and feasibly strengthen the examination on personnel in medical health institutions at grassroots. Assessment results should be linked with fund appropriation and internal income distribution to let the assessment functions of guidance and motivation into full play.

The eighth one is to intensify propaganda and accept social supervision. All prefectures should intensify propaganda of the basic public health service project with the media of broadcast, television, newspapers and periodicals, distribute propaganda materials and short message platform, make urban and rural residents know service contents and policies for free service, summarize and popularize good practices and good experience in the project implementation of the basic public health service, and mobilize the masses to participate actively. Medical health institutions at grassroots should involve service contents of the basic public health into the range of open information and accept supervision from society and residents. The project implementation of the basic public health service relates to the health of thousands of families and it is a piece of groundwork for the establishment of the state's basic medical health system. We must make long-term planning, perfect system, strengthen implementation, do a practically good and effective job and lay a solid foundation for the overall development of all work of medical reform.

(Ji Chenglian)

7. Have a Clear Picture of the Situation, Serve the Overall Interests and Continuously Create a New Situation in Health News Propaganda

—A Speech Given by Chen Zhu, Minister of Ministry of Health, at 2011 National Meeting on Health News (November 15th, 2011)

At the critical moment when people nationwide are earnestly studying and implementing the spirits of the important speech on "July 1st" by General Secretary Hu Jintao and the 6th plenary session of the 17th CPC Central Committee, and all medical workers throw themselves into medical reform, Ministry of Health, for the first time, holds a national conference on health news propaganda, which has a very important significance.

The main task of this conference is: to hold high the great banner of socialism with Chinese characteristics, adhere to Deng Xiaoping's theory and "three represents" as the instructions of important thoughts, thoroughly apply scientific outlook of development, study and implement the spirit of the 17th CPC National Congress, the 5th and the 6th plenary sessions of the 17th CPC Central Committee, conscientiously implement the requirements on health and propaganda work of the Party Central Committee and the State Council, summarize work experience of health news propaganda, be fully aware of the situation, clarify tasks, actively promote scientific development of health news propaganda, and make efforts to provide a powerful support of public opinions and the spiritual power for reform and the development of health undertaking.

Next, I'll speak out three points of opinions.

I. Unify Our Thinking, Build Consensus and Further Enhance Sense of Urgency and Consciousness of Health News Propaganda

Currently, China's national economic and social development has entered the "Twelfth-five Plan" period and the deepening of reform been in the stage of assaulting fortified positions, the new situation and tasks facing the reform and development of health undertaking require us to improve the understanding, unify our thinking and ceaselessly enhance the sense of urgency of news propaganda.

(1) Profoundly understand the important position and role of health news propaganda

Our Party has always attached great importance to news propaganda and Mao Zedong, Deng Xiaoping, Jiang Zemin, Hu Jintao and other CCP leaders made penetrating elaborations on the importance of news propaganda. It is stressed that news propaganda relates to the global work of the Party and the state, to the overall situation of reform, economic and social development and to the ever-lasting political stability. Chairman Mao had stated on many occasions that our Party has two teams: one is military and the other is civil. The military one refers to the barrel of a gun and its task is to destroy enemy's effective power; the civil one means pen holder and the task is to propagandize to the masses and organize the masses. Comrade Deng Xiaoping required that "propaganda and ideological work must be strengthened and mustn't be weakened". Comrade Jiang Zemin pointed out that "public opinion is ideological and political work, which relates to the future and destiny of our Party and our country." Comrade Hu Jintao stressed that "news propaganda relates to the global work of the Party and the state, to the overall situation of reform, economic and social development and to the ever-lasting political stability." The *Decision on Several Major Issues on Deepening Cultural Institution Reform and Promoting Greater Development and Prosperity of Socialist Culture* was examined, discussed and passed at the 6th plenary session of the 17th CPC Central Committee, which has just been held, deeply elaborates the great significance of promoting cultural reform and development under the new situation, illustrates the strategic plans for adhering to the development road of socialist culture with Chinese characteristics and striving to build a cultural power of socialism, puts forward the important policies of "five adherences" in the process of cultural reform and development, stresses the need to adhere to Marxist view of news, grasp the correct direction, improve the timeliness, authority, credibility and influence of public opinions, and indicates the direction in doing a good job in news propaganda.

Health news propaganda is an important part of our Party's propaganda on ideology and culture, an important duty and an important means and guarantee of public opinions for health department to serve people's health and the construction of socialist modernization. To do a good job in health news propaganda and bring the roles of correct orientation of public opinions into play benefits unity, stability and encouragement, the better construction and development of the Party's health position of ideological and cultural propaganda; reflects the Party's idea of people-orientation, power assumption for the people and maintenance of social harmony and stability; it also benefits the promotion of health culture construction, enhancement of health workers' cultural consciousness, sense of responsibility and sense of mission to boost morale, fix intents and gather strength; benefits the improvement in people's identity for health work and for the experience of medical service, the building of harmonious doctor-patient relationship and creation of a good social environment and atmosphere of public opinions for the reform and development of health undertaking. Historical experience tells us that sometimes, some places do not pay attention to health news propaganda, do not take the initiative to release information, do not respond to the questions of the masses, or accept media supervision. On the one hand, it directly affects health work progress and health industry image, on the other hand, the local problems affect the masses' trust in the Party, the government and social stability. Therefore, we must strengthen the sense of urgency and consciousness to do a good job in health news propaganda.

(2) The achievements in health news propaganda were fully confirmed.

Since the reform and opening-up, especially after the great victory of the battle against SARS and the weak conditions of health news propaganda, health system nationwide has worked sturdily, practiced bravely, explored aggressively, pioneered and innovated, accumulated experience ceaselessly, explored and obtained tremendous achievements in health news propaganda. Nowadays, health departments at all levels continuously improve the understanding of news propaganda, continuously strengthen the ability to work, so an increasingly important role of news propaganda in promoting the reform and development of health undertaking appears day by day and the status of the overall health work is constantly upgraded.

The first one is to constantly improve the working system of health news propaganda. In 2003, during the fighting against SARS, directed and supported by the news office of the State Council, Ministry of Health began to explore the construction of news release system and issued in succession the regulations and norms for epidemic information release, typical propaganda, and risk communication. All health administrative departments at provincial level established news release system, determined the fixed spokesmen, and released news regularly or irregularly. Health administrative departments at all levels and medical health units attached great importance to the construction of portal websites, and government information published through the websites increased year by year, which has acted as the main platform of health information release. Medical health units at city level established news release system in Beijing and Shanghai; News evaluation and incentive system were established in Tianjin and Hubei Province; News propaganda was covered in responsibility evaluation system of annual health work targets in Jiangxi Province and Shaanxi Province. These methods and measures effectively promoted the regularization, standardization and institutionalization of health news propaganda.

The second one is the rich and colorful activities of health news propaganda. In recent years, health administrative departments at all levels have actively strengthened the cooperation with media and carried out the rich and colorful news propaganda activities centering around the central work of health. Under the strong support of Propaganda Department of the Central Committee of the CPC and other departments, Ministry of Health planned the propaganda activities of "Pilot Reform in Public Hospitals", "Medical Reform in Progress", "Special Reports on Medical

Reform", and "Medical Reform at Grassroots". Beneficial explorations were made in all places. Anhui Province and Guangxi Zhuang Autonomous Region jointly started medical reform program with local mainstream media, focused on propaganda on benefaction to people from medical reform and dynamic of health work; Leaders from health departments in Jilin Province, Shandong Province and Yunnan Province perennially adhered to the participation in media hotline live activities of supervision on work styles of government officials, which enjoyed good reputation among the masses.

The third one is to gradually establish a risk communication mechanism for public health emergencies. In recent years, health administrative departments at all levels have carried out effective risk communication and actively guided public opinions closely related to health emergencies and the hot issues concerned by the masses. In prevention and control of epidemic situation of human infection with highly pathogenic avian influenza and H1N1 influenza A, medical rescues after Wenchuan and Yushu earthquakes and debris flow disaster in Zhouqu, and the handling of food safety and other public health events, Ministry of Health and health administrative departments in all places timely released information, responded to the public concern, explained questions and puzzles scientifically, and played a positive role in effectively dealing with emergencies. Fujian Province, Jiangxi Province, Henan Province, Hunan Province and other places accumulated experience on event disposal of public opinions. All places paid attention to healthcare communication in risk communication. Health departments and bureaus in Inner Mongolia, Liaoning Province, Heilongjiang Province, Ningxia, Xinjiang, and Xinjiang Production and Construction Corps cooperated with local mass media and started special columns on health knowledge; Zhejiang Province and Gansu Province explored to start official microblog to popularize health knowledge, and made communication and interaction with the public.

The fourth one is to set up good images of health industry through typical propaganda. Health administrative departments at all levels strengthened propaganda on models and introduced typical characters. Ministry of Health rolled out a number of major models: Wu Mengchao, Wang Zhongcheng, Wang Zhenyi, Qiao Shuping, Zheng Ziquan, Wang Zhengyan, Wang Wanqing and so on. In the selection activity of "Double Hundred" organized by the 11 ministries and commissions of Propaganda Department of the Central Committee of the CPC in 2009, 10 persons from health system were selected "Hero Model Character with Outstanding Contributions to the Founding of New China" and "Moving China Character Since the Founding of New China". Simultaneously, health administrative departments at all levels actively supported health publicity in a variety of forms of literature and art. The

TV play: Doctors' Benevolence supported by Health Bureau of Chongqing City and News Propaganda Center of Ministry of Health caused great repercussions in health industry and all sectors of society. Health departments and bureaus in Beijing, Tianjin, Shanghai, Sichuan and Gansu also actively explored to popularize advanced models in forms of film, television, drama and others.

The fifth one is that work mechanism for health news propaganda has taken shape. In 2004, Ministry of Health put news propaganda under centralized management by specialized department of ministerial news office, and in 2008, news propaganda center of Ministry of Health was established. Generally, all health administrative departments at provincial level have set up internal institutions in charge of news propaganda. Health Newspaper Office affiliated to Ministry of Health, People's Medical Publishing House, press and publication units, the responsible newspapers and periodicals brought the role of main position into full play, adhered to the glorious traditions, focused on the overall health situation of reform and development, conducted vigorous propaganda on health policies and measures, promoted academic progress, popularized health knowledge and made important contributions to the building of a good atmosphere of public opinions and social environment for health work. Health departments and bureaus in Beijing, Shanghai, Tianjin, Hebei and Gansu set up independent news propaganda divisions. Health news propaganda centers were established in Beijing, Jilin, Shanxi, Sichuan and Qinghai, and the full-time health news propaganda teams were formed. Health departments and bureaus in Jiangsu and Chongqing actively organized and launched trainings to effectively upgrade news propaganda of health system and risk communication ability.

In the practice and exploration of health news propaganda, we gradually accumulated and summarized some valuable experience, which was summed up in five aspects. The first one is to always adhere to the correct orientation, firmly establish political consciousness, consciousness of general situation, responsibility consciousness, and consciousness of position, constantly enhance political sharpness and political discriminability, adhere to main melody and ensure that health news propaganda always progresses in right direction. The second one is to always adhere to the service for the central work of health and play a positive role in promoting good and rapid development of medical health undertaking. The third one is to always adhere to the people-orientation, serve the people, be close to practice, life and the people, enhance pertinence and effectiveness of health news propaganda, and increase affinity, attraction and influence. The fourth one is to always adhere to the rules for news propaganda and health work, keep pace with times, reform and innovate, and make health news propaganda show characters of epoch, regularity and creation. The fifth one is to always strengthen leadership, clarify responsibilities, perfect system mechanisms and provide strong political guarantee and organizational guarantee for the healthy development of health news propaganda undertaking.

Achievements and progress in health news propaganda don't come easily so the obtained experience is quite precious. It is the result of the support and help from news propaganda departments and joint efforts from health system nationwide. Taking the opportunity, I, on behalf of Ministry of Health, express our heartfelt thanks to the departments in charge of news propaganda, sincere respect for press units and media reporters, and cordial greetings to health news propaganda workers nationwide!

Nevertheless, we must be acutely aware that health news propaganda also has many vulnerable spots and prominent problems, the main displays of which are that some departments and units failed to have the cognition of the importance and urgency of health news propaganda in the designated positions, especially the leaders' understanding didn't reach the designated position. There were loose organization, unsmooth system and mechanism, old ideas, poor consciousness of news propaganda and the inadaptable working methods for today's acquisition model of social information, channel of appeal reflection and the changes of news dissemination concepts. The existing problems didn't adapt to the changes of today's world situation, national conditions and conditions of the people, or coordinate with the need of the reform and development of health undertaking. And there was a great gap between the needs of the masses for health news dissemination and health knowledge popularization.

(3) Accurately grasp new situation and new requirements of news propaganda

The "Twelfth-five Year" is the important period in which a well-off society will be built in an all-around way, the key period when the development of health undertaking accelerates and the crucial period when reform is deepened. The new situation on health news propaganda puts forward new requirements, assigns new tasks and provides a broad space for fully developing our skills.

The first one is that economic and social development promotes health reform and development, which requires health news propaganda to actively guide public opinions. With economic and social development, scientific and technological progress and comprehensive strength enhancement nationwide, scientific development of health undertaking has more solid material foundation and condition security. In the *Twelfth-five Year Program Planning for National Economic and Social Development*, life expectancy per capita is, for the first time, subordinated to the main indicators of economic and social development. Party committees and governments at all levels gave unprecedented policy support and financial investment for medical reform and health work, and health work got social and public attention, which reflected the deployments of strategic decisions for the adherence of the Party and the government to scientific development, greater attention to protecting the livelihood of the people and the placement of health undertaking in a more prominent position. The important foundations of news consensus playing the guiding functions, and all health policies and measures being promoted into effect are sure to strengthen and improve news propaganda, speak thoroughly the background and basis for health policy making by the Party and government, explain clearly the aims and tasks, measures and methods, development and achievements, elaborate the interests and benefits of the masses of the people, and mobilize the masses to actively support and participate in health work.

The second one is to strengthen and innovate new responsibilities of health system given by social management. To strengthen and innovate social management is an important strategic task determined by the Party Central Committee from the overall situation of business development of the Party and nation by correctly grasping new changes and new features of domestic and international situations. Currently, in health field, there are still many contradictions and problems between the ability of medical service and people's growing health needs, development of medical security system and people's economic tolerance, the limited development of medical technology and infiniteness of patients' expectations, imperfect medical dispute resolution mechanism and people's appealing needs. These contradictions and problems will not self eliminate in the short term. If let them accumulate for a long time, they will intensify social contradictions and affect social harmony. Therefore, the effective channels to alleviate contradictions and strengthen social management are to strengthen and improve health news propaganda, interpret policies, respond to hot issues, listen attentively to the voice of the people, gather people's intelligence and bridge communications and understanding between health system and the society.

The third one is that the deepening of medical reform in crucial period requires health news propaganda to provide support of public opinions. Currently, with further promotion of medical reform, some deep system mechanism issues and more difficult problems come into play, and the deepening of medical reform is in crucial moment of assaulting fortified positions and overcoming difficult problems. All medical health workers urgently need a strong public opinion support and the spiritual impetus in order to further build consensus, boost confidence and throw themselves into medial reform. Simultaneously, the multi-level and diverse characteristics are present in people's demand for medical health, which puts forward higher request for medical health resource distribution, service mode transformation and medical security system. Some people expect too highly and hastily of medical reform, which needs correct guidance practically and realistically. To strengthen and improve health news propaganda is a powerful means to inspire health workers to take an active part in medical reform, serve people's health, and promote medical reform to follow the rules and develop scientifically.

The fourth one is that people have unprecedented attention to health and demand for the enhancement of health knowledge dissemination. With fast economic and social development and the ceaseless rise of living standard, good health has been the most important and urgent demand of the masses of people. And the masses' demands for the right to know, participation rights and expression rights for health work are more outstanding. The development of industrialization, informatization and urbanization, the fast changes of production method and life style, the frequent environmental pollutions and natural disasters, the still serious infectious diseases, the growing threat of chronic non-communicable diseases, the public health emergencies, the repeated events of food and drug safety as well as occupational disease hazard events have brought serious challenges to the health of the people. Research shows that public health literacy in our country is only 6. 48%, which is not consistent with the development, image and position of our country, and must be vigorously improved. The effective way to improve health literacy of the masses is to strengthen and improve health news propaganda, launch risk communication, popularize health knowledge and advocate healthy behaviors.

The fifth is that the profound changes of media communication modes and concepts require that health news propaganda must rapidly occupy the position of public opinions. Along with the rapid development of digital technology and network technology, Internet, mobile phone short message, microblog and the emerging media have become the important channels for people to get their news information and realize social communication. The application of 3G mobile phone makes it possible for everyone to be on the Internet anytime and everywhere and public opinions tend to be diversified. At the moment, the number of Internet users in China has reached 500 million and more than 50% of Internet users communicate, exchange and share information through social network. In some recent emergencies, emerging media has played an important role in releasing information, forming a focus and guiding public opinions. An inevitable requirement of improving the ability of public opinion guide under the new situation is to strengthen and improve health news propaganda and capture position of health opinions.

II. Scientifically Plan and Promote the Scientific Development of Health News Propaganda on the Overall Situation

To strengthen and improve health news propaganda is both an urgent and a long-term task. The current important work should be promoted urgently and the future strategic goal be made. Therefore, *Opinions on Comprehensive Strengthening and Improving Health News Propaganda (draft for comment)* was drafted by Ministry of Health, which was given to everyone as the material of the conference to be fully discussed by all places and units and be issued officially by Ministry of Health after collecting and absorbing advice from all sides. In the period of the "Twelfth-five Plan", health news propaganda should serve global situation, capture time theme, grasp correct orientation of public opinions, adhere to unity, stability and encouragement, build bridge for health system to contact with the masses and serve people, and provide intellectual impetus for all medical workers to throw themselves into medical reform and support of public opinions for the reform and development of health undertaking.

(1) To strengthen the overall positive guidance and typical propaganda and set up a good image of health industry

Since ancient times, medical practicing has been a respectable profession. In the new era, whether in daily work or in the rescue of disasters and accidents, all medical workers heal the wounded and rescue the dying, and make outstanding contributions in maintaining people's health and life safety. And a large number of outstanding figures have emerged. However, the particularity of the service in medical health institutions often becomes outbreak focus of social contradictions, and sometimes even arises in extreme forms. At the present critical moment of assaulting fortified positions and overcoming difficult problems in medical reform, propaganda on models in health industry is especially needed to be strengthened to promote healthy atmosphere, fight against injustice and maintain the image of the Party and the government. Propaganda on models plays the role in internal education and encourages all medical workers to throw themselves into medical reform, and sets up good image of the industry to the external to win the understanding and support of all sectors of the society and the masses of the people for health work. Propaganda on models should be combined with the activities of striving for the first and creating excellence in performances, "Three Goods and One Satisfaction", health cultural construction, and education of medical ethics and style so as to guide the Party members, cadres and all health workers to strengthen professional sense of honor, carry forward noble medical ethics, continuously improve the quality of medical treatment, take the measures of convenience and benefaction to people and make efforts to ameliorate people's experience in seeking medical care. All places and all units should actively win over the guidance and support of news propaganda departments, cooperate and work closely and jointly with the departments of news propaganda, personnel, Party committees, and departments checking unhealthy tendencies and malpractices. A number of advanced models are discovered, selected and established every year by means of news propaganda, grassroots recommendation, people's election, and organization selection. The study and propaganda are launched in the ways of report tour, media coverage, literary and artistic works so as to actively set up good images of health industry and medical workers.

(2) Further carry out the propaganda and report of the deepening of medical reform in a deep-going way and create a good atmosphere for health reform and development

The deepening of medical reform is a major policy decision by adhering to the people-orientation, scientific development by the Party Central Committee and the State Council, and powerful measure focusing on guaranteeing and improving the livelihood of the people. In the last two years, outstanding progress and positive results of the various reform tasks have been made. The propaganda on the deepening of medical reform must be well organized and developed to thoroughly popularize great measures made by the Party Central Committee and the State Council for the improvement in the livelihood of the people and the promotion of the coordinated development of the economy and the society. The progress and results of medical reform, the healthy and material benefits should be thoroughly popularized. The aggressive exploration and the accumulated valuable experience in medical practice of all places should be thoroughly propagandized. The selfless dedication to medical reform made by all medical workers and the advanced models by healing the wounded and rescuing the dying, and maintaining people's health should be thoroughly popularized. National health conditions, the chronicity, difficulty and complexity of medical reform, and rational expectations of medical reform from the society and the masses of the people should be given the in-depth propaganda. Propaganda can embody social consensus, boost confidence in reform and create a good atmosphere and social environment for the completion of the five key medical tasks and the implementation of the "Twelfth-five Year" plan. Attention should be paid to external health propaganda in order to objectively and comprehensively introduce great achievements in medical health undertaking in China, counterattack false reports by some western media and safeguard China's image in international public health field. At the moment of the completion of key tasks in the three-year in-depth medical reform, Ministry of Health and other departments jointly compiled the reports on the reform and development of health undertaking in China. This year,

Propaganda Department of the Central Committee of the CPC and other departments launched the activity of "Going to Grassroots Units, Changing Work Style, and Style of Writing". All health reporters went to the first line of medical reform investigating and interviewing, which formed a high tide in propaganda report on medical reform. The various localities should actively cooperate with the central media and coordinate with local media, further do a good job in health reports on the activity of "Going to Grassroots Units, Changing Work Style, and Style of Writing" and improve medical propaganda appeal and influence.

(3) Vigorously develop health news release and take the initiative of news transmission in hands

News release is the important content of news propaganda. Doing a good job in health news release can timely popularize health policies, laws and regulations, win over people's understanding and the support of all health workers, which is an effective method of guiding public opinions positively, and constructing sunshine government and service-oriented government. We should cooperate for the issue of major health policies and measures, organize and hold press conference and media communication conference to notify relevant situation, answer questions, and strive for information release at regular time and in regular places. We should also actively set agenda, plan publicity activities and improve dominance and effectiveness of information distribution, combining with major news and important activities in health industry and the hot issues commonly concerned by the people. We should innovate information release forms and improve pertinency and accessibility of information distribution, basing on different characteristics of contents and objects of information release. Attention should be paid to policy understanding in propaganda, the train of thought with profundity and in an easy-to-understand approach, and in popular and easy-to-understand language. Official website of health administrative departments and institutions should be perfected with health informatization construction so as to keep the authoritativeness and seriousness, strengthen the readability and interactivity and make the official website the important platform for information release at the same time. Communication with news media must be strengthened to actively introduce health work, positively cooperate with media to carry out publicity reports and provide convenience for interviews and researches.

(4) Attach great importance to emergency risk communication and improve the guiding ability of public opinions

With occasional emergencies in health field in recent years, timely and vigorous risk communication has benefited the proper resolution of crises and stabilized social emotion. The hot issues of public opinions must be timely found out, trend of public opinions be mastered, and analysis, research and judgment carried out by means of monitoring media reports, Internet information and 12320 public health hotline. In health emergencies involving in the respective jurisdictions and institutions, the mechanism of public health emergencies, local health administrative departments under unified leadership of the local Party committees and the governments, in line with timely, accurate, open and transparent principle, released information first, expressing the attitude of health department to the event, relevant policies and knowledge, the learned situation, the work to be done, and the plans for the next step, and timely released the related information along with the progress of the event disposal. Attention must be paid to emergencies and medical rescue, moving deeds of medical health workers be explored, publicity and reports on advanced figures strengthened and the influence of health news propaganda expanded. The supervision of public opinions must be treated correctly, the situation of public opinions involving in respective jurisdictions and institutions be timely investigated and verified, the investigation information and the future improvement of the solid case must be released in time, the false case be clarified in time and the problem must be limited or solved within their jurisdictions so as to make the influence of negative public opinions reduce to minimum. The emerging field of media and public opinions must be attached great importance to, the understanding and communication on social conditions and public opinions be learned through new media so as to answer questions and explain puzzles and properly channel public sentiments. The voice and comments of health system must be well organized in order to constantly improve risk communication and guiding ability of public opinions, and try hard to form the online positive strength of public opinions.

(5) Promote the deepening of information publicity in health industry and provide better public services for the masses

The openness of government affairs is the important content of news propaganda while news propaganda is the effective method to strongly promote the openness of government affairs. The principle of "Publicity is a rule and privacy is an exception" must be followed in order to do a good job in the openness of public health affairs. The government information which is not involved in state secrets, commercial secrets, personal privacy and effect on social stability, should be actively and timely opened to the public and the information basing on application for openness should be actively and prudently handled. The openness of administrative affairs in centers for disease control, health supervision departments, blood stations and other units of medical health service must be promoted according to *Management Method of Information Publicity in Units of Medical Health Service* and with the promotion of effective openness of hospital affairs. Ministry of Health will promptly improve the related policies and systems, express requirements to strengthen the publicity of administrative affairs of national health system and the construction of 12320 hotline for public welfare of health, further promote the openness of health affairs and deepen health service of administrative affairs.

(6) Continuously carry out dissemination of health knowledge and effectively enhance health literacy of the public

Health news propaganda is inseparable with health education. The popularity of health knowledge lies in the organic combination of health education involved in news propaganda and news release with necessary health knowledge. Publicity and popularization of health knowledge must be enhanced, healthy and civilized way of life be advocated, public health literacy upgraded, public discrimination ability of health information intensified, and people's health level improved. The spread of the knowledge related to health must be done with the issuing of major policies, the publicity of key work, "bringing cultural, scientific and medical services to rural areas", daily health activities and the handlings of emergencies. The spread form of health knowledge must be innovated, a batch of expert team of popularization of health science be trained according to plans, all medical health workers be encouraged to open blog and microblog to popularize health knowledge, introduce medical risks scientifically, guide the people to seek medical care rationally, and improve the ability and level of prevention and healthcare of the people.

Ⅲ. Strengthen the Leadership, Promote Comprehensively and Make Efforts to Create a New Situation in Health News Propaganda

Health news propaganda is global and strategic work with strong relation to policy and high sensitiveness, involving wide field and multiple levels so that powerful measures must be taken to realize the overall advancement in health news propaganda.

(1) Strengthen the organization and leadership

Administrative departments at all levels and in medical health institutions must maintain a high level of political sensitivity, fully understand the importance and difficulty of health news propaganda, enhance sense of responsibility, sense of mission and sense of urgency, place health news propaganda in an important position of global work and feasibly strengthen organization and leadership. The mainly responsible comrades from all localities and all units are the first responsible persons for news propaganda, who take the overall responsibility for news propaganda in their own localities and units, and the comrades in respective charge should take the concrete responsibility and handle the work personally. Health news propaganda must be placed on important agenda with special study, planned, deployed and implemented together with other health work. The work target responsibility system for news propaganda must be built as an important content of supervision and assessment on health work, which is in way of layer-to-layer implementation to ensure the actual effects. The working systems of top leaders taking the overall responsibility for news propaganda, departments of news propaganda taking the lead and responsibility, all departments making joint efforts to administrate, the relevant units offering effective support must be built to make health news propaganda a sustainable project of top leaders and all the personnel.

(2) Strengthen organizational construction

Health administrative departments at provincial level and in the rather large medical health institutions must continuously perfect the system of news spokesman, win over the support from the department of staffing management, and establish working body specially centralized into the administration of health news propaganda. The establishment of news release system must be vigorously promoted in administrative departments of public health at prefecture level, and medical institutions, institutions for disease prevention and control, health education institutions, health supervision agencies and blood centers (blood stations) at prefecture level or above so as to explore the establishment of news release system in health administrative departments and medical health agencies at or above the county, and make the leaders who are politically strong, professionally proficient, correct in style and familiar with comprehensive work the news spokesmen. By the end of 2012, news release system above prefecture level had been established and perfected, by the end of 2013, news release system covering health administrative departments and institutions at or above county level will have been initially set up, and by the end of 2015, news release system will be more perfect.

(3) Strengthen contingent construction

Contingent construction of health news propaganda must be strengthened and trained in order to adjust the cadres with good political thought, outstanding comprehensive quality, strong ability of writing, oral communication and solid style into news propaganda team. Cadres of health news propaganda must be cared, the mechanism for training, selection, evaluation and motivation be set up to inspire all people to always stay in positive and active state and high morale and contribute their intelligence and wisdom to health news propaganda. The concept of participation in publicity by all people in the whole system must be formed, and the forces inside and outside the industry be fully coordinated to build a health news propaganda team with health system as the core, supported and cooperated by the relevant departments and all sectors of society. Health news propaganda cadres should be designedly chosen to participate in business training to continuously improve their professional skills and working ability. Ministry of Health planned to train news spokesmen team at provincial level in the next two years and all provinces should pay close attention to the training for news spokesmen from health administrative departments and medical health institutions at levels of city and county.

(4) Make more investment

News publicity needs large manpower, financial and material resources as a basic guarantee. Therefore, all localities and all departments, according to the requirements of health news propaganda, must positively win financial support, and enroll expenditures for health news propaganda into budget to ensure normal business work. Social capital investment in health news propaganda must be actively encouraged and the enthusiasm of every respect be fully mobilized. Simultaneously, fund supervision must be well done to improve the utilization efficiency.

Health news propaganda is a significant, hopeful, arduous and challenging job. We must study and carry out earnestly the 6th plenary session of the 17th CPC Central Committee, and comprehensively strengthen and improve our work with more profound understanding, more open thinking, perfect mechanism, more forceful measures so as to comprehensively strengthen and improve our work, incessantly create a new situation in health news propaganda, provide health reform and development with the support of public opinions and the spiritual power, and make new greater contributions to the safeguard of people's health!

(Ji Chenglian)

8. To Speed up the High-Quality Medical and Health Personnel Training with an Emphasis on the Cultivation of General Practitioners in order to Provide a Powerful Guarantee for the Improvement of National Health Level

—A Speech Delivered by Health Minister Chen Zhu at the National Medical Education Reform Work Conference (December 6, 2011)

Distinguished Vice-chairman Han Qide, Minister RMB Yuan Guiren and comrades,

The national medical education reform work conference that was held jointly by the Ministry of Education and the Ministry of Health in 2008 has played a positive role in promoting the reform and development of medical education of our country. Currently, our country is entering the development period of the Twelfth Five-Year Plan. Therefore, the strategic position of science, technology and education is further being highlighted; scientific and technological advances and innovation is becoming a crucial prop to speed up the transformation of the pattern of economic development; improving the quality and capacity of our workers is providing a major guarantee for the transformation of the economic growth pattern.

Our country has intensified the strategic layout of reinvigorating China through science and education and strengthening the nation through human resource development and have successively formulated and implemented the National Medium-and Long-Term Plan for Scientific and Technological Development, the National Medium-and Long-Term Plan for Education Reform and Development and the National Medium-and Long-Term Plan for Human Resource Development; Reform of the pharmaceutical and healthcare systems and reform of education are being further deepened. Today, the Ministry of Education and the Ministry of Health is holding the national medical education reform work conference again to implement the spirit of the important speech delivered by General Secretary Hu Jintao at Tsinghua University's Centennial, to implement the national education plan and talent development plan and Opinions of the CPC Central Committee and the State Council on Deepening the Reform of the Medical and Health Care System, to implement Guidance of the State Council on the Establishment of a General Practitioner System, to promote close integration of reform of medical education and reform of the pharmaceutical and healthcare systems, and this is of great significance. State Councilor Liu Yandong has made special and important instructions on this conference, further clarifying the theme of this conference and pointing out the direction of reform and development of medical education; Vice-chairman of the Standing Committee of the National People's Congress Han Qide has squeezed time out from a busy schedule to attend the meeting in person and will deliver an important speech, of which we must earnestly study and implement the spirit. Just now, Comrade Guiren has delivered three important opinions on behalf of the Ministry of Education. Comrades, please study and implement them earnestly. Next, I will talk about three opinions on behalf of the Ministry of Health for your reference.

I. Unifying thinking and fully understanding the importance and urgency of vigorously promoting the comprehensive reform of medical education and speeding up the training of high-quality medical and health personnel.

The medical and health care cause constitutes an important of national economic and social development, which is closely related to the health and well-being of the broad masses of people all over the country. Talents are the first resource of medical and health care cause and medical education is the major guarantee for the construction of health personnel. Exploring the development road of medical education with Chinese characteristics and raising the overall quality of the training of medical and health talents are our sacred historical missions and one of the central tasks of the reform and development of education and health cause.

First, the objective requirement of deepening the reform of the pharmaceutical and healthcare system is to promote the reform of medical education and to speed up the training of high-quality medical and health personnel.

In 2009, the Party Central Committee and the State Council issued Opinions on Deepening the Reform of the Medical and Health Care System; thereafter, our country's medical and health care cause has entered a crucial stage of reform and development. Deepening the Reform of the Medical and Health Care System is a major practical action of deeply implementing the Scientific Development View, a major livelihoods project to guarantee health of the entire people, and a major development project to coordinate and promote the economic and social construction and expand domestic demand. Since 2009, under the strong leadership of the Party Central Committee and the State Council and through joint efforts of all regions and departments and all sectors of society, the reform of the pharmaceutical and healthcare system has achieved initial success. First, the coverage of the basic health insurance system has been dramatically widened. The population covered by basic health insurance has reached about 95% of the total. Second, the grass-roots health service delivery system has been significantly strengthened. More than 2000 county-level hospitals and more than 30,000 grass-roots health care institutions have been transformed and reconstructed. The plan for construction of grass-roots medical staff with an emphasis on general practitioners has been launched and implemented. Third, equalization of basic public health services has made new progress. National basic public health service programs and major public health service programs have been carried out across the country. Fourth, the Essential Drug System and public hospital pilot reform have been advanced in an orderly way. The Essential Drug System has been implemented in all government-run grass-roots health institutions. Fifth, the financial assistance in medical and health care cause has been increasingly intensified. The proportion of personal health care expenditures in total health expenditure has been continuously declining. Residents' medical expenses burden has been lightened to some extent.

As the reform of the pharmaceutical and healthcare system deepens, some structural problems have become increasingly prominent. Among these, the time-lag problem of the construction of pharmaceutical and healthcare staff is particularly striking, which has become a major restraining factor in deepening the medical reform. Currently, there are four prominent problems in our country's construction of medical staff. The first one is insufficiency of talents. Compared with Europe, America and other developed countries, the gap of licensed doctors and registered nurses per 1,000 people remains relatively large, China being close only to middle-income countries. The second is the quality and competence needs to be improved. In 2010, among the rural health technical personnel, only 14.3% have a bachelor's degree or above and only 3.9% have senior professional and technical titles. In many health clinics in towns and townships, there is a severe shortage of personnel who are competent in medical and health services and many normal routines couldn't be carried out and the configuration of some medical equipment couldn't give full play to efficiency. The third is the structure and distribution is still unreasonable and the gap of personnel distribution between urban and rural areas and regions is obvious. The fourth is the policy environment of medical education and talent training needs to be further improved; in particular, the safeguard measures of attracting and stabilizing grassroots health personnel urgently need to be strengthened. We should carefully study the above-mentioned issues and search for effective measures, paths and methods to crack the tough problems of medical reform.

Second, promoting the reform of medical education and speeding up the training of high-quality medical and health personnel is the main task for the implementation of national medium-and long-term plans for education and talent development.

Since the foundation of New China, our country has established a relatively complete system of medical education and trained large quantities of high-quality medical and health talents. Ever since the reform and opening up, our country's medical education cause has been further developed. Along with the economic and social development, the masses of people have had increasingly higher expectations and demands for medical and health services, however, high-quality medical and health talents are the important guarantee for living up to their expectations and meeting their demands. How to build a medical education system that consists of college education, after-graduation education and continuous education with Chinese characteristics and to innovate talents training mode proceeding from our national conditions and being closely adapted to demands and respecting for laws and application-oriented and drawing on international helpful experiences is a major task for the implementation of national medium-and long-term plans for education and talent development.

National medium-and long-term plans for education and talent development has made strategic arrangements for education, giving priority to the development of talents, and deepening reform. National medium-and long-term plans for education development has established the development goals for lifelong education system. In 2005, the Ministry of Education and the Ministry of Health have established an inter-ministerial coordination mechanism for the macro management of medical education, and have conducted regular communication and consultation over major issues including the reform and development of medical education and supporting health care reform and development, and have achieved remarkable results through mutual support and cooperation. Some provinces and cities have established coordination mechanisms between the education and health departments or bureaus in succession, which have produced positive effects. Since the start-up and implementation of medical reform, these two ministries have been cooperating even more closely. In October last year, the Ministry of education and the Ministry of Health jointly issued Opinions on Jointly Building University Medical Schools (Departments and Centers) that are Subordinated to Ministries, and decided to jointly build a first batch of 10 university medical schools subordinated to ministries, and issued 10 items of detailed measures in 5 aspects which have achieved initial success. Some departments will report the progress in the afternoon, which would provide beneficial experience for further strengthening the work of joint building. The two ministries will also carry a pilot project of jointly building local medical colleges with provincial governments and strengthen the national overall planning of medical education. Now, the Ministry of Education and the Ministry of Health decide to jointly implement the comprehensive reform program of clinical medical education and the training program of outstanding doctors, to standardize professional medical education, and to promote the reform and development of college medical education, to train excellent medical graduates, and to establish the general practitioner system and the standardized training system for resident doctors which specify the standardized path for the training of qualified doctors. The concerted efforts of the Ministry of Education and the Ministry of Health have embodied not only the close integration of the reform and development of medical education and health undertaking but also the overall consideration of the construction of an integrated system of college education, after-graduation education and continuous education. The National Medium-and Long-Term Plan for Human Resource Development lists the national health talent security project as one of 12 major talent projects and lists professional talents of clinical medicine, public health, nursing and pharmacy, etc. in the category of talents urgently needed in the key fields of social development and also put forward the detailed development goals. The above-mentioned strategic arrangement have highlighted the importance and urgency of training high-quality pharmaceutical and healthcare talents and have also pointed out a clear direction to struggle for the reform and development of medical education. The relevant work arrangements of the Ministry of Education and the Ministry of Health have reflected the organic link between educational reform and medical reform.

Third, establishing the general practitioner system is an important measure to promote the medical education and speed up the training of high-quality medical and health talents.

Last year, the world-famous medical journal The Lancet published an article titled *Health Professionals for a New Century: Transforming Education to Strengthening Health Systems in an Interdependent World* that was co-authored by 20 internationally famous medical educationists. The article summarizes the experience in medical education over the past century and envisions the revolution of medical education in the next century. A hundred years ago, the Flexner Report in America promoted the integration of science into the medical system, thus boosting the development of modern medicine. Currently, a new revolution is brewing in medical science, with the leading change in the community-based health promotion. The establishment and implementation of the general practitioner training system has become the core of this new revolution. General practitioners are a type of important inter-disciplinary medical talents, offering integration services mainly at the primary care level such as preventive health services, common and frequently-occurring disease treatment, referral, patient rehabilitation, chronic disease management and health management, known as the "gatekeeper" of residents' health. This training goal requires the organic integration of quality and ability in many aspects including occupation ethics, humanistic accomplishment, discipline integration and practice ability. Domestic and foreign medical practice reveals that whether large quantities of qualified general practitioners can be trained, whether grass-roots health care teams can be established, whether grass-roots health care services that put prevention first and is characterized by the integration of prevention and treatment can be provided, and whether the medical and health service system of first diagnosis at grass-roots level, two-way referral and top-down coordination can be formed will have a close bearing on the effective prevention and control of major diseases, the rise of level of people's health and the reasonable control of medical expenses and will truly embody the public welfare of health undertakings with Chinese characteristics. Currently, qualified general practitioners in our country are in severe short supply. There are only more than 80,000 medical practitioners who are registered in general medical section accounting for 4.3% of the total number of medical practitioners. In the countries and regions that attach importance to grass-roots health care, general practitioners generally account for more than one third or even half of the total number of doctors.

In July this year, the State Council issued Guidance on the Establishment of a General Practitioner System (hereinafter referred to as Guidance) offering an all-round top-layer design of the general practitioner system with Chinese characteristics. It requires the basic realization of 2-3 qualified general practitioners in both urban and rural areas per 10,000 inhabitants by 2020 and adaptation to the basic medical and health service demand of the masses. We should be fully aware of the significance of the establishment of general practitioner system and make vigorously training qualified general practitioners a major task for our country's medical education and construction of the team of health talents at present and for a very long time to come. In all regions and all relevant departments, the effective implementation of this task should be given great importance and resource guarantee including insufficient financial and material resources and policies should be provided.

II. Highlighting priorities and actively promoting the training of grass-roots health talents with an emphasis on general practitioners

Reforming medical education and speeding up the training of high-quality pharmaceutical and healthcare talents should put emphasis on the implementation of Guidance and the speeding up of the training of high-quality general practitioners. Therefore, attention should be paid to the work of the following aspects.

Firstly, having a comprehensive grasp of the design process of general practitioner training system

The Guidance has offered an all-round top-layer design of the general practitioner training model with Chinese characteristics and established the general practitioner train system of "one model, two paths, three unifications, four channels". "One model" is a model that will gradually standardize training general practitioners in "5+3" mode, that is, the first 5 years of clinical undergraduate education, plus 3 years of standardized general practitioner training. "Two paths" refer to the gradual transition of the two paths of standardized training after graduation and postgraduate education of master's degree program in clinical medicine to the unified path of standardized training after graduation. "Three unifications" are to unify the method and content of general practitioner standardized training, to unify practice access conditions of general practitioners, and to unify the criteria for conferment of degrees in general medicine. "Four channels" refer to 4 main approaches to train general practitioners in the transitional period — first, vigorously implementing the job-transfer training of grass-roots on-the-job doctors; second, intensifying skills training directed at general practitioners; third, raising educational levels of grass-roots on-the-job doctors; fourth, encouraging hospital doctors to work at the grass-roots level.

Secondly, deeply understanding the significance of the "5+3" model of general practitioner training

The practice indicates that standardized training after graduation is the indispensable way to a qualified general practitioner, which makes a general practitioner become a real "gatekeeper" of all residents' health; more than 80% of residents' health problems can be effectively dealt with in communities.

The medical education in China is multi-leveled, in which different lengths of schooling coexist and the construction of after-graduation medical education and continuous medical education system still need to be improved. Undergraduate medical students are lacking in systematic and standardized training process of clinical abilities and will directly engage in the clinical work of diagnosis and treatment after graduation. Thus, clinicians, particularly those in grass-roots health care institutions, often fail to deliver high service level and competence and fail to obtain a universal trust among residents. Quite a few health problems of minor ailments that should have been solved at grass-roots level are treated as big diseases, thus leading to rapid increase of medical expenses and excessive expansion of the size of large hospitals.

To establish the "5+3" model of general practitioner standardized training is a major reform of our country's practitioner training system. It can constantly dispatch high-quality clinical talents to grass-roots health institutions, provide people with comprehensive and convenient basic medical care and health services, promote the rational division of labor and cooperation between grass-roots health institutions and city hospitals, and ease people's concerns about "health care being too difficult and expensive".

Thirdly, looking forward to the future, establishing and improving the general practitioner standardized training system

In order to speed up the establishment of unified and standardized general practitioner training system, relevant departments of the State Council have currently been studying and formulating without any delay the supporting policies and measures including the standards of general practitioner standardized training, base standards, base identification, management measures and measures for conferment of master's degree in general clinical medicine under the guidance of the general framework of the Guidance. Different regions should pay attention to the following aspects in promoting this task:

First, emphasis should be put on overall planning. Based on conscientious investigations and studies, the demand and competence of general practitioner training of the local area should be analyzed conscientiously and feasible phase-by-phase training plans should be formulated. The year 2012 will be the first year of the formal implementation of standardized general practitioner training system. Hopefully, different regions would concentrate efforts, make plans without any delay, and elaborate the deployment, for getting off to a good start.

Second, emphasis should be put on policy guarantee. General practitioner training is a systematic project, which involves many fields including educational training, personnel management and financial input. Health and educational administrative departments at all levels should take the initiative to coordinate relevant aspects, fulfill the disbursement of relevant training grants and treatment guarantee of practitioners in training, and set about to establish a vigorous general practitioner management system and employee incentive mechanism creating conditions for general practitioners to keep their mind on grass-roots level health services. The practice of some regions indicates that an appropriate solution to problems of training work, employee incentive mechanism and treatment in training through overall planning is the major guarantee and key factor for the smooth implementation of standardized training.

Third, emphasis should be put on capacity building. To train qualified general practitioners, setting up the service concept for general practice is the basis and mastering the standardized and solid capacity for clinical medicine and public health is the core of the task. To strengthen the capacity building of general practitioner training, the following two points should be paid attention to in particular. The first is to launch without any delay the selection and construction of general practitioner training base. The medical institutions that conform to requirements and that are rich in teaching experience and earnest in general practitioner training should be given priority to be integrated into the category of training base construction; high-quality educational resources within education system should be fully absorbed and made good use of, especially the affiliated hospitals and teaching hospitals of medical colleges; input should be increased constantly with the support of construction project of general practitioner training base issued by the country; the infrastructure and skills training center that are indispensable to the training should be improved; formation of the base network that adapts to the needs and requirements should be speeded up and training capacity should be expanded. The second is to strengthen the building of general practice teaching staff. The training of general practice concept and the clinical and didactic teaching method should be carried out for clinician-teachers on the training base. The clinician-teachers should be supported and encouraged to undertake the clinical and didactic teaching tasks of general practitioners. The teaching training of teaching staff on grass-roots practice base should be strengthened on clinical training base in order to make the teaching staff competent for the clinical and didactic teaching task. Our country will also start the implementation of the training project of general practice teaching staff in due time to support the training work.

Fourth, emphasis should be put on control of the training quality. Training quality is the core of general practitioner training work. Medical colleges, particularly the key medical colleges should attach more importance to the development of the discipline of general practice, and strengthen the construction of clinical community bases and public health bases, and establish close cooperation mechanism, and build a basic platform for medical education. The training bases should practically carry out the work of training-quality control, and establish management system, implement management responsibilities, and meanwhile, strengthen management of the training process, earnestly fulfill the task of implementation and evaluation of training, thus ensuring that qualified general practitioners can be trained. During concrete implementation, successful experience and beneficial practice of foreign countries should be more widely used for reference. For instance, the average life expectancy Cuba, as a developing country, has reached 78 years old that is at the same level as US, in which general practitioners play a major role. The general practitioner training system in Cuba is the close integration of basic education and clinical practice. Community health service centers not only undertake the task of grass-roots medical and health service, but only serves as the basic platform of medical education. Medical students enter community health service centers in their freshman year, which embodies the close integration of basic medical education and grass-roots health practice and enhance their ability to communicate with people and encourage them to establish ideal and belief of taking root in grass roots.

Fourthly, staying firmly rooted in the present, training general practitioners through various channels at the present stage

The shortage and low quality of general practitioners is the present-day bottleneck of improving grass-rooms medical and health service system. In order to alleviate the current contradiction between the urgent need of general practitioners at grass-roots level and the long period of standardized general practitioner training, the Opinion puts forward four main approaches to train qualified general practitioners through various channels in the recent period, which include two projects of implementing the job-transfer training of general practitioners in the central and western regions in three consecutive years and free training of medical students ordered and oriented by rural areas, being supported by the Central Finance.

The job-transfer training of general practitioners is the transitional measure to solve the shortage of general practitioners at the present stage and the main channel of training general practitioners in the recent period. For more than a year of the implementation of job-transfer training, through the on-demand, split-ranging and tutorial-system training methods, the basic theory and practical skills of grass-roots trainees have been improved considerably; also, many trainees have established fixed relationship with clinician-teachers so that they can get timely technical problem-solving guidance provided by the tutors in base hospitals when they finish the training and return to grass roots, which helps to raise the level of grass-roots service. The free training project for medical students ordered and oriented by rural areas reflects the Country's care and support for the training of health talents in rural areas of the central and west of China, providing free higher medical education for students who aspire to take root at grass-roots level and offer medical and health service for fellow countrymen. Since the implementation of the project, departments including health, education, development and reform, human resources and social security, finance at all levels have closely cooperated with each other and successfully accomplished the task of recruiting and training of 2010-2011. Next, the achievements should be consolidated and problems that have been encountered should be studied and solved in time to ensure the smooth implementation of the project. Medical colleges that engage in this work should attach importance to improving the quality of training.

Currently, our country is still at the primary stage of socialism and fall behind developed countries in terms of economic and social development and meanwhile the development between urban and rural areas and between different regions is lopsided. Therefore, the Opinion has put forward some transitional measures. For instance, in the present transitional stage, on the premise of strict control of the proportion, the "3+2" model can be adopted for 3-year-medical-college graduates who work in the less-developed rural areas. That is, they can be registered as assistant general practitioners after receiving 2-year training of clinical and public health skills after graduation. The Ministry of Health is now studying and formulating the relevant training model and the guiding training content without any delay. Different regions should adjust measures to local conditions and implement the work of training.

Fifthly, exploring to establish the resident doctor standardized training system

The after-graduation medical education that is based on resident doctor standardized training is an indispensable phase in training qualified clinicians. Since the promulgation of the Provisional Measures for Clinical Resident Doctor Standardized Training by the Ministry of Health in 1993, hundreds of hospitals in 27 provinces, autonomous regions and municipalities across the country have implemented resident doctor standardized training and currently the enrollment scale per year has reached more than 20,000 people. Beijing, Sichuan, Tianjin, Jiangsu, Fujian and other areas have made profitable practices in the aspects including the improvement of training model, the strengthening of training management and the expansion of training scale, while Shanghai has promoted the construction of resident doctor standardized training system on the whole and has made breakthrough progress in the aspects of training management, security mechanism and cohesion of the academic degree system.

To establish the resident doctor standardized training system is a major reform of our country's medical education. Strict and standardized training can make medical students become qualified clinicians with quality and competence being guaranteed, thus making people satisfied and providing solid foundation for the development of medical and health staff and help those with both political integrity and professional competence develop the potential of growing to be subject-leading talents. During the process of deepening the reform of country-level public hospitals, implementing resident doctor standardized training can lay a solid foundation of talents to ensure "serious diseases out of country". Establishment of this system can also promote the building of the clinical diagnosis and treatment ability of hospitals in remote cities (prefectures) of the central and west of China, thus reducing the referrals of patients to the regions outside.

The Ministry of Health and the Ministry of Education have attached great importance to the building of resident doctor standardized training system and have currently collaborate with many departments to study and formulate without any delay the Guidance on the Establishment of Resident Doctor Standardized Training System. To improve the resident doctor standardized training system and speed up the training of qualified clinicians, the following principles should be paid attention and adhered to. The first is government playing the leading role and overall planning. Government at all levels should play a leading role in the implementation of resident doctor standardized training, and relevant departments should coordinated closely according to the segregation of duties and give full play to the function of social organizations of the profession. According to the principle of territorial management and based on the regional health planning, the scale and division of disciplines of resident doctor standardized training within the planned regions and the overall arrangement including the distribution of urban and rural areas and regions should be planned as a whole and coordinated. The second is providing macroscopical guidance and unifying standards. National health administrative departments take charge of providing macroscopical guidance on the organization and implementation of resident doctor standardized training and unifying the establishment of training model, training standard and management system. The third is highlighting key points and making overall plans and taking all factors into consideration. General practitioner training should be focused on and the training of grass-roots-level clinicians should be exerted efforts on. Meanwhile, various specialist training model (3+X) should be explored and improved; relevant professional training should be further extended based on 3-year intensive training, thus improving our country's after-graduation medical education model. The fourth is improving system and providing security. The institutional model, system mechanism and supporting policies should be gradually improved. The input guarantee policy of public finance, in particular, should be improved and the financing channels should be widened to embody the public product attribute of resident doctor standardized training. The fifth is improving competence and guaranteeing quality. The construction of training bases and teaching staff should be strengthened with the combination of public hospital reform and the ability of resident doctor standardized training should be raised gradually. Management of the training process should be put emphasis on and training quality should be guaranteed.

III. Making overall plans and taking all factors into consideration and earnestly implementing various kinds of health talent educational training

The key of whether our country's health talent team can meet the demands of medical reform and adapt to the challenge of population ageing and the change of disease spectrum lies in whether the quantity and quality of health talents can live up to the requirements of the development of health undertakings. In April this year, the Ministry of Health issued the National Medium- and Long-Term Plan for Medical and Health Talent Development (2011-2020), which puts forward the basic idea of "increasing the total quantity, raising the quality, adjusting the structure. Different regions should strengthen overall planning and carry out classified implementation, promote the educational training of various types of health talents as a whole and succeed in training a team of medical and health talents that has appropriate quantity and scale, excellent quality and competence and reasonable structure and distribution, according to this requirement.

Firstly, strengthening the continuous medical education of health personnel and training qualified talents on positions

It is a lifelong learning process of the growth and cultivation of medical and health talents. Continuous medical education is an important component of the lifelong medical education system in our country. The work of continuous medical education should target at raising the on-position service ability of health personnel as a whole, and further improve the system and innovate the mechanism and strengthen the construction of training system and expand the coverage of continuous medical education and incorporate various health personnel training into continuous medical education management, according to the principles of "overall planning and coordination, classified guidance, teaching based on demands, pursuit of practical results". The first is to put time and energy into reform of the content of continuous education, strengthening the butt joint between supply and demand and teaching based on demands and enhancing the pertinence and practicability continuous education activities, with post competency as the core. The second is to put time and energy into reform of the means of continuous education, strengthening the construction of distance education resources and encouraging the development of various kinds of distance medical education and alleviating the contradictions between work and study of medical personnel, especially the grass-roots trainees. The third is to put time and energy into construction of continuous education resources, integrating resources of training bases and teaching staff and forming a training network with reasonable layout and division of labor. The fourth is to put time and energy into management of continuous education, strengthening overall planning and coordination and classified guidance and reducing repeated training and raising the training quality.

In order to increase the effectiveness of on-job education training of medical personnel, with the vigorous support of the financial departments of the State, the Ministry of Health has set about to integrate the major and special medical reform projects of health personnel training from transfer payment by the Central Finance and adjusted the issuing method of major and special medical reform projects and increased capital investment since this year. Different regions should practically attach importance to the overall planning of training and actively explore to establish a working model of "combining centralization and decentralization" and gradually realize "four overall plans" in the aspects including the objects, content, time and approach of training to guarantee the quality and effectiveness of training.

Here, I want to put particular emphasis on strengthening the education training of rural doctors. Rural doctors are in closest touch with the vast majority of rural residents, undertaking the service function as "net bottom" of the rural medical and health service system and being able to function effectively at the grass-roots level of vast rural areas under practical circumstances. Health administrative departments in different regions should strengthen the education training of rural doctors according to the requirements of the Guidance of the General Office of the State Council on further Strengthening the Building of Team of Rural Doctors. The rural doctor regular on-job training system should be strictly implemented; clinical practice skills and general medical knowledge and informationization training should be strengthened with an emphasis on basic public health service and basic medical care; appropriated technology should be mastered; diagnosis and treatment behavior should be standardized. Target training should be provided for rural doctors who take the examinations for the qualifications of a licensed (assistant) doctor, thus making more rural doctors meet the qualifications for licensed (assistant) doctors. The effective approaches to strengthening the building of rural doctor reserve forces should be explored and the team of rural doctors should be improved and gradually trained to be licensed assistant doctors. The documents that were submitted to this conference for advice include the National Rural Doctor Education Plan (2011-2020) and the Twelfth Five-Year Plan for Continuous Medical Education. Comrades, please study them earnestly and set forth your opinions.

Secondly, making overall plans on the training of other health talents to meet the diversified talent demand

The first is to strengthening the training of talents in shortage and in urgent need. Currently, professional talents specializing in public health, nursing and pharmacy, etc. are in urgent need owing to the development of health undertaking, with the talent breach being huge. Professional training of the existing personnel should be enhanced in a planned way and with emphasis, and the shortage of talents on related positions should be solved through training to strengthen their professional knowledge and skills. Meanwhile, relevant medical colleges and schools should be guided to adjust the structure of academic disciplines and expand the enrollment and training scale of the urgently-needed talents according to specific conditions, thus increasing the talent supply. Since this year, the Ministry of Health has begun to implement the development project of professional talents in urgent need and by 2015, 370,000 various types of talents in shortage and urgent need will have been trained. The second is to strengthen the training of high-level medical and health talents. To train and bring up a batch of excellent medical talents with international competitiveness concerns the technology breakthrough of major diseases and health issues and concerns the seize of the commanding height of international biomedical science and technology and concerns the cultivation and development of the strategic emerging industries. A batch of high-level, innovative, interdisciplinary medical and health talents and innovative teams should be attracted and trained through the implementation of scientific research projects including major and special science and technology projects in the field of national population health and other relevant science and technology programs and through the construction of bases including national and department key laboratories and key disciplines, thus practically embodying the organic integration of project implementation, base construction and talent training. Opening up should be further expanded; international communication and cooperation platform should be actively constructed; earnestly implement the national overseas high-level talent introduction plan (One Thousand Talents Plan); well construct the innovative and entrepreneurial bases for overseas high-level talents; introduce a batch of scientists, leading entrepreneurial talents and innovative teams with international influence. Selection systems including "Middle-aged Expert with Outstanding Contribution of the Ministry of Health" and "Chinese Medicine Master" should be further improved to encourage high-level talents to stand out and improve continuously. By 2015, high-level professional talents will have been trained and introduced.

Thirdly, strengthening the training of talents of Chinese medicine and bringing into full play the characteristic advantages of Chinese medicine

Practices of the long-term development of Chinese medicine in our country indicate that Chinese medicine is very popular among ordinary people and plays an irreplaceable role in our country's medical and health service system, owing to its definite curative effect, relatively low cost and in particular the unique advantage of "preventive treatment of disease". Different regions should explore how talents of Chinese medicine can play an effective role in grass-roots medical and health care institutions such as community and township health centers and bridge the gap between the training of talents of Chinese medicine and the requirements of economic and social and profession development. Practices indicate that famous doctors and masters of Chinese medicine have grown out of the constant accumulation of clinical experience. The inherent laws of disciplines of Chinese medicine and the growth laws of talents of Chinese medicine should be abided by, with "emphasis on classics, proficiency in humanities, early practice, more clinic". We should intensify reforms of the training model and talent training mechanism of Chinese medical colleges and schools and strengthen training of students' inheritance ability and clinical thinking of Chinese medicine. The educational system of the succession of teachings from a master to his disciples should be further improved and the training of talents of Chinese medicine at grass-roots level and talents of Chinese medicine integrated with Western medicine should be strengthened. The "three famous" (famous doctor, famous department, famous hospital) strategy should be actively implemented and inheritance of the academic experience of Chinese medical experts and the clinical experience of experienced Chinese medical experts at grass-roots level should be carried out. During the period of the Twelfth Five-Year Plan, we will implement the project of Chinese medicine inheriting and innovative talents and train 85,000 Chinese medical talents, technical backbone personnel of clinical Chinese medicine and experienced academic successors of Chinese medicine at grass-roots level.

Fourthly, strengthening education of medical culture and medical ethics and training medical workers to satisfy the people

Culture is the soul and blood of a nation and is the inner foundation on which a nation relies for survival and development. The Sixth Plenary Session of the 17th CPC Central Committee that was held lately conducted a monographic study on the issue of socialist culture construction. Medical culture, as an important component of social culture, is both extensive and profound and both munificent and voluminous. Our country's medical culture mainly stems from three aspects. The first is the concept of "great physician of excellence and sincerity" of traditional medicine; the second is the humanistic spirit of western medicine; the third is the revolutionary humanitarianism along with the development of the liberation cause of New China and the construction of socialism. Medical ethics that was born synchronously with medical culture is the moral code of medical personnel from generation to generation in country and has become the spiritual impetus of the vast majority of health personnel to march forward courageously and sacrifice themselves in rescuing others under the threat of major infectious diseases and in the quake fighting and disaster relief combat. While deepening medical reform and exploring new models of the development of public hospitals, we should vigorously strengthen the construction of medical culture and raise the quality of civilization across the profession and train medical and health talents to satisfy the people. The first is to strengthen education of medical ethics and inherit the virtue of "doctors are healers with benevolent hearts". Higher requirements should be put forward to clinician-teachers who influence students by their own example; training bases should establish good surroundings of medical ethics to edify students. The second is to put emphasis on system construction. Qualitative and quantitative evaluation indicator system of medical ethics, particularly evaluation from patients, should be explored to establish. The third is to strengthen positive publicity and education and to promote righteousness of the profession and to vigorously scout for, set up and publicize advanced models and to lead the whole society to respect the medical laws and understand medical personnel and form a good social atmosphere of public opinion.

Comrades, reform of medical educations concerns the effective implementation of two national strategies of revitalizing China through science and education and reinvigorating China through talent development, and concerns the realization of two goals of the reform of national education and the reform of medical and health system, and concerns the implementation of three National Medium-and Long-Term Plans for science and technology, education and talents. Therefore, Health administrative departments at all levels should reform with keen determination, and pioneer and innovate, and further improve the macro-management and macro coordination mechanism of the two ministries, and join efforts to study and solve the bottleneck problems of medical education reform and medical and health system reform, and promote the education reform and medical reform in an in-depth and coordinating way, according to the important guiding spirit of Comrade Liu Yandong of "vigorously promoting the comprehensive reform of medical education and exploring the developing road of medical education with Chinese characteristics and conduction medical education to satisfy people". The pioneering spirit of comrades of different regions and departments should be fully promoted; creative practice and exploration should be encouraged; the implementation of pilot work in different regions should be pushed forward; energy and resources should be centralized to make great efforts to problems of reform and development; experience should be summed up in time to establish and improve relevant systems. Let's make arduous efforts to create a team of medical and health talents with lofty morality, profound attainments, exquisite skills, strong sense of social responsibilities and rich in innovative spirit! Let's make new and greater contribution to improving the overall health level of Chinese people!

(Chen Ying, Song Yang)

9. A Summary Speech Delivered by Secretary of the CPC Party Committee and Vice-Minister of the Ministry of Health Zhang Mao at 2011 National Health Work Conference (January 7th, 2011)

Comrades,

The conference has been held over two days and it will be closed today. The meeting has conveyed and studied the important instructions of Comrade Li Keqiang and Comrade Chen Zhu has made work report which reviewed the health work during the Eleventh Five-Year Plan period and the year 2010 and made overall deployments of health reform and development in the Twelfth Five-Year Plan period and put forward specific arrangements for health work of the year 2011 in accordance with the spirit of the fifth Plenary Session of the 17th CPC Central Committee and the requirements of the Central Economic Working Conference. The conference has solemnly commended representatives of excellent rural doctors across the country. During this conference, we have had heated discussions over Comrade Chen Zhu's work report and some major issues about health reform and development. Just now, all group leaders have delivered speeches on behalf of the comrades who attend the conference, which highly appreciated the work report made by Minister Chen Zhu and also reflected our clearer understanding of the situation and tasks that we are faced with and the full confidence that we have in fulfilling tasks of this year, and set forth some questions and feasible suggestions. All conferees showed unanimous agreement in their speeches that they will earnestly implement the spirit of this conference and comprehensively accomplish the recent high priority tasks of health reform and open up a new situation for the scientific development of health service. The conference has been convened successfully and has achieved expected goals of unifying thought, uplifting spirits, understanding situations and clarifying tasks and will certainly exert positive influence on the fulfillment of health work of this year and even of the Twelfth Five-Year Plan period.

Next, I would like to set forth some opinions on implementing the spirit of the fifth Plenary Session of the 17th CPC Central Committee and the requirements of the Central Economic Working Conference and on making overall arrangements of the health work.

I. Implementing the spirit of the fifth Plenary Session of the 17th CPC Central Committee and upholding the scientific outlook on development to direct health work

The fifth Plenary Session of the 17th CPC Central Committee has deliberated on and passed *the Opinion of CPC Central Committee on the Twelfth Five-Year Plan of national economic and social development* and has defined the development objectives and the major tasks in our country's Twelfth Five-Year Plan period. The Plenary Session pointed out that we should put more emphasis on ensuring and improving people's livelihood and take ensuring and improving people's livelihood as the fundamental starting point and foothold of accelerating the transformation of the mode of economic development, which point out the clear direction for speeding up the reform and development of the medical and health services. The important task of the national health system at present and in the next period to come is to unify the thought of the vast majority of cadres and workers' to live up to the spirit of the Plenary Session and to condense strength to implement various missions that the plenum has put forward.

The Plenary Session explicitly points out that the theme of the Twelfth Five-Year Plan is scientific development, which indicates distinctive features of our age. In studying and implementing the spirit of the Plenary Session, the health system must highlight the theme of scientific development, and grasp the main line of accelerating transformation of the mode of economic development, and integrate the nature and the characteristics of the health service and the current situation and tasks that we are faced with, and make the most of the fruitful results and the successful experiences of reform and development of health services in the Eleventh Five-Year Plan period, to keep the guiding ideology, development purposes, development modes, and major working thought highly consistent with the major decisions of the Central Government and the requirements of scientific development.

(1) Adhering to people foremost and grasping the law of health development. The fundamental goal of our country's socialist health service is to serve for people's health and all the health work must be launched centered on ensuring health rights and interests of people and maintaining fairness and justice of the society. We should see not only considerable achievements the health development has made but also quite a few aspects of the health work that fail to satisfy the vast majority of people. The health service has not yet satisfied the increasing health needs of ordinary people; thus, we should still make long-term and strenuous efforts to truly render people the safe, effective, convenient and inexpensive health services. To achieve scientific development of the health service, we must consistently adhere to the non-profit nature of public medical and health care, and adhere to the guideline of

the basic health work that puts prevention first, highlights the rural areas and pay equal attention to Chinese and western medicine, and adhere to the principle of the government leading, the whole society participating and all the people receiving benefit, and insist on deepening medical reform, and resorting to the basic medical care and health system to solve prominent issues, and lay the foundation for achieving people-oriented scientific development in the field of health service.

(2) Insisting on making overall plans and taking all factors into consideration, and pushing forward the comprehensive, balanced and sustainable development of health service. The fifth Plenary Session of the 17th CPC Central Committee puts emphasis on the comprehensive, balanced and sustainable development, which is entirely consistent with the reality of health development. To achieve scientific development of health services, the first requirement is that the health administrative departments at all levels, especially the leading comrades, should increase their abilities to grasp major issues, to scheme overall situation, and to make overall consideration. We should voluntarily integrate health work into the overall situation of macro economy and social development and give full play to the role of health work in promoting economic development and social progress. We should grasp the overall situation of health work, be adept in making overall consideration of the health work from the perspective of "macro health" and promote the comprehensive development of health services by building the basic medical care and health system. Currently, we should make overall plans and coordinate the building of four major systems in combination with the health reform, including public health services, medical care, medical security and drug supply security. The change of the reality of unbalanced development should be accelerated through guaranteeing the basic, strengthening grass roots and establishing mechanism; the development gap in development between urban and rural areas and between different regions should be solved. We should give full play to role of traditional Chinese medicine and western medicine, which are considered as "one body with two wings" of our medical and health service, and promote the coordinated development of Chinese medicine and western medicine. The stage characteristics of the national conditions and development should be precisely grasped; the relationships between current benefits and long-term benefits and between partial benefits and overall benefits should be taken into overall coordination and successfully handled. We should strengthen macro-control, and guide demands reasonably, and work in a down-to-earth manner and within our capabilities, and exert our utmost, so as to promote the sustainable development of the health service.

(3) Putting efforts in transforming the mode of health development and pushing forward the healthy development of health service.

The fifth Plenary Session of the 17th CPC Central Committee points out that accelerating transformation of the mode of economic development is a profound reform in the economic and social field of our country, which must penetrate the whole process and various fields of the economic and social development. In terms of the issue of transforming the mode of health development, Minister Chen Zhu has made a thorough expatiation in his work report, and here I would like to add some views. Over sixty years of development, our country has built up a health service system that functions relatively perfect and spreads all over urban and rural areas and has initially laid the foundation for the realization of the health work objectives in the new period. Currently, we should integrate seizing opportunities for development with innovating the concept and mode of development, and make efforts to achieve sound and rapid development. The relationship between the denotation and connotation of development should be handled properly; necessary development scale and speed should be maintained; the total health resources should also maintain its corresponding growth as the demands for national health increase; resources should be allocated to the fields and links that play essential and decisive role in the development of health service; stress should be laid on developing public health, urban and rural grass roots, the central and western regions and the fields of new services that the transformation of the mode of medical science requires; new technology that the scientific and technological progress of medical science has brought, especially the advanced technology with low cost and favorable effects should be developed. At present and even in the forthcoming period, we should attach great importance to the connotation construction, and promote the innovation of management system, compensation mechanism, operating mechanism, and service mode through deepening the reform, and strive to improve personnel quality, service quality, service efficiency and management level with persistence, and put more emphasis on promoting self-construction and improving the overall quality and efficiency of the health system by the means of legalization, informationization and so forth. I hope that comrades of the health departments at all levels could give more thought and conduct more research more on such major issues as transformation of the mode of health development, to make it truly reflected in the practice of health reform and development.

II. Clearly recognizing the current situation and taking the improvement of people's livelihood as a major mission of the health work

General Secretary Hu Jintao points out at the 20th collective learning activity of the 17th Political Bureau of the CPC Central Committee that the medical care and health service is closely linked to the health of millions upon millions of people, the happiness of thousands of households, the economic development and social harmony and a nation's prospect and future, which is a livelihood issue of great significance. Both the fifth Plenary Session of the 17th CPC Central Committee and the Central Economic Working Conference put solving the problems of people's livelihood in a prominent position. Comrades of health departments at all levels must clearly understand this important issue that is put forward in the process of economic and social development.

Currently, from the perspective of the people's livelihood, the situation of the health work we are faced with is not optimistic. Our country is in the period of rapid industrialization and urbanization; the ageing process of population is accelerating; the patterns of production and life are changing rapidly; and health problems are becoming increasingly complicated. On the one hand, the harm of the infectious diseases remains serious; the threats of chronic non-communicable diseases intensify continuously; the public health emergencies appear constantly; the events of the food and drug safety and the occupational disease hazard take place occasionally, which bring about severe challenges to people's health. On the other hand, people's expectations on health and demands for health care are increasing, and the improvement of security system and service standards have been paid unprecedented attention to. All of those changes mentioned above put forward newer and higher requirements for the adjustment of resource distribution, the improvement of public health services and regulatory functions, the raising of the capacities to provide medical care and health services, the transformation service mode and the construction of health security system. Properly solving the problems of people's livelihood in field of health has become an important mission of health work at the present stage.

Although it has not been long since the new round of medical reform was launched, we are still delighted to see that some phased achievements brought by the reform have already made the ordinary people reap the real benefits, and the deepening of medical reform has been continuously pushing forward the improvement of people's health condition. We must closely integrate the demands of improving people's livelihood made by the Party Central Committee and the State Council with the mission of deepening the medical reform, and firmly establish the awareness of people's livelihood, and take the viewpoints of the ordinary people as the ideological basis for improving people's livelihood.

— Taking people's health demands as the fundamental driving force to push forward the medical reform. All the policy and measures of medical reform begin with and serve for people's health demands. The Central and local governments have formulated and issue a series of supporting documents in succession centered on the recent five high priority tasks and have specified the relative policies for implementation. Comrades in all localities reported that there still exist various difficulties and problems in the process of policy implementation. It is unavoidable to encounter with difficulties and obstacles in the process of reforming and improving the original system and mechanism. We must make it clear that as long as a policy meets the requirement of the interests of people or corresponds to the real situation, it is a good policy and we should carry it out with perseverance. The difficulties in the process of implementing policies should be solved gradually by strengthening the communication and coordination between government leaders and departments and by formulating concrete operation methods and measures in accordance with the real situation. Over more than a year, promoting the construction of the basic drug system has brought us a lot of inspirations. Many difficulties were indeed encountered with at the beginning of the construction of the new system, which includes not only the recognition problems and policy supporting and actual operation problems; however, provinces (autonomous regions, municipalities) including Beijing, Tianjin, Shanghai, Anhui, Jiangxi, Shaanxi, Gansu, Ningxia have insisted on unshakably guaranteeing people's basic pharmaceuticals by establishing the basic drug system, and removed disturbances, and met difficulties head-on, and carried out work creatively proceeding from actual conditions, and achieved full coverage of basic drug system in the government-run grass-roots health care institutions in a short period of time. Thus, the burden of people's medical bills has been significantly reduced and the ordinary people have experienced the benefits brought by the policies in person.

— Considering whether the ordinary people have reaped benefits or not as the basic standard to determine the success or failure of the reform. To judge whether the medical reform has been crowned with success or not, there should also exist a standard. This standard is not simply applied to see how many infrastructure constructions have been implemented or how many new instruments have been increased but to see whether the general public have truly reaped benefits and whether their health conditions have been improved continuously. Recently, the Standing Committee of the National People's Congress has organized a special inquiry into deepening the work of the medical reform, which also focuses attention on the effects of medical reform in terms of the benefits people have received. The leading cadres at all levels of the health system should establish correct view of political achievements, and proceed from the benefits of people when thinking, making decisions and working, and consider whether people have reaped benefits or not as the "gauge" to measure the effectiveness of the work that has been conducted, and keep the developments of health service always consistent with the people's health benefits. To make people reap benefits, essentially speaking, is to bring inexpensive service and convinience to the people. The pilot project of treating children's serious diseases, which has implemented in the regions including Hunan and Jiangxi, is a good example to follow. In order to solve the problem of treatment costs that ordinary people can hardly afford, Hunan province has implemented free surgical treatment for rural children with congenital heart diseases under the new rural cooperative medical care system (NRCMS), and has exempted 90% of the treatment costs for families with children suffering from leukemia, which are jointly undertaken by NRCMS and serious illness assistance fund. Jiangxi province has implemented free treatment for children suffering from leukemia in urban and rural areas across the whole province, which is undertaken jointly by NRCMS, serious illness assistance fund and provincial financial fund, and carried out pilot projects of free treatments for children with congenital heart diseases in five cities with subordinate districts. The diseased children have received timely treatment and the cost burden has been reduced substantially, so that the beneficiary families deeply appreciate the favorable policies of medical reform formulated by the Party and government. It illustrates that health work is by no means simple technical work, but significant work of society, livelihood and politics instead, which plays a special role in maintaining the flesh-blood ties between the Party and ordinary people.

— Taking raising people's health level as the ultimate goal of health reform and development. The reform of medical and health system involves multiple interest groups and there could be different thoughts and points of entry to solve the problems. No matter what kind of thoughts it is, as long as it implements measures of reform closely centered on the most concerned, the most immediate and the most realistic interest issues of people, it will gain people's recognition. Counties including Zichang, Shenmu in Shaanxi province have carried out varieties of explorations and practices in this respect. Zichang county has comprehensively pushed forward the reform with the breakthrough of strengthening the non-profit nature of the public medical care and health services, and with the core of increasing input and transforming system and mechanism; Shenmu county has increased input and made the entire population enjoy equal access to medical security, with the entry point of establishing the medical security system for all people with urban-rural integration. In terms of the effects, different modes of reform have all made the ordinary reap remarkable practical benefits, and if these modes continue to operate, they will be bound to raise people's health level continuously.

After fulfilling the three-year tasks of medical reform, we will conduct comprehensive assessments of the results of medical reform under the unified arrangements of the medical reform office under the State Council, assessing not only the fulfillment of specific task objectives, but also the effects on improving livelihood and raising the level of the residents' health. All localities should attach more importance to the assessments in this aspect as well.

Ⅲ. Formulate the Twelfth Five-Year Plan of the health work scientifically

During the Twelfth Five-Year Plan period, the health work has achieved great accomplishments, especially made significant strides in deepening the reform of medical care and health system. The period of the Twelfth Five-Year plan is a crucial 5-year period of building a well-off society in all-round way that serves as a connecting link between the preceding and the following, and it is the crucial period of deepening reform and opening-up and accelerating the transformation of the economic development mode. Deeply understanding and precisely grasping the new situation and characteristics that the health work is faced with and scientifically formulating the Twelfth Five-Year plan of the health service is of great significance in continuing to seize and making the most of the important strategic opportunity period of health reform in our country and pushing forward the healthy development of the health service and raising the level of people's health.

Minister Chen Zhu has set forth the overall goals, basic thoughts and main tasks of the Twelfth Five-Year health reform and development in his work report. As for the planning and formulation, I would like to make several more requirements.

(1) Setting the planned objectives and indicators scientifically. During the Twelfth Five-Year Plan period, the overall objective of the health work is still to realize equal access to the basic medical care and health services. Within this overall objective, we should put forward the goal indicators in accordance with reality and the task indicators in several fields; we should take the average life expectancy, infant mortality, maternal mortality and the proportion of personal health expenditure of residents in national total health expenditure, which are internationally recognized and comprehensively reflect the level of health work and social and economic development, as the important goal indicators of the Twelfth Five-Year health plan, and strive to list them in the comprehensive national and regional Twelfth Five-Year comprehensive plans. Meanwhile, an array of quantifiable planned task indicators should be put forward in the major fields of health reform and development including medical security, major disease control and basic preventive health care, medical services and drug supplies, health resources allocation and social health management; implementation of various tasks should be directed with the indicator system which is scientific and reasonable, in accordance with reality and can be appraised. All the localities should attach great importance to studying and determining the planned goal indicators, and carry out baseline survey, and accurately grasp the current

situation and the major contradictions and the prominent issues that need to solved of the local health development, and specify the tasks, and set various objectives and indicators of the Twelfth Five-Year plan in a matter-of-fact manner, according to the requirements of health work by the Party Central Committee and the State Council and the practical situation of all the localities.

(2) Focusing on the objectives with the short-term and long-term integration and setting up the plans of projects and actions. The major plans of projects and actions are important means of implementing the tasks of the Twelfth Five-Year Plan. During the Eleventh Five-Year Plan period, we spent two years carrying out a strategic research named "Healthy China 2020", which conducted a prospective study on the development trend based on the analysis of prominent issues including major diseases, focus groups and health risk factors, and proposed a series of health action plans with long-term and short-term integration, goal-oriented tasks and good cost-effectiveness, and also proposed major projects to strengthen the weak links including basic public health, grass-roots medical and health care services, major disease control. As far as we know, quite a few regions also carried out strategic studies in this aspect, and gain valuable research results. I hope all the localities transform these achievements into specific contents while formulating the plans, and make them become a powerful grip for implementing the planned tasks.

(3) Putting emphasis on institutional innovation and mechanism transformation. Institutional innovation and mechanism transformation are the powerful impetus to promote health development. To formulate the Twelfth Five-Year Plan, we should adhere to deepening medical and health system reform as the core, and push forward the establishment and improvement of coordinated and unified medical and health management system, scientific and reasonable health input mechanism, high-efficient and standardized medical and health institution operating mechanism, the medical and health talent training mechanism and science and technology innovation mechanism with a long-term focus. Rapid and sound development of the health service would be achieved through the innovation of systems and mechanisms.

(4) Making effective communication and coordination. Health plans are concerned with the interests thousands of families and with various aspects of economic and social development; the process of formulating plans needs the understanding and support of governments, relevant departments and all sectors of the society. We should report to the local government leaders without delay the major goals, measures and action plans, and actively notify the situations, communicate thoughts, strive for conditions and get support from relevant departments. We should enhance the scientificity and transparency in the plan formulating process; the major thoughts and projects should be discussed and demonstrated by experts; major goals and indicators

should be formulated based on a wide range of opinions from various aspects from the inside and outside of the system. Specialized plans in health-related fields should be formulated in accordance with the overall plan of the local Twelfth Five-Year Plan for economic and social development and in combination with the Twelfth Five-Year Plan for health service, thus making various plans coordinated on the whole and practically feasible.

I hope that national health system will take the plan formulating process as the process of unifying understanding of the major issues of health reform, the process of reaching consensus on the future development goals of health service and the process of pushing forward the scientific, democratic decision, law-based decision making, and practically succeed in depicting the blueprint of the Twelfth Five-Year Plan for health development.

IV. Making efforts to solve the highlight and difficult problems, and continuously pushing forward the health reform

The year 2011 is the third year of fulfilling the recent tasks of health reform established by the State Council. In combination with the five high priority tasks of the health reform, I would like to put emphasis on several more issues.

(1) Putting emphasis on standardizing the bidding and procurement of basic drugs and implementing the zero-profit policy in basic drug sales in the aspect of improving national basic drug system. The Party Central Committee and the State Council take the improvement of basic drug system as one of the two key points that should be attached great importance to in health reform this year. Since the implementation of national basic drug system, remarkable progress and initial results have been achieved, but there have also emerged some problems that should be solved urgently, mainly the problems of bidding and procurement and zero-profit sales. If they were not solved in time, these problems would directly affect the establishment and implementation effects of basic drug system.

On the bidding and procurement of basic drugs. At the end of 2010, General Office of the State Council issued *the notice about printing and distributing the guiding opinion on establishing and standardizing the basic drug purchasing mechanism in the government-run grass-roots medical and health care institutions*, which clarifies the general ideas, major measures and work requirements of establishing and standardizing the basic drug procurement mechanism and formulates a series of measures in the aspects of procurement platform construction, bidding standardization, supply and distribution, electronic supervision and so forth and puts forward specific requirements for "quality linked up with price" and so forth. The health administrative departments of different provinces (autonomous regions and municipalities) should earnestly comprehend the spirit of the document, and do well in interpreting and publicizing, and practically implement requirements of the document in collaboration with relevant departments, and make efforts to establish a long-effect mechanism to standardize the bidding and procurement of basic drugs.

On the zero-profit sales of basic drugs. According to the situation of monitoring and supervising of medical reform, although some regions have been equipped with and put into use basic drugs in the government-run grass-roots medical and health care institutions, they fail to implement zero-profit sales. Here, it needs to be clarified that the zero-profit sales policy is the core content of implementing the basic drug system and is the important means and path to reform the mechanism of "subsidizing medical services with drug sales" and reduce the medication burden of the ordinary people. Without the implementation the basic drug zero-profit sales policy, the basic drug system has not yet been practically implemented. According to relevant regulations of the basic drug system, the 307 kinds of basic drugs promulgated by the country and the drugs supplemented by different provinces (autonomous regions and municipalities) should all implement the zero-profit sales. Some regions have not implemented the basic drug zero-profit sales policy for the supplementary drugs and have been carrying out "dual-track" price system, which fail to conform to the rules of the basic drug system. I hope these regions would analyze the reasons, and supervise the implementation of relevant supporting policies and management measures, to ensure the overall effect of the implementation of the policies.

(2) Speeding up the pilot reform of public hospitals. Since the start-up of the pilot reform of public hospitals in 2010, quite a lot feasible practice and experience have already been explored and summarized; the layout and structure of public hospitals in pilot cities have begun to be adjusted and optimized; the hospitals have begun to improve in the aspects including safety and quality, cost-effectiveness and service efficiency; the pilot reform work has received active response from medical staff and the general public. Lately, the Party Central Committee and the State Council have required putting the pilot reform of public hospitals in a more prominent place and speed up and push forward the reform, which makes a major deployment in accordance with the overall situation of health reform.

The public hospitals in our country undertake most of the tasks of clinical diagnosis and treatment for urban and rural residents, which are the major places of diagnosing and treating the difficult and severe diseases and the common and frequent diseases for the general public, and also shoulder important social responsibilities including promoting the development of medical science and technology, training medical and health talents, supporting grass-roots health institutions and providing medical treatment in response to major emergencies. For a period of time, the problem of difficulties and high expense in medical care, which has aroused strong resentment among the general public, has mainly focused on large public hospitals. Meanwhile, the reform of public hospitals plays a significant role of restricting and supporting for the other four tasks of the reform tasks; if the public hospital reform failed to keep pace with the reforms in other fields, the general public would hardly feel the obvious overall effects of health reform. Therefore, we must comply with the general situation of the development of health reform, and adapt to the eager expectation of ordinary people, and firmly implement the decision made by the Party Central Committee and the State Council, and practically speed up the pilot reform of public hospitals.

According to the deployment of the State Council's leading group for medical and health care reform, the Ministry of Health has studied and drafted *the key work arrangements on the pilot reform of public hospital in 2011*, and widely consulted the opinions from all walks of life, which will be formally issued after further amendment and perfection. Minister Chen Zhu has specified the major tasks of speeding up the pilot reform in the work report and hope that health administrative departments at all levels will unswervingly follow the spirit and unified deployment of the Central government, and practically take speeding up the pilot reform of public hospitals as the emphasis of health reform work of this year, through elaborate organization and implementation. We should not only widely popularize the reform measures with consensus, practice, effects and experience as soon as possible to reflect the social effects of public hospital reform, but also dare to meet difficulties head-on, reform with keen determination, and insist on the direction of public hospital reform, and carry out more in-depth exploration into some major system and mechanism issues related to public hospitals in the pilot cities, and summarize the experience in time. We should integrate implementing the measures for the convenience and benefits of people with pushing forward the comprehensive reform and exploring to solve the problems of system and mechanism, thus making both of them support and promote each other, to form sustaining inner impetus and establish a long-effect mechanism. To provide convenience and benefits for people is the goal of the comprehensive reform and the comprehensive reform is the impetus to provide convenience and benefits for people. During the process of speeding up the pilot reform, we should strengthen the overall planning and coordination between different departments, and divide labor with individual responsibility, and formulate and implement various policies of public hospital reform, and strengthen positive publicity and guidance of public opinion, in particular, reasonably guide the psychological expectations of the general public, and create a favorable atmosphere of public opinion and external environment for speeding up the pilot reform of public hospitals. The hospital internal management should be practically strengthened; strong measures should be taken to effectively restrain the excessively rapid increase of medical expense.

(3) Putting emphasis on strengthening refined management and further raising the level of fund supervision and operation, in terms of improving the new rural cooperative medical care system (NRCMS). In recent years, the fund-raising ability of the NRCMS has improved constantly, which has made the level of benefits that rural residents could reap increase continuously and has played increasingly important role in ensuring that rural residents receive medical care and treatment, easing the burden of medical expenses, reducing illness-related poverty and promoting social development of rural areas. With the expansion of the insurance coverage and the enhancement of insurance level of the NRCMS, the health service demands of rural residents have been gradually released and the operation and expenditure pressure of the New Rural Cooperative Medical funds has been increased accordingly, therefore, great importance should be attached to guaranteeing the safe and effective operation of funds. On the one hand, all the localities should scientifically measure and calculate the amount of funds that has been used in 2011, and improve compensation schemes, standardize the use of funds, and increase the efficiency of fund utilization, thus making the utmost of the New Rural Cooperative Medical funds in medical reimbursement for the rural residents who participate in the NRCMS and preventing the risk of overspending. On the other hand, the supervision and management of the New Rural Cooperative Medical funds should be further strengthened. There are large quantities of rural residents who have participated the NRCMS; the designated medical institutions have multiple service points and a wide range to cover; the management agencies have weak capacities; with the gradual expansion of the insurance coverage, new approaches should be adopted and great efforts should be made to realize effective supervision and management and completely eradicate loopholes. All the localities should continue to establish and perfect the NRCMS management agencies, and enplenish the power of supervision and management, and speed up the construction and improvement of the New Rural Cooperative Medical information network system, and improve the means of supervision and management, and enhance the capacities of supervision and management. We should actively push forward entrusting qualified commercial insurance agencies to participate in the management of handling the New Rural Cooperative Medical funds.

In the year 2011, our country will once again increase the subsidy standard of the NRCMS; thus, health departments should fulfill related tasks in collaboration with relevant departments, according to the unified requirements.

(4) Giving priority to the comprehensive supporting reform and the construction of talent team in grass-roots medical and health care institutions, in terms of

improving the grass-roots medical and health care service system. With the advancement of reform, the facilities and conditions of grass-roots medical and health care institutions have been improved significantly; some supporting economic policies have been implemented gradually; problems of the reform of internal operation mechanism and the construction of talent team have become increasingly prominent. This year, efforts should be made to intensify strength in the comprehensive reform of grass-roots medical and health care institutions and the talent construction.

The first is to push forward the comprehensive reform of grass-roots medical and health care institutions in all-round way. the experience and practices in Anhui provinces and other regions should be popularized; the non-profit nature of the government-run grass-roots health care institutions should be strengthened; reform of the personnel system and the distribution system should be deepened; effective accountability, competition and incentive mechanisms mechanism should be established; grass-roots medical and health care institutions should be guided to take the initiative to transform operation mechanism; the quality and efficiency of services should be increased; the function of undertaking basic public health services and the diagnosis and treatment of the common diseases and frequent diseases should be brought into full play. The key to the comprehensive supporting reform is the reform of compensation mechanism; if the reform of compensation mechanism fails to be put in place, other supporting reforms will hardly be pushed forward smoothly. In order to ensure the smooth operation and development of grass-roots medical and health care institutions, General Office of the State Council has printed and issued *the Opinions on establishing and improving the compensation mechanism of grass-roots medical and health care institutions,* further specifying the compensation policies for grass-roots medical and health care institutions. All the localities should earnestly implement the spirit of the document, and allocate government special subsidies to grass-roots medical and health care institutions including expenditure for development and construction, grants for basic public health services, subsidies for public health emergencies and personnel expenditure, and adjust the charging items and the medical insurance payment policy, and implement subsidies for recurrent balance of payment, and establish stable compensation channels and methods, and form a long-acting compensation mechanism, and ensure the effective operation and the healthy development of grass-roots medical and health care institutions and the reasonable treatment for the vast majority of grass-roots medical personnel and rural doctors.

The second is to strengthen the construction of grass-roots health talent team. The shortage of talents at grass-roots level is not a new problem; however, with the advancement of various medical reform work, more and more tasks need to be undertaken by grass-roots medical and health care institutions, and the requirements become higher and higher, and the talent problems become more and more prominent. All the localities should proceed from the reality and successfully implement various policies and measures on grass-roots talent team construction of the medical reform scheme and strive for practical results. Currently, relevant departments under the State Council are formulating relevant documents of establishing the general practitioner system; once issued, these documents should be earnestly implemented. I also hope that all the localities continue bold exploration, and innovate the systems and methods for grass-roots health talents, who could be introduced, retained, made good use of and improved, and continuously create fresh experience.

(5) Putting emphasis on system management and balanced advancement in terms of promoting gradual equalization of basic pubic health services. Management responsibility for equalization of basic public health services should be strengthened and management level should be raised. Different departments have reached a widespread consensus on public health services, with policies and measures being specified, support coming from all walks of life, funds being guaranteed by the governments. To implement tasks in this field, health departments at all levels undertake major responsibilities. Whether the work in this field could achieve favorable results or not directly reflect the competence and level of the health system of its own. We must clearly realize that arduous efforts should be made to provide basic public health services for all of the urban and rural residents and to gradually achieve equalization and to implement major public health projects that are featured by wide coverage and heavy workload. We should adopt a down-to-earth attitude to explore the feasible service approaches and working methods. The measures for equalization of basic public health services have been implemented for two years; health departments at all levels should summarize experience and establish a whole set of systems that clarify the division of responsibilities, decompose tasks reasonable, provide standardized and orderly services, conduct efficient organization and management and make strict performance appraisal, from the perspective of forming long-acting working mechanism, and practically raise the management and service level of equalized basic public health services, thus making this system benefit people's health continuously.

Great emphasis should be put to the imbalanced advancement of public heath service tasks. Based on the monitored results, different projects of public health services have made imbalanced progress. While traditional projects including health education, preventive vaccination, infectious disease prevention and control, maternal and child hygiene in some regions have been operating according to the original service contents and modes, the newly added projects including elderly health care, chronic disease management, holergasia management have been making slow progress, and some projects have even not yet been widely carried out. Although some regions have set up residents' health archives, these archives have not be used sufficiently. The monitored results also indicate that the development of public health services between different regions has also been imbalanced and the differences have been relatively significant. The reasons that give rise to the above-mentioned problems are multi-fold. To solve these problems, the first is to put emphasis on pushing forward this basis system, and strengthen management, and adhere to down-to-earth working style; the second is to strengthen coordination and cooperation between different departments and form joint force; the third is to adjust and replenish personnel who are engaged in public health services, and intensify professional training, and improve the work level; the fourth is to strengthen appraisal and supervision, and find out and solve prominent problems without delay. Equalization of basic public health services is a project of institutional building in medical reform, which is of utmost significance and is related to the national long-term health benefits; therefore, health departments at all levels should shoulder historical responsibilities and make this system benefit all of the urban and rural residents with the least delay possible.

V. Innovating working methods and improve working styles

Tasks of reform and development are arduous and complicate, which test the decision-making ability and executive capacity of health departments at all levels, particularly the leading comrades, and also test the cohesion and combat effectiveness and working capability of the health system. The situation requires us to innovate working methods, improve working styles and increase working efficiency.

(1) Strengthening monitoring and supervision and implementing the task and target responsibility system of medical reform. To monitor and supervise the progress of medical reform and various health work is an effective way of monitoring the progress, summarizing the experience, discovering the problem, supervising the implementation and also an embodiment of the innovation of working methods in medical reform. Since the launch of medical reform, the Ministry of Health has established the monitoring and supervision system of progress made in medical reform to monitor the quarterly progress and report the monitoring results to health departments in all localities in time according to the rank ordering of task and locality. This practice has produced positive results in promoting the implementation of tasks of medical reform and has great attention and identification in all localities. This year, the Ministry of Health will continue to carry out this task based on improving the indicator system, standardizing organization and management and improving the

quality of statistics. Different provinces (regions, cities) should also take advantage of the existing statistical information system to establish monitoring platform and to implement and continuously improve the monitoring and supervision over the medical reform in prefecture-level cities and counties.

In May of 2010, the leading group of the Ministry of Health for medical reform signed responsibility certificates with directors of the health departments and bureaus of all provinces (regions, cities) and directors of relevant departments of the Ministry of Health, thus clarifying their respective annual tasks. After signing the responsibility certificates, all provinces (regions, cities) and relevant departments of the Ministry of Health have earnestly studied and formulated annual implementation schemes according to the requirements of the responsibility certificates and assign tasks to different levels of government, thus providing strong guarantee for the smooth implementation of the tasks. By the end of the medical reform year, that is the end of March this year, the health departments of all provinces (regions, cities) and relevant departments of the Ministry of Health will have made evaluations according to the responsibility certificates, and implemented the accountability system, and circulate a notice of commendation for those that have accomplished the tasks successfully, and investigate and affix the responsibility for those that haven't fulfilled the tasks appropriately. All in all, I hope all responsibility units should practically fulfill the commitments.

(2) Improving ability of communication and coordination and forming joint effort to promote reform. The wider the field that the health work and tasks of reform have involved, the more the ability of communication and coordination we have to improve. Practice indicates that strengthening cooperation of government departments and forming joint working efforts under the leadership of the government is a major guarantee to implement tasks of medical reform. The leadership system of medical reform in which the central and many local departments have engaged also created favorable conditions for coordination and communication among different departments. Within this coordination mechanism, health departments should proceed from the whole situation, take the initiative at work, analyze progress of the tasks without delay, find out prominent problems, take the advice of relevant departments, put forward suggestions to the medical reform leading group in due time, build consensus, formulate policies and measures to solve problems and promote the work, and make efforts to create a favorable working atmosphere of mutual respect, mutual support, timely communication and cooperation among different departments.

Currently, the main problems that exist in the execution of funds for the medical reform are as follows: first, the overall progress of the execution of funds for the medical reform fails to live up to the requirements for progress formulated by financial departments; second, the local supporting funds couldn't be achieved sufficiently and funds for project implementation are in shortage; third, the scheme design of part of the projects is not scientific and reasonable enough. Health departments should take the initiative to coordinate with relevant departments, and practically improve the efficiency of allocation of funds for medical reform, and strengthen supervision of capital, and speed up funds execution. After the allocation of the Central funds for medical reform, the Ministry of health will issue the management plans for relevant tasks of medical reform with 10 working days; after receiving the plans, health administrative departments at province level should take the initiative to coordinate with the financial departments at the same level within 10 working days to issue specific plans for project implementation to relevant lower-level departments or project implementation units at the same level. Performance appraisal should be strengthened and the system of the arrangement and appropriation of funds linking up with the implementation of tasks should be established. Long-acting supervision mechanism should be improved; the supervisory role of many aspects including audit institutions, social intermediary organizations and the general public should be given full play; efforts of joint supervision and inspection by health and financial departments, etc. should be strengthened; progress of funds allocation and project implementation should be accelerated; funds security should be guaranteed; the efficiency of capital utilization should be raised.

(3) Strengthening investigation and study and summarizing and popularizing experience. Policies and tasks of medical reform should be implemented eventually at grass-roots level; difficulties and problems in medical reform are mainly reflected at grass-roots level; working experiences are often created at grass-roots level. Leading comrades of health administrative departments at all levels should establish the system of contact points for medical reform, and go grass roots more often to conduct investigation and study, and put more time and energy into investigating the real truth, giving the feasible advice and handling concrete affairs in a down-to-earth manner. Leading comrades should take the initiative to make friends with the cadres and ordinary people at the frontline, and be adept in looking at problems from their perspective and taking their advice and work collaboratively to study and solve problems in practical work. Beneficial experience and practice created by grass-roots units that conforms to the spirits of medical reform and withstands the test of practice and can be universally applied should be found out without delay and summarized and further popularized; the function of advanced areas in policy guidance, experience demonstration and pace setting should be brought into full play. The propaganda work of and communication of information for medical reform should be

strengthened; the role of mass media should be given full play; reform experience and progress should be publicized in time; particularly through the publicity of results of medical reform, the whole society would get to know and get involved in and support the medical reform, thus continuously building up the confidence in reform.

(4) Arousing the enthusiasm of medical personnel and bringing into full play their role as the major driving force in medical reform. The vast majority of medical personnel are the backbone force in health reform and development, on which the accomplishment of tasks of medical reform and realization of targets of medical reform mainly depends. The important speech delivered by General Secretary Hu Jintao at the 20th collective learning activity of the 17th Political Bureau of the CPC Central Committee fully appreciates the spirits of the vast majority of medical staff who cherish their posts and devote wholeheartedly to their work and fully appreciate the significant contribution made by the medical staff who improve people's health. It is the obligatory responsibility of governments and health administrative departments at all levels to take good care of and to well stabilize and develop this team. The first is to establish and improve a more feasible and effective talent training mechanism and to form a favorable talent growth environment for excellent talents to stand out. The resident doctor standardized training system and the general practitioner training system should be improved and implemented; more suitable talents should be trained for grass roots to enrich the medical and health care team at grass-roots level; the basic medical and health service demand of the ordinary people should be satisfied. Medical staff should be encouraged and supported to continuously upgrade their own quality and raise their service level through various ways including further study and clinical research. Conditions should be actively created and construction of talent echelon should be strengthened, with an emphasis not only on the training of grass-roots health talents but also on the training of top talents who lead the development of medical science. The second is to care for the vital interests of medical staff, and to establish a scientific and reasonable incentive mechanism, and to actively and steadily push forward the reform of the compensation mechanism and income distribution system of medical institutions to make the income of medical staff link up with the quality and quantity of work and satisfaction of people, and to gradually establish an income distribution system that corresponds with the value of medical labor and adapts to the level of economic and social development. This year, pilot reforms in public hospital will universally put into practice measures that benefit people including high-quality nursing, which is bound to increase the working intensity and pressure of medical personnel. Thus, health departments should report to government leaders without delay and strive to put forward explicit policies and measures in the aspects including reasonably increasing the staffing of medical personnel especially of

the nurses at the clinical frontline, increasing the technical service income of medical personnel and implementing corresponding treatment and subsidies. The third is to vigorously publicize the target, tasks and various requirements of medical reform within the health system, and to lead medical personnel to closely integrate their duties and medical reform tasks and give full play to their subjective initiatives to contribute ideas and exert efforts for medical reform and make dedications in the aspects including innovating mechanism, strengthening management, improving service and for the convenience and benefit of people. The fourth is to optimize the practice environment and conditions for medical staff and to build a healthy and harmonious doctor-patient relationship. The mechanism for third-party mediation in medical dispute should be established and the medical liability insurance and medical treatment unexpected injury insurance should be actively developed. The activity to establish "peaceful hospital" should be carried on and medical disturbance should be severely punished to protect the legal rights and interests of medical staff.

(5) Establishing a risk assessment mechanism of social stability for major issues in the health system. Establishing a risk assessment mechanism of social stability for major issues in the health system is an important measure to resolve social conflicts and maintain social stability, and is of great significance in raising consciousness of health administrative departments and medical institutions at all levels and of various kinds to defend the rights and interests of people's health and in ensuring healthy development of medical and health services and realization of the target of medical reform. Currently, health administrative departments and medical institutions at all levels and of various kinds should implement risk assessment for the major policy decisions, the important policy adjustment, the key working measures, formulation of major projects and management of public affairs that concern people's health rights and vital interests in the aspects including legitimacy, rationality, feasibility, security, controllability, in accordance with the principle of "who is in charge is who takes responsibility is who makes decision is who makes evaluation", and gradually form a long-term effective mechanism. The medical reform involves adjustments of complicated interest relations and different interest subjects may have different understanding and reaction to policies and measures of medical reform; thus, improper treatment may also give rise to new conflicts and contradictions and even unstable factors. Therefore, the possible problems that might be triggered should be predicted in advance before the full implementation of some measures of medical reform and preventive measures should be taken to guard against possible troubles. Establishing a risk assessment mechanism is a new task; health departments in all localities must attach highly importance and strive to prevent and reduce unstable factors in society at the source, thus creating a harmonious internal and external

environment for health reform and development.

VI. Strengthening the Party building and provide political guarantee for the healthy and sustainable development of health reform and health services

The 17th Central Committee of the Party has made overall arrangement of the new and great project of the Party building that is propelled by spirit of reform and innovation in an all-round manner. Deepening the implementation of studying and practicing the Scientific Outlook on Development and activities of striving for excellence in performance are important measures of carrying out this overall arrangement and strengthen and improve the Party building under new circumstances. In order to fulfill various recent tasks of deepening medical reform on schedule, the Party building should be practically strengthened and the role of the Party organizations as the core of leadership in deepening medical reform and promote the scientific development of health services should be given further play.

(1) Integrating activities of striving for excellence in performance and medical reform and providing impetus to fulfill tasks of medical reform. Since May of 2010, the Party organizations of all levels in the national medical and health system have insisted on the integration of striving for excellence in performance with implementing tasks of medical reform and with the central task within their own units, and carried out activities of striving for excellence in performance in an all-round and in-depth manner, and created a large amount of beneficial experience and practice, achieved remarkable phased results, according to the unified arrangements and requirements of the Central Government.

This year, health departments of all levels should further deepen the implementation of activities of striving for excellence in performance according to the unified the arrangements. Focusing on the center and promoting the work should continue to serve as the foothold; implementation of activities of striving for excellence in performance and fulfillment of tasks of medical reform should be more closely integrated; efforts should be put in improving the competence of leading groups and Party members who hold leading positions at all levels; the scientific development of health services and the medical reform should be guaranteed to make solid progress. The goal, theme, method and carrier of the activities should be determined in accordance of the practical health services, tightly focusing on deepening the medical reform; the vast majority of Party members and cadres and workers should be led to make commitments, fulfill commitments and strive for excellence in performance keeping a foothold on positions.

(2) Strengthening construction of Party organizations at grass-roots level and

bringing into play their role as combat fortress in fulfilling major tasks of health service. On the whole, Party organizations in national health system have been comparatively well constructed, however, the Party building of medical and health units at grass-roots level still needs to be further strengthening, in the face of arduous tasks of deepening medical reform. The health system should improve the construction of grass-roots Party organizations and promote innovations in Party building at grass-roots level and enhance the vitality of the team of grass-roots Party members who hold leading positions, in accordance with reality, under the leadership of local Party committees and with the support of organization departments. Construction of the Party organization itself should be strengthened; awareness of Party members should be raised; the Party spirit exercise should be intensified; cohesion and combat effectiveness of Party organizations should be enhanced. The leading cadres at grass-roots level should bring into full play the leading role as backbone and the vast majority of Communist Party members should bring into full play the vanguard and exemplary role, thus contributing to the fulfillment of the central task of health system and to commemorate the 90th anniversary of the CPC with excellent results.

(3) Strengthening construction of medical ethics and strive to form a good atmosphere of learning from the advanced model and competing to be the advanced model. Medical ethics is an important indicator of the evaluation of health services and the examination of purpose and consciousness by the general public and should be paid constant attention to. Recently, the Central leading comrades have made important instructions, requiring more emphasis on construction and strengthening of medical ethics in combination with deepening the medical reform. National health system should earnestly implement the spirit of the Central Government and put construction of medical ethics in a more prominent position, with close integration of the promotion of central task and the strengthening of construction of spiritual civilization, to obtain further achievements based on the previous work. The assessment system of medical ethics should be earnestly implemented; medical and health service level should be raised; medical ethics should be improved; the professionalism of having heart go out to people's health and caring for patients' life should be built; medical and health workers should be encouraged and led to devote to their duties with a keen sense of responsibility. The anti-corruption construction of health system should be promoted in an in-depth manner; centralized procurement of drugs and medical equipment should be further standardized; construction of ethics across the health profession should be vigorously strengthened; commercial bribery in the field of drug procurement and sales should be governed in an in-depth manner; efforts should be put in solving the prominent problems that threatened people's interests

in medicine purchase and sale and the medical services; construction of spiritual civilization across the profession should be promoted.

Here, it should be especially emphasized that we must further strengthen construction of the punishment and prevention system against corruption and firmly establish the ideological and moral line of defense against corruption and degeneration. Recently, phenomena including demanding kickbacks in the field of medicine purchase and sale and receiving red packets during medical services have aroused wide public concern. These behaviors have severely injured the interests of patients and corrupted the image of the health team, exerting extremely unfavorable influence on the healthy atmosphere of deepening medical education that is being formed gradually and in which we have put enormous efforts. Different regions should learn by analogy in combination with the cases that have happened and deepen implementation of one activity of education of ethics across the profession and clean politics, and investigate strictly the accountability of and punish with due severity the black sheep and criminals who have severely injured people's interest. To rectify the evil trends across the profession is a long-term task that needs constant attention. Health administrative departments at all levels must keep a cool head and a clear sense of right and wrong, never slackening investigations and punishments of the behaviors of taking advantage of the authority for improper benefits during work owing to the existing problems of health institutions in the aspects including compensation policy and personnel distribution system. As for the former, great efforts should be put to solve the problems gradually through reform; as for the latter, we should fight resolutely without any mercy.

We should be adept in discovering and establishing advanced role models. Advanced deeds and role models have emerged in large numbers in the health system at various periods of revolution and construction of our country. We should take the opportunity of striving for excellence in performance, and establish advanced role models around us and publicize their advanced deeds, and push forward a batch of typical role models on behalf of the advanced images of health system to the whole country, and guide and educate the vast majority of Party members, cadres and workers to learn from, adore, strive to be and catch up with and surpass role models. Since last year, different regions have put emphasis on discovering and publicizing advanced role models and have achieved positive results. The health system in Sichuan province has vigorously carried out the activity of "learning from Yang Yong, working as safeguard, competing for contribution and made efforts in activities of striving for excellence in performance to mold the "four-have" cadres who have stamina in persisting in scientific development, have thoughts in planning scientific development, have passion in promoting scientific development and have contribution in realizing scientific development. Provinces and cities including Beijing, Tianjin, Hebei, Shanxi, Shanghai, Zhejiang, Shandong and Guangdong have discovered and established a batch of advanced role models who are fulfilling their duties and making selfless dedication through various forms such as public selection, medium publicity, touring report, not only helping the vast majority of Party members set goals and direction and voluntarily fulfill their duties according to the standard of role models but also helping to win the understanding and support for medical and health services by people from all walks of life. This year, health system across the whole country should carry out the selection activity of "excellent Party members and excellent Party affair workers, advanced grass-roots Party organizations" in an in-depth manner, and promote the overall rise of ideological, moral and working level.

Finally, I would like to set forth some opinions on implementation of the spirit of this conference.

First, doing well in reporting and communication. I hope that comrades would report the spirit of this conference and priority tasks of this year to the Party committee and government leaders in time when returning back, and introduce information to medical reform leading group and relevant departments in local areas, striving to win over the attention and support of the Party committee and governments and the assistance and coordination of relevant departments.

Second, conveying and studying the conference spirit earnestly. Health work conferences in local areas should be held in different regions with the least possible delay to convey the spirit of national health work conference and make respective and practical arrangements for the fulfillments of various tasks of this year.

Third, putting great emphasis on the implementation of work. Arrangements of priority medical reform work of the year 2011 will soon be issued. In all localities, priority tasks and loopholes in local areas should be put great emphasis and implementation schemes and work arrangements should be refined according to the overall requirements, for early arrangement, early start-up and early implementation.

Fourth, guaranteeing fulfillment of the annual task of medical reform. After this conference, different provinces (regions, cities) should compare the responsibility certificates signed with the State Council and the specific tasks of local health departments according to the latest monitored results of the progress of medical reform, and make an overall analysis earnestly, and pinpoint the distance and insufficiency, and make the most of the three-month period of time, and make persistent efforts, striving to guarantee the fulfillment of annual working target by the scheduled time.

Comrades, in the period of the 12th Five-Year Plan, our country is facing a rare historic opportunity of health reform and development. The health system across the whole country should unite closely around the CPC Central Committee with Comrade Hu Jintao as General Secretary, earnestly implement the spirit of the fifth Plenary Session of the 17th CPC Central Committee, further study and practice the Scientific Outlook on Development, proceed with confidence, keep up our spirits, forge ahead with determination, make solid progress in our work, comprehensively deepen reform of the pharmaceutical and health care systems, speed up establishment of the basic medical and health care systems, promote the scientific development of the health cause, and strive to realize the goal of providing basic medical and health care services for all people and improve the quality of health of the whole nation!

(Song Yang, Chen Ying)

10. A Speech Delivered by Secretary of the Party Group of Ministry of Health and Vice Minister of Health, Zhang Mao, on Accelerating Comprehensive Reform in Medical Health Institutions at Grassroots at a Teleconference (May 26, 2011)

The purpose of the conference is to carry out and implement the national work conference spirit of medical reform of this year and the important instructions of Vice Premier Li Keqiang, further comb problems, act appropriately to the situation, concentrate to assault fortified positions and overcome difficulties and accelerate comprehensive reform in medical health institutions at grassroots. Just now, comrades from Anhui Province, Heilongjiang Province and Sichuan Province made very good introductions of their experience respectively, which embodied the reform spirit of subjective initiative, setting their wits to work, braveness in exploration, and positive conduct in all prefectures in the implementation of the national policy of medical reform. In his speech, Comrade Sun Zhigang elaborated the importance and urgency of the comprehensive reform at grassroots, focused on grasping advantageous opportunities, seizing the key links and implementing goal responsibility. I could not agree more with him. Next, I'll speak more suggestions.

I. Deepen the Understanding of the Importance and Urgency of the Comprehensive Reform in Medical Health Institutions at Grassroots

(1) Acceleration of the comprehensive reform in medical health institutions at grassroots is the important guarantee for carrying out the state's basic drug system.

The establishment of the state's basic drug system is a comprehensive reform, including multiple links of basic drug selection, production, circulation, and use, which involves the two lines of drugs and medical institutions, and the purpose is to benefit the masses of people. When the basic drug supply system is asked to be reshaped, new requirements for various mechanisms of subsidy, personnel and income distribution in medical health institutions at grassroots were raised as well. The acceleration of the comprehensive reform in medical health institutions at grassroots completely breaks the old developing mode of "subsiding hospitals with drugs" in medical health institutions at grassroots and the establishment of a new dynamic mechanism for maintaining public welfare, mobilizing initiative, guaranteeing sustainable development acts the key to ensure the implementation of the state's basic drug system, and the foundation of establishing the basic medical health system with Chinese characteristics. Currently, our national basic drug system progresses very fast, which urges the corresponding reform in medical health institutions at grassroots so to accommodate the developmental situation of the basic drug system and feasibly reduce the burden of seeking medical treatment for the masses of people.

(2) The acceleration of the comprehensive reform in medical health institutions at grassroots is the internal requirements of "safeguarding the basic, strengthening the grassroots and establishing the mechanism".

At the national work conference on deepening reform this year, Vice Premier Li Keqiang stressed once again that "safeguarding the basic, strengthening the grassroots and establishing the mechanism" is the basic principle and the train of thought on development, and the center of gravity for medical reform, which required us to make the basic outstanding, focus on key work and ensure the sustainability. The service in medical health institutions at grassroots covers the widest areas, involves the most people and it is one of the important carriers of the implementations of all tasks in medical reform. Starting with the implementation of the state's basic drug system, we should make the establishment of new mechanism as the important task, establish management system and operation mechanism in medical health institutions at grassroots, reflecting public welfare by means of the comprehensive reform on procurement mechanism of the basic drugs, input compensation mechanism and personnel distribution mechanism, mobilize enthusiasm of medical workers, improve service ability and service quality and turn the state's input in medical reform into the benefits enjoyed by the masses of people.

(3) The acceleration of the comprehensive reform in medical health institutions at grassroots is the important link to ensure the overall realization of the goals of medical reform.

The goal of deepening medical reform is to provide the basic medical health system as a public product for all the people and make everybody enjoy the basic medical health service. Medical reform needs to have priority of promotion at different stages and the fairness must be dealt with before everything. Currently, the reform has been in the stage of overall implementation in which fortified positions are assaulted and difficulties overcome. The difficult point and the main direction of the attack this year is the implementation of the basic drug system and the establishment of new operation mechanism in medical health institutions at grassroots, and the reform in public hospitals. If the mechanism construction of the comprehensive reform in medical health institutions at grassroots is not focused on and the new breakthrough is not made in some key fields, the basic drug system will not be truly set up at grassroots, the masses of people will not get the benefit from the reform, the reform will not be in a benign orbit and it will be very difficult to finish the tasks of medical reform.

II. Deepen Analysis and Judge Correctly the Situation of the Comprehensive Reform in Medical Health Institutions at Grassroots

Now, all prefectures are positively promoting medical reform and some good practices and good experience have been created. Comrade Zhigang personally went to 18 provinces to make investigations, the other comrades and I from Ministry of Health have been to many places to learn about the situations, on which we made analyses and judgment with the collected data from monitoring system of medical reform. Comrade Zhigang has just mentioned that medical reform nationwide is generally progressing smoothly with good momentum. However, mechanism building obviously lagged behind, and particularly, the comprehensive reform at grassroots remarkably lagged behind the coverage expansion of the basic drug system.

By the end of March, in 31 provinces (regions and cities) and Xinjiang Production and Construction Corps, the basic drug system had been practiced in 82% medical health institutions at grassroots run by the governments, and the whole coverage at grassroots had been realized in 16 princes and cities of Anhui, Tianjin, Ningxia and others. The basic drug system is also practiced in nongovernmental medical health system at grassroots and the pilot village clinics in Chongqing, Shandong, Qinghai and other places.

Although the state's basic drug system is practiced in most prefectures according to the state's requirements, there is still a lot more to do in the establishments of new drug procurement mechanism, new subsiding mechanism, new personnel mechanism, and new income distribution mechanism. From the establishment of new drug procurement mechanism, all provinces should have distributed new documents of drug procurement and the schemes for implementation by the end of last year according to the document requirements of the state's office, and finished the centralized procurement in one procurement cycle. But until now, only 14 provinces distributed the concrete methods in accordance with the requirements, 6 of which initiated the centralized procurement, the other provinces haven't yet issued the related documents. Though some provinces have issued the related documents, the related policies and measures, the requirements of technical operation haven't been implemented and quantity purchase has not been practiced, which meant a great distance from the specified schedule and the concrete requirements, low enthusiasm, emotions of fear, anxiety of pressure and challenge, the unwillingness to confront the problems at deeper level and the necessity for the improvement. From the comprehensive reform in medical health institution at grassroots, 25 provinces have issued the standards for staffing sizes in township health centers and institutions; the recruitment of hospital president has been practiced in 40.7% township health centers, and post employment been practiced in 70.3% township health centers run by the governments and 60.1% community health service centers. Performance salary has basically been cashed in 18 provinces, the proportion of the authorized medical health institutions practicing performance salary at grassroots run by the offices of the governments is 52.5%, the top five are Anhui Province, Heilongjiang Province, Shaanxi Province, Fujian Province and Yunnan Province with performance salary practice exceeding 90%, but the performance salary practice in the last five provinces has not reached 30%. In general, all prefectures did a lot of work in promoting the comprehensive reform in medical health institution at grassroots and the establishment of new operation mechanism, and obtained certain achievements. However, there is a great distance from the requirements of the Central Government and of medical reform task, especially the expectations of the masses of people and a large number of medical workers. Some prefectures haven't made or issued the related policies and measures while others distributed the related documents but the promotion advances slowly. Still others haven't issued measures for the implementation *of Opinions on Establishing and Perfecting the Subsiding Mechanism in Medical Health Institutions at Grassroots by General Office of the State Council*. Therefore, multi-channel subsidies can not be effectively implemented, full specified amount of appropriate subsidies can not be timely made. The reform of medical insurance payment progresses slowly, which impacts institution operation and the enthusiasm of the staff members. The reform of personnel system and distribution system in some provinces lags behind, the distribution system is unreasonable, the examination is not quite standardized and the effective restraint and incentive mechanism are not sufficient. The integrated management of rural health service has not been launched in some places, township health centers don't have enough managerial methods for financial revenues and expenditures, drug distribution and personnel allocation of village clinics. Rural linkage of the basic drug system is not realized in other places, resulting in the prices in village clinics higher than those in township health centers and it is difficult for farmers to get benefits from medical reform in the neighborhood.

Three categories of the situations about the progress and the problems in the promotion of the basic drug system in all places and the comprehensive reform in medical health institutions at grassroots can be roughly divided. The first one is that the comprehension of the policy and documents is in place, the direction is clarified, the leadership is powerful, the fast deployment and implementation is made according to the requirements of annual tasks, the organization is thorough, the measures are appropriate, all work of the comprehensive reform is completely coordinated and promoted and the reform achievements are striking. The second one is that the comprehension of the policies and the spirits of the documents is not deep enough, the direction is not quite clear, the overall consideration is not careful, the methods are not many, some of the "compulsory exercises" are done with the propulsion of single project, the comprehensive reform is not practiced and the new mechanism is not established. The third one is that the understanding is not sufficient, the enthusiasm is not high, there is emotion of fear, everything stays at the research level, and the reform progresses slowly and lags behind obviously. From the whole country, the proportion of the latter two cases is big, which, from one side, reflects the complexities and urgency of the reform. The experience from the regions with good work progress is summarized, particularly, the experience introduced at today's conference by Anhui Province, Heilongjiang Province, Sichuan Province and others. We think that there are three points are worth learning and using for reference by all places. The first one is that the Party Committees and the governments should attach great importance, and all departments cooperate closely. Because the main leaders from these places understand the polices and requirements of medical reform deeply, fully realize that the core of medical reform is the innovation of system mechanism and judge soberly the importance, urgency and complexity of the task, they pay great attention to the related work, concern themselves with it, make deployment personally, and the comrades in charge also take serious responsibility, strengthen the implementation, which forms a strong system of organization and leadership. Spontaneously, these prefectures have realized that the comprehensive reform in medical health institutions at grassroots is a systematic project so the Party committees and the governments established working mechanism of coordinated linkage, all the related departments of development and reform, health, finance, personnel and society, and staffing size take their own responsibilities, and cooperate whole heartedly, which guarantees forcefully the good implementation of the tasks of the comprehensive reform in medical health institutions at grassroots. The second one is to grasp the reform spirit correctly and clarify the contents and requirements of mechanism building. These prefectures didn't understand that the reform is simply to increase investment, nor satisfied with fundamental construction and hardware improvement but study and understand the spirits of national working conference on medical reform and the speech by Vice Premier Li Keqiang, realize that mechanism innovation is the core contents of the comprehensive in medical health institutions at grassroots. In accordance with the overall construction of new drug procurement mechanism and new subsiding mechanism, they establish new personnel mechanism and new income distribution mechanism with the purpose of maintaining public welfare, mobilizing enthusiasm, and ensuring the new mechanism for sustainable operation. They also fully realize the internal relations between these mechanisms so they make considerations planned as a whole, comprehensive planning, and coordinated promotion. The third one is innovate thinking, and explore courageously the appropriate reform paths and methods. Going down to the units at grassroots for investigation and research is a good way to feasibly understand and concretely implement the tasks of the comprehensive reform at grassroots. In promoting the comprehensive reform in medical health institutions at grassroots, these prefectures focus on in-depth investigation and research, full argumentation, and grasp comprehensively work situation and difficulties in local places, organize the relevant departments to study and use good methods in other provinces as reference, combine with local realities, innovate the train of thought directing at the existing problems, practice and explore courageously, make appropriate reform paths and methods, plan and arrange carefully, operate elaborately, and ensure the steady promotion of the comprehensive reform. The experience is feasible and effective so all the places are expected to make a careful control study, detect the existing prominent problems and hold on to the implementation of the key links.

Ⅲ. Assault Fortified Positions and Overcome Difficulties, and Make an All-out Promotion of the Comprehensive Reform in Medical Health Institutions at Grassroots

This year is the year of assaulting fortified positions in medical reform, time is tight, and the tasks are heavy. In order to complete the annual tasks of medical reform and the recent work targets of medical reform in the next three years, and then to lay a good foundation for achieving the work targets of medical reform in the Twelfth five-Year Plan, we must recognize the situation, keep up our spirits, go all out to assault fortified positions and overcome difficulties. Next, I'm going to put forward some requirements for the feasible promotion of the comprehensive reform in medical health institutions at grassroots.

(1) Put the understanding of the promotion of the basic drugs system and the comprehensive reform in medical health institutions at grassroots in place, which is the touch task to be completed in all places this year. The arrangements for this year's medical work clarified the provisions in the promotion of the basic drug system and the comprehensive reform in medical health institutions at grassroots. The great significance of the work promotion for the overall situation of medical reform was emphasized at national working conference on medical reform and the clarified deployment was made. Vice-premier Li Keqiang has made the important instructions in his speeches at the conferences for many times, and now we are holding the special video-telephone conference on the work promotion, which demonstrates our determinations for the work promotion of the Central Government. We must fully understand that the work can't be delayed and it should be done early rather than late. Documents for subsiding mechanisms of medical health institution at grassroots have been issued, policies and measures have been clarified, and the conditions for the overall promotion of the comprehensive reform in medical health institutions at grassroots have been ready. The increase of the input in medical funds by the country has provided a rare opportunity for the work promotion. If we don't start early, the opportunity will be missed and the reform will be in passivity. What's more, the later we start the work, the more input will be increased and the original interests pattern and original mechanism will be fixed, thus the reform cost and reform difficulty will be increased and the reform results will be counteracted by the old mechanisms or all our previous efforts be wasted. In addition, we must fully understand that the work is feasible and effective. Although reform promotion has brought us unprecedented new problems and new challenges, and with the reform deepening, more contradictions will be touched involving deeper interest adjustment, there have already been clearer and clearer reform ideas, trains of thought and working methods, the practice in some places has shown the work is feasible and effective, all prefectures have offered more and more precious experience for reference. Therefore, we shouldn't have too many concerns and the fear of emotions. If we can clarify the direction, get out of this mess, strengthen the leadership, intensify organization, arrange carefully, take powerful measures, we can promote the comprehensive reform, enhance the vitality in medical health institutions at grassroots and let the masses of the people enjoy the achievements of medical reform.

(2) Take targeted measures according to practical situations. We should use the experience and methods in other provinces for reference and launch the comprehensive reform suitable for local places in medical health institutions at grassroots in accordance with the practice of all places. We should clarify main

problems, and take targeted strategies and measures. In the places with rather obvious reform effects of the overall coordinated promotion of the comprehensive reform, the key work is to solidify and expand reform achievements, the evaluation on all links of reform should be made, the effective methods and experience for reform be summarized and expanded, the results be constantly solidified and expanded, measures taken actively, new situations, new problems and new mechanisms be set up firmly and operated healthily. For the places with uneven reform advancement, the key work is to form the joint effort and promote coordinately. The importance of coordination in the comprehensive reform planned as a whole must be fully understood and the trigger of the new and unnecessary conflicts be prevented. Train of thought should be made clear, the problems be located, the unified planning and the comprehensive coordination be strengthened, reform direction and key breakthroughs be clarified, the most feasible solutions be put into effect and the promotion of the work which hasn't been carried out should be fastened. For the places with slow development and obvious hysteresis, the thoughts should be unified for the enhancement of work. Particularly, for the places with unissued relevant documents or only the documents, the train of thought must be extended and the work be intensified to do all one can to catch up or the advancement of national medical reform will be hampered. Therefore, we will strengthen the guidance, supervision and inspection on these places from the national level.

(3) The tasks of reform should be refined and carried out seriously. In fastening the whole coverage of the basic drug system at grassroots, all places, in principle, should have realized the whole coverage of the basic drug system by the end of September. The places with conditions should be encouraged to involve village clinics and the nongovernmental medical health institutions at grassroots into the basic drug system. In the accelerating establishment of the standardized procurement mechanism, with *The Guiding Opinions on the Establishment and Standardization of the Basic Drug Procurement Mechanism in Medical Health Institutions at Grassroots* as a starting point, the systems like the centralized purchasing system at provincial level should be practiced, the standardized drug procurement mechanism be established, the relevant policies and the requirements for technical operation be implemented, transparent operation and sunny operation be adhered to so as to ensure that the safe and effective basic drugs with reasonable prices are timely provided. In the feasible implementation of subsiding policies, and according to the requirements of the documents by the State Council, the offsetting of special subsidy by the financial departments was brought into play, the reasonable subsidy was provided for village clinics and medical health institutions at grassroots practicing the basic drug system, the important subsiding function of medical insurance payment was put into effect,

the steady, long-term effective multi-channel subsiding mechanism was established in medical health institutions at grassroots with active coordination and effective cooperation. In addition, starting from the key point, the existence and development of village clinics should be supported to ensure a strong net bottom of medical health service system at rural grassroots. In the reform promotion of personnel system and income distribution system, the establishment of staffing size should be completed as soon as possible, on this basis, scientific posting, personnel employment and post competition be practiced; And the staffing mechanism of fixed staffing size and post with unfixed personnel, promotion and demotion, and coming and leaving be practiced. Spontaneously, the system of performance salary in medical health institutions at grassroots practicing the basic drug system should be put in place, synchronizing the reform on income distribution system by adhering to the optimal pains to optimal return, and widening differences in personal income so as to mobilize staff enthusiasm. In the establishment of evaluation and incentive mechanism of medical health institutions at grassroots, all places should fasten the formation of performance evaluation methods for the comprehensive quantification examination in accordance with the indexes of management performance, the quantity and quality of basic medical service and public health service, the satisfactory degree of service object, health status of the residents and so on. Talent training for medical health institutions at grassroots must be intensified. The relevant policies should be perfected to make targets and plans for the training of general practitioners as the focal point, all kinds of education training programs planned as a whole be implemented, security measures strengthened, the shortage of grassroots talents be solved in the mechanism, the management ability enhancement, especially the ability of policy understanding and implementation of the leaders in medical health institutions at grassroots be focused on in order to ensure that medical reform policy is put into effect. In short, various influences brought by benefit pattern adjustment must be attached great importance to so that in-depth and meticulous work is done well, and smooth conversion mechanism and smooth running of the institutions are ensured.

Finally, I'll take the opportunity to make some concrete requirements for health system.

Ministry of Health should allow the full play of subjective initiative. In 67 working indexes of 17 tasks of medical reform this year, Ministry of Health will take the lead in 46 indexes and cooperate in 18, which is the main battlefield of medical reform. Health administrative departments at all levels are the main organizers, pushers and practitioners while medical workers are the important force to realize the reform goals. In the case of supporting policies and government investment in place, the work of health departments relates to the success or failure of medical reform. At the working conference of medical reform of this year, Vice-premier Li Keqiang made a special emphasis on the important roles of the main battlefield of health departments and the main force of medical workers in his speech, which inspired all the medical departments. In the promotion of the basic drug system and the comprehensive reform in medical health institutions at grassroots, health administrative departments at all levels and all medical workers should keep up the spirits, strengthen the sense of responsibility and the sense of mission, throw themselves willingly and voluntarily into reform promotion, orderly promote all work, coordinate planned as a whole and cooperate closely. The comprehensive reform at grassroots, covering a wide range and having great influence, asks for the cooperation from all sides. Proceeding from the whole situation, health departments, whether taking the lead in work or cooperating with other departments, should have the clear awareness of the urgent medical situation, improve ideological understanding, keep the spirit to make progress, improve work style, actively contact and coordinate with the relevant departments, strengthen coordination and communication, carefully listen to the opinions of all the relevant departments, build consensus, solicit support, jointly promote the comprehensive reform at grassroots and establish a new operation mechanism. They should also clarify responsibilities and implement tasks. Health departments at all levels should refine and decompose tasks of medical reform, know well the responsibilities of medical health institutions of all kinds at all levels, the implementation progress and the measures for rewards and punishments. The main leaders from health administrative departments at provincial level should take the command personally to realize, quantize and refine work plans, carry out the responsibilities to each person. Risk assessment mechanism must be established and perfected, public opinions and feelings be paid close attention to, the related preplans be done well. Simultaneously, performance evaluation must be strengthened, regular supervision and inspection of work implementation progress, quantity completion and service quality be organized.

Comrades, the basic drug system and the comprehensive reform in medical health institutions at grassroots relate to the whole situation of medical reform, and to the fundamental interests of the masses of people. We believe that as long as our understanding is in place, the leaders pay attention to, the measures are powerful, do real practice and solid work and let everyone's intelligence into full play, we can build up a new operation mechanism of maintaining public welfare, mobilizing enthusiasm, and ensuring sustainability and realize all goals of medical reform.

(Ji Chenglian)

11. Strengthen and Improve Health News Propaganda to Provide the Development of Health Reform with Strong Support of Thought and Public Opinion

—A Speech Given by Zhang Mao, Secretary of the Party Group of Ministry of Health and Vice Minister of Health, at 2011 National Meeting on Health News (November 15, 2011)

The national work conference on health news propaganda is held under the situation of further study of the spirit of the 6th plenary session of the 17th National Congress of the CPC by health system nationwide. This conference signifies in mobilizing and encouraging national health system to seriously carry out and implement the spirit of the session, building a good social atmosphere for reform promotion, and providing better service for people's health, socialism and the overall work situation of the Party and the state.

This morning, Minister Chen Zhu made an important speech, taking all the progress and development in health news propaganda into retrospect, analyzed deeply the situation facing us and made the overall deployment of the work in next period. The leaders from the office of the Central Government for External Propaganda introduced the situations and tasks of news propaganda in our country. Just now, health departments from Beijing, Shanghai, Hubei and Gansu, offices of health newspaper, and Peking Union Medical College Hospital made speeches at the conference. Learning good experience from each other and using good practice for reference benefit us in doing a better job in health news propaganda.

Next, I'll speak some suggestions.

I. Firmly Grasp the Correct Orientation of Public Opinion with the Guidance of the Spirit of the 6th Plenary Session of the 17th National Congress of the CPC

The time for the holding of the 6th Plenary Session of the 17th National Congress of the CPC is the 90th anniversary of the founding of the Communist Party of China, which is a significant conference held in the key period of the comprehensive construction of a well-off society and the crucial period of deepening reform and opening up, and accelerating the transformation of economic growth mode. Comprehensive analysis of the current situation and tasks was made at the session, and *Decisions of Several Major Issues on Deepening Reform of Cultural System and Promoting Great Development of Socialist Culture by the Central Committee of the Communist Party of China (hereinafter referred to as Decisions)* was examined, discussed and approved. General Secretary Hu Jintao made an important speech at the session, reviewed and analyzed the work of the Political Bureau of the Central Committee in the past year, profoundly elaborated culture reform and development in the new situation, and made clear requirements on carrying out and implementing the spirit of the session and on doing a good job in all work of the Party and the state. *The Decision* approved at the session made the overall summarization of the rich practice and precious experience in culture reform and development of our country, studied several key issues of the deepening reform of culture system and the promotion of great development and prosperity of socialist culture, put forward the guiding ideology, important policies, target tasks, policy measures, which bears great and far-reaching significance in taking new victory of comprehensive construction of a well-off society and creating a new situation of socialist cause with Chinese characteristics. We must study carefully, understand deeply and fully carry out.

News propaganda is the main channel for culture transmission, lies in special status of the cultural development and plays an important role. Attaching great importance to propaganda and ideological work is fine tradition formed in the practice of revolution, construction and reform for a long time, and also a big advantage of the socialism with Chinese characteristics. *The Decision* at the session emphasized that Marxist view of journalism must be adhered to in the work of news and public opinions, the correct direction be firmly grasped, continuing unification, stability, encouragement and positive publicity be given priority to, mainstream public opinion be extended, and the propaganda on the Party's claims be popularized, promotion of social upright, understanding of social situation and public opinions, guiding of social hot issues, proper channeling of public sentiments in the supervision of public opinion be brought into full play to protect people's rights to know, to participate, to express, and to supervise. Correct guidance of public opinion is the good fortune to the Party and the people, while the wrong guidance of public opinion is the disaster to the Party and the people. As the integral part of propaganda and ideological work of the Party, the correct guidance of public opinion in health news propaganda must be firmly grasped, unification, stability, encouragement and positive publicity be given priority to, themes be made chanted, and voluntary fighting done well so that health news propaganda can serve the construction of health culture, the reform and development of health undertaking, and people's health consciously and actively, and common ideological and moral base for the unity and struggle of health system nationwide be constantly solidified.

(1) Health news propaganda should serve the construction of health culture

Based on the overall layout of the cause of socialism with Chinese characteristics, the *Decision* at the session makes the key study and deployment of culture construction related to economic construction, political construction and social construction.

On making the deployment of the promotion of culture reform and development, the *Decision*, first of all, stresses the promotion of the construction of socialist core value system, explicitly proposes to involve the socialist core value system into the whole process of the construction of national education, the construction of spiritual civilization and the Party construction, which goes through all fields of reform and opening up, and the construction of socialist modernization, is reflected in the creation, production and broadcast of the spiritual and cultural products. Socialist core value system must be adhered to in leading the social ideological trend and the unified guiding ideology, common ideal and belief, strong spiritual power and the basic moral norms must be formed in the whole Party and the whole society.

As an important field of social development and construction, health relates closely not only to the overall situation of economic and social development but to the health of the masses. The concept of health culture we proposed includes industry core value, industry mission, shared vision, medical spirit and professional ethics, whose contents interrelate, interpenetrate, and promote mutually, which is an organic and unified whole, rich ideological and cultural achievement obtained by the cadres and workers in health system in the long-term practice, and an important foundation and spiritual home of the development of health undertaking. China's health undertaking has profound cultural background and rich cultural resources and its development, basing on inheriting the tradition and incorporating things of diverse nature, embodies in unceasing extension and innovation, particularly, in expanding and inheriting the fine tradition of the Chinese medicine, absorbing and integrating the culture results of western medicine, inheriting and carrying forward revolutionary humanitarianism with Bethune spirit as core, to which new connotation is constantly added with time progress and the development of medical practice. Whether it is "virtue of great physician" in traditional medicine or patients first in western medical humanistic thought or healing the wounded and rescuing the dying in revolutionary humanitarianism, they share the common core—people oriented, which is reflected in the respect for life value of people and the attention to physical and mental health of people. It requires that health industry makes the maintenance of public welfare, attaching most importance to people's interests, and guarding health rights of the people the core connotation of culture construction; all medical workers possess a high level of medical technology, noble medical ethics and warm hearts to serve people wholeheartedly; all medical workers adhere to the pursuit of truth and scientific spirit, have the courage to undertake medical service, dare to be the first, make bold innovation in the practice of medical health, have the courage to break through in climbing the peak of medicine and relieve pain for patients. For quite some time, all medical workers always maintain and safeguard the rights of the people's health as the highest mission, cherish posts and devote wholeheartedly to work, work hard, and make important contributions to the improvement of people's health. Facing SARS, H1N1 Influenza A and other grave infectious diseases, earthquake, debris flow and other natural calamities, medical workers are always at the front, sacrifice themselves in rescuing others, make the interpretation of the professional beliefs with sweat, blood and even life, reflect the noble medical ethics and good working style, and demonstrate elegant demeanour and image of people's health guard. Currently, there are phenomena of favoring profit, like focusing on medical technology and ignoring humanistic care, focusing on hardware and environmental improvement and ignoring software and service quality or even excess prescription and over medical treatment. We must attach great importance to and bring the main channel of news propaganda in the broadcast of industry culture into play, increase the positive publicity, find the model deeds and typical experience of all medical health workers in seeing patient as relatives, relieving the pains for patients, and maintaining the health of the people, explore the pursuit of the value and the professional spirit of medical staff in healing the wounded and rescuing the dying, making perfection more perfect and diligently studying profession, set up the model for the industry, show the spirit style and features of health team, shape a good image of the medical staff, motivate and arouse service enthusiasm of all medical workers for people's health.

(2) Health news propaganda must serve the reform and development of health undertaking

The deepening of medical health system reform is the important decision made by the Central Party Committee and the State Council, a major project of people's livelihood benefiting more than 1,300,000,000 and a cosmopolitan problem. Our Party and the Government attach great importance to it, the whole society is concerned about it and the masses of people eagerly look forward to it. Vice-premier Li Keqiang pointed out in his speech at this year's national working conference on deepening medical health system reform that propaganda on medical reform must be carried out in a planned way and with focuses, the vigorous propaganda of the significance of medical reform, and the policies and strategies be strengthened, the results of medical reform and the benefits obtained by the masses of people be publicized, social expectations be reasonably guided, good experience, good practice and good model be actively promoted so that all walks of the society understand, support and participate in the reform. Since the start of medical reform two years ago, we, centering around safeguarding the basic, strengthening the grassroots and establishing the mechanism, have seized the three difficult tasks of promoting the basic medical insurance for all people, establishing the basic drug system, carrying out the pilot reform in public hospitals, pushed all the work sturdily, and obtained the positive results of medical reform. Health news propaganda must center around the difficult and key tasks of medical reform, publicize good experience and good practice in carrying out medical reform tasks in all places and all departments, advanced character and advanced model of medical personnel and medical health institutions at grassroots, active participation in medical reform and care about medical reform by the people, and the respect for medical staff by the people and the benefits of the people from medical reform in order to create a social atmosphere and the environment of public opinion in favor of assaulting fortified positions and overcoming difficulties in medical reform, instigate and cheer for the gradual realization of everyone's enjoying the basic medical health service.

This year is the starting year of the "Twelfth-five Year" Plan. According to the overall deployment covered in the outline of national "Twelfth-five Plan", we seize the hour to study and compile the "Twelfth-five Year" Plan for the development of health undertaking and medical reform programming in the period of the "Twelfth-five Year" Plan. These two plannings cover difficult and key tasks of deepening medical reform, and the deployment and requirements for the promotion of health undertaking development. Therefore, we should enhance propaganda, further unify our thinking, form consensus, make reform go down to the grassroots and into the hearts of the people, provide a strong public opinion support for the reform and development of health undertaking and create favorable conditions for further deepening medical reform and realizing scientific development of health undertaking.

(3) Health news propaganda must serve the improvement of people's health

Right until now, in China, GDP Per capita has reached $4000. The masses of people have more expectations on the improvement in people's living standard and quality and they pay more and more attention to medical treatment and health problems. In a certain sense, if there is no health there will be no better-off life. Life is the most precious to man. Our party, adhering to the people-orientation and governing for the people, must solve the problem of seeking medical treatment for the people and meet their demand for good health. Maintaining people's health and life safety and making health rights of the people realized, maintained and developed is the starting point and foothold. In news propaganda, we must focus on people's new expectations, new demands, the problems of being financially difficult and poverty due to diseases among urban and rural people of poverty, the feasible problems of difficult in seeking medical care and costly in seeing a doctor, press close to reality, life and the masses of people, and constantly intensify affinity, emotional appeal and influence. And we must make the communication of the basic health knowledge, health consciousness improvement and the guidance of the scientific way of life the key contents of propaganda, medical institutions at all levels the base and window for propaganda and popularization of health knowledge, guide all patients to understand medical science scientifically and rationally, share a correct view on the particularity, high technology, risk and limitation of medical service so as to promote more harmonious doctor-patient relationship.

II. Strengthen and Improve Health News Propaganda and Improve the Timeliness, Authority, Credibility, and Influence of Direction of Public Opinion

Truthfulness and accuracy is the life of news and the important source of strengthening the credibility and influence of news propaganda; Correct guidance is the soul of news and the fundamental guarantee of strengthening the guidance and authority of news propaganda. Health news propaganda in the new period is to adhere strictly to the requirements and deployment of the Central Government, strengthen and improve the positive publicity, the propaganda of socialist core value system, objectively analyze and judge health public opinion, correctly guide hot issues of health work, start from the problems of seeking medical care concerned by the people, solve problems and explain puzzles scientifically, and build consensus effectively. In the current and the future period, health system nationwide should rely on the People's Daily, Xinhua News Agency, China Central Television and other mainstream media, make the Ministry of Health web site, "Health", "China's Health" the main positions, pay attention to and make good use of new media, use a variety of means and media resources, and construct a new pattern of coordination planned as a whole, with clear responsibilities, complementary functions, wide coverage and highly efficient health news propaganda.

The first one is to strengthen positive propaganda, and give full scope to the main theme. With medical reform advancing into abyssal region, the strongly reflected problem of seeking medical care by the masses of people has been in the period of assaulting fortified positions and overcoming difficulties. News propaganda must center around the difficult and key points of medical reform, further research psychological characteristics and accept habits of all kinds of audience group under the new situation, combine closely what we advocate with what people need, speak thoroughly the background, basis and target of forming health policies concerned by the masses of people, make clear of tasks, measures, progress and results of health reform development, make people's benefits from medical reform understood, reflect the correct direction in the report of news facts, make more reports on vivid practice of medical reform and more healthy life style of the people, and new look of medical health institutions at grassroots, develop social consensus in people's communication and interaction, defuse maximumly the negative factors and create harmonious atmosphere.

The second one is to strengthen the guidance models, and encourage the morale of the team. Health industry is directly at the front line of the service for the people and endless advanced models emerge in health system, of whom are the great masters of medicine with smashing skills and ethics: Lin Qiaoya, Zhang Xiaoqian, Wu Mengchao, Wang Zhongcheng, Wang Zhenyi and others, and the respected medical workers at grassroots: Zhao Xuefang, Ye Xin, Wu Dengyun, Deng Qiandui, Lan Yun and others. Health news propaganda must combine model propaganda with health culture construction, education of medical ethics and styles, the activities of creating the first and striving for the excellence and "three goods and one satisfaction", bring the model guidance into play, guide the Party members, cadres and all medical workers to strengthen professional sense of honor, fulfill their duties, create the advanced, strive for the best based on post and constantly improve service consciousness and service level. Combining with the activity of "going to the grassroots, turning working style, and changing writing style" launched by news units, health news propaganda must launch incentive plan for health communication, interchange the roles of journalists and medical health workers, organize reporters to go down to the grassroots and reality, interview and write the reports on the advanced models at medical health front of grassroots and the improvement in the conditions of seeking medical care for the people. Health administrative departments at all levels must strive for guidance for news propaganda from competent departments, vigorously seek the support of the news media, set up a work mechanism for model selection and setting up, training, learning and propaganda, and form joint effort for model propaganda through the close cooperation with departments of news propaganda, personnel, party committee, style rectification within the system. With multi channels of media report, recommendation at grassroots, election by the masses of people, organized selection, all places should find out, select and set up a group of advanced models, launch the activities of learning and propaganda, and form a strong positive public opinion on health industry by means of touring reports, media propaganda, organized interview, selection and commendation.

The third one is to strengthen risk communication and maintain social harmony and stability. The 20-word policy of "timeliness and accuracy, publicity and transparency, orderly opening up, effective management and correct guidance" is the effectively summarized experience from the long-term practice of emergency news reports. The emergency mechanism for news release for emergency health news must be constantly perfected, emergency information release be well done, risk communication strengthened, the mechanism for emergency reports and public opinion guidance perfected, effectiveness improved and transparency increased.

Credit maintenance must be adhered to, coordinated development of credit consciousness, image consciousness, communication consciousness and benefit consciousness be strengthened, timely, accurate, open and transparent information be released, public communication be done in a fair and honest attitude and a bridge between the government and the society set up. The timing, tempo and intensity of the public opinion guidance must be well grasped, health policies and measures be propagandized by using health topics, and significant public events concerned by the people, the arrangement of the masses' benefit and the real difficulties be made clear, the prospect of problem solutions explicated, a good image of the government shown, thus, the people will enhance the trust and confidence in the Party and the government. The honest, responsible, open and transparent image of the government can be reflected and enhanced by means of the propaganda on health crisis disposal. Currently, China is in the special stage of economic and social transition, all kinds of social contradictions highlight. Because of the particularity of the medical industry, many social contradictions concentrated in medical health field burst out and even emerge in extreme forms. Health news propaganda must report every grave issues at critical moments, release authority information in the first time, severely condemn violence and crime, effectively protect the lawful rights and interests of the medical staff, expand the positive influence of information, and suppress the spread of noise and undesired sounds.

The fourth one is to strengthen the cultural innovation and consolidate the fields of public opinion. Compared the people's concerns about health undertaking with the importance of health undertaking in social life, the production and creation of health culture produces is relatively weak, which shows that there is still a lack of good products of medical health, and there are few products of high quality with wide spread, big influence and retainment worthiness. We should attach great importance to it and enhance guidance. We should also vigorously promote innovations of idea, system and mechanism, content-form, communication means, type of business and continuously improve style of leadership, organizational ways, working mode and management style so as to make health news propaganda better reflect epochal character, grasp regularity and be full of creativity. In the innovation of propaganda contents, they must keep pace with times, center around health pace, promote all literary and art workers in every field to go to the frontline of medical health, discover news materials on medical reform practice, and create the outstanding works reflecting the rich contents of medical health work. The innovation of ways and methods, new forms, new methods and new ways easily accepted by the masses of people must be actively explored and practiced so much so that the style of writing on the news materials provided to the media must be improved, lively language be used, more fresh and moving stories be reported, and short and highlighted articles written with the characteristics of ideology, guidance, knowledge and readability so as to enhance the affinity and appealing of news information. In the innovation of propaganda methods, the full use of the traditional modes and carriers of transmission of newspapers, radio, television must be made, special importance to the use of the Internet, mobile phones and other emerging media be attached, the online ideological consensus position be initiatively taken, and the right to speak and initiative of network public opinion be firmly grasped.

Ⅲ. Strengthen the Leadership of the Health News Propaganda and Create a Good Atmosphere for Health Reform and Development

Firstly, to strengthen the publicity of the spirit of the Session, and unify thought and action to the central decision and deployment. Currently, the study, propaganda and carrying out General Secretary Hu Jintao's important speech and the Decision of the Plenary Session must be taken as the first political task in current health news propaganda, the thought of the whole system be unified into the spirit of the Plenary Session by means of profound and sturdy propaganda, and wisdom and strength condensed to the deployment of the Session. The vigorous propaganda on the following must be enhanced in accordance with the requirements of the Circulation on the study, propaganda and carrying out the spirit of the Plenary Session by the Central Government: the reform and opening up, especially the great achievements and valuable experience since the 16th CPC National Congress, the strategic position of cultural construction in the general layout of socialist undertaking with Chinese characteristics, the responsibilities of the Party in the construction of socialist culture with Chinese characteristics, the overall goal of the construction of socialist culture power, the important policy for the construction of socialist culture with Chinese characteristics, the important viewpoints, the series of important tasks, and major measures proposed at Plenary Session, the warm response and positive evaluation on the Plenary Session by health system, the actual action and concrete results in carrying out all the spirit of the Plenary Session and promoting cultural reform and development by all places and units, the further improvement in the ideological understanding, strengthening of national pride, industry confidence and professional pride so that the cadres and the masses of health system are always filled with an enterprising spirit. The forces must be further organized to seriously study scientific connotation, accurate expression, transmission path, and propaganda carrier under new situation. Theoretically, the significance and important content of strengthening health culture construction must be explicated so that health culture can embody

Chinese excellent cultural tradition, the spirit of the age of reform and innovation, and socialist core values system. Also, fruitful results of health cultural development in all places must be condensed, and tangible policies and measures be proposed to guide all places to do a good and solid job in health culture construction. A series of activities of propaganda and education on health culture must be launched, combining health ethics education with spiritual civilization construction, and with the carriers of explanation and publicity, seminar and symposium. A group of bases must be constructed on the basis of relics sites of health culture, exhibition halls and museums for health culture propaganda and education. The battle field for cultural propaganda and education with health publication medium group as the core must be created and health cultural transmission system be made more powerful by taking the system reform in the publication units of books and the nonpolitical newspapers by the Central Government as an opportunity. Popular forms of cultural works of books, films, and TV programs on health themes and on the advanced models and the touching stories as the prototype must be supported and created so that socialist core values system can take the lead in health culture construction and everyone consciously participates in the long-term unremitting health culture construction culminates in the whole system, cultural consciousness and cultural confidence of all medical workers can be improved by gathering strength, boosting their spirit and inspiring the fighting spirit in order to provide strong spiritual power for the healthy development of public health undertaking.

Secondly, to strengthen leadership, establish and perfect the system mechanism of health news propaganda. The working mechanism of the top leader taking the overall responsibility for news propaganda, news propaganda departments taking the lead and duty, all departments working with joint efforts and the relevant units giving effective support is formed. The organization construction must be attached great importance to, the organizations with independent staffing size, specializing in the centralized administration of health news propaganda, be established to provide working funds and material guarantee. Health news propaganda must be included in the general plan for health reform and development, which, together with the key tasks should be studied, deployed, organized, implemented, supervised, and examined. The results of news propaganda must be involved in the evaluation system of the scientific development of health undertaking and be made an important basis to judge the achievements of leading bodies and leading cadres. The working mechanism of internal teamwork, external cooperation, and the upper and lower joint efforts in health news propaganda must be established, mechanism of labor division and cooperation in health news propaganda and the consultation mechanism for key news propaganda in all the units be established, which center around health, make regular study and deployment and complete the tasks with joint efforts. Network of health news propaganda must be established and perfected for the benefit of mutual cooperation and communication, and more unobstructed, faster and more efficient communication for information. Communication and cooperation among departments in charge, news media and health industry associations must be enhanced for mutual circulation, report status, experience exchange and the common research on the problems. The official websites of health administrative departments and organizations must be perfected, combined with health informatization construction, whose authority and seriousness must be kept, readability and interactivity be intensified so as to make the websites the important platform for news propaganda.

Thirdly, to strengthen news release and build up the network guided by public opinions. News release is the most effective way to expound health policies, publicize the information of government affairs, spread health knowledge, access to and understand social information and people's will, guide public opinion and accept social supervision. Currently, news release system has been established in national and provincial administrative departments of public health, and some large-scale medical health institutions, which should be further developed and improved. News spokesman, the contents issued, way of news release, release procedure, and limits of authority for news release must be clarified, and routinization, standardization and institutionalization of news release must be realized. The top leader responsible for news release should take feasible responsibility, the leading bodies do the special study and deployment, and make the assisting responsible leaders familiar with the work of news spokesman. News conference on grave news in health industry, important activities, the sensitive and hot issues commonly concerned by the people should be organized and held to circulate the relevant information, communicate information concerned by the media, answer questions, and strive for information release at fixed time and point. The working systems of theme propaganda, reports on key activities, emergency release, focused interview at grassroots, collection and feedback of public opinions and clarification of misleading information must be established and perfected to guarantee that a set of rules are strictly followed.

Fourthly, to strengthen contingent construction and provide powerful guarantee for news propaganda. If health news propaganda goes up to another new step, the team will be the foundation and the talent is the key. A talent team of health news propaganda with reasonable structure, combination of part-time and full time, and energy must be built up by standing from the present, thinking in a long-term view and meeting the requirements of firm political position, good quality, taking root at the grassroots and serving the people. News spokesman and full-time news publicity team are the strong forces in news propaganda, and they should have comprehensive and high quality, be familiar with the rules of health work and news propaganda rules. It is urgent that the talents be equipped and trained. News reporters are the most active power of health news propaganda, and they should combine "going to the grassroots, turning working style, and changing writing style" with medical reform, do more interviews and writings on living stories about medical reform and health work at grassroots. In recent years, there have emerged a number of high-quality professional and cultural workers in health system, and they should exert their social influence to serve health news propaganda and people's health. Health news propaganda is the work of high specialty, involving the fields of sociology, communication, public relation, and law. Therefore, we should be good at gathering a group of expert advisor teams, giving advice and suggestions, providing counsel and carrying out training. The mechanisms for talent cultivation and development, incentive and security must be perfected to honor and award the outstanding health news propaganda workers, create the talents growth environment of positive atmosphere and trend, harmony and endeavor, and comfortable fault-tolerance, and attract more talented people to join health news propaganda team.

Currently, China's reform and development of culture and health are facing a historic opportunity, the responsibility of health news propaganda is significant and the missions are glorious. Let us work together, seize the opportunity, make expansion and innovation, do a good job in health news propaganda, create a new situation of health news propaganda, and create a good atmosphere of public opinions and social environment for health reform and development!

(Ji Chenglian)

12. Carry through the Main Theme, Implement the Main Thread and Promote the Sound and Fast Development of the Undertaking of the Traditional Chinese Medical Science and Medicines in the 12th Five-Year-Plan Period

—A Working Report Given by Wang Guoqiang, Vice Minister of the Ministry of Health and Concurrently Chief of the State Administration of Traditional Chinese Medicine (TCM) at the 2011 National Working Conference on Traditional Chinese Medicine (January 13, 2011)

Comrades,

This year's National Working Conference on Traditional Chinese Medicine is a very important meeting held at a critical period of deepening the medical and health reform and comprehensively carrying through and implementing *the Several Opinions of the State Council on Supporting and Promoting the Development of TCM Undertaking* (hereinafter referred to as *Several Opinions)* and also a new period for the development in the 12th Five-Year-Plan period. The State Council attached great importance to the opening of the conference and Li Keqiang, member of the Standing Committee of the Political Bureau and Vice Premier, made an important instruction specially in which he fully affirmed the achievements made in the development of the undertaking of traditional Chinese medical science and medicines in past five years and put forward ardent hopes and requirements for the work. At the National Health Working Conference that is just closed, Chen Zhu, Minister of the Ministry of Health and Zhang Mao, Secretary of the Party Group of the Ministry of Health also spoke highly of the achievements in the work of traditional Chinese medical science and medicines in their speeches and explicitly raised new tasks and requirements. Minister Chen Zhu will come to the conference and deliver an important speech tomorrow. We must earnestly learn and fully understand leaders' speeches and implement them comprehensively.

The theme of this year's National Working Conference on Traditional Chinese Medicine is to thoroughly carry through the spirit of the 17th National Congress of the Party, the 3rd, 4th and 5th Plenary Session of the 17th Central Committee of the Party, the Central Economic Working Conference and the National Health Working Conference and under the guidance of the important thought of Deng Xiaoping Theory and the Three Representatives, study and practice the Scientific Outlook on Development deeply, retrospect and summarize the developmental achievements gained in the undertaking of the traditional Chinese medical science and medicines in the 11th Five-Year-Plan period and the working progress in 2010, correctly understand the situation and tasks facing the reform and development of the traditional Chinese medical science and medicines, with taking the promotion and realization of scientific development of the undertaking of the traditional Chinese medical science and medicines as the main theme and fully carrying through *the Several Opinions* in deepening the medical and health reform as the main thread, clarify the general ideology, objectives and tasks of the development in the 12th Five-Year-Plan period, make deployment for the key work in 2011, seize opportunities and make efforts to promote the sound and fast development of the undertaking of traditional Chinese medical science and medicines in the 12th Five-Year-Plan period.

Next, I'm to talk about my opinions on three aspects for your discussion.

I. New achievements in the development of the undertaking of the traditional Chinese medical science and medicines in the 11th Five-Year-Plan period and new progress in the traditional Chinese medical work in 2010

(1) New achievements gained in the development of the undertaking of the

traditional Chinese medical science and medicines in the 11th Five-Year-Plan period

The 11th Five-Year-Plan period is a period that is of significant importance in the history of the development of traditional Chinese medical science and medicines. The remarkable characteristics of the traditional Chinese medical science and medicines in these five years are that more importance was paid to people and people's needs, overall planning, coordinative development and methods of innovation in mechanisms and transformation of ideology. Breakthroughs have been made in many respects and remarkable achievements have been gained.

In the past five years, a new situation was created for the reform and development of traditional Chinese medical science and medicines. The Party and state paid more attention to traditional Chinese medical work and the Report of the 17th National Congress of the Party emphasized "attaching equal stress to traditional Chinese medicine and Western medicine" and "supporting the development of the undertaking of the traditional Chinese medical science and medicines and the undertaking of ethnic minority medicine". The State Council established the inter-ministerial coordinative mechanism for traditional Chinese medical work and issued the *Several Opinions*, which served as a milestone for the development of traditional Chinese medical science and medicines. The *Law of Traditional Chinese Medicine* was listed in the legislative plan of the 11th Session of National People's Congress, which represented that the legislation of the traditional Chinese medical science and medicines was brought into the legislative agenda of our country. Full play of the role of traditional Chinese medical science and medicines was attached importance in deepening the medical and health reform and traditional Chinese medical work was included in the five pieces of the key work. Relevant central and local departments gave more support to the traditional Chinese medical science and medicines in planning, projects, funds and policies and governments at all levels increased the investment from 4.14 billion RMB Yuan in 2005 to 10.97 billion RMB Yuan in 2009, up by 165%. Local Party committees and governments paid unprecedented attention and offered unprecedented support to traditional Chinese medical work. 22 provinces (autonomous regions, cities) issued policy documents on the support and promotion of the development of the undertaking of the traditional Chinese medical science and medicines and the management systems for the traditional Chinese medical science and medicines were also strengthened,there being 12 assistant department-level administrations nationwide.

In the past five years, a new ideology was set up for the reform and development of the traditional Chinese medical science and medicines. On the basis of China's basic national conditions, the summary of our country's development practices and the use of foreign development experience as reference, the Party Central Committee raised the Scientific Outlook on Development and established an ideology that development should be people-oriented, rely on people and its benefits should be shared by people. The 17th National Congress of the Party put forward explicitly the new requirements for the comprehensive construction of the well-off society and the goal of everyone's share of the basic medical and healthcare service and gave high priority to the development of the undertaking of the traditional Chinese medical science and medicines. In the past five years, the whole system of the traditional Chinese medical science and medicines throughout the country firmly established the consciousness and ideology of wholehearted service for people's health, took the satisfaction of people's need for the service of the traditional Chinese medical science and medicines as the starting point and supreme goal for the work, unified the understanding, adjusted the train of thought for the development, created working methods, made reforms in operating mechanisms, intensified weak links and improved service effectiveness. Generally speaking, traditional Chinese medical work exemplified the scientific people-oriented development ideology which is the ideological foundation for the new achievements in the past five year's work and significant spiritual wealth deserving our serious review and promotion.

In the past five years, a new train of thought was established for the reform and development of the traditional Chinese medical science and medicines. On the basis of review on the beneficial experience and successful exploration in the development of the undertaking of the traditional Chinese medical science and medicines since the founding of new China, especially, since the reform and opening up, the State Council formulated the *Several Opinions* which further clarified the guiding ideology, basic principles, overall train of thought, policy measures and key tasks and defined the new train of thought for the comprehensive and coordinative development of medical treatment, health protection, education, scientific research, industry and culture. By system innovation and policy guarantee, efforts were made to solve the key problems in systems, mechanisms and policies that affected and restricted the development of the undertaking of the traditional Chinese medical science and medicines so that the role of the traditional Chinese medical science and medicines could be brought into full play and people's health rights could be maintained. The *Several Opinions* is a guiding document that points the way for the development of the undertaking of the traditional Chinese medical science and medicines.

In the past five years, a new method was created for traditional Chinese medical work. Under the guidance of the Scientific Outlook on Development and with the collection of wisdom from all parts and unceasing improvement of the capacity for strategic thinking, dialectical thinking and innovative thinking, the working system and for traditional Chinese medical work were explored and established, involving integrative thinking, systematic operation, interaction of the micro, medium and macro levels and scientific development. The working system and operating mechanism focused on "putting people first", attached importance to the service for people' health and constructed an organic interaction of micro, medium and macro levels and dynamic development. It clarified that on the micro-level, efforts should be made to enhance service so as to be good at ideology, right protection, capacity, methods and effects; on the medium level, management should be strengthened so as to promote the implementation of the tasks of traditional Chinese medical work and on the macro-level, regulation and control should be enhanced and a forceful safeguard mechanism should be established. Under the guidance of this working system and operating mechanism, key problems that affected the operation of the system and restricted the development of the undertaking of the traditional Chinese medical science and medicines were found out accurately and efforts were made to perfect systems, mechanisms and policies and fully understand positions of each piece of work in the three levels and the role of the interaction, which energetically promoted the implementation of the working tasks of the traditional Chinese medical science and medicines.

In the past five years, new progress was made in the development of the undertaking of traditional Chinese medical science and medicines. Firstly, the service system of traditional Chinese science and service capacity were strengthened tremendously. From the end of 2005 to that of 2009 (the data of 2009 are based on the survey on the basic status quo of traditional Chinese medicine), hospitals of traditional Chinese medicine increased from 3,009 to 3299, up by 9.6%; hospital beds increased from 315 thousand to 449.3 thousand, up by 42.6; patients of inpatient department increased from 226 million person times to 328 million person times, up by 44.96% and discharged person times rose from 6.1153 million to 12.08 million, up by 97.54%. Secondly, the service of health protection of traditional Chinese medicine developed rapidly. The health engineering of "preventive treatment of diseases" was carried out and initial results in the service of health protection were gained in 103 medical institutions that launched the pilot of the service of "preventive treatment of diseases". Thirdly, the capacity for the prevention, treatment and emergency response to major serious diseases with the traditional Chinese medical science and medicines improved obviously. The construction of 615 state-level key specialties (treatment of special diseases) and 3,453 rural specialties with the characteristics of the traditional Chinese medical medicine was carried out and clinical effectiveness was further heightened. The traditional Chinese medical science and medicines played a unique role in the prevention and treatment of major serious diseases such AIDS, Influenza A (H1N1), hand-foot-and-mouth disease, etc. and the emergency response to contingencies and remarkable achievements were made. Fourthly, positive progress was made in the inheritance and innovation of the traditional Chinese medical science and medicine, a great number of offices being built for the inheritance of the experience of famous veteran experts in the traditional Chinese medical science and medicines; their academic thinking and experience in clinical diagnosis and treatment being organized and a system for famous veteran TCM experts' successors to get degrees in clinical medical majors being established. The construction of 16 clinical research bases of the traditional Chinese medical science and medicines and ethnical medicine was initiated; the construction of clinical research system for the prevention and treatment of infectious diseases and chronic non-infectious diseases with the traditional Chinese medical science and medicines was carried out and 108 key laboratories and 388 Class III laboratories were set up. Great achievements were made in the scientific research of the traditional Chinese medical science and medicines, 24 of which won the second prize of National Science and Technology Progress Award and 3 won the second prize of National Award for Technological Invention. Fifthly, the construction of talent contingent of the traditional Chinese medical science and medicines was further strengthened. Students of colleges and universities of the traditional Chinese medical science and medicines rose from 385 thousand in 2005 to 527 thousand in 2009, up by 36.9% and key disciplines constructed increased from 93 to 323. Cultivation of high-level talents and training of grassroots medical workers were strengthened intensively so that quality of the talents in traditional Chinese medical science and medicines improved obviously. The first selection of "National Honored Great Master of Traditional Chinese Medicine" was conducted and produced good social effects. Sixthly, the cultural construction of the traditional Chinese medical science and medicines created a new situation and the activity of "the Traditional Chinese Medical Science and Medicines in China" was carried out deeply, popularizing the knowledge and publicizing the culture of the traditional Chinese medical science and medicines. 41 projects of traditional Chinese medical science and medicines were listed into the National Intangible Cultural Heritage List and TCM acupuncture and moxibustion was listed into the Representative List of the Intangible Cultural Heritage of Humanity. Seventhly, the undertaking of ethnic minority medical science and medicines developed significantly. At present, there are 203 hospitals of ethnic minority medicine in China and 14 colleges and universities carry out the medical education of ethnic minority. The industry of ethnic minority medicines developed rapidly and there are 906 categories of medicines all together, which did positive contributions to people's health and economic development of minority nationality regions. Eighthly, the process of legislation, standardization and informationization of the traditional Chinese medical science and medicines was accelerated. The legislative process of the *Law of Traditional Chinese Medicine* was accelerated and currently, there are 26 local laws and regulations on traditional Chinese medical science and medicines throughout the country. 27 national standards and 221 industrial standards were issued; 4 national standardized technical committees of the traditional Chinese medical science and medicines were formally set up and the standardized system framework of traditional Chinese medicine was initially formed. Breakthroughs were made in the work of international standardization and the International Standard Organization (ISO) established the Technical Committee of Traditional Chinese Medicine (tentative name) with its secretariat set up in our country. Traditional Chinese medicine and some other traditional medicines were brought into the International Classification of Diseases and Code (ICD-11) for the first time. The informationizaed level of the traditional Chinese medical science and medicines was further improved. Ninthly, the international influence of the traditional Chinese medical science and medicines was further heightened. Agreements including cooperation in the traditional Chinese medical science and medicines signed by foreign governments with our country increased from 53 to 91 and agreements on cooperation in the traditional Chinese medical science and medicines specially rose from 22 to 48. Products of traditional Chinese medicines and service trade of the traditional Chinese medical science and medicines developed steadily and a development situation involving all directions, multi-layers and wide range of areas was basically formed.

In the past five years, all the medical workers of the system of the traditional Chinese medical science and medicines did new contributions to the maintenance and improvement of people' health. In the past five years, the whole system of the traditional Chinese medical science and medicines stood the tests of the destructive earthquake in Wenchuan, Sichuan Province, Influenza A (H1N1) and other major contingents. When people needed them, they were fearless of dangers and difficulties, responded quickly, did their utmost to rescue and treat patients, brought the characteristics and superiorities of the traditional Chinese medical science and medicines into full play and effectively protected people's life and health. In the important events such as Beijing Olympic Games and Shanghai World Exposition, the traditional Chinese medical science and medicines played a unique role in medical security. Medical workers of the system of the traditional Chinese medical science and medicines throughout the country worked hard in ordinary workplaces for the maintenance of people's health, made selfless devotion and did positive contributions. It has been proved that the whole system of the traditional Chinese medical science and medicines is one that can serve people with superb medical skills, noble ethics and great working capacity and deserves our respect and trust.

Comrades, after five years' hard work, we have accomplished main objectives and tasks in the 11th Five-Year Plan smoothly and the traditional Chinese medical science and medicines have played an important role in the promotion of the coordinated development of economy and society and the maintenance of people's health.

(2) New progress made in traditional Chinese medical work in 2010

1)*The Several Opinions* issued by the State Council was carried through and implemented deeply and new progress was made. Last year, we strengthened communication and coordination with relevant departments and formulated and perfected policies concerned. All the localities made relevant measures more specific and practicable in accordance with the actual local realities and 9 provinces (autonomous regions, cities) issued special documents for support and improvement of the development of the undertaking of the traditional Chinese medical science and medicines, including Jilin, Shanghai, Fujian, Hainan, Yunnan, Tibet, Gansu, Henan and Chongqing.

More funds were invested into the traditional Chinese medical science and medicines. In 2010, the Central Finance allocated 5,243 billion RMB Yuan of special funds to the construction of 16 state-level TCM clinical research bases, 41 prefecture-level, city-level and above key TCM hospitals, 147county-level TCM hospitals and the construction of the capacity for traditional Chinese medical service. It is the year that the Central Finance invested the largest amount of funds since the founding of new China. All the localities also further increased the investment.

The construction of administrative organizations was further enhanced. A leading group with the municipal government leader taking the lead was set up in Shanghai for the development of the undertaking of the traditional Chinese medical science and medicines, there being offices responsible for the development under it and all the districts and counties were required to establish corresponding organizational systems. Zhejiang Provincial Administration of Traditional Chinese Medicine was transformed from a internal office under the Provincial Health Department to a division directly under the leadership and management of the Provincial Health Department, the leader of the Provincial Administration of Traditional Chinese Medicine being with a higher rank and the Administration being with more staff quota. Guizhou Provincial Administration of Traditional Chinese Medicine increased divisions and staff quota.

New progress was made in compensatory mechanisms for the service of the traditional Chinese medical science and medicines. Shaanxi Province required clearly that basic salaries of all the staff members of county-level TCM hospitals should be fully budgeted; Henan Province demanded that on the basis of the establishment of quota for staff and posts and the performance evaluation, the basic income of TCM technical personnel in county-level and township medical institutions should be guaranteed. It was ruled in Ningbo City of Zhejiang Province, that financial subsidies should be rendered to government-run hospitals according to the standard of 8 RMB Yuan for the reception of each patient in the outpatient department and 15 RMB Yuan each day for each hospital bed in the inpatient department. Gansu Province increased the subsidiary standard for hospital beds of public TCM hospitals and the TCM department of general hospitals to 1.5 times of that of comprehensive hospitals.

Policies on Chinese herbal preparations in medical institutions were further perfected. Jointly with the Ministry of Health and the State Food and Drug Administration, the State Administration of Traditional Chinese Medicine formulated the *Opinions on Strengthening the Management of Chinese Herbal Preparations* which simplified the procedures of examination and approval, expanded the scope of preparations and better adapted to the development of the traditional Chinese medical science and medicines.

2) The whole system of the traditional Chinese medical science and medicines actively participated in the reform of medical and health system and the role of the traditional Chinese medical science and medicines was brought into fuller play

In 2010, according to the general deployment of the State Council and the arrangement for health work, the system of the traditional Chinese medical science and medicines positively promoted the implementation of the working tasks for deepening the medical and health reform, attached importance to solution to the problems in systems and mechanisms that restricted the play of the role traditional Chinese medical science and medicines and new progress was made.

In the construction of the basic medical security system, attention was paid to the guidance of offering and utilization of the service of the traditional Chinese medical science and medicines. Most of the provinces worked out policies on increase of the percentage of reimbursement and decrease of the lowest payment for hospitalization reimbursement of the expenses of the traditional Chinese medical science and medicines in the new rural cooperative medical care. Jilin Province required the basic urban medical insurance to decrease the lowest payment for hospitalization reimbursement in TCM hospitals and increase the percentage of the payment for the items of diagnosis and treatment of traditional Chinese medicine. Yunnan Province decreased the percentage of self-payment for TCM services for those participating in medical insurance.

In the construction of the essential drug system, the principle of putting equal stress on traditional Chinese medicine and western medicine was put into effect. The Administration of Traditional Chinese Medicine and the Ministry of Health together formulated the guide and guiding principles for clinical application of Chinese patent drugs. All the localities actively coordinated and did well the work of supplement, provision and application of the essential traditional Chinese medicines. Heilongjiang Province ruled that governments compensated rural and urban medical and health institutions 25%~30% of the total price of Chinese traditional medical herbal pieces. Tibet Autonomous Regions took Tibetan drugs as a main supplement to the essential drugs and the supplements amounted to 480 kinds. 124 kinds of patent drugs were added to the essential drugs in Guangdong Province, which accounted for more than half of the supplements.

In the construction of grassroots medical and health system, grassroots service networks of traditional Chinese medical science and medicines were strengthened. 369 county-level TCM hospitals were brought into the Central Government's key project of support and construction; basic standards for TCM department of township hospitals were issued and management regulations and basic standards for the clinics with Zuo Tang Yi (doctors of traditional Chinese medicine practicing medicine) were drawn up. All the localities positively explored effective ways and methods for the consolidation and perfection of grassroots TCM service networks. Anhui Province carried out the pilot of unified management of county, township and village medical work and Fujian Province conducted the project of the intensification of the construction of TCM department in township health care centers.

In the construction of the basic public medical and health service system, techniques and methods of health prevention and protection of traditional Chinese medicine were positively applied and the application of the traditional Chinese medical science and medicines was regarded as a part of the performance evaluation. Changning District of Shanghai City took the prevention and health protection of traditional Chinese medicine as an item of public health service and rendered fund subsidies. Gansu Province required all the disease prevention and control institutions to set up department of traditional Chinese medicine and offer TCM prevention and health protection service.

In the pilot of the reform of public hospitals, efforts were made to explore systems and mechanisms beneficial to full play of the characteristics and superiorities of the traditional Chinese medical science and medicines. In the pilot work of the reform of public hospitals, Anhui Province carried out the pilot of the classified compensatory mechanism in hospitals of traditional Chinese medicine. The State Administration of Traditional Chinese Medicine issued TCM clinical pathways and schemes of diagnosis and treatment for 42 categories of diseases, including orthopedics and traumatology, and were carried out as pilot.

3) Capacity for the service of the traditional Chinese medical science and medicines was further improved

With focus on improving rural specialties with the characteristics of traditional

Chinese medicine and popularizing appropriate techniques of the traditional Chinese medical science and medicines, urban and rural service capacity at the grassroots level was further improved. The activity of the construction of national advanced grassroots units in traditional Chinese medical work was carried out and the first 18 rural advanced units and 13 advanced communities were named. The First National Symposium on Folk Medicine and Non-Governmental TCM Medical Work was held, which promoted the development of folk and non-governmental TCM work.

New achievements were gained in the work of emergency response to contingents and the prevention and control of major serious infectious diseases with the traditional Chinese medical science and medicines. After the occurrence of the violent earthquake in Yushu, Qinghai Province and the severe mudslide in Zhouqu, Gansu Province, the State Administration of Traditional Chinese Medicine and the TCM administrations of provinces of Qinghai, Gansu and Sichuan set up medical teams rapidly and sent them to disaster areas to participate in rescue and treatment. Traditional remedies and Chinese medical preparations of traditional Chinese medicine (Tibetan medicine) were used extensively and played a unique role. Continuous efforts were made to prevent and control Influenza A (H1N1) and hand-foot-mouth disease and promote the pilot project of AIDS prevention and treatment with the traditional Chinese medical science and medicines.

The activity of "Year of TCM Hospital Management" was deepened and the quality and safety of the medical service were further heightened. Results of evaluation showed that all-level TCM hospitals further understood the direction and objectives for the development and paid more attention to the play of the characteristics and superiorities of the traditional Chinese medical science and medicines as well as the quality and safety of the medical service. 11 guidelines were issued for the construction and management of clinical departments and TCM nursing work of TCM hospitals.

Traditional Chinese medical work in general hospitals was also pushed forward unceasingly. The *Opinions on Conscientiously Strengthening the TCM Work of General Hospitals* was put into effect and special attention was given to the working requirements for traditional Chinese medical work in the formulation and revision of the basic standards for second-grade and tertiary general hospitals and the standards for the examination and evaluation of county-level general hospitals. The State Administration of Traditional Chinese Medicine, the Ministry of Health and the Health Bureau of the PLA Logistic Department jointly selected 103 general hospitals as the demonstrative units of traditional Chinese medical work.

There were remarkable results in the service of TCM prevention and health protection. The Third Summit Forum on "Preventive Treatment of Diseases" was held successfully. Evaluation on the service effectiveness of prevention and health protection of "preventive treatment of diseases"—improvement in health condition and service satisfaction was conducted and results showed that health condition of those people receiving the service of "preventive treatment of diseases" were improved.

4) New achievements were made in the construction of talent contingents of the traditional Chinese medical science and medicines. Reform in the education of colleges and universities of traditional Chinese medicine was promoted rapidly and the joint construction of TCM colleges and universities by the Ministry of Education and the State Administration of Traditional Chinese Medicine was pushed forward. The *Program for the Construction of Key Disciplines of Traditional Chinese Medicine* was formulated, which offered support to the construction of 107 key TCM clinical disciplines.

Cultivation of high-level talents and grassroots medical personnel was attached importance. Chongqing City selected 25 high-level talents and invested 3 million RMB Yuan and strived to cultivate a group of famous experts in the traditional Chinese medical science and medicines. Hubei Province carried out the activity of the election of "great TCM master" and "famous TCM master", which created an atmosphere in the society that famous experts in traditional Chinese medical science and medicine came forth in large numbers. Last year, 24 thousand village doctors participated in the secondary education of the major of traditional Chinese medicine and nearly 10 thousand TCM doctors received the standardized training of general practitioners of traditional Chinese medicine. By ways of the admission of TCM college and university students with reduced scores of the national entrance examination, oriented distribution after graduation and government subsidies, Henan Province cultivated the talents of the traditional Chinese medical science and medicines for rural areas specifically.

Continuing education of the traditional Chinese medical science and medicines was further enhanced. 694 state-level continuing educational projects were implemented and 273 State-Administration-level superior disciplinary continuing educational bases, 30 urban communities and 45 rural demonstrative bases for the training of knowledge and skills of the traditional Chinese medical science and medicines were elected. Almost all the localities set up three-level continuing educational bases, namely, provincial, municipal and county-level. Appraisal of professional technical personnel such as those specializing in Gua Sha (a popular treatment by scraping the patient's neck, chest or back) and preparation of traditional Chinese medicines was initiated.

5) New development was achieved in the inheritance and innovation of the

traditional Chinese medical science and medicines. The construction of clinical research bases of traditional Chinese medicine was promoted; professional construction plans of 16 bases was approved; cooperative mechanisms and expert working system were established; cooperative research on the characteristics and superiorities in the prevention and treatment of 14 kinds of diseases with the traditional Chinese medical science and medicines and key clinical problems was conducted. The National Research Center for Infectious Disease Prevention and Control with TCM and 41 key research laboratories of the prevention and control of infectious diseases with the traditional Chinese medical science and medicines were designated.

Fundamental research on the inheritance of the traditional Chinese medical science and medicines was further intensified. The collation of 400 kinds of important ancient literature was done and offices for the inheritance of clinical experience and academic ideology of 181 famous veteran experts in the traditional Chinese medical science and medicines were constructed. The comprehensive service platform of famous veteran TCM experts' clinical experience and academic ideology was established and the *Extract from Inheritance and Research on the National Honored Great Masters of Traditional Chinese Medicine was* publicized.

The pre-preparation for the general survey on the resources of Chinese medicinal materials was accelerated. Fundamental work such as technical regulations for the survey, classification and codes of the resources, monitoring and services of the main resources based on remote sensing data from our country's autonomous satellites was started. The special project for the development of high-tech industries of traditional Chinese medicines carried out jointly by the State Administration of Traditional Chinese Medicine and the State Development and Reform Commission ran smoothly.

6) The work of ethnic minority medicine and the integration of traditional Chinese medicine and western medicine were further enhanced. Jointly with the State Ethnic Affairs Commission, the Ministry of Health and the State Food and Drug Administration, the State Administration of Traditional Chinese Medicine issued the *Implementation Plan on Recent Priorities in National Ethnic Minority Medicine (2010-2012).* 150 pieces of literature with the characteristics of ethnic minority medicine and 140 techniques of diagnosis and treatment were collated and researched and it was the first time that a large-scale collation and research were carried out at national level. 16 key disciplinary construction sites of the ethnic minority medicine were designated. The first re-election of the Chinese Association of Minority Medicine ran smoothly at the expiration of the term, which laid foundation for the better play of the role of "bridge" and "bond". All the ethnic minority areas actively promoted the development of ethnic minority medicine in local areas in accordance with the actual

local conditions.

The integration of traditional Chinese medicine and western medicine was pushed forward steadily. Working guidelines was drafted for hospitals of traditional Chinese medicine and western medicine and evaluation indexes and systems were discussed and worked out so as to promote the construction and development of hospitals of traditional Chinese medicine and western medicine. All the localities further enhanced the construction of talents specializing in the integration of traditional Chinese medicine with western medicine. Jiangsu Province held postgraduate training classes for doctors of western medicine to study traditional Chinese medicine for four years successively in order to promote the improvement in the structure of professional technical staff of traditional Chinese medicine and western medicine in medical institutions. By three forms of education, namely, education of popular science, education with record of formal schooling and education of postgraduate course, Shandong Province held the training of "medical staff of western medicine studying traditional Chinese medicine" in all the TCM hospitals.

7) The cultural construction of the traditional Chinese medical science and medicines was deepened continuously. The activities of "the Traditional Chinese Medical Science and Medicines in China" in Xinjiang Uygur Autonomous Region, the Xinjiang Production and Construction Corps and Arctic frontier stations of military camps were organized. The three-year activity came to a successful end and a grand meeting of summary and commendation was convened in Beijing last September. The activity of "the Traditional Chinese Medical Science and Medicines in China • Science Popularization Week" was carried out throughout the country and at the same time, a new round of activities with the theme of "entering village, entering community, entering family" were launched. Experts' lecture tours of popular science on traditional Chinese medical culture were organized and people from all walks of life took an active part in the actives. The activity of "traditional Chinese medicine entering schools" was carried out in Beijing, Shanxi and Heilongjiang, which was very popular with students and teachers. A booklet of "The Traditional Chinese Medical and Medicine Make Us Healthier" was compiled in Shanghai, publicizing the traditional Chinese medical science and medicines to the visitors to Shanghai World Exposition and citizens and gained good results. Hubei Province issued "Guidelines on Designing the Image for the Cultural Construction of TCM Institutions" to promote the simultaneous implementation of cultural and infrastructural construction.

Breakthroughs were made in the application to the Representative List of the Intangible Cultural Heritage of Humanity. Last November, TCM acupuncture and moxibustion was listed formally into the Representative List of the Intangible Cultural Heritage of Humanity, which shows the recognition of the international community to

China's traditional medical culture. Moreover, two ancient books of Huang Di Nei Jing (Emperor's Inner Canon) and Ben Cao Gang Mu (Compendium of Materia Medica) were selected into the Asia-Pacific Memory of the World Register.

Increasing efforts were made to propagandize the traditional Chinese medical science and medicines. With focus on the central work, the role of major media was brought into play and pieces of news were reported timely so that industrial spirits were boosted and industrial image was fostered.

8) The legislation, standardization and informationization of the traditional Chinese medical science and medicines were promoted solidly. Phased progress was made in the legislation of the traditional Chinese medical science and medicines. With the efforts of the whole system, the first *Law of Traditional Chinese Medicine (Draft)* was finished last year and now is submitted to the Ministry of Health. Progress was also made in local legislative work. Shenzhen issued the *Regulations of Shenzhen Special Economic Zone on Traditional Chinese Medicine* and Inner Mongolia revised and issued new local regulations. The construction of the standardization and informationization was accelerated. Regulations for technical operation of TCM prevention and health protection were issued; national standards and industrial standards were examined and approved; 42 bases for the research and popularization of the standardization of the traditional Chinese medical science and medicines were designated and the work of research and popularization was strengthened. The *Nomenclature and Location of Auricular Points* won the second prize of 2010 China Standard Innovation Award. The compilation of the contents concerning the traditional Chinese medical science and medicines in the *Plan for Major National Informationized Construction* was organized and informationized level of the whole system was heightened obviously. The supervision and management on the traditional Chinese medical science and medicines were strengthened; monitoring of false and illegal TCM advertisements and false websites of medical institutions of traditional Chinese medicine was intensified and those publicizing false and illegal medical advertisements were punished according to law.

The survey on the basic status quo of the traditional Chinese medicine was finished smoothly. This is the first survey that has been carried out throughout the country since the founding of new China and all-level administrations of traditional Chinese medicine strengthened the organization and leadership for the survey conscientiously, deployed carefully, promoted solidly and guaranteed the working speed and data quality. So far, the draft of reports on the investigation and analysis and the demonstration nationwide have been basically finished.

9) Foreign exchange and cooperation in the traditional Chinese medical science and medicines were deepened unceasingly. Multilateral-cooperation in the traditional Chinese medical science and medicines was further consolidated and developed. In

close cooperation with the World Health Organization (WHO), the implementation of the *Resolution of Traditional Medicine* adopted in the 62nd World Health Assembly (WHA) of the WHO was promoted and efforts were made to take an active part in the formulation of the part of traditional medicine for ICD of WHO (International Classification of Diseases of the World Health Organization). Cooperation with the International Organization for Standard was enhanced and support was offered to the holding of the first conference by the Secretariat of the Technical Committee of Traditional Chinese medicine (ISO/TC 249). Areas of bilateral cooperation were expanding further. Cooperation in traditional Chinese medical science and medicines was brought into the framework of 2010 China-US strategic and economic dialogue and working mechanisms were established. Conferences on the cooperation with France, Singapore, etc. in the traditional Chinese medical science and medicines were held successfully. Good job was done to promote the Confucius Institutes to propagandize traditional Chinese medical culture; last June, Vice-Chairman Xi Jinping attended the opening ceremony of the Confucius Institute at Royal Melbourne Institute of Technology, Australia and fully affirmed the way of the integration of the teaching of the traditional Chinese medical science and medicines with that of Chinese.

The exchange and cooperation in traditional Chinese medical science and medicines with Hong Kong, Macao and Taiwan were strengthened continuously.

The First High-Level Coordination Meeting of the Mainland, Hong Kong and Macao was held and the cooperative mechanism of the three places was set up. The traditional Chinese medical science and medicines were brought into medical and health cooperative agreements of the two sides of the Taiwan straits and a group was formed to promote the traditional Chinese medical work of the both sides. In cooperation with relevant departments and localities, the "Cross-Strait Forum" and the "Cross-Strait Seminar on Traditional Chinese Medicines" were held successfully and the cross-strait cooperation in the traditional Chinese medical science and medicines was deepened.

10) The activity of "striving to excel in the performances" gained actual effects. According to the deployment of the Party Central Committee and actual conditions of the system of the traditional Chinese medical science and medicines, the activity of "striving to excel in the performances" was carried out with the general objective of "pushing forward scientific development, promoting social harmony, serving people, strengthening grassroots organizations" and the general carrier of actively participating in deepening the reform of the medical and health system, deeply carrying out and implementing the State Council's *Several Opinions*, continuously improving the capacity for inheritance and innovation, making efforts to solve the

problems that restricted the development of the traditional Chinese medical science and medicines and providing high-quality medical services for people. Since the beginning of the activity, numerous characteristics, effective methods and experience were created. With focus on the enhancement of the characteristics and superiorities of TCM public hospitals and the prosperity and development of traditional Chinese medical culture in our country's capital, efforts were made in Beijing to serve people and promote social harmony. Guangdong Hospital of Traditional Chinese Medicine combined China's traditional culture, the Party's fine working style and modern managerial systems organically, as a result, cultural construction of the hospital was promoted and the characteristics and superiorities of the traditional Chinese medical science and medicines were brought into play. Chongqing Hospital of Traditional Chinese Medicine put forward the "frontline working method' and the Party members carried out the three steps of "self-evaluation, public evaluation and public notification", which was fully affirmed by Vice-Chairman Xi Jinping. It is a consensus and act of all the staff members of the system of the traditional Chinese medical science and medicines that by the activity of "striving to excel in the performances", they shall make the broad masses who deeply love the traditional Chinese medical science and medicines more satisfied with their work.

Our achievements gained in the past five years are attributed to the correct leadership and scientific decision of the Party Central Committee and the State Council, great importance and energetic support given by all-level Party committees, governments and all relevant sectors, active concern and enthusiastic participation of all the people from all walks of life in the society and the broad masses and especially attributed to the solidarity, coordination and hard work of the broad medical workers of the system of traditional Chinese medical science and medicines. Here, on behalf of the State Administration of Traditional Chinese Medicine, I would like to take this chance to express my sincere gratitude and heartfelt respect to you, all the participants of the meeting and hope you to convey my greetings to the Party and government leaders and relevant sectors in all the localities and the medical workers in the system of the traditional Chinese medical science and medicines throughout the country.

Comrades, what have been gained in the past five years are hard-won; the experience accumulated is valuable and the cultural and ethical wealth created has a far-reaching influence. It has been proved that past five years is a period that the system of the traditional Chinese medical science and medicines renewed thinking and firmly established new ideology, the one that the whole system emancipated the minds, clarified the new train of thought for development and put forward new measures, the one that the whole system was bold in practice, exploration and creation of new working methods, the one that more attention was attached to overall planning and coordination and efforts were made to create a new situation for the comprehensive development of "six in one" (combining medical service, health protection, scientific research, education, industry and culture of traditional Chinese medical science and medicines into one), the one that the traditional Chinese medical science and medicines had an increasingly profound international influence and made new progress in the world and the one that the whole system strived to do solid work and did new contributions to the safeguard of people's health and the development of economy and society.

Review the work in the past five years, we deeply realize that if we want to clarify the train of though and objectives for development, we must persist in the guidance of the Scientific Outlook on Development, comply with and serve the overall situation of the development of economy and society and the development of the medical and health reform; if we want to be trusted and supported by people, we must insist on people-oriented principle and take the satisfaction of people's need for the service of the traditional Chinese medical science and medicines as the fundamental starting point for the development of the undertaking; if we want to maintain and develop the characteristics and superiorities, we must persist in the dialectical unity of inheritance and innovation and give priority to the original thinking of the traditional Chinese medical science and medicines; if we want to promote the comprehensive and harmonious development of the undertaking of the traditional Chinese medical science and medicines, we must insist on overall planning and push forward the development in an all-round way; if we want to ensure the implementation of the central policies in all the localities and realize the unity and coordination of the development of the traditional Chinese medical science and medicines, we must stick to giving full play to the enthusiasm of the Central Government and local governments and fully respect the initiative of all the localities; if we want to pool the strength and make achievements, we must be realistic and pragmatic, do solid work and unceasingly strengthen the self-construction of the system. What I talk about is the basic experience accumulated in the development of the undertaking of the traditional Chinese medical science and medicines in the 11th-Five-Year Plan period, which embodies everyone's wisdom and sweat, so we shall make efforts to continue and ceaselessly enrich and develop it in future practice.

II. Carry through and implement the spirit of the 5th Plenary Session of the 17th CPC Central Committee, seize opportunities, meet challenges and scientifically plan for the development of the undertaking of the traditional Chinese medical science and medicines in the 12th Five-Year-Plan period

(1) Understand thoroughly the new situations and demands that are faced with

the development of the undertaking of the traditional Chinese medical science and medicines

The 5th Plenary Session of the 17th CPC Central Committee is a very important conference held at the key period of the comprehensive construction of the well-off society and on the strenuous stage of deepening the reform and open up and accelerating the transformation of the patterns of economic development and it is an important one that summarized the past, planned for the future and defined the development direction and objectives. The *Suggestions of the Party Central Committee on Making the 12th Five-Year Plan for National Economic and Social Development* (hereinafter referred *to as Suggestions)* put forward the guiding ideology, development objectives and main tasks for the 12th Five-Year Plan and is the basic train of thought and program of action for national economic and social development in the next five years. The *Suggestions* took the safeguard and improvement of people's livelihood as the basic starting point and supreme goal for accelerating the transformation of the patterns of economic development, which fully embodies the Party Central Committee's concern about people's lives and shows the prominent position of the safeguard and improvement of people's livelihood in the promotion of our country's national economic and social development and the maintenance of social harmony and stability.

The *Suggestions* put the acceleration of medical and health reform in a very important place and raised explicitly that according to the requirement of "guarantee of the basic medical and health system, intensification of grassroots medical and health institutions and construction of mechanisms", we shall increase financial investment, deepen the reform of medical and health system, arouse medical personnel's enthusiasm, provide the basic medical and health system for all the residents as public products and give priority to the satisfaction of people's needs for the basic medical and health care. The *Suggestions* made a comprehensive deployment for the reform in medical and health system in the next five years and emphasized "sticking to putting equal stress on traditional Chinese medicine and western medicine and supporting the development of the undertaking of the traditional Chinese medical science and medicines". Currently, the environment for the development of the undertaking has changed a lot and we are faced with a period of important strategic opportunities.

Firstly, deep implementation of the Scientific Outlook on Development provides a theoretic safeguard for the acceleration of the development of the undertaking. The Scientific Outlook on Development views the realization of human being's comprehensive development as a fundamental objective and health is the foundation for the comprehensive development of human being. The traditional Chinese medical science and medicines play a unique role in the maintenance and promotion of people's health and concern everyone's immediate interests. Since the 17th Party's Congress, the full implementation of the Scientific Outlook on Development, the quickening acceleration of the social construction with focus on the improvement of people's livelihood and more importance attached to the undertaking of the traditional Chinese medical science and medicines provide a theoretic safeguard for the acceleration of the development of the undertaking of the traditional Chinese medical science and medicines.

Secondly, deep promotion of the reform of medical and health system and issue and implementation of the *Several Opinions* provide policy support for the development of the undertaking. The *Opinions of the Party Central Committee and the State Council on Deepening the Reform of Medical and Health System* put forward clearly that we shall stick to the principle of putting equal stress on traditional Chinese medicine and western medicine and give full play to the traditional Chinese medical science and medicines. The *Several Opinions* summarized briefly and scientifically the policies and guidelines on the traditional Chinese medical science and medicines since the founding of new China, fully showed the Party' and state's policy-making location for the development of the undertaking and put forward explicitly policy requirements and security measures, which provides policy support for the comprehensive, coordinative and sustainable development of the undertaking of the traditional Chinese medical science and medicines.

Thirdly, rapid development of economy and society serves as an economic support for the development of the undertaking. Since the reform and opening up, especially the extraordinary five years of the 11th Five-Year-Plan period, our country's comprehensive national powers kept strengthening continuously; financial income increased unceasingly and investment in the traditional Chinese medical science and medicines rose substantially. It can be predicted that the rapid and steady growth of our country's economy, gradual perfection of social security system and more attention paid to the safeguard and improvement of people's livelihood shall provide a more forceful economic support for the development of the undertaking of the traditional Chinese medical science and medicines.

Fourthly, the broad masses' trust in and need for the traditional Chinese medical science and medicines lay a social foundation for the development of the undertaking. A special survey result by the Horizon Research Consultancy Group shows 90% of the masses pay attention to the traditional Chinese medical science and medicines; 88% have the experience of getting access to them and 53% are willing to choose the treatment of the traditional Chinese medical science and medicines or the combination of traditional Chinese medicine and western medicine firstly when they are ill. The result fully indicates that in modern times, the broad masses have deep feeling and great trust in the traditional Chinese medical science and medicines, which lays a social foundation for the development of the undertaking of the traditional Chinese medical science and medicines.

Fifthly, changes in the medical mode and goals provide good opportunities for the development of the undertaking of the traditional Chinese medical science and medicines. Currently, the medical mode transforms to a biology-psychology-society mode while medical goals are also adjusted. Now the goals are "prevention of diseases and impairments, maintenance and improvement of health level". The holistic view and the characteristics and superiorities of attaching importance to individualization, humanization and "preventive treatment of diseases" in the traditional Chinese medical science and medicines coincide with the transformed medical mode and adjusted medical goals, which provides good opportunities for the play of the characteristics and superiorities of the traditional Chinese medical science and medicines.

Sixthly, concern and attention of the international community provide a broad space for the development of the undertaking. In modern times, it is still an arduous task for human beings to prevent and treat diseases and many countries are renovating and paying close attention to the role and value of traditional medicine. The international community's positive changes in the cognition of the traditional Chinese medical science and medicines and the acceptance and application of the traditional Chinese medical science and medicines by more and more peoples in different countries provide a broad space for the development of the undertaking of the traditional Chinese medical science and medicines.

Facing the good opportunities for the development, we shall also be fully aware of the difficulties and problems in the development of the undertaking of the traditional Chinese medical science and medicines. The first is that the characteristics and superiorities of the traditional Chinese medical science and medicines are not fully played and service areas are to be further expanded. Although with our joint efforts in recent years, the unfavorable situations have been improved and the traditional Chinese medical science and medicines play an important role particularly in the rescue and treatment of some contingents and the prevention and treatment of major serious diseases, it can be found from the results of the survey on the status quo that many TCM hospitals haven't fully played the characteristics and superiorities; few items of medical service are carried out and medical facilities are equipped adequately. Service items with TCM superiorities such as prevention, maintenance of health, health protection and rehabilitation lag behind, which can't meet people's need for health. The second is that inheritance and innovation shall be pushed forward energetically. We haven't done enough work in the exploration and development of the connotation of the original thinking of the traditional Chinese medical science and medicines, haven't done enough work in theoretical and technical innovation on the basis of the original thinking, haven't done enough work in the research on inheritance on the basis of famous veteran experts' experience and classic ancient literature and haven't done enough work in innovation and development by use of the scientific and technological achievements. Methods of research and evaluation and standardized systems suitable to the characteristics of the traditional Chinese medical science and medicines haven't been set up and independent innovative systems meeting the needs of the times haven't been formed. The third is that due to the weak foundation for the development of the traditional Chinese medical science and medicines, continuous efforts shall be made to fully implement and perfect the policies that support and promote the development of the undertaking. Results of the survey on the status quo show that only 59% of grassroots medical and health institutions are able to offer the service of the traditional Chinese medical science and medicines; the infrastructure and conditions of TCM hospitals need further improvement; TCM hospitals are under the high pressure of survival and development; there is an outstanding problem of imbalanced development between urban and rural areas and between different regions; defined policies on the support and promotion of the development haven't been fully implemented and some policy requirements need further perfection. The fourth is that the construction of the managerial system of the traditional Chinese medical science and medicines shall be strengthened. In spite of the intensification of the construction of the managerial system in recent years, generally speaking, we are still weak in management, especially in some cities and counties, lack of managerial institutions and professionals leads to difficulties in research and implementation of policies, industrial management and guidance, implementation and supervisory management of projects and so on, which can not meet the needs for the development of the undertaking and progress in the work.

We shall attach great importance to these difficulties and problems, enhance our sense of mission and sense of responsibility, seize the current favorable opportunities and energetically push forward the development of the undertaking of the traditional Chinese medical science and medicines otherwise; we may miss the opportunities and lose the achievements we have gained. We must forge ahead and overcome difficulties with greater determination, courage and energy, firmly hold on to the key task of promotion and realization of the scientific development of the undertaking, closely center on the mainline of full implementation of the *Several Opinions* in deepening the reform of medical and health system, clarify the train of thought for development, tackle difficult problems, make innovation in development patterns and improve development quality.

Firstly, we must insist on scientific development and pay more attention to overall planning and coordination. The theme of the 12th Five-Year Plan defined by the Party Central Committee is scientific development and the development of the traditional Chinese medical science and medicines shall also center closely on this theme. We shall do a good job in the overall planning of the coordinative development between the undertaking of the traditional Chinese medical science and medicines and health cause, economy and society and increase the rate of contribution to the construction of the well-off society in an all-round way. Efforts shall be made to comprehensively plan the coordinative development of medical treatment, health protection, scientific research, education, industry and culture and realize the renovating development of the undertaking of the traditional Chinese medical science and medicines. Importance shall be attached to the overall planning of the coordinative development of urban and rural areas so as to improve the accessibility to the service of the traditional Chinese medical science and medicines. We shall strive to comprehensively plan the development of the traditional Chinese medical science and medicines and the expansion of the international influence, pay more attention to the development of the traditional Chinese medical science and medicines, make each other promote mutually and realize a "win-win" situation.

Secondly, we shall emancipate our minds continuously and pay more attention to the innovation in mechanisms. Many years' practices in the traditional Chinese medical science and medicines have shown that irrational systems and mechanisms are the key factors that affect the play of the characteristics and superiorities and restrict the development of the undertaking. If we want to realize the sound and rapid development of the undertaking of the traditional Chinese medical science and medicines in the 12th Five-Year-Plan period, we must further emancipate our minds and renovate development ideology, tackle difficulties and make efforts to promote the innovation in systems and mechanisms in order to make them better embody the characteristics of the traditional Chinese medical science and medicines, accord with development laws, reflect development trends and meet the needs for development.

Thirdly, we must transform the development pattern and pay more attention to the characteristics and superiorities of the traditional Chinese medical science and medicines. At present, the disease pattern of our country is changing rapidly; if we are to realize the sound and rapid development of the undertaking in the 12th Five-Year-Plan period, we must respond to this change and transform the development pattern rapidly, changing it from the disease-treatment pattern to a comprehensive pattern of diseases prevention and treatment that attaches importance to both diseases treatment and prevention, health protection, maintenance of health and rehabilitation; from paying attention only to the single development of TCM hospitals to the joint development of multi-form medical and health institutions such as TCM hospitals, clinics, etc.; from paying attention only to the expansion of the scale of TCM hospitals to both appropriate attention to continuous expansion of the scale and greater attention to the construction of the characteristics and superiorities and the perfection of service functions and from a development situation invested only by governments to a diversified development situation involving both governments' investment and non-governmental sectors' investment.

Fourthly, technical support must be intensified and more attention must be paid to inheritance and innovation. Inheritance and innovation is not only the internal impetus for the development of the traditional Chinese medical science and medicines, but also the key for the traditional Chinese medical science and medicines to maintain vitality. Without technical support, development of TCM theories, improvement of clinical effectiveness, progress in industrial technology and formulation of public policies can't realize, so we shall persist in the original thinking of the traditional Chinese medical science and medicines and on the basis of fully understanding the essential properties and maintaining the characteristics of the traditional Chinese medical science and medicines, explore new methods, conduct new practice and strive to make new breakthroughs in the traditional Chinese medical science and medicines. We shall continuously enrich and develop the theoretic system by innovation in knowledge, unceasingly improve service capacity and technical level by innovation in techniques and make efforts to increase the impact of technical progress on the development of the undertaking.

(2) Plan scientifically, clarify tasks and promote the new development of the undertaking of the traditional Chinese medical science and medicines in the 12th Five-Year-Plan period

The 12th Five-Year-Plan period is a critical period for the overall and coordinative development of the traditional Chinese medical science and medicines, so we must make scientific judgment, keep abreast of the situation and development trend and fulfill the formulation of the 12th Five-Year Plan for the development of the traditional Chinese medical science and medicines. In accordance with the spirit of the 5th Plenary Session of the 17th CPC Central Committee, the train of thought for the development program and results of relevant research, I'll talk about some basic opinions on several problems in the formulation of the 12th Five-Year Plan for your discussion and reference.

On the general objective for the development of the undertaking of the traditional Chinese medical science and medicines in the 12th Five-Year-Plan period. By 2015, managerial systems and operational mechanisms of the traditional Chinese medical science and medicines will be more scientific and rational; TCM medical service and the emergency response system will be more perfect; TCM prevention and health protection service system will be basically constructed and service capacity will be improved remarkably. The quality of the talents in the traditional Chinese medical science and medicines will be improved greatly and the structure will be more reasonable. The system of inheritance and innovation will be established initially and remarkable achievements will be gained in inheritance and research. The level of industrial development of traditional Chinese medicines will be further heightened and the construction of the industrial system of modern Chinese medicines and the capacity for industrial innovation will be enhanced. Forms of the culture of the traditional Chinese medical science and medicines will be more diversified and cultural resources will be more effectively exploited and utilized. Legislation for the traditional Chinese medical science and medicines will be realized; the standardized system will be further perfected and informationized level will be further improved. More significant progress will be made in international exchange and cooperation; the dominant position of the traditional Chinese medical science and medicines in international traditional medicine will be consolidated and strengthened and the comprehensive and coordinative development of medical treatment, health protection, scientific research, education, industry and culture will be basically realized.

On the basic train of thought for the development of the undertaking of the traditional Chinese medical science and medicines in the 12th Five-Year-Plan period. With the Scientific Outlook on Development as the guidance for traditional Chinese medical work, promotion and realization of the scientific development of the undertaking as the major task, full implementation of the *Several Opinions* of the State Council in deepening the medical and health reform as the mainline, perfect systems and mechanisms, comply with development laws, maintain and develop the superiorities and characteristics, with focus on accelerating the promotion of the inheritance and innovation of the traditional Chinese medical science and medicines and the perfection and improvement of grassroots service system and capacity, accelerate the development of TCM preventive and healthcare service and the talent cultivation of the traditional Chinese medical science and medicines, strengthen the construction of legislation, standardization, informationzation and intensify supervision and management. We shall enhance coordination, make efforts to gain support and promote the comprehensive, coordinative and sustainable development of the undertaking of the traditional Chinese medical science and medicines.

On the key tasks for the development of the undertaking of the traditional Chinese medical science and medicines in the 12th Five-Year-Plan period.

—Strengthen the construction of the service system of TCM medical treatment, prevention and health protection. Focus shall be on the promotion of the construction of county-level TCM hospitals in order for them to reach the standards, the fulfillment of the standardized construction of the department of traditional Chinese medicine and the dispensary of traditional Chinese medicines in township and community health care centers and the improvement of the service capacity of village clinics and community health service stations. Efforts shall be made to promote medical institutions of traditional Chinese medicine and grassroots medical and health institutions to carry out preventive and healthcare service; exploitation in techniques and products shall be strengthened; service items shall be diversified and service specifications shall be perfected. Investment of non-governmental sectors shall be encouraged and guided to run TCM medical and preventive and healthcare service institutions so as to form a diversified situation of running hospitals.

—Strengthen the construction of the capacity for emergency response to and rescue and treatment and the networks of the prevention and treatment of major serious diseases with the traditional Chinese medical science and medicines. We shall perfect the working mechanisms and the networks of emergency response with the participation of the traditional Chinese medical science and medicines, build some clinical bases for the prevention and treatment of infectious diseases with the traditional Chinese medical science and medicines, promote the construction of the departments of the traditional Chinese medical science and medicines in hospitals for infectious diseases and basically establish the networks of the prevention and treatment of infectious diseases with the traditional Chinese medical science and medicines. The construction of key specialties (treatment of special diseases) and the specialties with the characteristics shall be intensified and cooperative networks of the prevention and treatment of major serious diseases with the traditional Chinese medical science and medicines shall be established. Mutual complement of traditional Chinese medicine and western medicine shall be pushed forward so as to bring each other's superiorities into full play and promote the integration.

—Promote the inheritance and innovation of the traditional Chinese medical science and medicines. Offices for the inheritance of famous veteran TCM experts' experience and TCM academic schools shall be constructed and ancient literature on traditional Chinese medicine shall be collated systematically. The construction of TCM clinical research bases and the clinical scientific research system of the prevention and treatment of infectious diseases and chronic non-infectious diseases with the traditional Chinese medical science and medicines shall be enhanced and the system of the inheritance and innovation of the traditional Chinese medical science and medicines shall be initially formed. Efforts shall be made to make breakthroughs in the explanation for the scientific connotation and the theoretic and technical innovation of the traditional Chinese medical science and medicines and also in the construction of the methodology and standardization system suitable to the traditional Chinese medical science and medicines.

—Intensify the construction of the talent contingents of the traditional Chinese medical science and medicines. Reform in the education of colleges and universities of the traditional Chinese medical science and medicines shall be promoted and the construction of key specialties shall be strengthened. Post-graduate education shall be carried out and standardized training for TCM resident doctors shall be enhanced. Master-disciple education shall be promoted and continuing education networks shall be perfected. Efforts shall be made to intensify the cultivation of high-level clinical talents and accelerate the cultivation and training of grassroots talents. Professional education shall be developed and training on technical skills and appraisal on some types of jobs peculiar to the industry of the traditional Chinese medical science and medicines shall be conducted. Talent incentive mechanisms shall be set up and optimized.

—Push forward development level of the industry of traditional Chinese medicines. W shall fully do well the work of the general survey on the resources of Chinese medicinal materials, gradually set up the monitoring system and accelerate the construction of the genetic germplasm repository. Research and application of key techniques in the production of traditional Chinese medicines and that of genuine medicinal materials shall be strengthened; TCM-related health industries shall also be developed.

—Accelerate the development of the undertaking of ethnic minority medicine. We shall strengthen the construction of the infrastructure of ethnical minority hospitals and the ethnic minority department of grassroots medical institutions in ethnic minority regions. Higher education of ethnic minority medical science and medicines shall be developed and talent cultivation shall be strengthened. Exploitation and inheritance of ethnic minority medical science and medicines shall be enhanced and the development and application shall be supported.

—Prosper and develop the culture of the traditional Chinese medicine and medicines. We shall develop and make good use of the cultural resources of the traditional Chinese medical science and medicines, set up networks to popularize the knowledge and culture, build some publicity and education bases and develop some creative products of science popularization. The national museum of the traditional Chinese medical science and medicines shall be built and the work of the protection and inheritance of the intangible cultural heritage of the traditional Chinese medical science and medicines shall be well done.

—Intensify the construction of the legislation, standardization and informationization of the traditional Chinese medical science and medicines.

The construction of the law system of the traditional Chinese medical science and medicines shall be promoted. Efforts shall be made to basically establish the standard system for the traditional Chinese medical science and medicines, set up the standardized research centers and the implementation and popularization bases and optimize the supporting systems for the standardization work. We shall perfect the electronic public service system for government affairs concerning the traditional Chinese medical science and medicines, set up systems of information statistics, optimize the construction of the system of information system of TCM hospitals and basically realize interconnection between the information on the traditional Chinese medical science and medicines and the information on medicine and health and the resource sharing.

—Push the traditional Chinese medical science and medicines to have greater international influence. Cooperation with foreign governments and international organizations shall be consolidated and expanded and non-governmental exchange and cooperation shall also be developed. We shall enhance the overseas propaganda for the culture of the traditional Chinese medical science and medicines and also promote the trade of services and products. Efforts shall be made to promote the internationalization process of the standard of the traditional Chinese medical science and medicines. Moreover, cooperation with Hong Kong, Macao and Taiwan shall be deepened and its unique role in the expansion of the international influence shall be brought into full play.

The above mentioned contents are the general consideration for the key tasks and the contents of the 12th Five-Year Plan for the development of the undertaking of the traditional Chinese medical science and medicines and all the localities shall put forward planning objectives, train of thought for development and working priorities in accordance with the actual local situations. All the localities shall closely integrate the formulation of the 12th Five-Year Plan, the implementation of *the Several Opinions* and local health development plans together and promote the work in a down-to-earth way.

III. Fully do well the work of the traditional Chinese medical science and medicines in 2011

This year is the first year of the 12th Five-Year-Plan period and also the key year for the full implantation of *the Several Opinions*. So, it is of significant importance for us to do well the work in 2011.

(1) With taking deepening the medical and health reform as a good opportunity, efforts shall be made to promote the full implementation of *the Several Opinions*

Policy measures put forward in the *Several Opinions* were well carried through and implemented in the past two years, but some policy requirements shall be made more specific and practicable and importance shall be attached to the implementation. This year is the last year for us to finish the recent five key tasks of the medical and health reform and the Party Central Committee determines to well construct the essential drug system and carry out the reform of public hospitals. We must seize this great opportunity, take the establishment and perfection of policy measures concerning "support and promotion" as the acting point and earnestly solve systematic and mechanic problems that affect and restrict the development of the undertaking of the traditional Chinese medical science and medicines. In the implementation of the essential drug system, with focus on the perfection of policies on the application of essential traditional Chinese medicines, efforts shall be made to strengthen the propaganda for essential traditional Chinese medicines, consolidate and expand the range and intensify the allocation and management in the application of the medicines. Selection of medicines for *the National Essential Drug List (for provision and use of other medical and health institutions)* shall be fulfilled and research shall be conducted on quality standards and prices, guarantee of production and supply and management of the allocation and application of Chinese traditional medical herbal pieces. In the pilot of promoting the reform of public hospitals, with focus on the establishment of systems and mechanisms beneficial to the play of the characteristics and superiorities of the traditional Chinese medical science and medicines, we shall carry out the pilot of financial compensation for traditional Chinese medical service, promote the implementation of TCM clinical pathways and explore ways of reform in the payment for the service, such as quota charging according to specific diseases and so on. In the construction of the promotion of the basic medical security system, efforts shall be made to implement the policies on the increase in the percentage of compensation for relevant expenses on the traditional Chinese medical science and medicines in the overall-planning scheme of the new rural cooperative medical care and the rise in the percentage of reimbursement for traditional Chinese medical service items in the basic urban medical insurance. In the promotion of the equalization of public healthcare service, importance shall be attached to carrying out traditional Chinese medical service and in performance evaluation on the basic public health service, evaluation on the service of the traditional Chinese medical science and medicines shall be well done and the pilot work that supports the basic public health service of the traditional Chinese medical science and medicines shall be pushed forward. In the construction of grassroots medical and health service system, we shall conduct research on the allocation of TCM resources and the planning for the construction the personnel specializing in the traditional Chinese medical science and medicines in grassroots medical and health institutions and do a good job in the renovation and construction of county-level TCM hospitals and the construction of the department of traditional Chinese medicine and the dispensary of traditional Chinese medicines in township and community health care centers and health service centers.

(2) With focus on urban and rural grassroots medical and health institutions, make efforts to heighten the capacity for the service of the traditional Chinese medical science and medicines

The first is to enhance the guidance and management on urban and rural medical work, organize and conduct the evaluation, carry out the pilot of the construction of comprehensive service regions of the traditional Chinese medical science and medicines in grassroots medical and health institutions and organize the training on the traditional Chinese medical science and medicines for leaders of county (city) health bureaus. The second is to make greater efforts to popularize appropriate techniques, do a good job in the construction of training bases, enhance teacher training, carry out hierarchical and classified popularization, intensify the supervision and guidance on the work and the evaluation on the effects, explore incentive mechanisms that encourage the application of appropriate techniques and improve the effects of popularization and application. The third is to intensify the construction of grassroots talents, attach importance to village doctors' education with record of formal schooling in the major of traditional Chinese medicine and continuously promote the work of bringing the personnel with special skills and techniques into the management of village doctors in rural areas. The fourth is to do well the work of the construction of key specialties (treatment of special diseases) with the characteristics of the traditional Chinese medical science and medicines in rural areas, carry out the construction of the clinical cooperative centers that have superiorities for the treatment of certain diseases with traditional Chinese medicine, work out and popularize TCM clinical diagnostic and therapeutic schemes and clinical pathways. The fifth is to strengthen the management of TCM hospitals and carry out deeply the activity of "management year of hospitals of traditional Chinese medicine"; revise basic standards and evaluation standards of medical institutions of traditional Chinese medicine, perfect systems of evaluation, monitoring, pre-warning and warning; enhance TCM nursing work and organize and initiate the engineering of qualified demonstrative nursing service. The Sixth is to further enhance the work of the traditional Chinese medical science and medicines in general hospitals, focus on the promotion of standardized construction of the departments of the traditional Chinese medical science and medicines and put basic service demands into effect. The seventh is to attach importance to the exploitation and collation, summary and improvement, popularization and application of folk medicine and drugs, formulate and perfect relevant policy measures that enable the personnel with special skills in folk medicine and drugs to play their role.

(3) With taking the intensification of the construction of inheritance and innovation as the hold, efforts shall be made to improve the capacity for scientific research on the traditional Chinese medical science and medicines

Firstly, inheritance and innovation in the traditional Chinese medical science and medicines shall be promoted. The collation and publication of the third batch of 400 ancient books on traditional Chinese medicine shall be fulfilled; the information database and the list of rare ancient books shall be set up and the general survey and registration shall be conducted in good time. Research-type inheritance of famous veteran TCM experts' experience shall be intensified unceasingly and the results shall be refined and popularized and research on the fundamental theories shall also be strengthened. Literature on ethnic minority medicine shall be well collated; some important pieces shall be emended, noted and publicized and appropriate techniques in ethnic minority medicine shall be selected and popularized. Secondly, the constitution of the clinical scientific research system shall be enhanced. With focus on the construction of national TCM clinical research bases, the construction of scientific and technological capacity and the platforms shall be intensified and open and cooperative mechanisms shall be established. Organizational patterns and operating mechanisms of the scientific research system for the prevention and treatment of infectious diseases and chronic non-infectious diseases shall be perfected and the close integration of clinical work and scientific research shall be pushed forward. Connotation construction of key research labs shall be deepened and key units, particularly enterprises of traditional Chinese medicines with superior resources and characteristic techniques shall build research labs. Thirdly, transformation and popularization of scientific research achievements shall be promoted. The role of technology-transfer organizations shall be brought into play and the scientific research achievements in the treatment of major complicated and difficult diseases, common diseases and in TCM acupuncture and moxibustion, traditional Chinese medicines etc. shall be summarized and popularized. Jointly with the State Development and Reform Commission, we shall continuously carry out the special project of high-tech industrial development of modern Chinese medicines and push forward the improvement of technological level of the industry. Fourthly, the general survey on the resources of traditional Chinese medicines shall be promoted; plans shall be perfected and implemented and the construction of the genetic germplasm repository of traditional Chinese medicines shall be intensified. Fifthly, efforts shall be made to plan and demonstrate major scientific and technological projects, strive to get national scientific and technologic supporting programs in the

12th Five-Year Plan and conduct community-oriented integrated research. With focus the research of major basic theories, special projects of traditional Chinese medicine in the National Basic Research Program (973 Program) shall be organized and carried out continuously. Continuous attention shall be paid to special industrial projects and research on the prevention and treatment of chronic non-infectious diseases shall be deepened. Sixthly, organizational and managerial patterns and mechanisms of science and technology shall be perfected; management on the quality of scientific research shall be strengthened; public platforms of scientific and technologic information service, ethic reviews on clinical researches and so on shall be constructed and expert consulting system shall be established and optimized.

(4) With focus on the cultivation of high-level talents and grassroots medical personnel, efforts shall be made to improve the quality of the talent contingents of the traditional Chinese medical science and medicines

The first is to strengthen the high-level talent cultivation and master-disciple education, do a good job in the inheritance of the fourth batch of veteran TCM experts' academic experience, excellent TCM clinical talents' research projects, the cultivation of academic pacesetters and the construction of offices for the inheritance of the experience of famous veteran TCM experts and TCM academic schools. The second is to promote job-transfer training for general practitioners majoring in traditional Chinese medicine and well organize the standardized training for resident doctors of TCM hospitals. The third is to enhance the construction of key disciplines, formulate and carry out the *Medium- and Long-Term Program for the Construction of Key Disciplines of Traditional Chinese Medicine*, do a good job in the implementation of the new round of the construction of key disciplines and push forward the construction of the sharing management platform. The fourth is to promote the development of vocational education of the traditional Chinese medical science and medicines and do research on the formulation of policy measures on transforming secondary schools and vocational colleges to institutions carrying out vocational education; standardize the training on technical skills for some types of jobs peculiar to the traditional Chinese medical science and medicines and do well the work of appraisal on professional techniques and skills. The fifth is to strengthen the continuing education of the traditional Chinese medical science and medicines, play the role of the continuing education bases of the disciplines with the superiorities of the traditional Chinese medical science and medicines and the urban community and rural demonstrative training bases of TCM knowledge and skills and ceaselessly increase the quality and coverage of the continuing education.

(5) With taking the active participation in the prevention and treatment of infectious diseases and the response to and rescue and treatment of public health

contingents as the entry point, efforts shall be made to improve the capacity for the prevention and treatment of infectious diseases and response to and rescue and treatment of public health contingents with the traditional Chinese medical science and medicines

The first is, on the basis of further improvement of the mechanism of the participation of the traditional Chinese medical science and medicines in response to health emergences, to intensify the construction of the medical emergency response system and build a team with remarkable basic skills, a wealth of clinical practices and experience and mastery of knowledge and skills concerning the prevention and control of infectious diseases and emergency rescue and treatment. The second is to do a good job in the construction of clinical bases of the prevention and treatment of infectious diseases with the traditional Chinese medical science and medicines and heighten the capacity for the prevention and control and the emergency rescue and treatment of infectious diseases of TCM hospitals. The third is to perfect technical programs for the prevention and treatment of major serious diseases and the emergency rescue and treatment of public health contingents, accomplish national major special projects of infectious diseases, enhance the construction of clinical scientific research system for response to newly-emerging and emergent infectious diseases and perfect emergency response networks and response mechanisms of scientific research for the participation of the traditional Chinese medical science and medicines in the prevention and treatment of major serious diseases. The fourth is to continuously do well the work of the prevention and treatment of infectious diseases such as influenza, hand-foot-mouth disease, etc. and the implementation of the task for expansion of the scale of AIDS treatment with traditional Chinese medical science and medicines.

(6) With taking the health engineering of "preventive treatment of diseases" as the prop, efforts shall be made to develop preventive and healthcare service of traditional Chinese medicine

We shall review the health engineering of "preventive treatment of diseases" comprehensively, do a good job in the evaluation on the service effects and promote the implementation of the engineering earnestly. The first is, with the construction of the supply system of preventive and healthcare service of traditional Chinese medicine as a foundation, to expand pilot and focus on the promotion of regional pilot work. The second is, with the perfection of the technical system of preventive and healthcare service as the starting point, to further strengthen the research and development of service technical methods and products, establish service items, work out service regulations and explore ways of offering oriented service of "preventive treatment of diseases" in the treatment of chronic diseases. The third is, with the perfection of relevant policy measures as the acting point, to formulate managerial systems for preventive and health care institutions and personnel, explore methods and measures that organically unite preventive and healthcare service with public health service and do researches on the establishment of service items, charging standards, medical insurance policies and other incentive measures. The fourth is to intensify propaganda and knowledge popularization and promote the broad masses to further understand the ideology of "preventive treatment of diseases" and the knowledge on the prevention and health protection of traditional Chinese medicine.

(7) With taking deepening the activity of "the Traditional Chinese Medical Science and Medicines in China" as the platform, efforts shall be made to promote the propaganda for the culture of the traditional Chinese medical science and medicines

The first is to further construct "the Traditional Chinese Medical Science and Medicines in China", deeply carry out the activity of "the Traditional Chinese Medical Science and Medicines in China • Entering Villages, Communities, Families", push forward the service to go down to the grassroots and benefit the broad masses. The second is to intensify the construction of networks that spread the knowledge and culture of the traditional Chinese medical science and medicines, well construct culture and education propaganda bases, organize experts' lecture tours for scientific popularization of the culture of the traditional Chinese medical science and medicines and promote the development of creative products of scientific popularization of the culture. The third is to push forward cultural construction of traditional Chinese medical institutions and carry out the pilot work of the cultural construction of TCM hospitals. The fourth is to perfect the news release system, timely release major news concerning the industry, strengthen the cooperation with mainstream media, do a good job in positive guidance of public opinions and expand the impact of the traditional Chinese medical science and medicines on the society. The fifth is to do well the work of the protection and inheritance of the intangible cultural heritage of the traditional Chinese medical science and medicines and make greater efforts to protect the items in the National Intangible Cultural Heritage List.

(8) With taking the acceleration of the construction of legislation, standardization and informationization as the foundation, efforts shall be made to promote the standardized construction of the traditional Chinese medical science and medicines

The first is to accelerate the legislative process of *the Law of Traditional Chinese Medicine*, do thorough research on major and key issues, cooperate actively with the Ministry of Health in the fulfillment of the revision and perfection of the draft and strive to report it to the State Council as soon as possible after the consideration of the Ministry of Health. The second is to accelerate the standardized construction, work out and implement programs for the development of standardization in the 12th Five-Year-

Plan period, research and decide the framework of the standard system, enhance the organization and guidance on the formulation of standards by the China Association of Chinese Medicine and relevant groups, perfect standardized managerial systems and working mechanisms, promote the construction of standard research and popularization bases (pilots) and perfect the supportive systems. The third is to accelerate informationizd construction, organize the formulation and implementation of the programs for the development of informationization, participate in medical and health informationized construction, strengthen the formulation of information standards and regulations, enhance the training and popularization of information technology and push forward the sharing of public health information resources. The fourth is to further enhance supervision and with focus on the regulation of TCM service market, perfect supervisory mechanisms, improve supervisory methods and heighten supervisory level.

(9)With focus on high-level international cooperation and exchange in the traditional Chinese medical science and medicines, efforts shall be made to promote the traditional Chinese medical science and medicines to go to the world more extensively

The first is to carry out research on the international development strategy of the traditional Chinese medical science and medicines and clarify the train of thought for development, objectives and tasks and working priorities in the new era. The second is to fully realize the strategic position of standardization in the promotion of the traditional Chinese medical science and medicines to go global, lay a solid foundation for the internationalization of the standardization of the traditional Chinese medical science and medicines, intensify cooperation with the World Health Organization (WHO), the International Standardization Organization (ISO) and so on,participate actively in the formulation of the International Classification of Diseases of WHO for the part of traditional medicine and offer active support to the work of the Secretariat of the Technical Committee of Traditional Chinese medicine of ISO. The third is to strengthen the cooperation with the United Nations Educational, Scientific and Cultural Organization (UNESCO) and strive to list ancient books on traditional Chinese medicine into the Memory of the World Register; put "Nanning Declaration" into effect, promote the cooperation between China and the Association of Southeast Asian Nations (ASEAN); enhance the coordination with the European Union (EU) and push forward the traditional Chinese medical science and medicines to enter EU market. The fourth is to intensify bilateral cooperation, put governmental agreements into effect and deepen the cooperation with America, France, Singapore and so on; meanwhile, strengthen and give guidance to people-to-people exchange and cooperation. The fifth is to promote international cooperation in scientific research on the traditional Chinese medical science and medicines and centering on key diseases of national clinical research bases and the construction of standards for traditional Chinese medicines, strengthen the exchange and cooperation in introduction of new technology, research on methodology, standards for traditional Chinese medicines, etc.. The sixth is to continue the overseas propaganda for the culture of the traditional Chinese medical science and medicines and explore forms and ways of international exchange in the culture of the traditional Chinese medical science and medicines. The service trade of the traditional Chinese medical science and medicines shall be promoted in trade negotiations. The seventh is to strengthen the construction of foreign cooperative bases and international-oriented expert contingents. The eighth is to deepen the exchange and cooperation with Hong Kong, Macao and Taiwan, carry out the agreements of the mainland and Hong Kong, Macao and Taiwan on the traditional Chinese medical science and medicines and promote the development of TCM medical service in Hong Kong, Macao and Taiwan. Cross-strait cooperative agreements shall be put into effect and substantial progress shall be pushed forward.

(10) The activity of "striving to excel in the performances" shall be carried out deeply

Strengthening the Party building and striving to excel in the performances is a political impetus and organizational guarantee for the sound and rapid development of the undertaking of the traditional Chinese medical science and medicines. We shall closely center on deepening the medical and health reform and carrying through the *Several Opinions* and carry out the activity of "striving to excel in the performances". The first is to enhance study and understanding, unify our ideological thinking with the working deployment and requirements of the Party Central Committee and Party Group and lay a solid ideological foundation for the deep implementation of the activity of "striving to excel in the performances". The second is, in accordance with the actual situation of the implantation of the tasks of the medical and health reform and the *Several Opinions*, to carry out the activity of medical workers' public commitment, leaders' comment and common people's evaluation to arouse Party members' and cadres' enthusiasm for the fulfillment of their responsibilities and make the broad masses more satisfied with the work of the traditional Chinese medical science and medicines. The third is to propagandize and carry forward the advanced models and outstanding deeds of the system and create a good environment, in which everyone competes in study, work and dedication and everyone learns from models, catches up with models and strives to be models. The fourth is, in accordance with the construction of learning-type Party organizations and "construction in three respects", strive to heighten all-level leading groups' and Party leaders' capacity and level for putting people first and governing for the people and ensure the scientific development of the undertaking of the traditional Chinese medical science and medicines.

Comrades, fulfillment of this year's traditional Chinese medical work is of significant importance for the full implementation of the *Several Opinions* and creation of a sound environment for a good start of the development in the 12th Five-Year-Plan period. Let's closely unite around the Party Central Committee with Hu Jintao as the General Secretary, unify our thinking, activate our spirit, make bold changes and innovations, do solid work, make efforts to open up a new prospect for the work of the traditional Chinese medical science and medicines and greet the 90th anniversary of the founding of the Communist Party of China with greater achievements.

(Zhao Yinghong)

13. An Address Delivered at 2011 Work Conference of National Food and Drug Supervision and Management

—By Shao Mingli, Commissioner of State Food and Drug Administration (January 13, 2011) (Excerpts)

In the following parts, I'll dwell on three aspects on behalf of the Party Group of the State Food and Drug Administration.

I. Summary on work in 2010 and review on work in the 11th Five-Year-Plan period

The year 2010 was the last year of the 11th-Five-Year-Plan period. The national food and drug supervisory and administrative system thoroughly implemented the important policies and deployments of the Party Central Committee and the State Council, forcefully strengthened food and drug supervision and administration, steadily carried out the campaign of Excellent Service, effectively strengthened the construction of the Party's working style and the clean government so that all the key work deployed at the beginning of the year was accomplished successfully. Firstly, we took the long view and worked well on the compilation of the 12th-Five-Year program. Active efforts were made to embody food and drug administration in the national overall planning. Consequently, *National Drug Safety Program (2011-2015)* was listed as the special program examined and approved by the State Council. All the localities endeavored to include food and drug safety into the local 12th-Five-Year programs with periodical major achievements. Secondly, we kept active yet steady and pushed forward the reform of supervisory and administrative system and mechanism. Efforts were made to implement the essence of the State Council leaders' instructions, strengthen follow-up instructions, get policy assistance, carry out the regulations on Major Responsibilities, Internal Organs and Personnel Staffing, obtain the relatively independent status for the institutions at the municipal and county levels, keep the team relatively stable and make sure the supervision and administration were not weakened. The construction of the team under the new system was accelerated. New duties of supervision on catering services, health food and cosmetics were initially fulfilled. Thirdly, we pooled our strength to fulfill the four key tasks of the supervision on the quality of essential drugs. Working plan for improving the quality standards of national essential drugs was formulated and implemented, sampling inspections covering all types of drugs were fulfilled, electronic supervision on essential drugs was started, the system of ADR (drug adverse reaction) monitoring, reporting and evaluating at the municipal and county levels were gradually completed and the supervision on the production, distribution and use of essential drugs was strengthened to ensure the quality safety of essential drugs. Fourthly, we endeavored to deal with the roots of the problems and pushed forward the special rectification on food and drug safety. The joint mechanism for anti-counterfeiting and rectification by multiple departments was consolidated and concentrated actions of cracking down on publicizing and selling counterfeit drugs via the internet was launched. Assisted by the police, many serious and major cases of counterfeit drugs were severely investigated and punished in Beijing, Guangdong, Zhejiang, Jiangsu, Shanghai, Heilongjiang, Hubei, Liaoning and Guangxi etc. , which effectively cracked down on the law violations and crimes and regulated drug market orders. Special rectifications on school canteens and construction site canteens were carried on, which purified the environment of catering services. Fifthly, we made all our efforts to safeguard the food and drug safety for the major activities. We successfully fulfilled the tasks of ensuring food and drug safety for Shanghai World Expo and Guangzhou Asian Games etc. and safeguarding disaster relief for Yushu earthquake in Qinghai and Zhouqu catastrophic flood and landslide in Gansu. Besides, the counterpart assistance for Tibet and Xinjiang were started in all aspects. China's vaccine regulatory system was assessed by the World Health Organization (WHO). All the achievements mentioned above laid a solid foundation for fulfilling the tasks of the 11th-Five-Year program and planning for the new development during the 12th-Five-Year-Plan period.

The 11th-Five-Year-Plan period was a truly extraordinary time in the course of the country's development. It was also the five years in which food and drug administrative departments at various levels conquered adversities and made progress bravely and remarkable achievements were made for food and drug supervision and administration. In the five years, the Party Central Committee and the State Council attached unprecedented importance to food and drug supervision and administration, the Party committees and governments at various levels provided unprecedented support and investment for food and drug supervision and administration, all sectors of the society paid unprecedented attention to food and drug supervision and administration and the food and drug supervisory and administrative system achieved unprecedented progress in emancipating the mind, serving the overall situation, innovating supervision and rectifying the market. Through unremitting efforts by the food and drug supervisory and administrative departments at various levels, new development was achieved for the cause of supervision and administration, and the situation of food and drug safety turned for the better, which greatly contributed to safeguarding and improving people's livelihood and pushing forward the balanced development of economy and society.

(1) The scientific concept of supervision and administration was established and applied, which determined the guidelines for food and drug supervision and administration. The guidelines for food and drug supervision and administration had direct influence on the basic requirements and the development orientation of supervision and administration. Since 2006, we have been analyzing and summarizing the success and failure in supervision and administration, investigating the root causes for the previous problems, getting the wits from the whole system together and, under the instruction of the Scientific Outlook on Development, we have come up with the requirements of establishing and practicing the scientific concept of administration. The essence and nuclei of the scientific concept of administration are to put people first, build the party for the interests of the people and exercise the governance for the people. The basic requirements of the scientific concept of administration are to promote carrying out government administration in accordance with the law, make policies scientifically and democratically, rely on technical support and ensure the team. The fundamental goal is to safeguard the food and drug safety for the public to promote the harmonious development of economy and society. It must be stressed out that in order to practice the scientific concept of administration, we must deal with the relationship between administration and development and the relationship between public interests and commercial interests properly and create the social environment that is safe for consumption and the market environment that is orderly for competition.

Guided by the scientific concept of administration, our minds are freer, our horizons are broader, our thoughts are more unified and our steps are more concordant. Pooling our minds and strength together, we have won two victories in rectifying market orders and strengthening the building of the team, which have won the recognition of the Party Central Committee and the State Council and the trust of the people so that food and drug supervision and administration is moving ahead for the new developments.

(2) The input into the construction of infrastructure and technical support system was increased so that the capability of food and drug supervision and administration was remarkably improved. During the 11th-Five-Year-Plan period, focusing on the grassroots and relying on the science and technology, remarkable achievements were made in the capability construction of supervision and administration. According to statistics, by the end of 2010, there had been 2,835 supervisory and administrative organs, 1,174 public institutions, 100% of the counties and 98.2% of villages had been covered by the rural drug supervisory net, 100% of counties and 93.8% of villages had been covered by the drug supply net, so that the administrative and technical supervisory system had come into being which covered both the urban and rural areas, horizontally covering the entire territory and vertically reaching the grassroots level.

The infrastructure for supervision and administration and the equipment for law enforcement were improved remarkably. During the 11th-Five-Year-Plan period, a total of 59.2 billion RMB Yuan was invested into improving the conditions of supervision and administration by finances at various levels, among which, the central finance invested 12.2 billion RMB Yuan, five times that in the 10th- Five-Year-Plan period. By the beginning of 2010, the whole system had possessed 4.01 million square meters of office buildings, 1.8 times that in 2005, 6.05 billion RMB Yuan of fixed assets, 2.3 times that in 2005, and 1.66 billion RMB Yuan worth of law enforcement equipment, 2.8 times that in 2005.

The construction of technical support system was strengthened remarkably. During the 11th-Five-Year-Plan period, the technical equipment for supervision and administration was improved, with 6,984 newly added pieces of various examining and testing equipment and devices, and 650,000 square meters of laboratories. The national action plan for improving drug standards was implemented steadily, with over 5,000 drug standards improved, *Chinese Pharmacopoeia* (2010) was issued and implemented smoothly and the drug standard system with *Chinese Pharmacopoeia* as the core was further improved. 571 standards for medical devices were formulated and revised. Besides, the construction of informationization was strengthened to promote the electronic supervision on drugs and improve the efficiency of supervision. Active efforts were made to participate in international communication and cooperation to gradually narrow the gap between us and the international advanced levels so that advancements were made towards internationalization of supervision and administration.

(3) Legal construction and system reform were pushed forward steadily and the long-term mechanism for food and drug supervision and administration was

improved. During the 11th-Five-Year-Plan period, the laws and regulations for food and drug supervision and administration were effectively improve. *Food Safety Law* was promulgated and implemented, several laws and regulations were formulated and revised, and fifteen departmental rules were issued successively so that a comparatively complete law and regulation system for supervision and administration has come into existence with laws and regulations as the basis and the departmental rules and regulatory documents as auxiliaries.

Reform on supervisory system was further deepened. On the basis of Three Separations (separation of administrative acceptance, separation of technical evaluation and separation of administrative approval) and Three System and One Construction (the system of the collective responsibility of the chief examiners, the system of publicizing examiners and the system of responsibility tracing for drug evaluation and approval and the construction of informationization), an administrative system for drug registration was established which is open and fair, normative and transparent and encourages innovation. The system of accredited supervisor and the system of qualified person were practiced, random inspections and on-site inspections were carried out and a stricter supervisory system for the quality of drug production was established. Monitoring on adverse drug reaction was strengthened, information reporting system was practiced and the mechanism of risk management was established. The opening of governmental affairs was expanded, and the mechanism of news releasing and information communication was improved. The principle of prevention first and combining prevention with emergency response was practiced and the emergency response mechanism was established with the goal of Early Detection, Early Reporting and Early Control.

In 2008, the State Council made major adjustments to the system of food and drug supervision and administration. Keeping the overall interests in mind and carefully implementing the essence of the reform by the State Council, food and drug administrations at all levels did a large amount of hard and detailed work in keeping stability, administrating by law and strengthening supervision and administration etc. Meanwhile, we emancipated our mind and improved the systems and mechanisms creatively. Cooperating with Hubei government, Hunan government, Chongqing government, Fujian government and Jiangxi government, State Food and Drug Administration initially explored on the new mechanism of comprehensive management under the new system. In Shanghai, Henan, Jilin, Guangxi, Changchun, Shenyang, Wuhan, Xi'an etc, we scientifically determined the institutions, personnel posts and duties in accordance with the local conditions and successfully fulfilled the task of system reform.

(4) Special rectifications were carried on and food and drug safety was getting for

the better. During the 11th-Five-Year-Plan period, food and drug administrations at all levels pooled the forces to carry out special rectifications with strict standards and measures, focusing on the hot issues and difficult issues such as A Drug with More than One Name, counterfeit application documents for drug registration, the spread of fake drug advertisements, non-drugs pretending to be drugs and illegal additives in health food and cosmetics etc. Monitoring net for drug abuse was established to control stimulants. Some serious food and drug safety incidents were severely investigated and punished, including Qieryao counterfeit drug event and the adverse drug reaction event of Clindamycin Phosphate Glucose injection (Xinfu event), Bioyee event of polluted Human Immunoglobulin (pH4) for intravenous injection and Sanlu Milk Powder etc., which effectively purified market order and consuming environment.

In the link of research and development, frauds were severely cracked down on to regulate the orders of registration and application. 36,000 application documents for drug registration and 31,000 application documents for medical device registration were verified. In the link of production, over 58,000 inspections were conducted including GMP certifications, follow-up inspections, random inspections and special inspections of quality system for medical device manufactures. Fourteen *Drug Production Licenses* were revoked, fifteen *Medical Device Manufacture Licenses* were canceled, and two hundred and seventy-five *Drug GMP Certificates* were recalled. Consequently, manufacturers' sense of quality safety was enhanced remarkably. In the link of circulation, comprehensive sampling inspections were conducted, illegal conducts like adjunct businesses were cracked down on, 350,000 illegal advertisements were monitored and transferred to police, 595 advertisement approval numbers were cancelled or recalled, 2,306 measures were taken to suspend the sales of illegally advertised products and 1,844 websites releasing illegal advertisements were transferred to the police or closed. Electronic supervisions were conducted on narcotic drugs, psychotropic drugs, blood products, vaccines and TCM injections. Publicity on safe drug-use was carried out to create a good social environment. With these special rectifications, the situations of drug safety were improving year by year.

While fulfilling the duty of comprehensive supervision on food and drug safety, we led the project of safe food, organized special rectifications on food safety, the investigation and punishments of serious incidents and emergency responses, actively explored the building of comprehensive evaluation and credit system for food safety, the building of demonstrative counties for food safety and its evaluation system to improve the comprehensive supervision mechanism for food safety. Since we took up the duties of supervision on catering service safety, health food safety and cosmetic safety, we have joined hands with relevant departments to make food safety rectifications for catering services and actively improve the supervision mechanism and system for food safety for catering services to forcefully enhance the construction of supervision team and capability. The examination and approval mechanisms for health food and cosmetics were improved, the technical approval standards were increased, supervision and inspections on production and management were intensified, monitoring on safety risks were conducted and remarkable achievements were made in the construction of technical support system and risk control system etc.

(5) The construction of the Party's working style and a clean government was strengthened so that the quality of the food and drug supervisory team was greatly improved. We always attached great importance to the construction of the Party's working style and a clean government and forcefully pushed forward the work on combating corruption and upholding integrity with the focus on constructing the system of punishing and preventing corruption. The campaign was launched to further study the Scientific Outlook on Development, focusing on solving the serious problems concerning Party's nature, Party's style and Party's disciplines etc, with which the people are most dissatisfied, and effectively enhancing the sense of exercising governance for the people. Eight Bans and Five Systems on practicing clean governance were formulated to regulate supervision. Decentralization of supervision and comprehensively open administration were pushed forward so as to address the roots of corruption. Violations and illegal cases were severely investigated and punished to educate the Party members and leaders and purify the supervisory team. We launched campaigns to encourage excellent service, publicize the advanced models around us, and spread the nobility represented by advanced individuals like Shi Junqin and advanced units to set up good profiles for the food and drug supervisory team.

The number of talents was increasing gradually and the comprehensive quality was improving gradually. According to statistics, by the beginning of 2010, the number of supervisory staff amounted to 68,000, among whom 75.7% were professionals and 65.8% were graduates or postgraduates, a remarkable increase compared with those in 2005. The scale of in-job-training reached new peak and model projects of training Top Leaders at the grassroots were carried out, which trained 792 directors-general of municipal food and drug administrations and directors-general of municipal institutes for drug control and 1,300 directors-general of county food and drug administrations. 248 national training workshops were conducted with 23,000 trainees. All the localities also conducted large-scaled, multi-layered and multi-channeled training for the staff. During the 11th-Five-Year-Plan period, we dealt with a series of serious events, major events and emergent events actively and appropriately. We effectively safeguarded the food and drug safety for the Celebration Ceremony for the 60th Anniversary of the Founding of the People's Republic of China, Beijing Olympic Games, Shanghai World Expo, Guangzhou Asian Games and Wenchuan massive earthquake. After the outbreak of pandemic H1N1influenza in 2009, we made elaborate planning and guidance and with the help of our technical storage for years, we completed the examining, testing, evaluating and approving for H1N1 vaccine in a comparatively short time so that our vaccine took lead in coming to market and achieving large-scaled safe vaccination. In 2010, while conducting large-scaled compulsory vaccination of measles vaccine for 110,000,000 people, we strengthened supervision throughout the whole process so that not a single quality safety incident occurred.

Strict and normative supervision and administration greatly promoted the sound development of the medical and pharmaceutical industry in China. In 2009, the gross output value of the entire industry exceeded 1,000 billion RMB Yuan and it was expected to exceed 1,200 billion RMB Yuan in 2010. Therefore, the safety, effectiveness and accessibility are effectively ensured for people's drug use.

Reviewing the 11th-Five-Year-Plan period, we have come to realize that to promote the scientific development of food and drug supervision and administration, we must endeavor to do the followings: firstly, we must be guided by the Scientific Outlook on Development, practice the scientific concept on supervision and administration, and adhere to putting people first and exercising governance for the people so as to ensure food and drug safety for the people and promote the sound and fast development of economy and society; secondly, we must adhere to administrating by law, strengthen the construction of laws, regulations and standardization, push forward making administrative affairs open and endeavor to construct a normative and transparent supervisory system to ensure the supervision and administration unified, efficient and authoritative; thirdly, we must keep on improving the capability of supervision and administration, focus on strengthening education and training for the leaders, strengthen the construction of technical support system and continuously improve the technicalization and informationalization of supervision and administration; fourthly, we must keep on reforming and innovating, actively adjust to the changes of environment and requirements of supervision and administration and while keeping development and reform in mind, deal with new problems in practice properly and try to solve new problems on our way; fifthly, we must adhere to the principle of attaching equal importance to reforming and combating corruption, change our working style, exercise our power cautiously and fulfill our duties correctly.

It is not easy for us to make these achievements and therefore the experience we have learned is especially precious. All the progress we have made in food and drug supervision and administration should be attributed to the wise leadership of the CPC central committee and the State Council, the powerful support of relevant departments including the media and the hard work of all the cadres and staff of food and drug administrative system nationwide. So now, on behalf of the Party Group of SFDA, I would like to express our sincere gratitude to all relevant departments and all sectors of the whole society who care for and support food and drug supervision and administration. Also, I would like to express our honorable respect to all the cadres and staff working diligently in the field of food and drug supervision and administration.

II. The situations and tasks we will be faced with during the 12th-Five-Year-Plan period.

The 12th-Five-Year-Plan period is very crucial for building a prosperous society in China comprehensively, deepening reform and opening-up and speeding up the transformation of the pattern of economic development. The 17th CPC National Congress, the third, the fourth and the fifth plenary sessions of the 17th CPC National Congress stressed time and again to ensure food and drug safety. All the food and drug administrative departments at all levels must fully understand and practice the essence of the Central Committee, carefully analyze the situations faced by supervision and administration, actively seize and make full use of the important opportunities for development, appropriately deal with various risks and challenges and try to improve food and drug safety.

Analyzing the situations home and abroad comprehensively, we can say with certainty that food and drug administration is still in an important period of strategic opportunities during the 12th- Five-Year-Plan period. Firstly, we are faced with an important opportunity to continuously strengthen supervision and administration. At present, GDP per capita in China has exceeded $4,000. Both the international experience and the domestic development show that the consuming structure of the public will keep on upgrading and the requirements for food and drug safety will grow rapidly during this stage of development. At the 5th plenary session of the 17th CPC National Congress, "scientific development" was defined as the theme of the 12th-Five-Year-Plan program, and it was demanded that safeguarding and improving people's livelihood be the aim and outcome of accelerating the changes of growth models and food and drug safety be an important part of social construction. The 6th plenary session of the 17th CPC National Congress especially stressed putting people first and exercising governance for the people, which created a favorable environment for us to get support from the Party committees and governments at various levels and continuously strengthen food and drug supervision and administration. Secondly, we are faced with an important opportunity to push forward scientific supervision and administration comprehensively. The 5th plenary session of the 17th CPC National Congress defined speeding up the transformation of the pattern of economic development as the major task of the 12th-Five-Year-Plan program. For the development in the future, more and more importance will be attached to scientific innovation and structure adjustment, and it will be possible to really solve the problems concerning the development of food and drug economy, i.e. the undue relying on the increase in numbers, comparatively extensive development models and comparatively low levels of development. As an important component of the modern industry system and strategic new industries, food and drug industry will be more and more powerful with rapid and sound development. We are able to play a more and more important role in improving standards, strengthening normalization, and leading innovation etc. We are able to push forward scientific supervision comprehensively and push forward scientific development with scientific supervision so as to achieve sound interaction between supervision and development and lay a solid foundation for the long-term development of food and drug safety. Thirdly, we are faced with an important opportunity to deeply regulate orders of drug production and circulation. The present is a crucial period of time for fully pushing forward the reform of medical and healthcare system. It has become the determination of the Party and the nation as well as a major task for the governments at all levels to establish and improve a system to guarantee drug supply with the national essential drug system as the base to ensure drug quality and safety. This makes it possible for us to adopt stricter supervision measures, push forward electronic supervision on drugs, improve the normalization of drug production and circulation and solve some deeper problems that hold back the development of supervision and administration. Fourthly, we are faced with an important opportunity to accelerate improving the internationalization of supervision and administration. With the globalization of economy, food and drug industry in China is evolving from the simple import and export trade in the past to more comprehensive and deeper opening up. International integration is accelerating with comprehensive and deeper international cooperation in the fields of basic research, clinical trial and production and supply of drugs. Food and drug industry is adopting the strategy of Going Global. We must take into account the changes of domestic situations and international situations, accelerate bringing our policies and laws, management norms and quality standards more in line with international ones, narrow the gap between China and the developed countries, have more say on supervision and administration internationally and better safeguard our national interests and people's rights of health.

While being faced with the opportunities, we must also be aware that the contradiction between people's rapidly increasing demands for food and drug safety and the comparatively backward levels of food and drug safety will be the main contradiction we will have to face in the 12th - Five-Year-Plan period or even a longer period of time. On our way forward, there still exist many problems and challenges: Firstly, the system and mechanism of supervision and administration are not perfect. The problems of incomplete structure and unbalanced regional development are still serious. The basis of supervision on catering services, health food and cosmetics are comparatively weak. The capabilities of ensuring food and drug safety at the grassroots and in the remote areas need to be improved. The division of supervision authority is not scientific and the efficiency of supervision needs to be improved. Secondly, the development level of the industry is not high in general. The scale of our food and drug industry is quite large, and some of our production capacities can rank first in the world, but our overall level is low, and so are the level of intensification and technology content. The integrity system of the society is not complete, manufacture and supply are not normative, and there are frequent frauds and circumventions of supervision. Thirdly, the construction of supervisory capability has fallen behind comparatively. Compared with the significant improvements in the infrastructure construction and the equipment of law enforcement, the problems of backward supervisory models, weak technical methods and insufficient top talents are even more serious. The quality of the cadres and the construction of working styles need to be strengthened and administration by law needs to be improved.

In general, we will be faced with unprecedented opportunities as well as severe challenges during the 12th-Five-Year-Plan period. So we must both seize and make full use of the opportunities and meet and overcome the challenges.

Taking into account the development tendency in the future and the existent work basis, we set forth the following main objectives for food and drug supervision and administration in the 12th-Five-Year-Plan period: to put food and drug safety under scientific supervision so as to resemble the international advanced levels, continue to strengthen ensuring food and drug safety and supervision on it and lay a crucial foundation for the long-term food and drug safety.

People's food and drug safety will be ensured by the effective system and mechanism. Supervisory institutions at the national, provincial, municipal and county levels will be further improved and accountability systems for catering service food safety, health food safety, cosmetic safety, drug safety and medical device safety will be fully practiced. The supervisory system will be more scientific, the division of authority will be more rational, and the operation of power will be opener so as to share supervision resources and improve the efficiency of supervision significantly.

The foundation for administration by law will be consolidated. The law and regulation system of food and drug supervision and administration will be improved. A technical specification and standard system has formed which covers catering service food safety and the supervision on health food, cosmetics, drugs and medical devices, the standards for drugs and medical devices will be the same as or resemble international advanced levels.

The system of technical support will be fully strengthened. A system of technical support will be set up which can meet the needs of supervision and administration and conforms to the real conditions in China and the tendency of internationalization of supervision and administration. The electronic supervisory network will be improved. A talent team for supervision will be primarily formed which is moderate in size, rational in structure and good in quality.

The quality and supply of drug will be significantly improved. The quality safety of essential drugs will be ensured. A monitoring network for ADR (adverse drug reaction) that covers both the urban and the rural areas will be established. A policy system for supervision will be completed that can ensure safety, regulate the market and encourage innovation so that remarkable achievements will be made in promoting industrial upgrading and scientific innovation.

To achieve the above objectives, we will have to fulfill the following main tasks:

(1) We will adjust to the new situations of supervision and administration and continue to enrich and develop the scientific concept of supervision in practice. Firstly, we will attach more importance to putting people first. We will keep the fundamental interests of the overwhelming majority of the people in mind, and make ensuring food and drug safety for the people the aim and outcome of all our work, trying all our efforts to protect and benefit the people effectively. Secondly, we will attach more importance to administration by law. We will set forth the goal of establishing a government of laws, keep on scientific and democratic legislation, forcefully promote normative, fair, civilized and efficient law enforcement and continuously strengthen supervision on law enforcement to ensure the full and accurate implementation of supervisory laws and regulations. Thirdly, we will attach more importance to scientific and democratic decision-making. The procedure of decision-making will be improved, the responsibility for decision-making will be strengthened, the decision-making for supervision will be more transparent, the reviewing-evaluation on decision-making will be strengthened and the supervision and check on the exercise of power will be strengthened as well. Fourthly, we will attach more importance to innovation in supervision and administration. Great efforts will be made to conduct scientific research on supervision and administration and promote theory innovation, system innovation, science and technology innovation and method innovation for supervision and administration so as to steadily improve efficiency during the process

of innovation. Fifthly, we will attach more importance to making supervision and administration more internationalized. We will initially adjust to the globalization of the economy and strengthen international communication and cooperation, especially with the supervisory departments in advanced countries in supervisory theories, examination and approval, check and authentication, inspection and testing and surveillance and evaluation etc.

(2) We will reform and better system and mechanism and continue to improve the efficiency of supervision and administration. Firstly, efforts will be made to strengthen the construction of regulations and rules and the system of standards. A framework of laws and regulations will be improved that covers the supervisions on drugs, medical devices, health food, cosmetics and catering services etc. Focusing on implementing and applying laws and regulations, active efforts will be made to construct correspondent auxiliary systems. The national system of drug standards and the system of standard management will be completed so that the standards for chemical drugs and biological drugs in *Chinese Pharmacopeia (2015 Edition)* will be the same as or resemble the international advanced level and those of TCM will lead the international standards. The management system for medical device standards will be completed. The standard system or technical requirements for the safety of health food and cosmetics will be completed. Efforts will be made to propel the establishment of standard system for food safety in catering services. Secondly, efforts will be made to establish the new mechanism of supervision and administration that is open and transparent, with smooth information communication and clear responsibility. Communication with relevant departments, enterprises and the public will be strengthened so that all the sectors of the society can have more chances to participate in supervision on food and drug safety. Active work will be done on the scientific publicity of food and drug safety. Reform on the system of administrative examination and approval will be deepened to intensify making government affairs open and making supervision more transparent. Efforts will be made to apply the responsibility system of "local government taking overall responsibility, supervisory departments taking their respective responsibility and the manufactures being the first person responsible". Thirdly, efforts will be made to form a new pattern of supervision and administration with optimized allocation of resources, complementary advantages and efficient operation. The sense of overall situation will be intensified for the whole supervisory system, the power for supervision will be scientifically allocated to dispatch supervisory resources rationally, and the system of authority division will be improved to give maximum play to the efficacy of the present staff, institutions and equipment. Technical support institutions will be completed and optimized so that we can share inspection information, examination and approval resources and the

techniques for inspection and testing to the maximum.

(3) We will seize the opportunities for development to continuously improve our capability of supervision and administration. Firstly, we will strengthen the construction of technical support system for supervision and administration. The focus will be on strengthening the construction of technical institutions of examination and approval, inspection and authentication, checking and testing and surveillance and evaluation etc. The checking and testing system for drugs and medical devices will be improved and the checking and testing system for catering services, health food and cosmetics will be established and completed. The construction of ADR surveillance will be strengthened focusing on improving the capability of ADR surveillance at the grassroots and the quality of reports. The construction of the supervisor team will be strengthened. Secondly, we will strengthen the construction of the interior management system. Active efforts will be made to introduce the modern concepts of management and comprehensively propel the construction of quality management system in the aspects of examination and approval, inspection and authentication, checking and testing and surveillance and evaluation etc. Thirdly, we will strengthen the construction of supervisory infornationalization. The first stage of the project of the national information system for drug supervision will be completed and the second stage of the project will be started. The construction of the national electronic supervisory system for drug will be completed. The construction of the information system for the supervision on health food, cosmetics and food safety for catering services will be started. Fourthly, the construction of the grassroots will be strengthened. We will try to get more support from the central finance, and more favor will be given to the grassroots, remote areas and minority ethnic areas in the arrangement of funds, project construction and technical assistance etc. so as to improve the conditions for law enforcement in all aspects, improve the quality of the team at the grassroots and achieve the balanced and harmonious development for the capability of ensuring food and drug safety.

(4) We will make great efforts to strengthen the construction of the team and adopt the strategy of training competent personnel as a priority. Firstly, we will complete the mechanism for supervising the construction of the personnel team. The incentive system for food and drug supervisory personnel will be completed. To meet the needs of supervision and administration, we will explore establishing the mechanism for the construction of supervisory institutions and personnel at the grassroots that is related with factors such as the population in the area, objects of supervision and size of supervision. Efforts will be made to get investment from the government finance to ensure that the average increase in the investment into supervisory personnel will be higher than the increase in supervision funds. Secondly, we will strengthen the

construction of education and training system. The reform on education and training for cadres will be deepened; education and training institutions will be established that can meet the needs of personnel construction and the system of subjects, courses and textbooks as well as the system of teacher team will be completed. Thirdly, we will carry out various trainings carefully. We will finish the new round of trainings for leaders of the provincial supervisory institutions and the new round of trainings for the persons in charge of the municipal and county level supervisory institutions. Training for the staff members of the institutions affiliated directly to the State Food and Drug Administration (SFDA) will be strengthened. We will vigorously develop on-line education. Fourthly, we will accelerate carrying out the program for cultivating international talents. We will try to meet the needs of the development of science and technology and the internationalization of supervision, strengthen cultivating talents who are in urgent need and demand, and pool all our strength to cultivate a galaxy of top experts and talents who can lead the scientific and technological development of supervision in China and are capable of participating in international supervision as well.

(5) We will focus on transforming the pattern of the economical development and lead adjusting the industrial structure. Firstly, efforts will be made to complete the drug supply system with the national essential drug system as the basis. We will seize the opportunity of implementing essential drug system to accelerate improving standards, strengthen the whole-process supervision on drug quality, and fully promote electronic supervision on drug to ensure the quality safety of essential drugs. Vigorous efforts will be made to promote the centralization of essential drug manufacture and supply to the excellent manufacturers to increase the centralization of drug industry. Secondly, efforts will be made to encourage the development of new drugs. We will implement and practice the national strategic deployments on the development of major new drugs, and, aiming at improving independent development of new drugs, explore and improve the examination and approval mechanism and strategy that encourage innovation with definite guide. Efforts will be made to strengthen the technical cooperation and communication with the colleges and universities, research institutes, drug manufacturers and local organizations. Efforts will be made to encourage the innovation and the second development of traditional Chinese medicines (TCM) and the minority ethnic medicines. Thirdly, efforts will be made to improve the technical specifications and the standards of product quality. The new *Good Manufacturing Practice for Pharmaceutical Products* will be fully carried out and *Good Supplying Practice for Pharmaceutical Products* will be revised and carried out. *Good Manufacturing Practice for Medical Devices* will be carried out comprehensively. We will go on carrying out the working plan for improving

standards to improve the standards for drugs and medical devices comprehensively and eliminate the outdated products. Fourthly, vigorous efforts will be made to give full play to the role of macro-control of the supervisory policies. To address the serious contradiction of the low level of industrial development, we will accelerate formulating and carrying out supervisory policies which support the superior and eliminate the inferior and propel centralization, complete the mechanism of market exiting and lead the industry to increase the core competitiveness.

Ⅲ. Arrangements on the key work in 2011

The year 2011 is the first year of the 12th-Five-Year-Plan period, and it is also the crucial period for us to accomplish the recent objectives of the reform on the medical and healthcare system. Thus, the tasks for food and drug supervision and administration are arduous and heavy. Taking into consideration the overall situations of supervisory system reform at present and the objectives and requirements for the 12th-Five-Year-Plan period, we will focus our attention on accelerating the establishment of the new working mechanism of supervision and administration that fits with the present system, pushing forward the reform and innovation on supervisory mechanism and system with more determination and more effective measures and fulfilling our responsibility for supervision and administration effectively to achieve progress in improving efficiency and synergy.

The leaders of the relevant bureaus will make detailed deployments on the work of this year concerning catering services, health food, cosmetics, drugs and medical devices etc. Here, I will emphasize some key work:

(1) We will determine the development strategy and objectives for the next five years with the compilation of the development program in the 12th-Five-Year-Plan period as the key task. All the departments and units must attach great importance to programming and try to have a successful start for devising the development program and accomplishing the development objectives. Firstly, we will implement and apply the essence of the fifth plenary session of the 17th CPC National Congress, take food and drug safety as the important contents, include it into the overall development of the local economy and society and endeavor to embody food and drug supervision and administration in the local overall programs. Secondly, we will, in line with the basis and conditions of supervision and administration in our jurisdictions, formulate the development objectives and task requirements corresponding to the development of economy and society. We must be provident and practical while determining our tasks, rather than blindly follow others' examples. Thirdly, we must determine the key projects and supporting measures. Efforts will be made to include the development

program for food and drug supervision and administration into the local specialized programs, work well on the compilation of the projects and ensure the funds to lay foundation for accomplishing the tasks of supervision and administration.

(2) We will ensure drug quality safety with the supervision on the quality of essential drugs as the key task. In line with the short-term objectives in three years of the medical and healthcare reform, all the departments and units will further strengthen leadership to accomplish responsibilities and effectively strengthen the supervision on essential drugs. Firstly, we will fulfill the task of electronic supervision on all type of drugs. By April 1, 2011, all types of essential drugs taking bids will have been under electronic supervision. There is no bargaining for the deadline and no change to our determination. All the localities must attach great importance and push forward the work unswervingly in strict accordance with the requirements. Secondly, we will strengthen the surveillance and evaluation on adverse drug reaction (ADR) of essential drugs. Efforts will be made to finish the construction of the reporting and evaluating system for ADR at the municipal level. *Methods on the Management of ADR Report and Surveillance* will be issued, therefore, we will endeavor to publicize and carry out it to fully strengthen ADR report and surveillance at the grassroots.

(3) We will improve the efficacy of food and drug supervision and administration with the construction of responsibility system as the key task. We must be aware that we are still at the special phase of the reform on supervisory system and the supervisory systems, supervisory duties and supervisory modes vary form place to place. Therefore, it is urgent that the new mechanism of supervision and administration be researched on and established that fits with the present system. This year, we will focus our attention on the following two tasks: Firstly, efforts will be made to promote the construction of responsibility system. In order to explore the experience on building the supporting system, management system and operation mechanism and accelerate establishing and completing the responsibility system for food and drug safety, eight provinces (municipalities) will conduct pilot on the construction of responsibility system for food and drug safety with the support of the local governments, i.e. Hubei, Hunan, Heilongjiang, Zhejiang, Jiangsu, Jiangxi, Chongqing and Ningbo. Besides, the campaigns of building demonstration counties for food and drug safety and demonstration projects for food and drug safety for catering services will be carried on nationwide and we will fully explore the working mechanism of carrying out the responsibility of the local governments, the departments and the manufacturers. SFDA will strengthen the guidance on the pilot units and provide necessary policies and funds. Meanwhile, all the localities will be encouraged to carry out pilots in accordance with their actual conditions to accumulate experience. Secondly, efforts will be made to propel the reform on the interior operation

mechanism of the supervisory institutions. Aiming at optimizing procedures, fulfilling duties and improving efficiency, we will accelerate the reform on the examination and approval systems for drugs, medical devices, health food and cosmetics. More efforts will be made to research on the division of authority on technical examination and administrative approval, on the definition and division of authority between SFDA and provincial food and drug administrations. Reform on the system of vaccine lot release will be pushed forward. Efforts will be made to optimize the allocation of supervision resources and improve the co-movement so that it will be possible to make the procedure more scientific and rational, seek accountability and improve efficiency significantly.

(4) We will further purify food and drug market orders with consolidating and expanding the achievements of rectification as the key task. Efforts will be made to create a fair, just and orderly market, lead the enterprises to accelerate transforming the patterns of economic development, and we will strengthen the quality control and attach more importance to technical innovation. Firstly, we will improve the foundation for the laws and regulations which propel industrial restructuring. Vigorous efforts will be made to assist relevant departments with the annual legislation on *Regulations for Supervision and Administration of Health Food and Regulations for Supervision and Administration of Medical Devices* etc. More efforts will be made to issue urgently needed regulations and regulatory documents for the management of drug standards, the management of medical device registration, the supervision and management of health food and cosmetics and the supervision and management of food safety operation specifications for catering services. We will assist the research and implementation of policies on industrial restructuring. Secondly, joining hands with other departments, we will carry on the forceful campaign of cracking down on counterfeit and substandard drugs. Some major and serious cases which brought about negative influence in the society and with witch the people were most dissatisfied were investigated and punished under public supervision. Continuous efforts were made to crack down on frauds on drug development and registration application. Thirdly, policy guidance was clarified to encourage drug innovation. Regulations for the examination and approval of health food, cosmetics, drugs and medical devices were strictly carried out and standards for examination and approval and reevaluation were improved to ensure the examination and approval can be finished by law and on time. Good work will be done on the publication, training and implementation of *Chinese Pharmacopeia (2010)* and the compilation of *Chinese Pharmacopeia (2015)* will be started. Emphasis will be put on the publicity, training and implementation of the new GMP of drugs. Efforts will be made to propel carrying out the major projects of new drug development and innovation.

Opinions on strengthening the management of TCM will be promulgated to guide the sound development of TCM industry.

(5) We will keep on improving the quality of the cadre team with strengthening education and management as the key task. Efforts will be made to cultivate a cadre team which can meet the needs of scientific development so as to provide talented personnel and intelligent support for the implementation of the development program in the 12th-Five-Year-Plan period. Firstly, we will earnestly implement CPC Central Committee's *Outline of Deeping Reform on Personnel System of Cadres Program (2010-2020)*, vigorously and steadily push forward the reform on the personnel system of cadres and complete the mechanism for selecting and promoting cadres to enhance the dynamic and vitality of the team. Secondly, we will fully implement *Outline of the National Medium and Long-term Talented Personnel Development Program (2010-2020)* and compile *Medium and Long-term Program of Food and Drug Supervisory Personnel Development* to establish the development strategy of talents first. Thirdly, we will earnestly implement the *2010-2020 Outline of Reform on Education and Training for Cadres* to intensify education and training for cadres. Good work will be done on training for members of the leader bodies of the provincial institutions, chief responsible persons of the administrative supervisory institutions at the municipal and county levels and the chief responsible persons of technical supervisory institutions at the provincial and municipal levels. Training for the supervisory teams for catering services, health food and cosmetics will be intensified. Plans for the cultivation of personnel in different fields will be made respectively. Plans for cultivating international talents will be implemented. The construction of licensed pharmacists will be strengthened and planning for the medium and long-term development and guidelines on the 12th-Five-Year-Plan for further education will be compiled. Efforts will be made to equip drug retail stores with licensed pharmacists.

(6) We will provide political motivation and organizational guarantee for supervision and administration with the campaign of Excellent Service and the construction of the Party's working style and the clean government as the key tasks. Efforts will be made to improve working mechanisms and strengthen the construction of the Party. With the theme of "Ensuring Food and Drug Safety with Scientific Supervision and Management", we will focus on the main tasks for food and drug supervision and administration to deepen the campaign of Excellent Service. We will give full play to the advanced models to encourage and guide the cadres and staff members to have firm confidence, activate the spirit and pool our mind and strength and endeavor to build the administrative organs which are committed to learning, operated by law, service-oriented, efficient and democratic.

More importance will be attached to the building of Party's style and a clean government and combating corruption to make new progress in combating corruption and upholding integrity for food and drug supervision and administration. In recent years, we have adhered to addressing both the symptoms and root causes and combining punishment and prevention and kept the forceful tendency of investigating and punishing cases of violating regulations and laws. Education has been more targeted and more practical and the construction of rules and regulations have been more rigorous, more scientific and more effective, both of which have ensured and promoted food and drug supervision and administration. But meanwhile, we must be keenly aware that there are officials and staff members who abuse the authorities, take bribes, ask for bribes or neglect their duties and there are cases of violations of laws or regulations. We must be keenly aware that the struggle against corruption will be long, complex and arduous so we can push forward combating corruption and upholding integrity with firmer confidence, more determined attitude and more powerful measures. The sixth plenary session of the 17th National Congress of the Communist Party has just concluded. Leaders at all levels, especially the top leaders of all the departments and units, must earnestly learn and deeply implement the essence of the session, especially the important speech delivered by General Secretary Hu Jintao so as to firmly set up and conscientiously practice the concepts of putting people first and exercising the power for the people and earnestly fulfill the political responsibilities of building the Party's style of work and the clean government and combating corruption. In accordance with the program for the development of punishment and prevention system, we will further carry out education on building the clean government, improve the system of the clean government, ensure the management of the Party members strictly, strengthen the auditing and supervision on the major projects and funds, promote the culture of the clean government, intensify the efforts to enforce disciplines and investigate violations of laws and firmly rectify all the misconducts that harm people's interests. Soon, SFDA will hold the work conference on building the Party's style of work and the clean government to transmit, study and practice the essence of the sixth plenary session of the CPC Central Disciplinary Commission and research and deploy specifically on work on building the Party's style of work and the clean government.

Comrades, the fifth plenary session of the 17th National Congress of the Communist Party has decided on the development program for the next five years. Therefore, we must earnestly implement and practice the essence of the CPC Central Committee. We must seize the opportunities, set higher aims and work elaborately on the development program and task deployment for supervision and administration during the 12th-Five-Year-Plan period. We will carry out all work effectively to promote the cause of food and drug supervision and administration into a new phase of development so that we can make greater contribution to celebrating the 90th anniversary of the founding of the CPC and promoting the building of the moderately prosperous society in all respects.

(Zhao Xuemei)

Part Ⅱ Policy and Statute

Order of the President of the People's Republic of China (No. 52)

The Decision of the Standing Committee of the National People's Congress on Amending the Law of the People's Republic of China on the Prevention and Control of Occupational Diseases, was adopted at the 24th session of the Standing Committee of the 11th National People's Congress of the People's Republic of China on December 31, 2011, is hereby issued and shall come into force on the date of issuance.

Hu Jintao, President of the People's Republic of China
December 31, 2011

1. *Law of the People's Republic of China on Prevention and Control of Occupational Diseases (Amendment 2011)*

Chapter I General Provisions

【**Article 1**】This Law is enacted, in accordance with *the Constitution*, for the purpose of preventing, controlling and eliminating occupational disease hazards, preventing and controlling occupational diseases, protecting the health and related rights an interests of workers, and promoting economic and social development.

【**Article 2**】This Law is applicable to activities conducted within the territory of the People's Republic of China to prevent and control occupational diseases.

For the purpose of this Law "occupational diseases" means the diseases contracted by the employees of an enterprise, a public institution and an individual economic organization (hereinafter all are referred to as the employer) due to their exposure in the course of work to dusts, radioactive substances and other toxic and harmful substances, etc.

The categories and catalogue of occupational diseases shall be determined, adjusted, and published by the health administrative department of the State Council in conjunction with the work safety administrative department and labor and social security administrative department of the State Council."

【Article 3】 In prevention and control of occupational diseases, the principle of putting prevention first and combining prevention with controlling shall be upheld, a mechanism of "responsibility of the employer, regulation by the administrative organs, industry self-discipline, participation by the employees, and supervision by the general public" shall be established, and categorized management and comprehensive control shall be implemented.

【Article 4】 The workers enjoy the right to occupational health protection.

The employer shall create the working environment and conditions that conform to the national norms for occupational health and requirements for public health and take measures to ensure that the workers receive occupational health protection.

Trade unions shall oversee the prevention and control of occupational diseases and protect the lawful rights and interests of employees according to law. When formulating or amending rules and regulations on the prevention and control of occupational diseases, the employer shall solicit the opinions of trade unions.

【Article 5】 The employer shall establish and improve the responsibility system for prevention and control of occupational diseases, in order to enhance management and raise the level in this field, and bear responsibility for the occupational disease hazards produced in the unit.

【Article 6】 The primary person in charge of an employer shall assume the overall responsibility for the employer's prevention and control of occupational diseases.

【Article 7】 The employer shall, as required by laws, undertake work-related injury insurance.

The administrative departments for occupational security under the State Council and the local people's governments at or above the country level shall conduct strict supervision and control of work-related injury insurance, in order to ensure that the workers receive social insurance for industrial injuries.

【Article 8】 The state encourages and supports the research, development, promotion, and application of new technologies, new processes, new equipment, and new materials which facilitate the prevention and control of occupational diseases and the health protection of employees and accentuates the fundamental research on the mechanisms and occurrence patterns of occupational diseases to elevate the scientific and technological levels in the prevention and control of occupational diseases; technologies, processes, equipment, and materials which are effective for the prevention and control of occupational diseases shall be actively adopted; and technologies, processes, equipment, and materials which cause serious occupational disease hazards shall be restricted in use or eliminated.

The state encourages and supports the construction of medical rehabilitation institutions for occupational diseases.

【**Article 9**】The State applies a supervision system for occupational health.

The work safety administrative department, health administrative department, and labor and social security administrative department of the State Council shall, according to the functions prescribed by this Law and the State Council, supervise and administer the prevention and control of occupational diseases across the country. Other relevant departments of the State Council shall, within their respective functions, supervise and administer the prevention and control of occupational diseases.

The work safety administrative departments, health administrative departments, and labor and social security administrative departments of the local people's governments at and above the county level shall, according to their respective functions, supervise and administer the prevention and control of occupational diseases within their respective administrative regions. Other relevant departments of the local people's governments at and above the county level shall supervise and administer the prevention and control of occupational diseases within their respective functions.

The work safety administrative departments, health administrative departments, and labor and social security administrative departments of the people's governments at and above the county level (hereinafter together referred to as the "departments of occupational health supervision and administration") shall strengthen communication and cooperate closely with each other and, according to their respective functions, legally exercise powers and assume responsibilities."

【**Article 10**】The State Council and the local people's governments at or above the country level shall formulated plans for prevention and control of occupational diseases, incorporate them into the national economic and social development plans and make arrangements for their implementation.

The local people's governments at or above the county level shall uniformly lead, organize, and coordinate work on the prevention and control of occupational diseases within their respective administrative regions, establish effective work systems and mechanisms for the prevention and control of occupational diseases, and uniformly lead and direct work in response to occupational health emergencies; and enhance their capabilities of preventing and controlling occupational diseases and related service systems and improve and implement the responsibility system for the prevention and control of occupational diseases.

The people's governments of townships, ethnic townships and towns shall, in accordance with this Law, support the departments of occupational health supervision and administration in performing their statutory functions.

【**Article 11**】 The departments of occupational health supervision and administration of the people's governments at and above the county level shall provide more publicity and education on the prevention and control of occupational diseases, disseminate knowledge on the prevention and control of occupational diseases, reinforce the employer's awareness of prevention and control of occupational diseases, and improve employees' awareness of occupational health and self-protection and ability to exercise rights to occupational health protection.

【**Article 12**】 The national occupational health standards regarding the prevention and control of occupational diseases shall be formulated and published by the health administrative department of the State Council.

The health administrative department of the State Council shall organize monitoring and special investigations on major occupational diseases and assessments on occupational health risks to provide a scientific basis for formulating occupational health standards and policies for the prevention and control of occupational diseases.

The health administrative departments of the local people's governments at and above the county level shall collect statistics and conduct survey and analysis on the prevention and control of occupational diseases within their respective administrative regions on a regular basis."

【**Article 13**】 Any entity or individual shall have the right to report and make accusations regarding violations of this Law. The relevant department shall handle such reports and accusations in a timely manner after receipt.

The units and individuals that have made outstanding contributions to prevention and control of occupational diseases shall be rewarded.

【**Article 14**】 The employer shall, as required by laws and regulations, strictly comply with the national occupational health standards and implement preventative measures against occupational diseases to control and eliminate occupational disease hazards at source.

Chapter II Preliminary Prevention

【**Article 15**】 The workplace, set up by the employer, where occupational disease hazards are produced shall, apart from fulfilling the conditions specified by laws and administrative regulations, meet the following requirements for occupational health:

(1) The strength or concentration of the factors of occupational disease hazards shall meet the national norms for occupational health;

(2) There are facilities commensurate with the prevention of occupational disease hazards;

(3) The production processes are arranged rationally and in conformity with the principle of separation the harmful from non-harmful processes;

(4) There are supporting health facilities such as locker rooms, bathrooms and a lounge for pregnant women workers;

(5) The equipment, tools, apparatus and other facilities meet the requirements for protecting workers' physiological and psychological health; and

(6) The workplace meets the other requirements specified by laws administrative regulations and the public health administration department under the State Council regarding the protection of worker's health.

【Article 16】 The state shall establish a declaration system for projects with occupational disease hazards.

Where an employer's work site has any occupational disease hazard factors as listed in the catalogue of occupational diseases, the employer shall truthfully declare the hazardous project to the local work safety administrative department in a timely manner and accept supervision.

A catalogue of categorized occupational disease hazard factors shall be formulated, adjusted, and published by the health administrative department of the State Council in conjunction with the work safety administrative department of the State Council. The specific measures for declaration of projects with occupational disease hazards shall be formulated by the work safety administrative department of the State Council.

【Article 17】 For construction projects, including projects to be constructed, expanded and reconstructed, and projects for technical updating and introduction, which may produce occupational disease hazards, the unit responsible for a construction project shall, during the period of feasibility study, submit to the public health administration department a preliminary assessment report on the hazards. The said department shall, within 30 days from the date the report is received, make a decision upon examination and inform the unit of the decision in writing. Where a unit fails to submit such a report to or obtain approval by the public health administration department after examination of the report, the authority concerned may not grant approval to the construction project.

The preliminary assessment report on the occupational disease hazards shall include the assessment of the occupational hazard factors that the construction project may produce and of the effects that such factors may have on the workplace and the workers' health, the defined category of the hazards and the measures to be taken for prevention of occupational diseases.

The measures for the categorized administration of occupational disease hazards in construction projects shall be formulated by the work safety administrative department of the State Council.

【Article 18】 The expenditure entailed by the facilities included in a construction project, for prevention of occupational diseases shall be incorporated into the budget of the project, and the facilities shall be designed, built and put into operation and use simultaneously with the main body of the construction project.

For a construction project with serious occupational disease hazards, the design of protective facilities shall be examined by the work safety administrative department, and construction may commence only after the national occupational health standards and health requirements are met.

Before the construction project is completed for inspection and acceptance, the construction unit shall assess the effect of the control of occupational disease hazards when the project is completed and ready for inspection and acceptance, the facilities for prevention of occupational diseases may be put into formal operation and use only after they pass the inspection by the public health administration department.

【Article 19】 Preliminary assessment of occupational disease hazards and of the effect of the control of such hazards shall be conducted by the occupational health technical service that is set up in accordance with law and is authenticated as qualified by the public health administration department of the people's governments at or above the provincial level. The assessment made by the said institution shall be objective and truthful.

【Article 20】 The state shall apply special administration to radioactive, highly toxic, and high-risk dust operations. The specific administrative measures shall be formulated by the State Council.

Chapter III Prevention and Control in the Course of Work

【Article 21】 The employer shall take the following measures for prevention and control of occupational disease:

(1) to set up or designate an institution or organization for occupational health control, and have it manned with full-time or part-time occupational health management personnel to be responsible for prevention and control of occupational diseases in the unit;

(2) to make plans for prevention and control of occupational diseases and programs for their implementation;

(3) to establish and improve the control system for occupational health and rules for its application;

(4) to keep files on occupational health and files on monitoring and protecting of the workers' health, and improve the practice;

(5) to set up and improve the system for monitoring and assessing the factors of occupational disease hazards at the workplace; and

(6) to make and improve preliminary plans for emergency rescue in accidents caused by occupational disease hazards.

【Article 22】 The employer shall ensure the funds required for the prevention and control of occupational diseases, shall not misappropriate such funds, and shall be liable for the consequences of insufficient funds.

【Article 23】 The employer shall have effective facilities for prevention of occupational disease and shall provide individual workers with articles for prevention of occupational diseases.

The articles for prevention of occupational diseases provided by the employer to individual workers shall meet the requirements for prevention and control of occupational diseases; otherwise, such articles may not be used.

【Article 24】 The employer shall give priority to the use of new technologies, new technologies, new equipment and new materials that are conducive to prevention and control of occupational diseases and to protection of workers' health, in order to gradually replace the technologies, techniques, equipment and materials that produce serious occupational disease hazards.

【Article 25】 The employer of a unit where occupational disease hazards are produced shall set up bulletin boards at eye-catching places to publish the rules and regulations for prevention and control of occupational diseases, the rules for their application, emergency rescue measures in accidents caused by occupational disease hazards, and the monitoring results of the factors of occupational disease hazards at the workplace.

At eye-catching places, alarming signs with warning descriptions in Chinese shall be put up at the operation posts where serious occupational disease hazards are produced. The descriptions shall clearly furnish the categories, consequences and prevention of and the emergency rescue measures for, the occupational disease hazards.

【Article 26】 At the workplace with toxic and hazardous substances where acute occupational injuries may occur, the employer shall have such places equipped with alarming devices, first-aid articles and washing equipment, and have emergency exit passages built and necessary risk obviating areas prepared.

For the workplaces exposed to radioactive substances and the transportation and storage of radioisotope, the employer shall install protective equipment and alarming devices, and make sure that the workers exposed to radioactive rays wear dosimeters for personal use.

With regard to the equipment for prevention of occupational diseases, emergency rescue facilities, and the articles to be used by individuals for prevention of occupational diseases, the employer shall have them maintained and overhauled regularly and have their properties and effects tested periodically, in order to keep them in normal condition. Without authorization, it may not have them dismantle or discontinue their use.

【Article 27】 The employer shall assign special persons to carry out day-to-day monitoring of the factors of occupational disease hazards and make sure that the monitoring system is kept in normal working conditions.

The employer shall, in accordance with the regulations of the public health administration department under the State Council, have the factors of occupational disease hazards monitored and assessed regularly at the workplace. The results of monitoring and assessment shall be kept in the unit's files of occupational health regularly reported to the local public health administration department and announced to the workers.

The factors of occupational disease hazards shall be monitored and assessed by the occupational health technical service institutions set up in accordance with law and authenticated as qualified by the public health administration departments of the people's governments at or above the provincial level. The monitoring and assessment made by the said institution shall be objective and truthful.

When discovering the factors of occupational disease hazards at the workplace do not conform to the national requirements for occupational health, the employer shall immediately adopt appropriated measures to keep them under control. If they still cannot meet the norms or requirements, the operation where such factors exist, shall be stopped. It can be resumed only after the factors are kept under control and meet the said norms and requirements.

【Article 28】 Occupational health technical service institutions shall legally conduct tests and evaluations of occupational disease hazard factors and accept supervision and inspection by the work safety administrative departments. Work safety administrative departments shall legally perform their duties of supervision.

【Article 29】 When providing the employer with the equipment that may produce occupational disease hazards, the supplier shall give a handbook in Chinese and put up alarming signs with warning descriptions in Chinese at eye-catching spots on the equipment. The descriptions shall clearly furnish the properties of the equipment, the possible occupational disease hazards it may produce, points for attention for safety operation and maintenance, protection against occupational diseases, measures for emergency rescue, etc.

【Article 30】 When providing the employer with occupational disease hazards producing chemicals, radioisotope or materials containing radioactive substances, the supplier shall give a handbook in Chinese. The handbook shall clearly contain the properties of the product, the main constituents, the hazardous factors present and the possible hazardous consequences, the points for attention for safety application, protection against occupational diseases, emergency rescue measures, and other particulars. On the package of the product there shall be eye-catching alarming signs with warning descriptions in Chinese. In the places where the materials mentioned above are stored, signs for dangerous goods or alarming signs for radioactive substances shall be put up at specified spots.

For chemicals pertaining to occupational disease hazards which are to be used or imported for the first time in the country, the user or importer shall, upon approval by the relevant department under the State Council, as required by State regulations, submit to the public health administration department under the State Council the report on the identification of the toxicity of the chemicals and the documents proving its registration with the department concerned or proving the approval for import.

Radioisotope, radiation devices and goods containing radioactive substances shall be imported in accordance with the relevant regulations of the State.

【Article 31】 No unit or individual may produce, deal in, import or use the equipment or materials which may produce occupational disease hazards and the use of which is prohibited by State decree.

【Article 32】 No unit or individual may transfer the operation that produces occupational disease hazards to another unit or individual that lacks the conditions for prevention of occupational diseases. No unit or individual that lacks the conditions for prevention of occupational diseases may accept any operation that produces occupational disease hazards.

【Article 33】 The employer shall know the occupational disease hazards produced by the technologies, techniques, equipment and materials it employs; if it conceals the fact that the technologies, techniques, equipment and materials produce occupational disease hazards and employs them, it shall bear responsibility for the consequences of the hazards.

【Article 34】 When signing with the workers labor contracts (including contracts of employment), the employer shall truthfully inform the workers of he potential occupational disease hazards the consequences in the course of work, the measures for prevention of such diseases and the material benefits, and it shall have the same clearly put down in the contracts; it may not conceal the facts or deceive the workers.

If, during the contracted period of time, a worker, because of change in work post or assignment, begins to engage in an operation with occupational disease hazards, which is not mentioned in the contact, the employer shall, in accordance with the provisions in the preceding paragraph, perform its obligation by informing the worker of the true situation and, through consultation with the worker, alter the related provisions in the original contract.

If the employer violates the provisions in the preceding two paragraphs, the worker shall have the right to reject the assignment where occupational disease hazards exist, and the employer may not thus cancel labor contract with the worker.

【Article 35】 The primary person in charge and the occupational health management personnel of an employer shall receive occupational health training, abide by laws and regulations on the prevention and control of occupational diseases, and legally organize the employer's prevention and control of occupational diseases.

The employer shall provide the workers with pre-service training in occupational health and regular in-service training in this field, in order to popularize knowledge about occupational health, urge on them the need to abide by the laws, rules and regulations on prevention and control of occupational diseases and the rules of operation, as well as to show them the correct way of using the facilities for prevention of occupational diseases and such articles for personal use.

Employees shall gain occupational health knowledge through studies, enhance their awareness of preventing occupational diseases, abide by laws, regulations, rules, and operating procedures on the prevention and control of occupational diseases, properly use and maintain occupational disease protective equipment and occupational disease protective items for personal use, and report any discovered risks of occupational disease hazard accidents in a timely manner.

If an employee does not perform the obligation specified in the preceding paragraph, the employer shall enlighten him on the need to do so.

【Article 36】 With regard to the workers who engage in operation exposed to occupational disease hazards, the employer shall, in accordance with the regulations of the public health administration department under the State Council, make arrangements for pre-service, in-service and job leaving occupational health checkups and inform the workers in writing of the results of the checkups. The expenses for occupational health checkups shall be borne by the employer.

No employer may assign to workers who have not received pre-service occupational health check-ups any jobs exposed to occupational disease hazards, nor assign to workers forbidden jobs. Workers whose signs of job-related injuries are shown by occupational health checkups shall be transferred from their original posts and proper arrangements shall be made for them. With regard to workers who have not received occupational health checkups before leaving their jobs, the employer may not cancel or terminate the labor contracts concluded with them.

Occupational health checkups shall be undertaken by the medical and health institutions approved by the public health administration departments of the people's government at or above the provincial level.

【Article 37】 The employer shall keep files on occupational health monitoring and protection for the workers and keep the files in good condition for a specified period of time.

In the file on occupational health monitoring and protection shall be recorded the worker's professional history, history of exposure to occupational disease hazards, the results of occupational health checkups and diagnosis and treatment of occupational diseases and other information related to his health.

When a worker leaves the employer, he shall have the right to ask for a copy of the file on monitoring and protection of his occupational health. The employer shall provide a truthful copy to him free of charge, and have it signed and sealed.

【Article 38】 Where an acute occupational disease hazard accident occurs or may occur, an employer shall immediately take emergency rescue and control measures and report the accident to the local work safety administrative department and relevant departments in a timely manner. The work safety administrative department shall, after receiving the report, organize investigation and disposition in a timely manner in conjunction with the relevant departments; and when necessary, may take temporary control measures. The health administrative department shall organize effective medical treatment.

With regard to the workers who are exposed to, or are likely exposed to, an accident of acute occupational disease hazards, the employer shall immediately make arrangements for their rescue and treatment, for health checkups and medical observation. The expenses thus entailed shall be borne by the employer.

【Article 39】 No employer may assign minors jobs that are exposed to occupational disease hazards, or assign women workers who are pregnant or breastfeeding babies jobs that are harmful to them and to the embryos and the babies.

【Article 40】 The workers shall enjoy the following rights of protection for their occupational health:

(1) receive education and training in occupational health;

(2) to receive services for prevention and control of occupational diseases, such as health checkups, diagnosis, treatment and recuperation;

(3) to know about the occupational disease hazard factors that may or are likely to exist at the workplace, the consequences of the hazards and the necessary measures to be taken for prevention of occupational diseases;

(4) to ask the employer to provide the facilities for prevention of occupational diseases that meet the requirements for prevention and control of such diseases, provide the workers with articles to be used personally for the same purpose and improve the working conditions;

(5) to criticize, report and accuse violations of the laws and regulations on

prevention and control of occupational diseases and acts that endanger the lives and health of the workers;

(6) to reject directions that are against regulations and coercive orders for doing jobs where the measures for prevention of occupational diseases are lacking; and

(7) to participate in the unit's democratic management of occupational health, and to put forward comments and suggestions about prevention and control of occupational diseases.

The employer shall ensure that the workers exercise the rights mentioned in the preceding paragraph. Any reduction of the workers' wages, welfare or material benefits, and any cancellation or termination of the labor contracts concluded with the workers, because the workers exercise their legitimate rights pursuant to law, shall be invalid.

【Article 41】 The trade union of an employer shall oversee and assist the employer in providing publicity, education and training regarding occupational health, be entitled to offer opinions and suggestions on the employer's prevention and control of occupational diseases, legally conclude a special collective contract on labor safety and health with the employer on behalf of employees, consult with the employer over issues raised by employees concerning the prevention and control of occupational diseases, and promote the resolution of such issues.

The trade union organizations shall have the right to demand rectification where the employer violates the laws and regulations on prevention and control of occupational diseases and infringes upon the workers' legislative rights and interests. When serious occupational hazards occur, they shall have the right to demand that protective measures be taken, or to raise suggestions to the government department concerned for adoption of compulsory measures. When an occupational disease hazard accident occurs, they shall have the right to participate in the investigation and handling of the accident. When they discover that the workers' lives or health are in danger, they shall have the right to make suggestions to the employer that arrangements be made for the workers to withdraw from the dangerous spot, and the employer shall take action immediately.

【Article 42】 The expenses which the employer, in compliance with the requirements for prevention and control of occupational disease, pays for prevention and control of occupational disease hazards, public health monitoring at the workplace, health monitoring and protection and training in occupational health shall truthfully be incorporated into the production cost in accordance with relevant State regulations.

【Article 43】 The departments of occupational health supervision and administration shall, according to their respective functions, strengthen their supervision and inspection on the employer's adoption of management measures for protection from occupational diseases and legally exercise powers and assume responsibilities.

Chapter IV Diagnosis of Occupational Diseases and Security for Occupational Disease Patients

【Article 44】 Medical and health institutions shall provide occupational disease diagnosis with the approval of the health administrative department of the people's government of a province, autonomous region, or municipality directly under the Central Government. The health administrative department of the people's government of a province, autonomous region, or municipality directly under the Central Government shall publish a list of medical and health institutions providing occupational disease diagnosis within its administrative region.

Medical and health institutions providing occupational disease diagnosis shall meet the following conditions:

(1) hold a Practicing License for a Medical Institution;

(2) have medical and health technical personnel appropriate for providing occupational disease diagnosis;

(3) have instruments and equipment appropriate for providing occupational disease diagnosis; and

(4) have effective quality management rules for occupational disease diagnosis.

No medical and health institutions providing occupational disease diagnosis shall refuse an employee's request for occupational disease diagnosis.

【Article 45】 An employee may seek occupational disease diagnosis at medical and health institutions legally providing occupational disease diagnosis at the place where the employer is located, at the place of the employee's registered permanent residence, or at the place of the employee's habitual residence.

【Article 46】 The criteria for the diagnosis of occupational diseases and the measures for such diagnosis and confirmation shall be formulated by the public health administration department under the State Council. The measures for confirmation of the grades for injuries and disabilities caused by occupational diseases shall be formulated by the labor security administration department together with the public health administration department under the State Council.

【Article 47】 In the diagnosis of occupational diseases, the following factors shall be analyzed comprehensively.

(1) the patient's occupational history;

(2) a history of exposures to occupational disease hazards and information on occupational disease hazard factors in the work site; and

(3) the clinical symptoms and the results of auxiliary examinations.

Where there is no evidence for denying a necessary connection between occupational disease hazard factors and a patient's clinical manifestations, the patient shall be diagnosed with an occupational disease.

The medical and health institution that undertakes the diagnosis of occupational diseases shall at least have three licensed doctors who are qualified for diagnosis of occupational diseases to make diagnosis collectively.

The certificate for diagnosis of occupational diseases shall be signed jointly by the doctors who participate in the diagnosis and be stamped with seal of the medical and health institution after its examination and approval.

【Article 48】 An employer shall truthfully provide the occupational history and history of exposures to occupational disease hazard factors of employees, test results of occupational disease hazard factors at work sites, and other information necessary for occupational disease diagnosis or identification; the work safety administrative department shall oversee and urge the employer to provide the aforesaid information; and employees and relevant institutions shall also provide information related to occupational disease diagnosis or identification.

Where an occupational disease diagnosis or identification institution needs information on the occupational disease hazard factors at a work site, it may conduct an on-site investigation of the work site or request the work safety administrative department to do so, and the work safety administrative department shall organize an on-site investigation within 10 days. The employer shall not refuse or obstruct the on-site investigation.

【Article 49】 Where, in the process of occupational disease diagnosis or identification, an employer fails to provide the test results of occupational disease hazard factors at a work site and other information, the diagnosis or identification institution shall, in consideration of the clinical manifestations and assistant examination results of an employee, the occupational history and history of exposures to occupational disease hazards of an employee, the personal statement of an employee, the routine supervision and inspection information from the work safety administrative department, and other information, arrive at a conclusion of occupational disease diagnosis or identification.

Where an employee raises any objection to the test results of occupational disease hazard factors at a work site and other information provided by the employer or the aforesaid information is not provided because of the dissolution or bankruptcy of the employer, the diagnosis or identification institution shall request the work safety administrative department to conduct an investigation, and the work safety administrative department shall, within 30 days after receiving the request, make a determination on the information in dispute or information on occupational disease hazard factors at the work site; and the relevant departments shall cooperate.

【Article 50】 Where, in the process of occupational disease diagnosis or identification, the parties dispute the employment relationship, type of work, post, or working hours when the employee's occupational history and history of exposures to occupational disease hazard factors are validated, they may apply to the local labor and personnel dispute arbitration committee for arbitration; and the labor and personnel dispute arbitration committee receiving the application shall accept it and render an award within 30 days.

The parties shall provide evidence for their own claims during arbitration. Where an employee cannot provide evidence relevant to his or her arbitral claims that is controlled or managed by the employer, the arbitral tribunal shall require the employer to provide such evidence within a specified time limit; and the employer shall assume any adverse consequences for failing to provide such evidence within the specified time limit.

An employee may file a lawsuit with the people's court against an arbitral award.

An employer may, within 15 days after the end of the occupational disease diagnosis or identification procedure, file a lawsuit with the people's court according to law against an arbitral award. During the lawsuit, the treatment expenses of the employee shall be paid from financial sources prescribed for occupational diseases.

【Article 51】 The employer and medical and health institutions shall report in a timely manner discovered occupational disease patients or patients suspected of occupational diseases to the local health administrative department and work safety administrative department. If an occupational disease is confirmed, an employer shall also report to the local labor and social security administrative department. The departments receiving such reports shall make dispositions according to law.

【Article 52】 The public health administration departments of the people's governments at or above the county level shall be responsible for the management of the statistic reports on occupational diseases in their own administrative areas and, according to regulations, submit the reports to the departments at higher levels.

【Article 53】 A party who has objection to the diagnosis of occupational disease may apply to the public health administration department of the people's government of the place where the medical and health institution is located for verification.

Where a dispute arises over the diagnosis of occupational diseases, the public health administration department of the people's government at or above the level of a city divided into districts shall, on the basis of the application filed by the party, make arrangements for a verification committee of occupational disease diagnosis to make a conclusion of the diagnosis.

Where the party is dissatisfied with the conclusion made on the diagnosis of occupational diseases by the verification committee of occupational disease diagnosis at the level of a city divided into districts, he may apply to the public health administration department of the people's government of a province, autonomous region or municipality directly under the Central Government for further verification.

【Article 54】 The verification committee of occupational disease diagnosis shall consist of experts of related professions.

The public health administration departments of people's governments of provinces, autonomous regions and municipalities directly under the Central Government shall have banks of related experts, and when it is necessary to verify a diagnosis of occupational disease under dispute, the party or the related public health administration department entrusted by the party may at random select some experts from the bank and appoint them members of the diagnosis verification committee.

The verification committee of occupational disease diagnosis shall, in accordance with the criteria for the diagnosis of occupational disease and the measures for such diagnosis for verification and of the diagnosis published by the public health administration department under the State Council, conduct verification of occupational disease diagnosis and issue to the party a certificate for verification of occupational disease diagnosis. The expense for such verification shall be borne by the employer.

【Article 55】 The member of the occupational disease diagnosis verification committee shall abide by professional ethics and be objective and impartial in verifying diagnosis, and they shall be held responsible accordingly. None of them may have contract with the party in private or accept any money or things of value or other benefits from the party. If any of them has an interest with the party, he shall withdraw.

When in handling a case the People's Court needs verification of occupational diseases, it shall select, for the purpose, experts from the bank of experts set up by the public health administration department of the people's government of a province, autonomous region or municipality directly under the Central Government.

【Article 56】 When the medical and health institution finds that a worker is suspected of being an occupational disease patient, it shall let the worker himself know it and inform the employer of the matter without delay.

The employer shall make arrangements for the patient suspected of occupational disease to be diagnosed. During the period of diagnosis or medical observation, the employer may not cancel or terminate the labor contract it concludes with the said patient.

The expenses incurred during the period of diagnosis and medical observation of the patient suspected of occupational disease shall be borne by the employer.

【Article 57】 The employer shall ensure that occupational diseases patients enjoy the occupational disease benefits prescribed by the state.

The employer shall, in accordance with relevant State regulations, make arrangements for patients of occupational diseases to undergo treatment, to recuperate and to receive regular checkups.

The employer shall transfer to other posts the patients of occupational diseases who are no longer suited for the jobs they are originally assigned, and make proper arrangements for them.

The employer shall give workers who are exposed to occupational disease hazards subsidies appropriate to the jobs they are doing.

【Article 58】 The expenses for diagnosis and recuperation of occupational disease patients and the social security for such patients who are injured and disabled shall be dealt with according to State regulations on work-related injury insurance.

【Article 59】 In addition to enjoying, in accordance with law, work-related injury insurance, the occupational disease patients who, according to related civil laws, still have the right to compensation, shall have the right to make a claim against the employer.

【Article 60】 Where an employee is diagnosed with an occupational disease but the employer fails to participate in the work-related injury insurance as required by law, the employee's medical and living expenses shall be assumed by the employer.

【Article 61】 When a patient of occupational disease goes to work in another unit, the material benefits he enjoys in accordance with law shall remain unchanged.

An employer undergoing any business split or combination, dissolution, or bankruptcy shall provide health examination for employees conducting operations with exposure to occupational disease hazards and appropriately settle occupational diseases patients according to the relevant provisions of the state.

【Article 62】 "Where the employer of an occupational disease patient no longer exists or the employment relationship of an occupational disease cannot be confirmed, the patient may apply to the civil affairs department of the local people's government for medical assistance, subsistence support, and so on.

The local people's governments at all levels shall, based on the actual local circumstances, take other measures to secure medical assistance and treatment for occupational disease patients in the preceding paragraph.

Chapter V Supervision and Inspection

【Article 63】 The departments of occupational health supervision and administration of the people's governments at and above the county level shall, in accordance with laws and regulations on the prevention and control of occupational diseases and national occupational health standards and health requirements, conduct supervision and inspection on the prevention and control of occupational diseases according to their respective functions.

【Article 64】 When performing its duties of supervision and inspection, the public health administration departments shall have the right to take the following measures:

(1) to enter the unit under inspection and the place exposed to occupational disease hazards, to get to know the situation, conduct investigation and take evidence;

(2) to consult or duplicate material related to violations of the laws and regulations on prevention and control of occupational diseases, and to collect sample; and

(3) to order the unit or individual that violates the laws and regulations on prevention and control of occupational diseases to discontinue violation.

【Article 65】 When an accident of occupational disease hazards occurs or there is evidence proving that the hazards may lead to occurrence of such an accident, the public health administration department may adopt the following measures to keep the situation under control:

(1) to order suspension of the operation that may lead to an accident of occupational disease hazards;

(2) to seal up for safekeeping the materials and equipment that has caused, or may lead to, the occurrence of an accident of occupational disease hazards; and

(3) to get people to keep under control the place where the accident of occupational disease hazards has occurred.

When the accident of occupational disease hazards or the hazardous situation has been kept under effective control, the public health administration department shall repeal the control measures without delay.

【Article 66】 When performing their duties in accordance with law, officials in charge of supervision and law enforcement shall show their papers of supervision and laws enforcement.

Officials in charge of occupational health supervision and law enforcement shall be devoted to their duty, impartial in enforcing laws and strictly abide by the norms for law enforcement; where the secrets of the employer are involved, they shall keep its secrets.

【Article 67】 When officials in charge of occupational health supervision and law enforcement performing their duties in accordance with law, the unit under inspection shall accept, assist and cooperate with the inspection; it may not refuse to do so or put obstacles in their way.

【Article 68】 When performing its or their duties, no public health administration department or its officials in charge of occupational health supervision and law enforcement may do any of the following:

(1) issuing to construction projects that do not meet the statutory conditions related certifying documents or qualification certificates or giving approval to such projects;

(2) failing to perform the duties of supervision and inspection where a construction project has obtained the related certifying documents;

(3) failing to take timely measures in accordance with law to keep the situation under control when discovering that in the workplace of the employer there exist occupational disease hazards that may lead to an accident; and

(4) other violations of this Law.

【Article 69】 The qualifications of official in charge of occupational health supervision and law enforcement shall, in accordance with law, undergo authentication.

The public health administration departments shall strengthen their contingents, raise their level of political and professional quality and, in accordance with the provisions of this Law and other related laws and regulations, establish and improve the system for internal supervision, in order to supervise and inspect how their officials enforce the laws and regulations and observe discipline.

Chapter VI Legal responsibility

【Article 70】 Where the construction unit, in violation of the provisions of this Law, commits one of the following acts, the public health administration department shall give it a disciplinary warning and order it to make rectification within a time limit; if it fails to do so at the expiration of the time limit, it shall be fined not less than 100,000 RMB Yuan but not more than 500,000 RMB Yuan. If the circumstances are serious, it shall be ordered to discontinue the operation that produces occupational disease hazards, or the department may request the related people's government, within the limits of its powers specified by the State Council, to order the unit to discontinue construction or close down:

(1) commencing construction without conducting a preliminary assessment of occupational disease hazards as required, without submitting a report on the preliminary assessment of occupational disease hazards, or without obtaining an approval from the work safety administrative department of the report on the preliminary assessment of occupational disease hazards;

(2) failing to have the facilities for prevention of occupational disease put into operation and use simultaneously with the main body of the construction project, as is required by regulations;

(3) commencing construction of a construction project with serious occupational disease hazards whose design for occupational disease protective facilities has not

been examined by the work safety administrative department or fails to meet the national occupational health standards and health requirements; and

(4) putting into use the facilities for prevention of occupational diseases without assessing the effectiveness of their control of occupational disease hazards, as is required by regulations, or without inspection and acceptance by the public health administration department or without passing the inspection;

【Article 71】 Any employer who, in violation of the provisions of this Law, commits one of the following acts shall be given a disciplinary warning by the public health administration department and shall be ordered to make rectification within a time limit; if it fails to do so at the expiration of the time limit, it shall be fined not more than 100,000 RMB Yuan:

(1) failing to keep files on the results of the monitoring and assessment of the factors of occupational disease hazards at the workplace, and to report and publish the results;

(2) failing to adopt the measures for prevention and control of occupational diseases, as specified in Article 19 of this Law;

(3) failing to publish the rules and regulations on prevention and control of occupational diseases, the rules for their application and the emergency rescue measures in accidents of occupational disease hazards as is required by regulations;

(4) failing to make arrangements for workers to receive training in occupational health and to take measures for guiding and urging individual workers to protect themselves against occupational diseases, as is required by regulations; and

(5) failing to submit information on the identification of toxicity of the chemicals which contain occupational disease hazards and are to be used or imported for the first time in the country, and the documents proving its registration with the department concerned and proving the approval for import, as is required by regulations.

【Article 72】 Where the employer, in violation of the provisions of this Law, commits one of the following acts, the public health administration department shall order it to make rectification within a time limit and give it a disciplinary warning, and may also impose on it a fine not less than 50,000 RMB Yuan but not more than 100,000 RMB Yuan:

(1) failing to submit timely and truthful report to the public health administration department on the project that produces occupational disease hazards, as is required by regulations;

(2) failing to assign special persons to carry out day-to-day monitoring of the factors of occupational disease hazards and failing to keep the monitoring system in normal working conditions;

(3) when concluding or altering labor contracts, failing to inform the workers of the true situation of occupational disease hazards;

(4) failing to make arrangements for occupational health checkups, to keep files on occupational health monitoring and protection and to inform the worker in writing of the results of the checkups; and

(5) failing to provide a copy of occupational health surveillance files according to the provisions of this Law when employees leave the employer.

【Article 73】 Where the employer, in violation of the provisions of this Law, commits one of the following acts, the public health administration department shall give it a disciplinary warning and order it to make rectification within a time limit; if it fails to do so at the expiration of the time limit, it shall be fined not less than 50,000 RMB Yuan but not more than 200,000 RMB Yuan. If the circumstances are serious, the said department shall order it to discontinue operation that produces occupational disease hazards, or the department may request the related people's government, within the limits of its powers specified by the State Council, to order it to close down:

(1) failing to keep the strength or concentrations of the factors of occupational disease hazards at the workplace from exceeding the national norms for occupational health;

(2) failing to provide facilities for prevention of occupational diseases and to provide such articles for personal use, or failing to provide the said facilities and articles that meet the national norms and requirements for occupational health;

(3) failing to maintain, overhaul and test the equipment for prevention of occupational diseases, the emergency rescue facilities and the articles to be used by individuals for prevention of such diseases, as is required by regulations, or failing to keep them in normal operation and use;

(4) failing to monitor and assess the factors of occupational disease hazards at the workplace, as is required by regulations;

(5) failing to discontinue work where the factors of occupational disease hazards exist, when such factors at the workplace still remain below the national norms and requirements for occupational health, even after treatment;

(6) failing to make arrangements for patients of occupational diseases or suspected patients of such diseases to receive diagnosis and treatment, as is required by regulations;

(7) failing to adopt emergency rescue and control measures immediately after the occurrence of an accident of acute occupational disease hazards or when such occurrence is likely, or failing to report such occurrence immediately, as is required by regulations;

(8) failing to put up alarming indications with warning descriptions in Chinese at

eye-catching spots of a post where serious occupational disease hazards are produced, as is required by regulations;

(9) refusing supervision and inspection by the departments of occupational health supervision and administration;

(10) withholding, forging, tempering with, or damaging occupational health surveillance files, test and evaluation results of occupational disease hazard factors at a work site, and other relevant information or refusing to provide information necessary for occupational disease diagnosis or identification; and

(11) failing to assume the occupational disease diagnosis or identification expenses and the medical and living security expenses of occupational disease patients according to the relevant provisions.

【Article 74】 Where the supplier that provides the employer with the equipment and materials which may produce occupational disease hazards fails to provide handbook in Chinese or alarming indications with warning descriptions in Chinese attached, as is required by regulations, the public health administration department shall order it to make rectification within a time limit and give it a disciplinary warning, and may also impose on it a fine not less than 50,000 RMB Yuan but not more than 200,000 RMB Yuan.

【Article 75】 Where the employer or the medical and health institution fails to report cases of occupational diseases or suspected cases of such diseases, as is required by regulations, it shall be ordered by the public health administration department to make rectification within a time limit and given a disciplinary warning and may also be fined not more than 10,000 RMB Yuan. If it practices fraud, it may also be fined not less than 20,000 RMB Yuan but not more than 50,000 RMB Yuan. The persons directly in charge and the other persons directly responsible may be demoted or dismissed from office in accordance with law.

【Article 76】 Where the employer, unit or individual, in violation of the provisions of this Law, commits one of the following acts, it shall be ordered by the public health administration department to make rectification within a time limit and may also be fined not less than 50,000 RMB Yuan but not more than 300,000 RMB Yuan. If the circumstances are serious, the department shall order it to discontinue the operation that produces occupational disease hazards or request the related people's government, within the limits of its powers defined by the State Council, to order the employer to close down:

(1) concealing the occupational disease hazards produced by the technologies, techniques, equipment and materials and employing them;

(2) concealing the truth about occupational health in the unit;

(3) failing to comply with the provisions of Article 23 of this Law in respect of the

workplaces with toxic and hazardous substances that may cause acute occupational injuries, workplaces exposed to radioactive substances and in respect of the transportation and storage of radioisotope;

(4) using the equipment or materials which may produce occupational disease hazards and the use of which is prohibited by State decree;

(5) transferring the operation that produces occupational disease hazards to another unit or individual that lacks the conditions for prevention of occupational diseases; or accepting the said operation by a unit or individual that lacks the said conditions;

(6) without authorization, dismantling or casing to use the equipment for prevention of occupational diseases or the emergency rescue facilities;

(7) assigning to workers who have not received occupational health checkups, workers who must avoid certain jobs, minors or women workers who are pregnant or breastfeeding babies jobs that are exposed to occupational disease hazards or that they must avoid; and

(8) giving directions against regulations or compelling workers to do jobs for which the measures for prevention of occupational disease are lacking.

【Article 77】 Any unit or individual that produces, deals in or imports the equipment or materials which may produce occupational disease hazards and the use of which is prohibited by State decree shall be punished according to the related laws and administrative regulations.

【Article 78】 Where the employer, in violation of the provisions of this Law, has caused serious harm to the workers' lives and health, the public health administration department shall order it to discontinue the operation that produces occupational disease hazards, or request the related people's government, within the limits of its powers defined by the State Council, to order it close down, and also impose on it a fine not less than 100,000 RMB Yuan but not more than 500,000 RMB Yuan.

【Article 79】 Where due to violation by the employer of the provisions of this Law, a major accident caused by occupational disease hazards occurred or other serious consequences ensued, if a crime is constituted, the persons directly in charge and the other persons directly responsible shall be investigated for criminal responsibility according to law.

【Article 80】 Anyone who, without obtaining qualification certificate for occupational health technical services, engages in such services, or any medical and health institution that, without obtaining approval, conducts occupational health checkup and diagnosis of occupational diseases, shall be ordered by the public health administration department to discontinue the illegal acts, and the unlawful gains shall be confiscated. If the unlawful gains amount to more than 5,000 RMB Yuan, he or it shall also be fined not less than two times but not more than 10 times the amount of such gains. If there are no unlawful gains or such gains are less than 5,000 RMB Yuan, he or it shall also be fined not less than 5,000 RMB Yuan but not more than 50,000 RMB Yuan. If the circumstances are serious, the persons directly in charge and the other persons directly responsible shall, in accordance with law, be demoted, dismissed from office or discharged as punishment.

【Article 81】 Any occupational health technical service institution or any medical and health institution for occupational checkups and occupational disease diagnosis that, in violation of the provisions of this Law, commits one of the following acts shall be ordered by the public health administration department to discontinue the violation immediately and be given a disciplinary warning, and the unlawful gains shall be confiscated; if the unlawful gains exceed 5,000 RMB Yuan, it shall also be fined not less than two times but nor more than five times the amount of the unlawful gains; if there are no unlawful gains or such gains are less than 5,000 RMB Yuan, it shall also be fined not less than 5,000 RMB Yuan but not more than 20,000 RMB Yuan; if the circumstances are serious, it shall be disqualified by the original certifying or approving authority; the persons directly in charge and the other persons directly responsible shall, in accordance with law, be demoted, dismissed form office or discharged; if a crime is constituted, criminal responsibility shall be investigated in accordance with law:

(1) engaging in occupational health technical services or conducting occupational health checkups and occupational disease diagnosis beyond the scope certified or approval;

(2) failing to perform the statutory duty in accordance with the provisions of this Law; and

(3) issuing false accreditation documents.

【Article 82】 Where a member of the verification committee of occupational disease diagnosis accepts money, things of value or other benefits from the party to a dispute over an occupational disease diagnosis, he shall be given a disciplinary warning, the money and things of value accepted shall be confiscated, he may also be fined not less that 3,000 RMB Yuan but not more than 50,000 RMB Yuan, he shall be disqualified for membership of the verification committee of occupational disease diagnosis and his name shall be removed from the bank of experts established by the public health administration department of the people's government of the province, autonomous region or municipality directly under the Central Government.

【Article 83】 Where a health administrative department or a work safety administrative department fails to report any occupational disease or occupational disease hazard accident as required, the administrative department at the next higher level shall order it to make correction, circulate a notice of criticism, and issue a warning to it; and if the department falsifies a report or withholds information in a report, the person in charge, the directly responsible chief, and other directly liable persons of the department shall be subject to the disciplinary action of demotion, removal from office, or expulsion according to law.

【Article 84】 Where a relevant department approves a construction project or issues a construction license in violation of Article 17 or 18 of this Law, the supervisory authority or the superior authority shall, according to law, take disciplinary actions against the directly responsible chief and other directly liable persons of the department from demerit to expulsion.

【Article 85】 Where a local people's government at or above the county level fails to perform its functions in accordance with this Law in the prevention and control of occupational diseases, causing the occurrence of a major occupational disease hazard accident in its administrative region with any serious social impact, the directly responsible chief and other directly liable persons shall be subject to disciplinary actions from major demerit to expulsion according to law.

Where a department of occupational health supervision and administration of a people's government at or above the county level fails to perform its functions prescribed by this Law, abuses its powers, neglects its duties, makes falsification, or practices favoritism, the directly responsible chief and other directly liable persons shall be subject to the disciplinary action of major demerit or demotion according to law and, if any occupational disease hazard accident or other serious consequence is caused, shall be subject to the disciplinary action of removal from office or expulsion according to law.

【Article 86】 Whoever commits a crime by violating this Law shall be subject to criminal liability according to law.

Chapter VII Supplementary Provisions

【Article 87】 The meanings of the following terms used in this Law are:

Occupational disease hazards refer to the various kinds of hazards that may cause occupational diseases to workers engaged in an occupation. The factors of occupational disease hazards include the various kinds of chemical, physical and biological factors existing in occupational activities and other occupational hazardous factors that come into existence in the process of operation.

Forbidden jobs mean jobs where, when workers are engaged in certain jobs or are exposed to certain factors of occupational disease hazards, they are more liable than the ordinary run of workers to occupational disease hazards or more easily suffer from occupational diseases, or their original diseases may become aggravated, or in the course of work their peculiar physiological or pathological conditions may induce diseases that may constitute a danger to other persons' lives and health.

【Article 88】 When occupational disease hazards occur in units other than the ones mentioned in Article 2 of this Law, the provisions of this Law may be applied mutatis mutandis in their efforts to prevent and control occupational diseases.

Entities using dispatched labor forces shall perform the obligations of the employer as prescribed by this Law.

The measures for the People's Liberation Army to apply this Law mutatis mutandis shall be formulated by the State Council and Central Military Commission.

【Article 89】 The supervision and administration of medical institutions' control of radioactive occupational disease hazards shall be conducted by the health administrative departments in accordance with this Law.

【Article 90】 This Law shall go into effect as of May 1, 2002.

2. *The Guiding Opinions of the State Council on the Establishment of the General Practitioner System*

(Abridged)

[2011] No. 23 issued by the State Council
July 1, 2011

3. *Notice of the General Office of the State Council on Printing and Issuing the 2011 Arrangement of the Pilot Work for the Public Hospitals*

(Abridged)

[2011] No.10 issued by the General Office of the State Council
February 28, 2011

4. *Guiding Opinions of the General Office of the State Council on Further Strengthening the Construction of Village Doctors' Contingent*

(Abridged)

[2011] No. 31 issued by the General Office of the State Council
July 2, 2011

Order of the Ministry of Health of the People's Republic of China (No. 79)

The Standardization of the Production Quality of Medicines (Revision of 2010) was discussed and adopted at the conference of the Ministry of Health on October 19, 2010 and now is hereby promulgated and shall come into force as of the date of March 1, 2011.

Minister Chen Zhu
January 17, 2011

5. *The Standardization of the Production Quality of Medicines (Revision of 2010)*

(Abridged)

Order of the Ministry of Health of the People's Republic of China (No. 80)

Detailed Regulations of the Implementation of Health Management for the Public Places was discussed and adopted at the conference of the Ministry of Health on February 14, 2011 and now is hereby promulgated and shall come into force as of the date of May 1, 2011.

Minister Chen Zhu
March 10, 2011

6. *Detailed Regulations of the Implementation of Health Management for the Public Places*

(Abridged)

Order of the Ministry of Health of the People's Republic of China (No. 81)

The Report and Administrative Measures for Adverse Reactions of Medicines was discussed and adopted at the conference of the Ministry of Health on December 13,

2010 and now is hereby promulgated and shall come into force as of the date of July 1, 2011.

Minister Chen Zhu
May 4, 2011

7. *The Report and Administrative Measures for Adverse Reactions of Medicines*

(Abridged)

Order of the Ministry of Health of the People's Republic of China (No. 82)

Administrative Measures for Recalling Medical Instruments (Trial Edition) was discussed and adopted at the conference of the Ministry of Health on June 28, 2010 and now is hereby promulgated and shall come into force as of the date of July 1, 2011.

Minister Chen Zhu
May 20, 2011

8. *Administrative Measures for Recalling Medical Instruments (Trial Edition)*

(Abridged)

(Wang Dian)

Part Ⅲ
Progress of Work

1. The Progress of Health Work in 2011

2011 is the year of assaulting fortified positions in the five key tasks of medical reform and the starting year of health progress in the "Twelfth-five Year Plan". Under the strong leadership of the CPC Central Committee and the State Council, national health system pooled the wisdom and efforts of everyone, planned the overall situation, paid attention to reform, promoted development and obtained significant achievements in medical reform and all health work.

I. The Tasks of Medical Reform Led by Ministry of Health

Ministry of Health took the lead in and undertook 46 projects of the 67 projects determined by the State Council, cooperated and completed 18 of them.

(1) The New Rural Cooperative Medical Care System

In 2011, the number of the population participating in the new rural cooperative medical care system nationwide was 832,000,000 and the participating rate was 97%. The proportion of self-paid medical expenses by the farmers who participated in the new rural cooperative medical care system dropped from 73.4% in 2008 to 49.5% in 2011, and medical expense burden was relieved obviously. End-stage renal disease and two cancers of women were added into the guarantee of the grave and special diseases in Jiangxi Province, Jiangsu Province, Liaoning Province, Hebei Province, Shandong Province, Chongqing City, Anhui Province, Hunan Province, Hubei Province, and Hainan Province and the guarantee was expanded to cover 20 diseases in Jilin Province. The pilot projects of supplementary insurance of the grave and special diseases and the purchase of commercial insurance were launched in Xinjiang Uygur Autonomous Region, Yunnan Province, Tibet Autonomous Region, Qinghai Province, Fujian Province and Hunan Province. Changshu City in Jiangsu Province and Lanshan City in Hunan Province to carry out the reform of payment. Inner Mongolia Autonomous Region and Shaanxi Province improved the level of the overall planning to city (alliance). Guangdong Province, Henan Province, Hunan Province and other (regions and cities) explored the management of the new rural cooperative medical care system handled by commercial insurance institutions. Jiangsu Province established stable growth mechanism in legislative forms to finance for the new rural cooperative medical care system.

(2) National System for the Basic Drugs

All prefectures made the implementation of the basic drug system the breakthrough and promoted the comprehensive reform in medical health institutions at grassroots planned as a whole. 16 provinces (regions and cities) of Anhui, Shandong, Hebei, Sichuan and Hubei completed a new round of procurement and the average price fell 30%. 11 provinces of Jiangxi and Zhejiang demanded the medical institutions above the second grade to prepare and use the basic drugs according to the regulations and proportion. Ningxia Hui Autonomous Region, Henan Province and other provinces (regions and cities) explored the centralized bid procurement of some high-value consumables. Anhui Province issued 30 articles of supplementary policies. 16 provinces (regions and cities) of Liaoning, Shaanxi, Qinghai and Xinjiang Production and Construction Corps practiced full employment in medical health institutions run by the governments at grassroots. Most provinces (regions and cities) like Heilongjiang Province basically cashed performance pay in medical health institutions at grassroots.

(3) Medical Health Service System at Grassroots

The transformation construction of the county hospitals, township health centers, village clinics, and community health service institutions as the key must be continuously promoted. Medical health talent construction focused on general practitioners at grassroots must be enhanced, job-transfer training for general practitioners, the free training for medical students according to order and orientation for rural areas and the recruitment of medical practitioners be carried out, the "Project of Rendering Aid to the Rural Health by Tens of Thousands of Doctors" was implemented continuously, subsidy policies for rural doctors be gradually implemented and social endowment problems be solved. Hebei Province recruited 2000 "village doctors of college students". Beijing City, Shanghai City and other provinces (regions and cities) practiced family doctor service. Inner Mongolia Autonomous Region explored the practice of the "small box engineering of health guarantee".

(4) Equal Access to the Basic Public Health Service

The basic public health service at urban and rural grassroots was extensively carried out. By the end of November, 2011, the electronic filing rate of the standardized health files of urban and rural residents has reached 55.3%; The numbers of pregnant and puerpera women, children of 0-6 years old, old people above 65 under health management reached respectively 14,540,000, 73,860,000 and 103,660,000;

The numbers of patients with high blood pressure, diabetes and serious mental disease under standardized management reached respectively 61,280,000, 16,680,000 and 2,790,000. In 2011, 515,000 poor cataract patients were given free vision recovery operation. Guizhou Province completed the project of hazard elimination of burning coal fluorosis one year ahead. All prefectures positively innovated the methods of public health service and management. Jiangxi Province, Qinghai Province and Tibet Autonomous Region (regions and cities) raised the matching proportion of provincial capital to reduce the grassroots burden. Beijing City, Hubei Province, Shandong Province and other provinces (regions and cities) started cross-department promotion project of social health. Jiangxi Province put the third party assessment mechanism of equal access to the basic public health service into trial use.

(5) Pilot Reform in Public Hospitals

17 national contact pilot cities, 37 provincial pilot cities and 745 public hospitals in 18 provinces (regions and cities) carried out comprehensive pilot reform and made comprehensive exploration into planning layout, management system, compensation mechanism, payment system, inner management, service improvement, supporting the grassroots and the encouragement of medicine operation by the society. All prefectures started with the enhanced service, and carried out a batch of reform measures of quick effect and easy to operate. Booking diagnosis and treatment, seeking medical care in certain period of time and qualified nursing service were vigorously carried out, and the pilot project of clinical pathway and electronic medical records in hospitals of the second and the third grades were launched. Booking outpatient rate in some hospitals of Beijing City reached around 40%. Beijing City, Hainan Province, Shenzhen City, Kunming City, Chengdu City, Luoyang City and others carried out the pilot project of physicians practicing at multiple sites. The 9 cities of Anshan, Zhenjiang, Wuhu and so on formed medical groups with distinctive features. The 5 cities of Shanghai, Beijing and others explored to establish medical associations. Shaanxi Province, Jiangsu Province, Zhejiang Province, Hubei Province, Shanxi Province and other provinces (regions and cities) started comprehensive reform in public hospitals at county level. Anhui Province, combining with medical insurance reimbursement policy, promoted payment according to diseases and preliminarily realized hierarchical diagnosis and treatment.

II. Prevention and Control of Major Disease, Health Emergency, Maternal and Child Health Care

(1) Disease Prevention and Control

Prevention and control measures for the key infectious diseases, like influenza, hand-foot-and-mouth disease, brucellosis and others must be effectively carried out and the legal infectious diseases of Class I and Class II be stabilized. The coverage of AIDS monitoring, testing and treatment, intervention, and the interdiction of maternal-neonatal transmission must be expanded. The number of AIDS patients tested and the number in anti-virus therapy increased by 16% and 37%, compared with the same period a year ago. 830,000 cases of tuberculosis were accumulatively detected and treated, and the cure rate of infectious tuberculosis was 93%. The morbidity of the key parasitic diseases, like schistosomiasis, was on a declining curve. The significant result in intensive immunization of measles vaccine was made, and the morbidity decreased from 25/1,000,000 in 2010 to less than 10/1,000,000. The imported wild poliovirus in Xinjiang was positively dealt with and 22,000,000 persons/times were given the intensive polio immunization. The elimination goal of iodine deficiency disorders was realized in 28 provinces (regions and cities) nationwide. Chronic disease prevention and control was continuously strengthened. 39 demonstration plots of comprehensive prevention and control for chronic diseases passed the examination and acceptance, and the action of healthy lifestyle for all people was carried on in 892 counties (prefectures). Early diagnosis and treatment, and the screening for 200,000 people with key cancers were made. Key construction projects of professional mental health institutions were practiced and national information management system for heavy mental diseases was established. Comprehensive intervention pilots for children of oral diseases in 25 provinces (regions and cities) were launched. Patriotic health campaign was carried out extensively and profoundly, the number of National Hygienic City (Region) and Hygienic Town increased, the connotation was upgraded and the staged achievements in urban and rural environmental improvement action were obtained. Monitoring of rural drinking water was intensified and the coverage was further expanded.

(2) Health Emergency

Linkage mechanism for the disposal of public health emergency by multiple divisions was perfected. A batch of contingency plans for public health emergencies were made, and the construction of core ability for emergency was enhanced. The construction tasks of 27 national health emergency teams of 4 categories were carried out. The strengthened training of managerial cadres, provincial teachers and backbones was enhanced. The adjustment of anti-terrorist health emergency reserve directory and material preparation were completed. Early warning, prevention and control of sudden and unexplained infectious diseases were reinforced. Plague prevention and treatment in key areas was continuously strengthened. Emergent anthrax incidents in Liaoning Province, Jilin Province, Inner Mongolia Autonomous Region and other places were positively responded. Quick reaction to international and domestic events, such as nuclear accident in Fukushima, Japan, "7.23" pile up of railway bullet train and so on was made.

(3) Maternal and Child Health

Maternity and child care system construction was vigorously promoted and 4.3 billion RMB Yuan was invested to support the basic equipment in maternal and child care institutions at county level of mid-west areas. The projects of "Reducing the mortality of pregnant and puerpera women and eliminating neonatal tetanus" were continuously carried out, comprehensive prevention and treatment of birth defects was promoted, free pre-marital medical check-up was extended, and prenatal diagnosis was carried forward. The construction of health education system was enhanced, professional training for personnel of health education was organized and launched, and health literacy promotion for citizens was promoted. Smoking ban in public places was launched, and no efforts were spared to promote the creation and construction of smoke-free medical health system. In 2011, the mortality of pregnant and puerpera women dropped to 26.1/100,000 and infant mortality rate to 12.1‰.

Ⅲ. Food and Drug Safety

(1) Long-term Mechanism and System Construction

National Drug Safety Planning was formulated, and the newly-revised management standardization of pharmaceutical production quality in 2010 was promulgated and implemented. The construction of drug electronic monitoring system was promoted, and the drug quality traceability and safety emergency management system was established and improved. Drug examination and approval mechanism was reformed. A complaint reporting center was organized and established. The construction of technical support system was feasibly strengthened. The action plan for improving drug standards was promoted. The information system of drug selective testing was established. Fast drug inspection technology was implemented. The monitoring and evaluation on drugs after marketing was intensified. The system of adverse drug reaction reporting and monitoring management was improved, the decision to deal with drugs of existing safety risks were timely made, drug safety propaganda was carried out in a deep-going way, and drug safety of the public was maintained. The two-year special rectification of drug safety was completely finished, and the fighting against the infringement of intellectual property rights, manufacturing and selling fake drugs, medical apparatus and instruments, and health care products was carried out in a deep-going way. Illegal drug advertisements were seriously administrated, and food and drug market order was standardized.

(2) Rectification of Food Safety

The specific project adding illegal non-food substances into food was carried out profoundly, and the lists of 64 non-food substances and 22 easily abused additives were publicized. A batch of food safety events concerned by the society was properly disposed, and the hot issues of the society were timely responded. The construction of technical regulations of food safety and standards were enhanced, 124 articles of national food safety standards were examined and approved and 21 articles were promulgated. 96 articles of food additive product standards were formulated, food additives, such as benzoperoxide were repealed, and the ban of bisphenol A in baby bottles was proclaimed. National food safety risk assessment center was organized and established, and monitoring system of food safety risks covered 244 places nationwide. Food safety problems found were circulated seven times successively to the departments, like the office of food safety committee of the State Council through active monitoring. Unlawful acts, such as illegal additives in food, health care food, and cosmetics were cracked down with concentrated efforts. The specific project of attacking unlawful acts of non-food addictives in catering service link was launched.

IV. Health Supervision and Law Enforcement

Routine health supervision and law enforcement was carried out in a deep-going way. 800,000 medical institutions/times were examined, and 41,000 unlicensed medical institutions/times were outlawed. 146,000 schools/times were supervised and examined. National monitoring network of urban and rural drinking water hygiene covering 620 counties (prefectures) of 110 prefectures were established, about 20,000 monitoring points were set up for general water quality survey supplied by civic governments, and 28,000 water supplying units were supervised and examined. Quantified and classified management was practiced in more than 500,000 public places. The supervision and inspection on centralized tableware disinfection was strengthened and the qualified rate of the sampled table ware was 86%. Special inspection on illegal blood collection and supply was continuously carried out. A batch of institutions of occupational disease diagnosis, prevention and control at prefecture and county levels were newly constructed to properly handle a batch of occupational hazard events, such as pneumonoconiosis and occupational poisoning. The relevant departments were united to launch occupational health survey nationwide. The pilot project of medical radiation protection monitoring was carried out in 17 provinces (regions and cities). The Central Committee of the Party input 5.6 billion RMB Yuan for housing construction and configuration of law enforcement equipment in more than 2,000 health supervision institutions at county level, and great achievements were made in the construction of health supervision system.

V. Work of Traditional Chinese Medicine

Several Opinions on the Support and Promotion of the Development of Traditional Chinese Medicine by the State Council was actively implemented in all prefectures, and the functions of traditional Chinese medicine in medical reform were brought into play. The ability construction of traditional Chinese medicine was launched in 1,814 hospitals of traditional Chinese medicine at county level, 58 hospitals of ethnic medicine at prefecture level and 88 hospitals of traditional Chinese medicine at prefecture level in the west part of China. Working mechanism for the handling of emergencies with traditional Chinese medicine, and prevention and treatment of new cases of infectious diseases was perfected. Health project of "preventive treatment of disease" was promoted and the preventive service of menu type for 10 chronic diseases was implemented. Guangxi Zhuang Autonomous Region issued policies to comprehensively promote the development of traditional Chinese medicine and ethnic medicine. Zhejiang Province, Fujian Province, and Shandong Province launched respectively pilot projects of prevention and treatment of chronic diseases with traditional Chinese medicine and integrated management. Gansu Province, Hebei Province, Zhejiang Province, Ningxia Hui Autonomous Region and other provinces (regions and cities) involved traditional Chinese medicine service into the basic public health service. Tianjin City, Beijing City, Shanghai City and other cities enhanced the construction of "House of National Doctor" to bring the characteristics and advantages of traditional Chinese medicine into play. The pilot project of general resource survey on traditional Chinese medicine was started. The appraisal on personnel with professional skills in specific industry of traditional Chinese medicine was promoted. The research results of inheritance of a group of old doctors of traditional Chinese medicine were refined and popularized, the establishment of inheritance studios of the famous and old experts of traditional Chinese medical science and medicine was promoted nationwide and the inheritance of traditional Chinese medicine was pushed ahead. Gansu Province elected 1,000 famous and old doctors of traditional Chinese medicine, and supported "the training of apprentices by teachers" to quicken talent training of traditional Chinese medicine. The constructions of key discipline of traditional Chinese medicine, vocational education and culture were strengthened. Tu Youyou, life-long researcher of China Academy of Chinese Medical Sciences, had the honor to win 2011 Lasker~DeBakery Clinical Medical Award, which embodied the potential value of traditional Chinese medicine. Internationalization of traditional Chinese medicine standards was promoted to further build the discourse power and dominant right of traditional Chinese medicine.

VI. Medical Quality and Safety, Service Supervision and Management

The activities of "Three Goods and One Satisfaction" and "Thousand Miles Tour of Medical Quality" were carried out in a deep-going way and the special rectification of clinical application of antimicrobial agents was launched. The supervision and management of clinical services, such as organ transplantation, and assisted reproductive techniques was intensified. The construction of medical centers in 110 regions in mid-west parts of China was launched, 316 construction projects of national clinical key specialty were evaluated and determined, and the construction of pre-hospital emergency system and department of pediatrics at prefecture level was enhanced. The clinical paths for 109 diseases were newly formulated and distributed. Standardized diagnosis and treatment of major diseases, like children's congenital heart disease, children's leukemia and others was implemented. Standardized diagnosis and treatment of 20 common diseases was started in medical institutions at grassroots.

Achievements were obtained in medical cost control. From January to November, 2011, according to comparable prices, the average expense for outpatient service and discharge fee in public hospitals rose 3.4% and 2.6% respectively, the amount of increase was significantly lower than those in the past two years. Fujian Province, Guangdong Province, Gansu Province, Ningxia Hui Autonomous Region, Zhejiang Province, Shanghai City and other provinces (regions and cities) feasibly enhanced the cost control efforts and accumulated valuable experience.

VII. The Construction of Health Informatization

The Central Committee of the Party and local places arranged special funds for health informatization to enhance the constructions of information system of the new rural cooperative medical care system, electronic health records and electronic medical records of the residents, remote consultation system, and regional health information platform. All local places, based on electronic medical records, optimized business process, and implemented the integrated service measures convenient for the people, such as outpatient service by appointment, diagnosis, treatment and payment, which were convenient for the masses to seek medical treatment. The remote consultation system of Xinjiang Uygur Autonomous Region was connected with those in 88 counties (cities) and the consultation quantity exceeded 20,000 cases. Shanghai City, Jiangsu Province, Zhejiang Province, Henan Province, Hubei Province, Jiangxi Province and other provinces (regions and cities) accelerated the construction of regional health information platform. And the functions of real-time updated electronic health records of the residents, patients' reservation by appointment, inquires of health files, performance evaluation on medical workers, supervision and management of medical health service had been realized.

Ⅷ. Other Health Work

The activity of creating the first and striving for the excellence was combined with the deepening of medical reform, the activity of carrier innovation was started, service for the people was made outstanding, the activity of "three goods and one satisfaction" was carried out in a deep-going way, and all tasks were vigorously promoted and implemented. The propaganda on health policies, results of medical reform, and advanced model in industry were strengthened, the hot issues of public opinions concerned by the masses were positively guided and the good atmosphere of public opinions for health work and medical reform was created with great efforts. The system construction for punishing and preventing corruption in health system was enhanced, and the mechanism construction for monitoring power operation was continuously carried out in a deep-going way in departments of health administration and law enforcement. Centralized drug procurement was vigorously regulated. Specific work of dealing with commercial bribery in the field of pharmaceutical sales and correcting unhealthy tendency of medical service were constantly solidified and deepened. The responsibility system for checking unhealthy tendencies and malpractices, and the appraisal system for medical ethics of medical workers were practiced. Risk assessment mechanism for social stability in health system, doctor-patient dispute mediation mechanism and the long-term mechanism of health petition letters and visits were established to conciliate contradictions and maintain stability. Health care for cadres was actively improved, and the level of health care was continuously upgraded. The life and health of veteran cadres were concerned and they were supported to give their advice and consultations.

The management of medical funds and finance were feasibly strengthened. The methods of fund allocation were renovated and the whole coverage of supervision and management of medical funds was promoted. New systems of financing and accounting were carried out. The planning outline for health undertaking in the "Twelfth-five Year Plan" period was formulated, regional health planning, large-scale medical equipment allocation and the basic construction management were continuously enhanced, and the centralized procurement of large-scale medical equipment and high-value consumables was promoted. Health supports in Xinjiang, Tibet and Qinghai were feasibly intensified, and the post-disaster restoration and reconstruction in Wenchuan, Yushu and Danqu were completed or promoted smoothly.

Medical Health Medium and Long-term Talent Development Plan (2011-2020) was formulated and talent engineerings, such as health talents at grassroots, outstanding talents of medical science, special talents in shortage, talents of traditional Chinese medical science and medicine and the standardized training for doctors were launched. Coordination of national medical education among ministries was intensified. The *Twelfth-five Year Plan for the Development of Medical Science and Technology* was formulated and implemented. The two major projects of science and technology of "Prevention and Treatment of Major Infectious Diseases of AIDS and Virus Hepatitis" and "Creation and Production of Major New Drug" were vigorously implemented, and the scientific and technological support of the results of research and development was further brought into play.

National and regional interaction and cooperation were extensively carried out. Concept and progress of medical reform in China was propagandized, international support of technology and funds was introduced for health development by means of diplomatic platforms, like international organizations, international conferences, multiple and bilateral activities and so on. The major global health actions were positively attended, which played an active role in promoting the prevention and treatment of chronic diseases, improving decisive factor for healthy society and promoting international food safety. International organizations were invited to make independent evaluation on health reform in China. China's vaccine supervision system had passed WHO's Pre-Accreditation. High-level dialogue and technical cooperation with developing countries, neighboring countries, and countries of emerging economy in health fields were enhanced. The construction and innovation of foreign aid medical team were strengthened. Deep health cooperation with Hong Kong and Macao, and health communication on both sides of Taiwan straits were constantly promoted.

(Ji Chenglian)

2. Support WHO Independent Evaluation on China's Medical Reform

Ministry of Health specially set up the supporting expert group of domestic health policies to fully support and coordinate WHO independent evaluation on China's medical system reform.

WHO expert group arrived in China in July, 2011, made policy interview with the comrades responsible for medical reform and the relevant persons in all administrative departments and bureaus, convened the symposium of experts and stakeholders, made the field investigation in Anhui Province and formulated report of independent evaluation (the first draft) at the beginning of September. The relevant ministries, commissions, and all administrative departments and bureaus affiliated to Ministry of Health put forward written amendment opinions on the draft of the report. In late September, WHO expert group arrived in Beijing again to listen to the feedback of all parties, and went to Zichang County, Shaanxi Province for the field investigation. On September 30th, WHO expert group completed the final assessment report. The evaluation supporting group of Ministry of Health organized the translation and checked the report.

(Ji Chenglian)

3. Promotion of Administrative Work according to Law

In accordance with the *Opinions on the Construction of Law-based Government by the State Council, the Implementation Opinions on the Carrying out the Opinions on the Construction of Law-based Government by the State Council by Ministry of Health* and work division scheme in the related administrative departments and bureaus were formulated, printed and distributed and the definite requirements for further intensification of administrative work in health system according to law were put forward. According to the requirements of Legislative Affairs Office of the State Council, the relevant materials of impartial, honest law enforcement and health administrative enforcement were submitted.

The spirit of video and telephone conference on further promotion of the reform of administrative approval system by the State Council was carried out. On November 21st, 2011, the meeting on ministerial affairs was held to study, examine and discuss work arrangements of Ministry of Health for the implementation of the spirit of the video and telephone conference. The clear-up work on the projects of health administrative examination and approval of the 6th batch must be well done: the would-be canceled and adjusted projects of health administrative examination and approval with signed *Letter of Confirmation* reported to the Office of Examination and Correction of the State Council; and the projects involved canceling, distribution, merger and adjustment to other relevant ministries and commissions. On December 16th, 2011, the Party Group Secretary of Ministry of Health, Zhang Mao and the Group Leader of Discipline Inspection in Ministry of Health, Li Xi presided over the leading group meeting on the reform of administrative examination and approval system of Ministry of Health. And they made definite requirements for the acceleration of the construction of Government Affair Hall of Ministry of Health, and the implementation of "One window for foreign service", combined with the reconstruction of Office Building of Ministry of Health. The administrative examination and approval procedures were continuously improved and the power operation of administrative examination and approval was standardized.

(Ji Chenglian)

4. WTO Work in Health Field in 2011

In 2011, a good job in WTO work in health field was continued, performance of WTO commitments in health field was promoted and the interests of the state were feasibly safeguarded.

The strategies of free trade zones were seriously implemented. We actively participated in China and Sweden negotiation on free trade zone, completed China and Australia market access negotiations relevant with medical service trade in the 16th and the 17th rounds of negotiations and timely adjusted price strategies according to the unified deployment of the State Council and the new situations in the negotiations. We cooperated with Ministry of Commerce and General Administration of Quality Supervision, made active coordination with Food and Drug Administration and Bureau of Traditional Chinese Medicine, and accomplished the preparations and attendance for the 22nd China-US Joint Commission on Commerce and Trade, and the joint meeting of technical trade measures.

The relevant departments were cooperated to make work planning for the relevant fields. We, together with 34 departments, like Ministry of Commerce, issued the *Outline of the Twelfth-five Year Planning for the Development of Service and Trade*, and put forward the development goals of medical service trade and the key work. We, cooperating with General Administration of Quality Supervision, formulated the *Twelfth-year Planning for the Field of National Technical Trade Measures* and put forward job objectives of China's technical trade measures.

According to WTO transparency requirement, the circulation and evaluation should be well done. In 2011, Ministry of Health circulated 165 national standards of food safety to WTO/SPS committees, and 1 standard to WTO/TBT committees. The experts were organized to study and reply about 150 pieces of evaluation opinions from other members, trade associations and international organizations, put forward the evaluation opinions on other WTO members (including probiotics species list of Thailand, EU's detection methods for marine biological toxin and so on) and maintain the health rights of the residents in China, and the economic interests of the relevant domestic industries.

The activities under WTO framework were substantively participated in and the interests of the state were maintained. We attended the 50th to 52nd regular meetings of WTO/SPS committees, participated in the discussion of the related trade rules, responded to the concerns of other WTO members with China's standards for distilled spirits and configuration wine, the usage criteria for food addictives and the limited quantity of food contamination, clarified the relevant problems and completed the tasks of meeting attendance and bilateral consultations. We joined in and responded to all WTO examinations and discussions, examined and discussed trade policies of EU members, put forward opinions of examination and discussion on WTO technical trade measures and promoted the solutions to some relevant problems. We cooperated with Ministry of Commerce to respond to and passed WTO's last SPS transitional examination and discussion on China and made previous preparations for WTO fourth examination and discussion on China's trade policies.

(Ji Chenglian)

Chapter I Disease Prevention and Control

1. Disease Prevention and Control in 2011

I. The Realization of Medical Reform Targets of Disease Prevention and Control by the Scheduled Time

The major projects and the projects of the basic public health service were positively carried out: In 2011, totally, 6,980,000 persons under 15 were resowed with hepatitis B vaccine; Stove changes in endemic areas of coal burning fluorosis were made in 211,000 households; Harmless sanitation toilets was built in 4,021,000 rural households, and 118%, 100% and 116% of the target tasks were completed respectively; More than 300 million agents/times of national immunization planning vaccine were given to children at appropriate age and the reported vaccination rate was above 90%, morbidity of the vaccine targeted diseases, such as whooping cough, diphtheria, hepatitis A, and epidemic encephalitis B decreased dramatically, the rate of Hepatitis B virus infection of the children under 5 was controlled below 5%, which reached WHO controlling objectives planned in Western Pacific Region in 2012; The numbers of the patients with high blood pressure and diabetes under the management were 61,280,000 and 16,670,000 respectively, and 81,750,000 people above 65 were given health examination; Paper health files were established for 2,220,000 patients of mental disease and the information of 1,500,000 patients with mental disease was input into database.

II. Further Consolidate Groundwork for Laws and Regulations, Policies and Measures

The draft of *Mental Health Act* has just been finished, examined and discussed at the first meeting of National People's Congress. The *Opinions on Strengthening and Innovating Social Management by the Central Committee of the Communist Party of China* definitely put forward the requirements of "the Establishment of the Working Mechanism for Early Warning, Treatment, Service and Management for Patients of Grave Mental Disease" and "Strengthening Social Psychological Service", which provides policy guarantee for mental health work. With the new situation of infectious disease prevention and treatment, the amendment of *Law on Prevention and Treatment of Infectious Diseases was* reported for examination and discussion, and the revision of *Implementation Plan for Health and Quarantine Regulations of Domestic Communication* was organized. *National Tuberculosis Prevention and Treatment Planning (2011-2015)* was issued by the State Council, China's *"Twelfth-five Year" Action Plan for AIDS Containment, Prevention and Treatment* was passed through examination and discussion by Working Committee on AIDS Prevention and Treatment of the State Council; *National Planning for Prevention and Treatment of Endemic Diseases (2011-2015)* has been reported to General Office of the State Council for retransmission; *National Planning for Leprosy Harm Elimination (2011-2020)*the *Outline of the Planning for the Key Projects of Comprehensive Schistosomiasis Treatment (2009-2015), China's Action Plan for Malaria Elimination (2010-2015),* and *Action Plan for Echinococcosis Prevention and Treatment (2010-2015)* were printed and distributed by multiple departments; *China's Planning for the Prevention and Treatment of Chronic Diseases (2011-2015) and China's Planning for Mental Health (2012-2015)* were under opinion soliciting from multiple departments; *Planning for the Construction of Vaccine Supply System* has been approved through examination and discussion by the State Council and retransmitted by General Office of the State Council. The study on the establishment of training system for public health physicians was started to clarify problems about responsibility orientation and training mode of public health physicians. *Provisions on the Management of Institution for Disease Prevention and Control and Guiding Opinions on Post Setting Management of Institution for Disease Prevention and Control* were organized and drafted in order to promote the ability construction of institution of disease prevention and control to fully perform their duties and strengthen personnel access and the responsibilities of work requirements.

According to the requirements of the *Opinions on Strengthening and Innovating Social Management* by the Central Committee of the Communist Party of China and the State Council, the organization and coordination of health service management for migrant people were feasibly well done, and disease prevention and control among migrant people was positively launched; The responsibilities of health service and management for overseas personnel were clarified and health service management was launched by cooperating with the relevant departments. The spirit of the joint meeting for rural workers by the State Council was actively implemented, the special study on health service for rural workers was carried out, and policy suggestions on health service for rural workers were formulated and proposed, which provided bases for further formulation of the relevant policies to solve the problems for rural workers. The relevant departments were positively coordinated, and orphan rescue and health education for the key groups of people of rural workers, migrant people, teenagers and women were continuously carried out.

Ⅲ. Steady Progress in the Prevention and Control of Major Diseases

In 2011, the epidemic situation of infectious diseases was general stable. The number of information systems of disease prevention and control in operation was 20, of which direct online report system of infectious diseases and public emergencies has been in smooth operation for 7 years, and the reporting quality and monitoring sensitivity were continuously improved. Statutory epidemics of infectious diseases were promulgated regularly every month, the information concerned by the society, like hand-foot-and-mouth disease and influenza was timely circulated and the real-time risk communication was carried out. Significant result in the reinforced immunization of measles vaccine was obtained, the morbidity in 2010 dropped from 25/1,000,000 to lower than 10/1,000,000, which laid the foundation for measles elimination. In 2011, AIDS testing of more than 84,000.000 people/times were done, and 140,000 drug addicts were given outpatient methadone maintenance treatment; Intervention coverage of high risk groups of people, such as illicit prostitutes and MSM increased 15% and 20% respectively. 900,000 TB patients were detected and treated, the curative rate of infectious TB patients stay above 90%, and the pilot projects of standardized diagnosis, treatment and management for TB resistant to many drugs were expanded to 18 provinces. Ministerial and provincial cooperation mechanism or technology supporting mechanism in high epidemic areas was established to vigorously promote the progress in leprosy harm elimination. The comprehensive strategies for schistosomiasis prevention and treatment by mainly controlling the source of infection were continuously promoted, malaria elimination was steadily promoted and reported cases of acute schistosomiasis and malaria dropped 93% and 41%, compared with those of last year; There were nearly 30,000 patients of echinococcosis under treatment. 28 provinces have reached the elimination goal of iodine deficiency disorders and 97.9% counties realized the elimination goal of iodine deficiency disorders; Drinking water safety problems were basically solved in endemic areas of moderate and severe fluorosis and stove changes in endemic areas of coal burning fluorosis poisoning was 92.6%; Water change in endemic areas of arsenic poisoning of drinking water and the potential villages found before 2004 was completely finished, and all measures for stove change in endemic areas of coal burning arsenic poisoning were implemented; The morbidity of Kaschin-Beck disease and Keshan disease was quite stable and controlled effectively. 39 districts and counties were awarded demonstration areas of national comprehensive prevention and control of chronic diseases, more than 40% of the districts and counties nationwide have launched the action of healthy lifestyle, and the number of tumor registration points was 193, covering 180 million people. 185,000 people were given diagnostic screening in the project of the early diagnosis and early treatment of cancer, and the treatment rate was 80%. Pit and fissure sealing for children was started in 25 provinces. 170 cities, and 766 districts and counties, basing on the requirements, have established management mechanisms for patients of grave mental disease, covering 391 million people. The imported polio epidemics was powerfully responded to, three rounds of strengthened immunization for children were launched everywhere in Xinjiang Uygur Autonomous Region, two rounds of intensified immunization for adults were given in five zhous in the south part of Xinjiang Uygur Autonomous Region and accumulatively more than 22 million people took vaccines.

(Ji Chenglian)

2. Significant Achievements in the Projects of Disease Prevention and Control Covered in the Deepening Reform of Medical Health System

I. Smooth Progress in Disease Prevention and Control of the Basic Public Health Service

From 2009 to 2011, disease monitoring system was constantly improved, 1,556 national monitoring stations were set up, and the trend of 25 kinds of infectious diseases and 4 kinds of vector organisms was instantly grasped. 100% institutions for disease prevention and control, 98% medical institutions above county level and 87% township health centers realized direct online report on epidemic situation of infectious disease and public health emergencies, and the quality of the reports and epidemic monitoring sensitivity increased year by year. State immunization planning projects were implemented and expanded, children at appropriate age were vaccinated, 339 million doses/times, 361 million doses/times and 385 million doses/times were vaccinated in 3 years respectively and inoculation rate of conventional vaccines was above 90%. The number of the patients with high blood pressure and diabetes under health management reached 61.28 million and 16.67 million respectively and the filing rate was 68.8%. 766 districts and counties in 170 zhous established management and treatment network with medical institutions of mental health as the main body, the comprehensive hospitals as auxiliary agencies, grassroots medical institutions in community and township as support, institutions of disease prevention and control as supplement, which covered 391 million people. Health files of grave mental diseases involved in national basic public health service were established and the number under the follow-up management was 2.786 million. 1.851 million children at appropriate age from 295 counties (districts) were given oral health examination and 1.091 million children at appropriate age were given pit and fissure sealing.

II. Comprehensive Implementation of Disease Prevention and Control in Major Projects of Public Health Service

In 2011, 6.98 million people nationwide were resowed with hepatitis B vaccine and 112% of the tasks were completed; Stove changes were finished in 211,000 households and 100% of the tasks were finished; Harmless sanitation toilets were built in 4.021 million households in rural areas and 116% of the tasks were fulfilled. From 2009 to 2011, accumulatively 68.32 million people were resowed with hepatitis B vaccine and 118% of the total tasks were completed, which increased the vaccination rate of hepatitis B of the people born from 1994 to 2001, protected the susceptible population, further reduced the infection rate of hepatitis B virus and the carrying rate of HbsAg in this group of people and accelerated the control process of hepatitis B. Stove changes were done in 1.689 million households, 104% of the total tasks were finished, which effectively controlled the indoor coal-burning pollution in endemic areas, improved ecological environment in endemic areas and sped up the pace of prevention and treatment of coal burning fluorine poisoning; Harmless sanitation toilets were built in 13.33 million households in rural areas and 121% of the total tasks were completed, which effectively prevented and reduced the occurrence of diseases, significantly improved the outlook of rural environment and health, helped the crowd cultivating health behavior and habits, promoted the spiritual civilization construction in the countryside and new rural construction, and got the recognition and welcome from the common people.

III. Profound Development of the Investigation and Study on Disease Prevention and Control in Medical Reform

In accordance with the spirit of *Circulation on Printing and Distributing Working System of Contacting Point of Medical Reform of Ministerial Leaders* by the Party Group of Ministry of Health, and *Working Scheme for Comprehensive Contacting Point of Medical Reform in Weifang City of Shandong Province* were studied and formulated. Led by the leaders from Ministry of Health, the relevant people went to Zhenjiang City of Jiangsu Province and Weifang City of Shandong Province to make the investigation and study of special projects on the development of the deepening of medical health system reform; 8 groups of investigation from disease prevention and control bureau went to 12 provinces to undertake the comprehensive investigation and study on the deepening of medical health system reform, disease prevention and control and patriotic health work; Forums on disease prevention and control and patriotic health work were held in dividing areas of middle and east regions, to listen to opinions and suggestions from all places. Simultaneously, the study on public health service system was positively carried out, the research reports on work program for disease control in medical reform covered in the "Twelfth-five Year Plan" were drafted, and the major projects of special needs and suggestions on medical reform were put forward, *Opinions on the Enhancement of Public Health Service at Grassroots (draft for comment)* was organized for the draft to fully promote the construction of disease prevention and control system combining prevention and treatment, and the implementation of all the tasks of disease prevention and control covered in medical reform.

(Ji Chenglian)

3. Study on Standardized Training for Physicians of Public Health

In 2011, Ministry of Health organized the study on standardized training for physicians of public health and made many rounds of researches on strategies and measures of system construction, the contents of the training system, the methods and contents of the training, the requirements and standards of base construction and other relevant matters. The drafts of *Guiding Opinions on the Construction of Standardized Training System for Public Health Physician, Implementation Plan for Standardized Training System for Public Health Physician and Base Construction Scheme for Standardized Training System for Public Health Physician* and other relevant documents for comment were preliminarily formulated.

(Ji Chenglian)

4. The Outline of Statutory Epidemics of Infectious Diseases Nationwide in 2011

In 2011 (from zero hour on Jan. 1st to 24 hour on Dec. 31st, 2011), the number of the reports on statutory infectious diseases nationwide was 6,320,099, the number of deaths was 15,802, the reported morbidity was 471.33/100,000 and mortality was 1.18/100,000.

In 2011, the total number of the incidence of statutory infectious diseases of Class I nationwide was 25, and the death number was 1; There was no incident or death report on infectious diseases of Class II, such as SARS and diphtheria, but there were reports on 3,237,533 cases of other diseases and 15,263 deaths. The reported morbidity of infectious diseases of Class I and Class II was 241.44/100,000 and the mortality was 1.14/100,000, 1.15% and 6.33% higher than that of 2010 respectively. The first five reported diseases were successively virus hepatitis, pulmonary tuberculosis, syphilis, bacterial and amebic dysentery, and gonorrhoea, accounting for 94.41% of the reported total incidence of infectious diseases of Class I and Class II. The first five reported deaths were successively AIDS, pulmonary tuberculosis, rabies, virus hepatitis and epidemic hemorrhagic fever, accounting for 97.56% of the total death reports of infectious diseases of Class I and Class II.

In the corresponding period, the reported case number of infectious diseases of Class III was 3,082,541, the death number was 538, the reported morbidity was 229.88/100,000, and the mortality was 0.04/100,000, 4.83% and 44.69% lower than those of 2010 respectively. The first five reported diseases were successively hand-foot-mouth disease, other infectious diarrhea, epidemic mumps, influenza and rubella, accounting for 98.70% of the reported total incidence of infectious diseases of Class III. The first three reported deaths were successively hand-foot-mouth disease, other infectious diarrhea and influenza.

Compared with that of 2010, the reported number of the incidence of infectious diseases of intestinal infectious diseases and respiratory infectious disease of Class I and Class II decreased to 4.73% and 2.38%, and the reported number of the incidence of infectious diseases of natural source and insect-born infectious diseases, blood source and sexually transmitted infectious diseases increased 1.31% and 4.66%. In intestinal infectious diseases, the number of hepatitis E increased. The number of cholera, hepatitis A, typhoid fever/paratyphoid fever, bacterial and amebic dysentery, and unclassified hepatitis decreased; In respiratory infectious diseases, there was no report on morbidity and mortality of SARS and diphtheria, but the reported number of scarlet fever, whooping cough and H1N1 influenza A increased slightly, the reported incidence number of measles, epidemic cerebrospinal meningitis and pulmonary tuberculosis decreased slightly; The incidence number of pestilence, dengue, malaria, leptospirosis, epidemic encephalitis B and rabies of natural source and insect-borne infectious diseases decreased slightly, there was 1 case of highly pathogenic avian influenza to human compared with that of 2010, and the reported number of epidemic hemorrhagic fever, brucellosis, anthrax and schistosomiasis increased at varying degrees; The reported incidence number of gonorrhoea of blood source and sexually transmitted diseases decreased slightly and the reported incidence number of AIDS, hepatitis C, syphilis and hepatitis B increased.

In 2011, there was 1 case report on pestilence, the death number was 1 and the reported incidence number and death number were 6 and 1, fewer than those of 2010; The total reported number of cholera was 24, and the reported morbidity was 0.0018/100,000, 84.75% lower than that of 2010; There was 1 case report of highly pathogenic avian influenza to human, the death number was 1 and the reported number of incidence and death were the same as those of 2010; The reported number of polio was 20, the death number was 1 and the reported cases were the overseas input caused by the infection of polio wild virus of Type I.

The First Ten Reported Incidence Number and the Death Number of Infectious Diseases of Class I and Class II in 2011 Nationwide

Ranking	Reported Disease	Reported Morbidity	Reported Disease	Death
1	hepatitis B	1,093,335	AIDS	9,224
2	tuberculosis	953,275	tuberculosis	2,840
3	syphilis	395,182	rabies	1,879
4	dysentery	237,930	hepatitis B	637
5	hepatitis C	173,872	hepatitis C	125
6	gonorrhoea	97,954	hemorrhagic fever	119
7	scarlet fever	63,878	syphilis	75
8	unclassified hepatitis	44,479	H1N1 influenza A	75
9	brucellosis	38,151	encephalitis B	63
10	Hepatitis A	31,456	neonatal tetanus	52

(Ji Chenglian)

5. The Substantial Progress in National Measles Elimination

In 2011, Ministry of Health authorized Health Development Research Center of Peking University and China CDC to make evaluation on measles elimination. The evaluation results show that the morbidity of measles decreased greatly, vaccination knowledge was further popularized, a significant result was made in the strengthened measles immunization and the masses of people were quite satisfied with the direct benefit from medical reform. However, the progress was disparate in different places and measles epidemics were quite grave in some provinces. To promote measles elimination in these places, General Office of Ministry of Health printed and distributed *Circulation on Measles Elimination This Winter and Next Spring,* demanded all places to follow the principle of making focal points standout, classifying guidance and advancing on the whole, comprehensively tamp conventional immunization of vaccination, launch strengthened immunization in key counties with higher morbidity of measles, carry out leak survey and resowing in other places, clear up immune blank, establish crowd immune barrier and block the spreading of measles virus. By the end of 2011, there have been 9,943 case reports of measles nationwide, 74% lower than that of 2010 (38,159 cases), the reported morbidity was 7.4/1,000,000, which was the lowest in history and the annual goals (5~10/1,000,000) specified in *Action Plan for National Measles Elimination (2010-2012)* were realized.

(Ji Chenglian)

6. WHO Started Verification of the Planning for Target Realization of Hepatitis B Control in China

In 2005, the 56th Session of WHO Committee of Western Pacific Region passed a resolution, requiring the member nations to control the infection rate of children under five with chronic hepatitis B virus under 2% in 2012. The realization of the planning target of hepatitis B was verified, the confirmation was done with epidemiological investigation of hepatitis B serum, and higher vaccination rate of hepatitis B maintained. In 2006, the result of epidemiological investigation of hepatitis B serum showed that national carrying rate of children under five with hepatitis B surface antigen was 0.96%, the whole process of vaccination rate of hepatitis B for children under 12 months old was above 93% and the rate of the prompt vaccination of hepatitis B vaccine for the first time was 82%. In 2010, the whole process of vaccination rate of hepatitis B was 93%, and the rate of the prompt vaccination was 91%. These data showed that the planning target of hepatitis B control was basically realized in China. In 2011, WHO Office of Western Pacific Region wrote to Ministry of Health, stating that the planning target of hepatitis B control was realized in China and suggesting that verification procedures be launched in China. In December, 2011, Ministry of Health applied to WHO for the launching of verification of the planning target of hepatitis B control in China.

(Ji Chenglian)

7. Progress in AIDS Prevention and Treatment in 2011

By the end of 2011, accumulative reported number of HIV-infected persons and AIDS patients was 444,712, of which 174, 399 were AIDS patients and the reported mortality was 93,003. In 2011, the reported total number of HIV-infected persons was 53,757 and the number of AIDS patients was 39,183.

The Party Central Committee and the State Council attached great importance to AIDS prevention and treatment, the Central Finance input more to AIDS prevention and treatment, and funds for AIDS prevention and treatment subsidized to local public health special funds by the Central increased from 2.06 billion RMB Yuan in 2010 to 2.2 billion in 2011. The member units of AIDS Prevention and Treatment Committee of the State Council actively carried out the spirit of *Circulation on Further Strengthening AIDS Prevention and Treatment (hereinafter Circulation),* combining with characteristics of the departments and their own responsibilities, cooperated closely, intensified the work and made obvious achievements in publicity and education, key crowd intervention, patient treatment, salvation, help and support.

The coverage of monitoring and detection was further expanded. In 2011, 1,888 spots of sentinel supervision were set up nationwide, so were 339 laboratories of corroboration and 14,305 laboratories of screening. All provinces had detection ability of CD4 cells and virus load and detection network expanded continuously to the grassroots. In 2011, more than 8,400 persons/times nationwide were given AIDS virus antibody detection, 30.3% more than that of 2010 and the newly-found case was 16.2% higher than that of 2010; More than 1.83 million persons/times voluntarily had syphilis detected at the points of detection and consultation and 47,000 persons were tested syphilis positive.

The coverage of antiviral therapy was further expanded. By the end of 2011, accumulative 156,000 patients were treated nationwide, the number of new patients was 150,000, 46,000 more than that of 2010 and the annual growth was 75.6%. 124,000 persons were under treatment, of whom 19,000 persons were taking the second line drugs. Accumulatively, there were 2,788 AIDS children nationwide, 2,322 of them were under treatment and 216 were taking the second line drugs. The ratios of the new patients surviving after 12 months treatment and adhering to treatment, follow-up visit, CD4 detection and the test of virus load were slightly higher, and the standardized treatment was significantly enhanced.

The coverage of comprehensive intervention was further expanded. By the end of 2011, 738 community clinics of methadone maintenance and 29 mobile medication cars were opened to the patients. Accumulatively, more than 344,000 drug addicts were treated, 16.6% more than that of 2010; In December, 140,000 persons were under treatment, 14.8% more than that of 2010. The rate of new AIDS infection of crowd addicted to drugs under community drug maintenance therapy was 0.31% in 2011, 26% lower than that of 2010. The monthly number of persons with needle exchange was about 42,000. 540,000 illicit prostitutes were intervened every month and the monthly rate of intervention was 68.0%, 15% higher than that of 2010. 198,000 people of MSM were intervened every month, the monthly rate of intervention coverage was 49.0%, 20% higher than that of 2010.

The coverage of blocking mother-to-child transmission was further expanded. In 2011, the prevention of AIDS mother-to-child transmission was launched in 1,156 counties nationwide, more than 870 pregnant and puerperal women were given AIDS virus antibody detection, and drug application proportion for maternal antiviral infection reached 74.1%. By the end of 2011, the rate of AIDS mother-to-child transmission dropped from 34.8% to 7.4%.

(Ji Chenglian)

8. China's AIDS Epidemic Joint Assessment Report in 2011

In 2011, Ministry of Health, UNAIDS and WHO made joint assessment on China's AIDS epidemic. Technical assessment was undertaken by health administrative departments and organizations at all levels and the relevant experts from American Centers for Disease Prevention and Control were invited for the participation. The epidemic assessment was done with Workbook mode as the basic method recommended by WHO and UNAIDS, and the estimated numbers of the new HIV-infection and deaths relating to AIDS were confirmed with EPP/Spectrum recommended by WHO and UNAIDS.

Epidemic assessment results showed that by the end of 2011, there existed 780,000 HIV-infected survivors and AIDS patients, the infection rate of the whole group was 0.058%, of which 154,000 persons were AIDS patients; In 2011, the newly-detected number of HIV-infected persons was about 48,000 and the death number related with AIDS was 28,000.

The assessment results showed that there were five characteristics of AIDS epidemic in China First, national AIDS epidemic was in low popular trend but the epidemic was serious in some places; Second, the numbers of HIV-infected persons and AIDS patients constantly increased but the case number of new infection remained low; Third, the former HIV-infected persons were successively in period of disease, and the numbers of case incidence and death increased; Fourth, sexually transmission was the main communication way and the proportion continuously increased; Fifth, there were diversified population of infection and the epidemic situation was complicated.

(Ji Chenglian)

9. The Implementation of Global Fund Projects Went through Great Waves and the Projects of the Second Round Would Terminate

On May 16th, 2011, with the reasons of low participation into prevention and treatment by China's social organizations and some problems about finance and management in project areas, the secretariats of global funds for AIDS, tuberculosis and malaria suspended appropriation for China's global fund projects, except the treatment for patients, without board discussion or prior notice. The comprehensive analysis of all parties showed that it related with the tremendous pressure brought by global finance crisis for raising money by global funds ($ 5 billion financing gap in 2010) and big differences in definitions of social organizations by China and global funds. After many efforts, global funds made public commitment in August to resume the appropriations for China's projects, and China got the first grant at the end of December. Project suspension and the delay in resumed appropriation had a strong impact on the prevention and control of AIDS, tuberculosis and malaria in China.

In November, 2011, the 25th Board of Global Funds decided that China, as a country of middle and high income among the group of 20 countries, would no longer had the qualification for applying the second phase of the projects and China's global fund projects of malaria, AIDS and tuberculosis would be terminated successively in June, December of 2012 and June of 2013. According to the estimation, the affected total amount for the prevention and treatment of the three diseases was 4.44 billion RMB Yuan, of which 1.7 billion RMB Yuan was for AIDS project, 2.05 billion RMB Yuan for tuberculosis and 690 million RMB Yuan for malaria.

(Ji Chenglian)

10. The 6th Experience Exchange Conference on China AIDS Prevention and Treatment of International Cooperation Project Was Held in Beijing

On October 31st, 2011, Ministry of Health, and China's Subcommittee of UNAIDS jointly held the 6th Experience Exchange Conference on China AIDS Prevention and Treatment of International Cooperation Project in Beijing. The theme of the conference was "Sharing Experience and Strengthening Cooperation". Delegates from the neighboring countries of Vietnam, Laos, Burma, Cambodia and Mongolia attended the conference. More than 600 delegates attended the conference and they were from some member units of Working Committee on AIDS Prevention and Treatment of the State Council, 42 international organizations, foreign non-governmental organizations, health administrative departments and bureaus of all China's provinces (autonomous regions and municipalities directly under the central government), centers for disease prevention and control and some social organizations. Minister of Health, Chen Zhu, Chairman of China's Subcommittee of UNAIDS, Mark Stirling, and the goodwill ambassador of WHO AIDS and Tuberculosis Prevention and Treatment, and propagandist of AIDS Prevention of Ministry of Health, Peng Li RMB Yuan attended the opening ceremony and made speeches.

Chen Zhu expressed that Chinese government attaches great importance to the leadership and coordination of AIDS prevention and treatment and continuously brings it into the track of legalized and standardized management. After years of effort, the mechanism of prevention and treatment of "Government Organization and leadership, individual departments taking their own responsibilities and joint Participation of the Whole Society" was initially established. The policy of "Four Frees and One Care" was fully implemented, the rapid increase of AIDS epidemic slowed down, the mortality decreased slightly and the effect of prevention and treatment appeared gradually. These achievements were inseparable with the continuous support of capital, technology and personnel from all international cooperation projects in the fields of AIDS prevention and treatment. Chen Zhu emphasized that as a responsible power, China would earnestly implement the solemn promise of "Containing and Reversing AIDS Epidemic by 2015", continue to strengthen international communication and cooperation, and make due contributions to achieving the millennium development goals globally and containing AIDS epidemic.

(Ji Chenglian)

11. National Planning for Tuberculosis Prevention and Treatment (2011-2015) Printed and Distributed by General Office of the State Council

In November, 2011, General Office of the State Council printed and distributed National Planning for Tuberculosis Prevention and Treatment (2011-2015) (hereinafter referred to as Planning), which was the fourth national planning for tuberculosis prevention and treatment formulated by China's government since the 80's of last century.

The Planning summarized comprehensively the great achievements in tuberculosis prevention and treatment during 2001-2010, made the profound analysis on current challenges in tuberculosis prevention and treatment, and put forward a series of new controlling indexes of the detection of TB patients and treatment management, compound preparation extension of fixed doses, laboratory ability construction at all levels, tuberculosis patient management among mobile population, tuberculosis prevention and treatment for resistance to many medicines, prevention and treatment of double infections of tuberculosis bacterium and AIDS virus and awareness rate of core TB information during the period of the "Twelfth five-Year Plan".

The Planning explicated the measures for prevention and treatment of early detection of patients, standardized management for patients, expanded the coverage of tuberculosis diagnosis and treatment for more drug resistance, strengthened the management for mobile patients, enhanced prevention and treatment for double infections, intensified propaganda and education and strengthened scientific researches.

In order to ensure the implementation of prevention and treatment, the Planning put forward comprehensive security measures for clarification of the responsibilities of the departments of health, development and reform, industry informatization, finance, science and technology, public security, administration of justice, civil administration, human resources and social security, food and drug supervision, and radio, film and television; The Planning put forward the principle of adjusting measures to local conditions, and classified guidance, and steady promotion. And the new service system of prevention and treatment for the gradual establishment of designated medical institutions, medical health institutions at grassroots, institutions for disease prevention and control with clear labor division, coordination and cooperation was set up. The Planning emphasized that funds for TB prevention and treatment should be involved in government budget and the input be increased gradually; The Planning initiated that all places should expand medical cost reduction range appropriately according to the actual conditions, and clarify medical expense of TB patients outside the payment scope of public health, which was paid in accordance with the relevant provisions of the basic medical security system; The contingent construction should be strengthened, the ability of prevention and treatment be upgraded, the production and supply of anti-tuberculosis drugs be enhanced, and the supervision and management be intensified.

(Ji Chenglian)

12. Core Information on TB Prevention and Treatment Issued by Ministry of Health (2010 Edition)

In order to promote a unified and standardized propaganda on the relevant policies and key knowledge points, Ministry of Health organized the revision on Core Information on TB Prevention and Treatment (2008 Edition) and issued Core Information on TB Prevention and Treatment (2010 Edition) in March, 2011. The core information was divided into two categories, of which 6 pieces to all groups of people were common core information popular and easy to understand for the popularization of the basic knowledge of TB prevention and treatment among society and the public; and the core information for the target population (heads of government, medical workers, patients, hermetic bondings, mobile population and teachers) was specifically for publicity and education among different objects.

(Ji Chenglian)

13. Nationwide Malaria Epidemic and the Progress in Malaria Elimination

According to the directly reported data from national network for infectious diseases, nationwide malaria epidemic continued to drop considerably in 2011, the total reported number of malaria cases was 4,158 in 31 provinces (regions and cities), of which more than 60% was the imported cases, 41.1% (7,433) lower than that of 2010. The reported morbidity was 0.03/10,000, of which there were 2,468 cases of vivax malaria,

1,437 cases of malignant malaria, 253 cases of unclassified malaria and 30 deaths.

The first five provinces with malaria incidence were successively Yunnan Province, Anhui Province, Jiangsu Province, Henan Province, and Sichuan Province, and the morbidity of the five provinces accounted for 66.5% of the total in China, of which there were 1,216 reported cases of malaria in Yunnan Province, accounting for 29.2% of the total number nationwide, 42.4% lower than that of 2010, and the morbidity was 0.26/10,000, 42.6% lower than that of 2010. There were 650 reported cases of malaria in Anhui Province, 65.2% lower than that of 2010, and the morbidity was 0.11/10,000, 64.1% lower than that of 2010. There were 373 reported cases of malaria in Jiangsu Province, 3.6% higher than that of 2010, and the morbidity was 0.05/10,000, 1.7% higher than that of 2010 and 95% were the imported cases. There were 324 reported cases of malaria in Henan Province, 63.8% lower than that of 2010, and the morbidity was 0.03/10,000, 63.6% lower than that of 2010. There were 200 reported cases of the imported malaria in Sichuan Province, 37.1% lower than that of 2010, and the morbidity was 0.02/10,000, 36.0% lower than that of 2010.

The year of 2011 was the second year in which the action plan for malaria elimination was fully implemented in China and all the measures for malaria elimination basing on case detection and epidemic point disposal were enhanced. The proportion of case with definite diagnosis and verification was significantly improved, the proportion of the cases with definite diagnosis in lab was 94%, and the unclassified cases accounted for 6%. With the epidemiological investigation on each case, 95.5% cases of malignant malaria were verified and the infection sources were confirmed, which provided the solid base for scientific disposal of the challenges of malaria elimination provoked by the imported cases, effective reduction of deaths from malignant malaria and the ultimate malaria elimination nationwide.

(Ji Chenglian)

14. Final Stage Assessment Results of the "Eleventh-five Year Plan" for National Key Endemic Disease Prevention and Treatment

To learn about the implementation of National Planning for Prevention and Treatment of Key Endemic Diseases (2004-2010) (hereinafter referred to as Planning) and comprehensively assess the achievements of prevention and treatment, in accordance with the requirements of assessment programs for the final stage of the Planning and basing on the completion of self assessment in all places, from September, 2010 to June, 2011, Ministry of Health took the lead in the final stage assessment on the Planning target implementation in all provinces (regions and cities) and Xinjiang Production and Construction Corps. The assessment result showed that by the end of

2010, 28 provinces (regions and cities) nationwide had reached the provincial stage objective of IDD elimination, and 97.9% of the counties (cities and districts) reached the objective of IDD elimination. The survey on high iodine regions of water source by taking township as the unit was completed, and iodized salt supply in high iodine regions of water source was stopped. The rate of stove improvement in areas of coal burning fluorosis pollution reached 92.6%, water improvement project in areas known as the medium and grave degrees of endemic fluorosis of drinking water was basically finished; The investigation on epidemic intensity and distribution of endemic fluorosis of drinking water was basically completed; The investigation on distribution areas of endemic arsenic poisoning was finished and measures of stove changes, arsenic dropping and water change in the known areas of the diseases were basically implemented; The detection rate of X ray positive of more than 99% of the children with Kaschin-Beck disease in key areas of serious diseases reached the controlling standards; Keshan disease was controlled effectively. The monitoring system for endemic diseases was basically perfected. In general, the planning targets of the key endemic diseases covered in the "Eleventh Five-year Plan" were reached nationwide.

(Ji Chenglian)

15. Ministry of Health Printed and Issued National Standardizations for Chronic Disease Prevention and Control to Further Standardize Chronic Disease Prevention and Control at All Levels

In March, 2011, Ministry of Health printed and issued National Standardizations for Chronic Disease Prevention and Control Nationwide (trial edition). The Standardization centered around the four categories of diseases doing serious harm to the residents in our country, such as cardiovascular and cerebrovascular diseases, malignant cancers, chronic respiratory diseases and diabetes. The responsibilities, tasks and working contents of chronic disease prevention and control in health administrative departments, institutions for disease prevention and control, medical health institutions at grassroots, hospitals, professional institutions of prevention and treatment were made clear from the seven respects of institution duties and personnel, work plan and implementation scheme, monitoring and investigation, intervention and management, information management, capacity building and comprehensive assessment. The Standardization formulated the provisions for work flow, assessment criterion and assessment method for key chronic disease prevention and control and provided technological support for the standardization of routine work for chronic disease in different institutions.

(Ji Chenglian)

16. High-Level Conferences on Chronic Diseases Were Held by the United Nations

The 66th high-level NCD General Assembly of the United Nations honored as the "Milestone of Chronic Disease Prevention and Control" was held from September 19th to 20th, 2011 in New York, UN member countries and the delegates from international organizations and non-governmental organizations attended the conference. Delegates from more than 130 countries gave speeches, including more than 30 heads of the states and heads of governments. Minister of Health, Chen Zhu led Chinese delegation of Ministry of Health, Ministry of Foreign Affairs, China CDC, Food and Health Bureau of Hong Kong attended the assembly. This assembly was another high-level health meeting after the special general meeting on AIDS problems. All parties at the meeting made the in-depth exploration into the situation of non-infectious disease prevention and control, economic and social consequences, national capacity building, international cooperation and others, and made a unanimous approval by consensus of Political Declaration of High-Level Meeting on Non-infectious Disease Prevention and Control. All parties thought that non infectious diseases constituted real challenges for both developed countries and developing countries, brought real effect on public health, economic development and social stability, and related to whether the deadline of millennium development goals would be met. The risk factors of non-infectious diseases involved the respects of life, food supply, and urban planning, which needed the concerted efforts from each department and the participation from the whole society. Through the efforts from governments of each country and the whole society, international communities should strengthen cooperation, reduce risk factors, create health promoting environment, improve the ability of health system, and meet the challenge to human brought by chronic diseases.

(Ji Chenglian)

17. Involvement of Harm Reduction to Children into the State Children's Development Goals in the Next Ten Years

With China's social and economic development, harm has become the main killer of children. National death investigations in 2004-2005 showed that the mortality caused by the harm to children of 1-17 years old was 25.1/100,000, accounting for 53.2% of the deaths of this cause among the children of the ages, which was the first death cause. The prevention and control of harm to children was of great significance in improving children's health. In 2011, the State Council issued the Outline for Children's Development in China (2011-2020) and expressly required "reduction of death and disability caused by the harm to children and 1/6 lower mortality caused by the harm to children under 18 lowered by taking the figure in 2010 as the base". The Outline required that in the next ten years "the action plan for comprehensive intervention of children's harm would be formulated and implemented by means of cooperation of multiple departments. Law enforcement, supervision and management were intensified, safe learning and living environment was created for children, and the major damages to children, such as drowning, injuries, traffic accidents were prevented and controlled". The indexes of harm reduction to children was involved into the outline of the state's children's development, which provided powerful target guidance and policy guarantee for the prevention of harm to children launched by all departments nationwide.

(Ji Chenglian)

18. Involvement of Psychological Health of Women and Children into China's Ten-year Outline of Development of Women and Children

In June, 2011, the State Council printed and distributed Outline for Women's Development in China (2011-2020) and Outline for Children's Development in China (2011-2020) (hereinafter referred to as Outline), in which 109 development goals, and their own policies and measures for health and education of women and children in the next ten years were determined. The promotion of psychological health for women and children was one of the major targets, policies and measures in health field.

The Outline made the "improvement in the awareness rates of the knowledge about women's psychological health and mental disease prevention" and the "reduction of children's psychological behavior problems and children's mental disease prevalence" the major health indexes of women and children. The Outline required that "women's mental health service must be improved. The service network of perfect functions covering cities and villages for the prevention and treatment of mental health and rehabilitation was established. Consultation and service according to women's physiological and psychological characteristics were launched. The trainings of mental health knowledge for mental health professional institutions and personnel from institutions of medical health were strengthened. Depression prevention, early detection and intervention for postpartum women and the public service network of children's psychological health" were launched. "Children's hospitals, special mental hospitals and the conditional institutions for the health of women and children set up children psychology department (outpatient) with specialist doctors. Schools were equipped with psychological counseling rooms and full-time teachers of mental health education. The training for specialized persons of mental health was launched". Psychological health of women and children was involved into the Outline for the first time and the concrete policies and measures were put forward.

(Ji Chenglian)

Section 1 Work Progress in China's Center for Disease Prevention and Control

1. Beijing's Seminar on Current Situation and Prospect of Global Tuberculosis Vaccines

From September 21st to 23rd, China's Center for Disease Control and AERAS, American Bill and Melinda Gates Foundation jointly held Beijing's Seminar on current situation and prospect of global tuberculosis vaccines. Totally, more than 230 experts in the research and development of tuberculosis vaccines from China, America, Europe and Africa and the scholars in the fields of tuberculosis foundation, medical treatment, prevention and treatment attended the conference.

The opening ceremony of the conference was presided by deputy director of China's Center for Disease Control, Yang Weizhong, who, together with Professor Thomas Evans from AERAS, and Professor Chris Wilson from American Bill and Melinda Gates Foundation, made the opening speeches. 37 foreign and domestic experts made special reports, covering the basic research of tuberculosis vaccines, studies on tuberculosis epidemiology, the screening of tuberculosis vaccine antigens and clinical verifications of TB alternative vaccine products of various types.

(Ji Chenglian)

2. Progress in TB Prevention and Control of China's Ministry of Health-the Gates Foundation

4 subprojects of the first round covered in China-the Gates' TB projects fully accessed to the implementation stage, and the overall progress went smoothly and passed the comprehensive audit given by the United States KPMG international accounting firm with a good audit result. The application for the projects of the second round was successful in November and the total funding was $23 million. The projects of the second round would be on the basis of those in the first round, integrate the verified new tools and new health service into a comprehensive mode and expand their application. Simultaneously, demonstration and evaluation on new tools were continued, the overall result evaluation and the appraisal on sustainable development

of the projects of the second round were made.

(Ji Chenglian)

3. Work Progress in National Measles Elimination

In 2011, *National Action Plan for Measles Elimination (2006-2012)*, strategies and technical measures defined in *National Action Plan for Measles Elimination (2010-2012)* were continuously implemented. In 2011, the accumulatively reported number of measles cases nationwide was 9,943, 74% (38,159 cases) lower than that of 2010, the reported morbidity was 0.74/100,000, the accumulatively reported death number was 10, 63% (27 cases) lower than that of 2010.

From March to May, 2011, measles epidemic rose in Xinjiang Uygur Autonomous Region, Gansu Province, Shaanxi Province, Sichuan Province, and Zhejiang Province. China's Center for Disease Control organized and held the seminar on measles epidemic in provinces of high incidence, analyzed the dangerous factors for measles incidence and discussed the countermeasures; Working conference and training classes on national measles monitoring were held to support measles elimination in the key provinces. From June on, experts were organized for many times to make comprehensive analysis, estimate the key counties and areas of measles elimination concerned in this winter and next spring, put forward strategies and measures for the key counties and areas and technical suggestions for further controlling measles transmission in 2012.

(Ji Chenglian)

4. Progress in Hepatitis B Prevention and Treatment Nationwide

China's Center for Disease Control actively launched the training of the knowledge about hepatitis B prevention and treatment and more than 1,000 medical workers from Shanghai City, Guangdong Province, Beijing City and Sichuan Province were trained. The Project Office of Ministry of Health and GAVI completed tasks covered in 125 million RMB Yuan of fund appropriation, such as leak survey and resowing, improvement in the rate of the prompt vaccination for the first time, informatization construction and the documentary film shooting in GAVI project and distributed more than 140,000 copies of propaganda materials of various kinds. The major special subject of science and technology "Research on the Strategies for China's Immunization Prevention of Hepatitis B Virus" went smoothly. In response to WHO initiative, Ministry of Health and China's Center for Disease Control held media communication meeting on "World Hepatitis Day" and academic exchange on July 28th,

2011, to improve the cognition of hepatitis prevention and treatment of the masses.

(Ji Chenglian)

5. Completion of the Compilation of China's Chronic Disease Report (Chinese and English editions)

With the support of Ministry of Health, China's Center for Disease Control organized the experts from National Cancer Center, National Center of Cardiovascular Disease, National Office of Encephalopathy Disease and completed both English and Chinese editions of *China's Chronic Disease Report (2011)* in April and October, 2011 respectively, which were distributed at the ministerial conference on healthy life style and chronic disease prevention and control held in Moscow in April and UN's meeting of high level on prevention and control of non-infectious diseases in September. *China's Chronic Disease Report* were also sent to the headquarter of WHO, China's Office of WHO, the United States CDC Office in China, international organizations and centers for disease control in all provinces nationwide.

(Ji Chenglian)

6. China-American Children and Family Cooperation Projects

15 years after the implementation of folic replenishment for Chinese women in the period of peri-conception, CFCS project mainly targeted the survey on influencing factors in the early stage of adult malignant tumors and other non-infectious diseases. China's Center for Disease Control played an active role in 3 tasks: No. 1. The completion of the training for investigators at the project points in Task 1. 25 investigators from Taicang City of Jiangsu Province and Leting County of Hebei Province were trained, family tracking location, questionnaire survey and body measurement were completed and the percentages of completion were 83.6% and 81.4%, which achieved the anticipated goals; No. 2. Successful holding of the planning meeting. The coordination and communication with US experts and experts from institutes of nutritious food were made, research plans and process were clarified, research plans, working manual and training materials in Task 2 were revised with the institutes of nutrition and food security, the budget was made at the project points with US party and the research agreement was repeatedly discussed, revised and improved; No. 3. Children leukemia cases were inspected in No. 1. Hospital of Suzhou City, Hospital for Children of Suzhou City and People's Hospital of Taicang City, the information was extracted and the research programs in Task 3 were revised.

(Ji Chenglian)

7. The Visit to the Institute for Parasitic Diseases Paid by Director-general of WHO Margaret Chan Fung Fu-chun

Upon the invitation of Ministry of Health, on July, 15th, a line of 6 people of Director-general of WHO Margaret Chan Fung Fu-chun and WHO representative in China, Micheal O'Leary visited the institute for parasitic diseases and had a discussion about bringing China's advantages of resources into further play and the service for global health with Director of China's Center for Disease Control, Wang Yu, Deputy Director General of Shanghai Health Bureau, Shen Yuandong, Associate Inspector, Wang Panshi, and President of Institute for Parasitic Disease Prevention and Treatment, Zhou Xiaonong, and put forward the concrete suggestions on utilizing China's advantages of resources and providing supports of public health and control of chronic diseases in developing countries, like Africa.

Margaret Chan Fung Fu-chun was quite satisfied with all the work of Institute for Parasitic Disease as "WHO cooperation center for malaria, filariasis and schistosomiasis" and wrote an inscription: "Continue to work hard and play a leading role around the world as WHO cooperation center for parasitic disease prevention and treatment".

(Ji Chenglian)

8. 2011 Annual Conference on Sino-US Cooperative Project of the Newly Detected and Reoccurred Infectious Diseases

From December 6th to 7th, 2011, 2011 annual conference on Sino-US cooperative project of the newly detected and reoccurred infectious diseases was held in Beijing. About 170 delegates attended the conference. They were delegates from the member units of project cooperation committees, the relevant leaders and delegates from China's Center for Disease Control, delegates from executive units of each subproject, delegates from project provinces, technical experts from American Center for Disease Prevention and Control and those from US projects in China, World Bank, WHO, United Nations Children's Fund, United Nations Food and Agriculture Organization, UK Department for International Development and other international organizations. The progress, achievements and influence of EID projects in 2011, the key cooperative projects and budgetary performance ($2.28 million for the performance in 2011 and $2.85 million for the performance in 2012) of America Center for Disease Control in the next 5 years, the annual plan in 2012 and project management were introduced at the meeting. The achievements in Sino-US EID projects of last year were confirmed and the related requirements for project performance and development in the future were put forward.

(Ji Chenglian)

9. Inauguration of WHO Research Cooperation Center for Participation and Reference of Global Flu

On October 29th, 2010, National Influenza Center was officially appointed as WHO Research Cooperation Center for Participation and Reference of Global Flu. On March 14th, 2011, inauguration of WHO Research Cooperation Center for Participation and Reference of Global Flu was held in Beijing. Health officials from Ministry of Health, WHO and 16 countries around the world attended the ceremony. Minister of Health, Chen Zhu and director of WHO Western Pacific Region, Shen Yingxiu unveiled the plaque for the Center. The Center was the fifth one in the world appointed by WHO and the first research cooperation center for participation and reference of global flu among developing countries.

(Ji Chenglian)

10. Overall Promotion of Partnership with American Center for Disease Control and Other Health Institutions

The mechanism for regular meetings and communication with the director of American Center for Disease Control was maintained; And new progress was made in project cooperation in the field of infectious diseases with American Center for Disease Control. For example, memorandum of Sino-US cooperation projects of the newly detected and reoccurred infectious diseases in the second five-year performance was renewed, and the research projects of Sino-US global AIDS prevention and treatment and China's health queues of children and family went smoothly; The cooperation in the field of chronic diseases was steadily promoted, office of Sino-US cooperation projects of chronic diseases was set up, and breakthroughs were made in pilot projects of behavioral risk factor supervision, high blood pressure prevention and control with limited salt in Shandong Province, the expansion of the training projects for field epidemiology and technical support in education of chronic diseases; The cooperation projects of tuberculosis and AIDS covered in China-the Gates Foundation was in the second phase of application; Folk cooperation in the field of high-end biological research was strengthened with US research institutions of science and technology, such as US Fred Hutchinson Cancer Research Center.

(Ji Chenglian)

Chapter II Patriotic Health Campaign

Patriotic Health Campaign in 2011

In 2011, in accordance with the requirements of *National Sanitation City (Region) Standard* and its administrative measures, National Patriotic Health Campaign Committee Office named in a concentrated way 35 new national sanitation cities (regions), reconfirmed 227 national s sanitation cities and towns, which were honored in a concentrated way at video and telephone conference held by National Patriotic Health Campaign Committee. Environmental health outlook in urban and rural areas was improved greatly by means of constantly solidifying and expanding creative achievements and bringing radiating and driving functions for rural environment into play. The establishment of healthy cities and towns was fully confirmed by governments at all levels and welcomed by the whole society. "Healthy Beijing", "Healthy Tianjin" "Healthy Chongqing", "Healthy Shandong" and "Healthy Hubei" have been the healthy strategies put forward by the governments of the provinces and cities, which were involved into all social policies and have become the working mechanism and system engineering advocated by the governments, supported by all departments, participated and managed with joint efforts by the whole society.

The action for healthy, clean and tidy environment in urban and rural areas nationwide was sturdily promoted to improve environmental health outlook in urban and rural areas by combining with the construction of new socialist countryside, adhering to the action target, taking powerful measures and bringing radiating and driving functions for rural environment into play. The monitoring and hygienical evaluation on drinking water quality in rural areas was enhanced, the construction of monitoring network for the improvement in drinking water quality in rural areas was perfected and 50,000 projects for centralized water supply were monitored. The monitoring of hazard factors to rural environment health was carried out in 14,000 villages to learn about health status and dynamic changes in rural environment.

(Ji Chenglian)

Chapter Ⅲ Health Emergency Response

Health Emergency Response in 2011

I. Clarifying the goals for the construction and development of health emergency response system during the 12th Five-Year-Plan period

The national 12th Five-Year-Plan program for the construction of health emergency response system was formulated, the overall goals and key projects for the health emergency response during the 12th Five-Year-Plan period were decided, health emergency response at the grassroots was included into the project of equalization of basic public health services and the contents of the major public health service projects were primarily decided. The key contents of the program for the construction of health emergency response system were included *in Outline of the 12th Five-Year-Plan for National Economic and Social Development, Outline of the 12th Five-Year-Plan for the Health Development, Program for Deepening the Reform of Medical and Health System during the 12th Five-Year-Plan Period, and Program for the Construction of National Emergency Response System (2011-2015).*

II. Propelling the construction of legislation and normalization for health emergency response

We organized the revision of *Regulations on Preparedness for and Response to Public Health Emergencies* and participated in the revision of *Law of the People's Republic of China on the Prevention and Treatment of Infections Diseases and Frontier Health and Quarantine Law of the People's Republic of China.* In order to effectively implement *International Health Regulations (2005),* we carried out evaluation on the nuclear capacities of *International Health Regulations (2005). Multiple-Department Coordinative Mechanism on Public Health Emergencies* was improved and meanwhile, the departmental coordinative mechanism on heath emergency response was established between the Ministry of Health and the Chinese Armed Police Force. Many pre-plans were formulated (or revised) including *National Emergency Pre-plan for the Outbreak of Influenza* and *Health Emergency Pre-plan of the Ministry of Health for Emergent Poisoning Events. Work Plan on the Construction and Evaluation of National Demonstrative Counties (Cities ,Districts) for Health Emergency Response* was printed and issued so as to strengthen the capability of health emergency response at the grassroots with the construction of the demonstrative counties (cities, districts) of health emergency response as the key measure. The expert consulting commission of the Ministry of Health on health emergency response to urgent events was established.

Ⅲ. Strengthening the prevention and control of acute infectious diseases

In order to guide the prevention of plague in all the localities, the Ministry of Health, the Commission of Development and Reform and the Ministry of Finance jointly issued *National 12th Five-Year-Plan for the Prevention and Treatment of Plague,* the Ministry of Health issued *National Diagnosis and Treatment Plan for Plague (for trial implementation)* and revised *National Plan for the Monitoring of Plague.* Surveys were made on the welfare and treatment of staff working at the high-risk positions in the institutions of plague prevention nationwide and efforts were made to assist the Personnel Department of the Ministry of Health to implement the policies on the welfare and treatment of relevant staff members. Work was done to propel the construction of national centers for plague culture in Qinghai, Yunnan and Jilin as well as the construction of national drilling base for plague prevention and control in Hebei. The epidemiological research on the key technique of plague was propelled, which included the research on the key techniques on the tracing of Yersinia pestis, the determination of boundaries for plague foci, various risk assessment and the risk assessment of plague foci in various places.

Special supervision and instruction were made on the prevention and control of H1N1 influenza, human infection with highly pathogenic avian influenza and SARS, timely analysis, research and judgments were made on the situations of prevention and control of the pandemics, measures on the prevention and control were put forward and relevant results were informed to all the provinces and relevant departments to guide the localities to strengthen prevention and control.

Ⅳ. Working effectively on health response to various emergencies

Prevention and control of plague in some key areas such as Yushu earthquake-hit areas were strengthened. Plague in Huang Yuan County, Xining, Qinghai Province and the pandemic of European H1N1 swain influenza were effectively dealt with, timely instructions were made on the public health emergencies including the outbreaks of anthrax in Liaoning, Jilin and Inner Mongolia and viral encephalitis in Fujian Province. Vigorous efforts were made to prevent the 0104 EHEC that broke out in Europe. We assisted the Center for Disease Control and Prevention of the Ministry of Health to organize the handling of polio outbreak in Hetian, Xinjiang. We guided Chinese Center for Disease Control and Prevention and health department in Yunnan

Province to conduct epidemiological survey and etiological study on the cases of sudden deaths for unknown reasons in Yunnan.

Efforts were made to guide the local health departments on providing medical and health relief for various accidents and disasters and safety events and providing medical and health guarantee for major activities. Health emergency responses were organized for a series of emergencies like Yingjiang earthquake in Yunnan, 7.23 train crash on the Yongtaiwen railway line, food poisoning events in Hetian, Xinjiang and Longxi, Gansu, the riot in Kashi, Xinjiang, and floods, droughts, and landslides etc. in some places. We coordinated and guided the health guarantee for Shenzhen Universiade and China-Eurasia Expo in Urumqi. We assisted the national emergency response office for nuclear events to finish work on health-related monitoring, situation evaluation, news releasing and guidance of public opinion on Fukushima nuclear leaking accident in Japan.

V. Starting risk assessment on public health emergencies

Management methods and technical guidance on the risk assessment on public health emergencies were formulated. Since April, 2011, national monthly risk assessment on public health emergencies had been started. Pilot on provincial risk assessment on public health emergencies was launched in Shandong, Zhejiang, Gansu, Shanghai and Hebei. Risk assessment on public health emergencies and the construction of relevant capacities were strengthened by means of such international cooperative programs as China-U.S. Cooperative Program on Emerging and Re-emerging Infectious Diseases etc.

VI. Strengthening the construction of national team for health emergency response

In 2011, the central finance allocated 320 billion RMB Yuan for the program of strengthening the construction of four types of twenty-seven national teams for health emergency response, i.e. the prevention and control of emergent infectious diseases, emergent medical rescue, the handling of emergent poisoning events and the handling of nuclear and radiation events. With the implementation of the program, the logos and the personal portable devices for health emergency response nationwide were unified and standardized, the provincial training for lecturers and key employees were conducted on the management of health emergency response, risk communication on health emergency response, the prevention and control of plague, risk assessment, medical rescue for emergency nuclear radiation events and health emergency response to emergent poisoning events. Consequently, all the localities improved their capability of responding to and dealing with health emergencies.

(Zhao Xuemei)

Chapter IV Food Safety, Health Supervision and Law Enforcement

1. Comprehensive Coordination for Food Safety and Health Supervision in 2011

In 2011, all work on food safety and health supervision was fulfilled in line with the deployments on deepening the reform of medical and healthcare system and the requirements of the national health work conference.

I. Food Safety

(1) Comprehensive coordination and rectification were made. Evaluation and examination on rectification were conducted to summarize the rectification in the past two years. Special actions were arranged for the health department to crack down on illegal additives in food, the joint working mechanism was established with the department of food safety, and the event of plastic DEHP found in Taiwan food was dealt with, which involved organizing emergency monitoring, timely release of relevant health knowledge and urging and supervising the localities to investigate the cases of plastic DEHP. Investigations into the cases of substandard milk powder were intensified and on-site investigations were made into the case of substandard milk powder in Yuzhong, Shanxi, and the event of Ruduobao substandard milk powder in Heilongjiang. We participated in the investigation into the event of Shuanghui ractopamine in Ji Yuan, Henan and the special rectification on ractopamine, and assisted the investigation into cases of rhodamine B found in hotpot flavoring in Guangdong, fake wine in Changli, Hebei, food poisoning caused by milk contaminated with sulphites in Pingliang, Gansu, the death of a male baby caused by suspected use of milk powder in Yunan and the suspected illegal adding of non-edible substances at the seafood markets in Jinan, Shandong, etc. The organization and coordination of food safety and safety guarantee for the 14th FINA World Championships and the 26th Universiade were fulfilled successfully. Research into safety of brick tea was made joining hands with relevant departments. We participated in the drafting of *National Program for the System of Food Safety Supervision and Management during the 12th Five-Year-Plan Period* and *Decision of the State Council on Further Improving and Strengthening Work on Food Safety.*

(2) Systems and mechanisms were improved. Leadership on food safety by the health system was further strengthened and the leading group for food safety of the Ministry of Health was established in charge of making deployments and overall instruction on food safety by the health departments nationwide, with the Minister of

Health, Chen Zhu, as the director of the group, the Deputy Minister of Health, Chen Xiaohong, as the vice director, and the eleven bureaus of the Ministry of Health (MOH), State Food and Drug Administration (SFDA) and three units directly affiliated to the MOH as the members. *The Ministry of Health's Measures for Implementing <Food Safety Law>* was formulated to standardize the procedure for the Ministry of Health to fulfill the duties. *Measures for Investigating and Punishing Food Safety Accidents* was drafted and submitted to the food safety office for coordination, *Measures for the Administration of New Source Food* was revised, *Measures for the Administration of Local Standards for Food Safety, Regulations on the Administration of Administrative Permits for Food-related New Products* as well as the regulations on their application and reception were printed and issued, *Norms on the Epidemical Surveys on Food Safety* Accidents was formulated, and *Circular on Strengthening the Investigation and Transference of Cases of Using Non-edible Substances for Food Production* was issued jointly with other six departments including the Ministry of Public Security.

(3) Work on food safety standards was strengthened. Firstly, laws and regulations as well as working rules for food safety standards were improved; *Plan for National Standards of Food Safety (2011-2015)* and *Norms for Follow-up Evaluation on National Standards for Food Safety* were drafted. The procedures for the drafting of the standards and the soliciting opinions of the standards were further improved for the open and transparent procedures. Secondly, the sorting and integration as well as the formulation (revision) of food safety standards were enhanced. Twenty-one national standards for food safety were promulgated, including some basic standards such as *Limits of Mycotoxins in Food, Limits of the Maximum Residue Fifty-four Pesticides Including Paraquat, Standards for the Use Food Additives, General Rules on Compound Food Additives, General Rules on Labels for Pre-packed Food,* and *General Rules on Nutrition Labels for Pre-packed Food* etc., and some standards for food products like *Honey, Frozen Flour and Rice Products* and *Stainless Steel Products,* etc. The standards mentioned above strictly regulated twenty-eight limit standards for six kinds of mycotoxins, 118 limit standards for fifty-four kinds of pesticides and the safe use of 2,314 additives. Besides, new standards for eleven kinds of food additives were formulated and promulgated including potassium iodate and standards for eighty-five kinds of food additives were assigned referring to the foreign standards. Thirdly, the announcement on strengthening the connection between the production license for food additives and supervision and administration was promulgated together with the General Administration of Supervision, Inspection and Quarantine of China to tighten the management of production license for food additives and vigorously explore the classified management system for food additives. Fourthly, work was done to accelerate the sorting out of standards for food packing materials. Consequently,

systematic sorting out was conducted for over 3,000 substances used for food packing materials submitted by the industry and the list of 107 resins for packing materials was announced. Fifthly, some out-dated standards were abolished. Zinc, bronze, iron and selenium were no longer managed as pollution indexes. The benzoyl peroxide and calcium peroxide were revoked as food additives, and the announcement also banned bisphenol A to be used for the production of feeding bottles. Sixthly, the management of the committee was stricter to further standardize the examination of standards. The committee held altogether eleven conferences of the directors and conferences of the subcommittees and examined and approved 125 standards. Seventhly, the publicity and implementation of the standards were strengthened, and efforts were made to reply to people's doubts and properly deal with public opinions. By means of press conferences, media communications and symposiums etc. we made introduction about the formulation and promulgation of standards. Efforts were made to deal with public opinions concerning standards for dairy products, frozen flour and rice products, stainless steel products, food additives, and nitrite in edible bird's nest etc. Eighthly, we took advantages of the host country of CCFA Codex Committee on Food Additives to strengthen the follow-up study on the international standards of food additives and push forward the synchronous development of our standards of food additives and the foreign standards.

(4) Risk monitoring and assessment were improved. Macro analysis and risk assessment were made on the result of national risk monitoring for food safety in 2010. The findings were reported to the State Council and all the localities and relevant departments and Vice Premier Li Keqiang made some important instruction on the report of the Ministry of Health. We organized the risk monitoring for food safety in 2011 and supervised its progress. We reported to the food safety office of the State Council and relevant departments seven times the potential risks of food safety that we had detected via monitoring and the food safety office of the State Council held multi-departmental conferences to study and deploy supervision and counter-measures. Documents were issued requiring the local governments to seriously investigate and effectively supervise the problems of illegally adding industrial dye into chili products detected via monitoring. We organized thirteen provinces (regions, cities), including Beijing and Guangdong etc. to make emergent monitoring on plastic DEHP, which provided timely clues to handling the event of plastic EDHP pollution. In accordance with the results of the monitoring and the situation of food poisoning in all the localities, timely pre-warnings were made to the whole country on food poisoning. The program of national risk monitoring for food safety in 2012 were formulated and issued. It was proposed that special attention should be paid to monitoring illegal additives in food, manufacturers and suppliers of food made by

small workshops, supplied at small stands and small restaurants in the rural trade fairs and places around schools and foodborne diseases. Working norms were drafted for reporting the results of risk monitoring and food safety risk assessment, data collection and exchange, quality control and sampling etc. Programs of prioritized risk assessment were carried out on aluminum, boron and formaldehyde in food. Study was made on the restrict value of cadmium in polluted rice that people in high-cadmium areas were exposed to and evaluation opinions were provided, which provided scientific evidence for the determination of standard value of cadmium restrict value in rice. Emergent evaluations were made on the hot issues that were the concerns of the whole society like Nestlé's Infant Rice Paste, Beef Extract, Poisonous Ginger, Fluorescent Whitening Agent, Lubricant for Soybean Milk Maker and Aflatoxin M1, etc. and authoritative information was release at proper time to respond to the concern of the whole society. Under the guidance of the State Commission Office for Public Sector Reform, the preparation for the national center for food safety risk assessment was finished. The council of national center for food safety risk assessment was inaugurated and an unveiling ceremony was held for its foundation on October 13, which propelled some provinces to accelerate the construction of technical support institutions of the provincial centers for risk assessment.

In order to assist the State Council Office for Food Safety to crack down on the violations of illegal adding in food, we went on studying and announcing the Blacklist for the illegal additives in food and the food additives liable to abuse and the testing methods for them. We promptly included seventeen kinds of phthalate esters (plastic EDHP) into the Blacklist and clarified the temporary restrict values. Thus, we had announced six batches of Blacklists, involving sixty-four kinds of illegal food additives and twenty-two kinds of food additives liable to abuse. Research on the testing methods for Recycled Gutter Oil was conducted, which provided technical supply for the State Council Office for Food Safety to crack down on the violation of producing cooking oil from Recycled Gutter Oil.

The construction projects of risk monitoring capability pilot for food safety were launched, with the focus on strengthening the capabilities of monitoring on illegal additives in food and radioactive substances in food and the initial monitoring and tracing for foodborne diseases. In order to effectively ensure the quality of risk monitoring for food safety, six national reference labs for the risk monitoring for food safety were built, i.e. labs on food additives in food, pesticide residue in food, mycotoxin in food , dioxin in food and heavy metals in food etc.

(5) Work on information and publicity was further strengthened. Training and implementation of *Measures for the Management of Food Safety Information Release* were organized, the national information net for food safety was established, *2010 Report*

on the General Situation of Food Safety in China was finished and the inter-departmental liaison system for the urgent report of food safety information was established. Acting on the requirements of *Outlines for the Publicity and Education of Food Safety (2011-2015)*, we issued circulars demanding all the localities to work well on the publicity and education of food safety in 2011 in line with their local realities. We carefully prepared and fulfilled all the work on the publicity week for *Food Safety Law* in 2011, participated in China Policy Forum-Food Safety in Action and held training workshops on food safety for the media. Timely responses were made to the issues that were the concerns of the whole society such as One Drop of Spice, the safety of hot pot flavoring, Different Standards Home and Abroad, Additives in Rice, etc.

II. Occupational Health

(1) Joint efforts were made to push forward the prevention and control of occupational diseases. In accordance with the system of joint inter-ministerial meeting for the prevention and control of occupational diseases, we assisted the State Administration for Work Safety in holding the second plenary session of the joint meeting. *Circular of the General Office of the Ministry of Health on Establishing the Leading Group of the Ministry of Health for the Prevention and Control of Occupational Diseases* was issued to establish the system of joint inter-departmental meeting within the Ministry of Health. Vice Minister of Health, Chen Xiaohong, led a joint supervision group composed of four departments to supervise and guide the prevention and control of occupational diseases in Guangdong Province and Jiangxi Province. In accordance with the instructions of the ministerial leaders, investigations were conducted into the event of pneumoconiosis in Gulang County, Gansu Province and the prevention and control of occupational diseases for migrant workers. We joined the joint inter-ministerial meeting for the disposal of municipal domestic wastes to assist in the prevention and control of occupational diseases for the sanitation workers.

(2) Surveys on occupational health were conducted. At the beginning of the year, joining hands with other nine departments, we held the video and telephone conference on launching the surveys, and issued *Circular on Conducting Surveys on Occupational Health* to make overall deployments of the surveys. The national leading group and office for the surveys on occupational health was founded and the working system was established.

(3) Laws, regulations and rules on occupational health were improved. We assisted the Education, Science, Culture and Public Health Committee of the National People's Congress, the Legislative Affairs Commission of the National People's Congress and the Central Committee of Chinese Peasants and Workers Democratic

Party in investigating and surveying the present situation about the prevention and control of occupational diseases; we organized relevant experts to make investigation into the present situation about the diagnosis and identification of occupational diseases in six provinces (cities) including Beijing, the report of which was submitted to the Legislative Affairs Office of the State Council; we attended three conferences held by the National People's Congress to exam and discuss *Amendment to Law on Prevention and Control of Occupational Diseases (Draft)* and organized the experts time and again to research into the opinions and suggestions proposed by the members of NPC Standing Committee on the definition of occupational diseases, the diagnosis of occupational disease and the standards of occupational health etc. In accordance with the ideas and principles of revising *Law on Prevention and Control of Occupational Diseases,* we initially revised the supporting regulations like *Measures for the Management of Occupational Disease Diagnosis and Identification* etc. Joining hands with relevant departments, we conducted investigations and surveys into the legislation on labor protection in scorching weather to push forward the formulation of *Rules of Labor Protection in Scorching Weather.*

(4) The construction of capability was strengthened. *Circular of the Ministry of Health on Effectively Fulfilling Duties and Further Strengthening Prevention and Control of Occupational Diseases* was issued. All the localities worked even harder so that the coverage of diagnosing institutions for occupational diseases at the municipal level reached 80%, and that at the county level reached 54%. Hence, the construction of occupational disease prevention and control system and capability was strengthened.

(5) Information report and publicity were strengthened. We organized the data collection, examination, summarizing and analysis for national occupational diseases in 2010 and the first half of 2011 and reported to the State Council the situations of occupational diseases. Joining hands with the Ministry of Human Resource and Social Security, State Administration of Work Safety and All China Federation of Trade Unions, we deployed the national publicity week for law on prevention and control of occupational diseases in 2011 with "Caring for Occupational Health for Migrant Workers" as the theme. Joining hands with All China Federation of Trade Unions, we distributed 100,000 *Booklets on Prevention and Control of Pneumoconiosis* to the high-prevalence areas and high-risk population of pneumoconiosis in thirty-one provinces (regions, municipalities) and Xinjiang Production and Construction Corps.

(6) Great efforts were made on the sentinel surveillance on key occupational diseases. Teachers' training workshops were held on the technical instruction and quality control for the implementation of *Technical Program for the Surveillance on Key Occupational Diseases.* The number of sentinel surveillances on occupational diseases increased from 72 in 2010 to 120 at present.

Ⅲ. Environmental Health

(1) National supervision and surveillance on drinking water hygiene was forcefully pushed forward. Firstly, work conference on national health supervision and surveillance on drinking water hygiene was held, at which the situation faced with and the prominent problems were analyzed and overall deployments were made on the work in the next stage on the health supervision and surveillance on drinking water hygiene. *Guiding Opinions of the Ministry of Health on Further Strengthening Supervision and Surveillance on Drinking Water Hygiene* was drafted. Secondly, the guarantee for drinking water hygiene was included into the items of basic public health services of the medical and healthcare reform and the weak aspects of supervision on drinking water hygiene was gradually improved by means of concentrated water supply in the rural areas, secondary water supply and tour inspections on safety of water supply for rural and urban schools. Thirdly, *Guarantee Plan for Safety of Urban and Rural Drinking Water (2011-2020)* was compiled, in accordance with which the construction of local capability of strengthening supervision and surveillance on drinking water hygiene was pushed forward. By now, the countersignature for the plan had been primarily finished by the National Development and Reform Commission, the Ministry of Environmental Protection, the Ministry of Housing and Urban-Rural Development and the Ministry of Water Resources. Fourthly, on the basis of summarizing the national pilot work on surveillance on urban drinking water hygiene, the national work plan for surveillance on drinking water hygiene was issued in 2011, which propelled the surveillance on drinking water hygiene nationwide, and the national surveillance net had been gradually established and completed. At present, the national surveillance net had covered thirty-one provinces, 110 cities above county level and 620 counties (county-level cities), with nearly 20,000 surveillance stations. Fifthly, surveys were conducted on the CDC's capability of surveillance on drinking water at various levels nationwide. Special investigations were made into the supervision and surveillance on the hygiene of urban and rural drinking water in eight provinces. Joining hands with the Ministry of Housing and Urban-Rural Development, we conducted general surveys on the quality of municipal water supply in over 1,200 cities nationwide. On the basis of these investigations and surveys, measures were researched on to ensure the overall implementation of *Hygiene Standards for Domestic Drinking Water* on July, 1, 2012.

(2) Supervision on public place hygiene was deepened. Firstly, training was conducted for over 400 key supervisors for public places on *Detailed Rules for Implementation of Regulations on the Management of Public Place Hygiene* to ensure that they could correctly grasp and understand the contents and essence of the

regulations. Secondly, supervision and sampling inspections were conducted on the ventilation systems of central air conditioning in swimming pools and public places and the results of the sampling inspections for swimming pools were notified to the whole society. Thirdly, the health norms and relevant technical requirements for the ventilation system of central air conditioning in public places were revised and perfected in accordance with the regulations of *Detailed Rules for Implementation* to improve supervision.

(3) Work on the licenses of disinfection products and water related products as well as the supervision and sampling inspection was strengthened. Firstly, the construction of examination and approval system was sped up. Secondly, the examination and approval procedures for licenses of disinfection products and water related products were revised. Thirdly, national supervision and sampling inspections were conducted on the disinfection products and water related products with license documents. Altogether 159 products by 99 manufacturers were sampled in twelve provinces (regions, municipalities) including Beijing. The supervision and inspection were focused on the consistency of actual production and the contents of the licenses and some of the products were tested. Of all the products sampled, thirty-nine products were found with inconsistency of the labels of the products and the contents of the licenses, thirteen were found with changed formulas and techniques, and ten products were found to be substandard. Next, the results of the sampling inspections would be notified, the substandard products would be announced and violations of laws and regulations would be investigated and punished by law.

(4) Work on environment and health was pushed forward prudently. Cooperating with the Ministry of Environment Protection and relevant departments and bureaus within MOH, we carried out the tasks involving Ministry of Health which were included in the 12th Five-Year-Plan for Comprehensive Prevention and Control of Heavy Metal Pollution. Firstly, we divided the tasks involving Ministry of Health which were included in the 12th Five-Year-Plan and then printed and issued them to relevant units. Secondly, we organized relevant experts from relevant departments and bureaus and Chinese Center for Disease Control and Prevention to sort out and research on the standards and normative documents concerning the biological test methods, judgment for health damage and treatment of five heavy metals, i.e. lead, mercury, cadmium, chromium and arsenic. Thirdly, we assisted the Ministry of Environment Protection in conducting the national surveys on environment and health in the key areas. We recommended experts to participate in drafting the technical plans for the surveys. Fourthly, joining hands with the Ministry of Environment Protection, we held the second session for the national leading group on environment and health.

(5) Supervision was carried out on the units of centralized disinfection for tableware. In accordance with the requirements of *Ministry of Health Program for Key Work of Food Safety in 2011*, the special supervision and inspection on the units of centralized disinfection for tableware were carried out nationwide from July to October 2011. According to the results submitted by twenty-nine provinces (regions, municipalities), altogether 44,719 health supervisors participated in the special supervision and inspection nationwide, 43,273 sets of disinfected tableware were sampled, 3,073 units of centralized disinfection for tableware were requested to rectify and 399 units were fined of over 620,000 RMB Yuan.

IV. Work on Radioation Health

(1) Vigorous efforts were made to respond to the accident of radiation leaking from the nuclear power plant in Japan. Radiation supervision on food and drinking water was stared in Beijing, Northeast, fourteen provinces (regions, municipalities) along the coast and eight provinces in the middle and western regions. *Questions and Answers-Medical Emergency Response to Nuclear and Radiation Accidents* was compiled to instruct the public on responding to the accidents of nuclear leaking. Efforts were made to assist the Ministry of Agriculture in carrying out monitoring on the radioactive contaminants of seafood.

(2) Supervision on the protection for radiological diagnosis and treatment was strengthened. Firstly, while carrying out the key supervision and inspection in 2011, we conducted surveys on the basic situations of protection for radiological diagnosis and treatment in the medical institutions nationwide. Secondly, special inspections were made on the campaign "Medical Quality on Long March"- the radiological protection in diagnosis and treatment. With the focus on radiological treatment, special supervision and inspection were made in ten provinces including Beijing and Xinjiang Production and Construction Corps, the results of which would be notified to the whole country. 2011 national special inspection would be made with the focus on radiological treatment, nuclear medicine and interventional radiology. Thirdly, the pilot on the monitoring net for medical radiation protection was pushed forward. On the basis of summarizing the experience from the nine pilot provinces in the previous year, the pilot was conducted in another eight provinces.

(3) The capability construction and radiation monitoring were strengthened. Firstly, personnel's training was strengthened and Jilin University and Suzhou University were entrusted to hold the national training workshops for supervisors on radiological health. National training workshops for the key supervisors on radiological health were held. Secondly, the institutional capability construction

was strengthened and 2011 assessments for the technical service institutions on radiological health were conducted. Thirdly, work related to the monitoring on the heath and hygiene for residents living around nuclear power plants was carried out. The monitoring on the radionuclide in food around the nuclear power plants was included in the 2012 assessment program for the food risk monitoring and the monitoring on the radionuclide in drinking water was included in the 2012 program for drinking water monitoring.

V. Supervision on the prevention and treatment of infectious diseases and health supervision on school

(1) Supervision on infectious diseases was conscientiously carried out. *Standards for the Daily Supervision on the Prevention and Treatment of Infectious Diseases* was implemented. Supervision on the prevention and treatment of infectious diseases was conducted in all aspects with the focus on the reporting of the pandemics of infectious diseases and the disposal of medical wastes and over 520,000 supervisory inspections on the prevention and treatment of infectious diseases were made for various medical institutions at various levels nationwide. Firstly, we responded immediately to the event reported by the media of illegal recycling of medical wastes at high prices in Jiangsu and timely notifications were made to the nearby provinces of Anhui, Shandong, Henan and Hunan etc., demanding relevant provinces to screen the potential hazards carefully to prevent the medical wastes from leaving medical institutions. Secondly, special inspections were made on the supervision on the prevention and treatment of infectious diseases in some provinces, thirty-one medical institutions were sampled and the serious problems found in the inspections and samplings were notified to the whole country. Thirdly, joint supervision on the investigation and punishment of "Black Cotton" was conducted with the departments of quality supervision, education, public security, industry and commerce and environment protection etc. and forty-eight units were sampled including schools, hospitals and units for the centralized disposal of medical wastes. Fourthly, personnel training was strengthened. Two national training workshops and on-site conferences for experience-exchange were held on the supervision on the prevention and treatment of infectious diseases and thorough surveys were made on the organization arrangements and their work on the prevention of infectious diseases at the provincial level nationwide.

(2) Supervision on school health was vigorously carried out. Firstly, *Circular on Strengthening Supervision on Prevention and Control of Infectious Diseases at School [MOH (2011), No 31]* was issued, demanding all the localities to regard schools as

the key areas for the prevention and control of infectious diseases and strengthen supervision on school health. In 2011, altogether 146,000 schools were supervised and inspected, which meant increasing the coverage of supervision. Secondly, the Ministry of Health and the Ministry of Education jointly carried out special inspections on school health. 192 primary and secondary schools in Heilongjiang Province were sampled and the results of the sampling were notified to the whole country. Thirdly, special investigations were made into the supervision on the prevention and control of infectious diseases and supervision on school health in Shanghai, Guangxi and Liaoning etc. and the seminar on supervision on school health of eight provinces (cities) was held in Liaoning. Fourthly, exploration and innovation on the modes and methods for supervision on school health were vigorously pushed forward in Guangxi, Liaoning and Hunan etc. Meanwhile, efforts were made to know about the construction of the supervisory team for school health nationwide and surveys were made on the organization arrangements and their work on the supervision of school health at the provincial health supervisory institutions and centers for disease prevention and control nationwide.

VI. Severer punishments were made to crack down on illegal medical practices and illegal collection and supply of blood

Firstly, the system of supervisory investigation for key cases was practiced. Cases were investigated and punished including the event of blood trader in Fangshan District, Beijing, the spread of illegal clinics in Huanan County, Heilongjiang, and the spread of illegal clinics in Fuchuan County in Guangxi Zhuang Autonomous Region etc. Secondly, joint supervisory inspections were made on the collection and supply of blood to urge the localities to fulfill relevant responsibilities carefully. Thirdly, *Circular on Further Strengthening Cracking Down on Illegal Medical Practice and Illegal Collection and Supply of Blood [MOH (2011) No 69]* was issued jointly with the Ministry of Public Security. Study was made to establish the system of joint conference, and the transference of cases was carried out to keep on effectively cracking down on the violations of laws and regulations like illegal medical practice and illegal collection and supply of blood.

VII. Construction of health supervisory system was pushed forward vigorously to regulate administrative law enforcement of health

(1) The construction of health supervisory system was pushed forward vigorously. Firstly, efforts were made to assist the National Development and Reform Commission

with the connection of programs on the construction of health supervisory system. In September, 2011, National Development and Reform Commission issued the investment plan of 2011 within the central budgets (first batch) for the programs on the construction of health supervisory system with an investment of 3.5 billion RMB Yuan for the construction of 2,150 health supervisory institutions at the county level. To assist the implementation of the programs, we compiled *Programs for the Construction and Development of the Health Supervisory System* and the instruction on the personnel posts, and organized experts to compile and issue *Reference Atlas for Standardized Construction of Health Supervisory Institutions.* National training workshops were held jointly with the Department of Planning and Finance to guide the localities to standardize the housing construction. Secondly, 2.1223 billion RMB Yuan was allocated by the central finance to the local finances as the subsidies for medical and healthcare reform to arm the health supervisory institutions at the county level in the middle and western regions with law enforcement equipment. The national special training on the construction of health supervisory institutions was held and relevant experts were organized to revise and issue *Equipment Standards for Health Supervisory Institutions (2011).*

(2) Vigorous efforts were made to push forward health supervision and coordination services. Health supervision and coordination were included into nation basic public health services, including the health supervision and coordination of information reporting of food safety accidents, consultation on occupational health, tour inspections on drinking water safety, school health and cracking down on illegal medical practice and illegal collection and supply of blood, and efforts were made to organize the formulation of service norms and technical norms for health supervision and coordination services. *Guiding Opinions of the Ministry of Health on Working Well on Health Supervision and Coordination Services* was printed and issued, which put forward requirements for all the localities to push forward supervision and coordination. Deployments were made on the national health supervision and coordination, which clarified the tasks and requirements and formulated methods for assessments.

(3) Vigorous efforts were made to aid Xinjiang and Tibet. Aid to Tibet was further strengthened and capable cadres were sent to take temporary posts in the health supervisory institutions in Tibet Autonomous region. Training workshops on the construction management of health supervisory institutions in Xinjiang and Tibet were held to strengthen the capability construction of health supervisory institutions as well as guarantee for food safety and the prevention and control of occupational diseases. In accordance with the needs of health supervision in Xinjiang, vigorous efforts were made to coordinate the health supervision center of the Ministry of Health and the capable local health supervisory institutions to offer partner

assistance to the health supervisory institute of Xinjiang Autonomous Regions and the health supervisory institute of the Production and Construction Corps, the health supervisory institute of Urumqi, and the health supervisory institute of Karamay and a brief meeting about the partner assistance was held in Urumqi to arrange the program of the partner assistance.

(4) Informationization of health supervision was strengthened. *Regulations on Management of Health Supervisory Information Reporting* was revised to strengthen the guidance on the operation of the national system for the health supervisory information reporting and the construction of the system. The third session of the leading group for the construction program of the national health supervisory information system was held to carry out the construction of the second stage program of the national system platform for health supervision. Joint supervisory investigations were made with the health supervisory center of the Ministry of Health on the construction of health supervisory informationization in nine provinces and cities including Tianjin, Hebei and Shanxi etc. and *Notification of the General Office of the Ministry of Health on Health Supervisory Information Reporting Nationwide from January to August 2011* was printed and issued. The construction of national system platform for health supervision was vigorously pushed forward. The system of health supervisory information reporting operated well nationwide, with 3,300 institution users of health supervisory institutions, 64,000 individual users of health supervisors, nearly five million reports of information on five types, i.e. occupational health, radioactive health, drinking water safety and school health etc. and the coverage of archive bank had covered over 99% units supervised nationwide.

(5) The management of the health supervisory team was forcefully strengthened. Firstly, the management system for personnel was further completed. *Methods for Management of Health Supervisors* was revised, which improved policies for the management of health supervisors from several aspects like personnel admission, definition of duties and management of assessment etc. Vigorous efforts were made to explore the implementation of the system of duty-classified management for health supervisors (originally called the system of classified supervisor management) and the draft for the system had been formed. Secondly, training for health supervisors was systematically planned. *2011-2015 National Training Program for Health Supervisors* was formulated. Overall planning was made on the training in the next five years. Besides, joining hands with relevant departments and bureaus, we vigorously pushed forward the identification of national training bases for health supervision. Joining hands with the health supervision center, we finished the first stage of development for the national on-line training platform for health supervisors and arranged the trial operation. Supervisors nationwide highly appraised the function of the platform

in improving the capability of the team. Thirdly, the national training workshop on health administration and law enforcement was held. Over 180 people attended the workshop, including directors of provincial departments in charge of health supervision, heads of relevant departments, heads of supervisory institutes etc. Vice Minister of Health, Chen Xiaohong, attended the workshop and delivered an important speech. Invited to the workshop were famous experts and scholars from Legislative Affairs Commission of the National People's Congress, Chinese Academy of Governance, Tsinghua University and Chinese Center for Disease Prevention and Control, who lectured on strengthening and innovating social management, administration laws, situations of food safety, giving play to the function of media and strengthening social communication etc. Fourthly, assessment was strengthened and performance management was launched. *Methods for Implementation of Performance Assessment for Health Supervisory Institutions (trial)* was formulated and issued to push forward performance assessment. Acting on the requirements, all the localities made detailed methods for assessment and put forward implementation plan and the *Methods* was implemented step by step.

(6) Law enforcement for health supervision was regulated in all aspects. Firstly, *Circular of the General Office of the Ministry of Health on Sorting out Duties for Food Safety and Health Supervision* was issued. Efforts were made to organize all the localities to sort out duties in all aspects to find out the weakness and eliminate the gaps in our supervision and administration. All the provinces had reported the results of the sorting out as required by the Circular and made suggestions on how to strengthen the fulfilling of duties subsequently. Secondly, inspection on law enforcement was strengthened. The national training workshop on inspection and meeting for exchanging experience was held, which was attended by over 300 people in charge of inspection above prefectural level. Training on inspection and exchange of work experience were carried out, which were highly praised. Meanwhile, circulars were issued to organize all the localities to make daily inspections and special inspections on the key links of power running and key work on law enforcement concerning administrative licensing. All the localities took active actions and made careful deployments so that anticipated results were achieved of the special inspections and the risks of law enforcement were effectively prevented and solved. Thirdly, the construction of relevant systems was strengthened. Over 800 normative documents involving food safety and health supervision were sorted out and inspected. In order to assist the implementation of *Administrative Coercion Law* and meet the needs of law enforcement in all the localities, we organized the revision of *Document for Administrative Law Enforcement on Health*. The construction of punishment and prevention system of corruption and work on rectifying unhealthy tendencies were

strengthened. Acting on the unified deployments of the Central Commission for Discipline Inspection of the CPC and Ministry of Supervision of PRC, we led in finishing the survey on the construction plan for the punishment and prevention system of supervision and administration on food safety.

(Zhao Xuemei)

2. China Successfully Elected Asian Executive Member of Codex Alimentarius Commission

In July 2011, China was elected Asian Executive Member of Codex Alimentarius Commission (herein after referred to as ACA) at the 34th Session of CAC. As Asian Executive Member, China would represent Asia to further participate in the meetings at the decision-making level, which would play an active role in promoting exchange and cooperation between China and other countries on standards of food safety and improving the influence of China in CAC. Besides, it would be of great importance to helping China to participate in various activities of CAC and learn from international standards on food safety.

(Zhao Xuemei)

3. 43rd Session of Codex Committee on Food Additives was hosted

From March 14 to 18, 2011, the Ministry of Health hosted the 43rd Session of Codex Committee on Food Additives in Xiamen, which was the fifth time that China had hosted sessions of Codex Committee on Food Additives since we became the hosting country of Codex Committee on Food Additives in 2006. The session was chaired by the Chairman of Codex Committee on Food Additives Dr. Chen Junshi (Professor of the Chinese Center for Disease Control and Prevention). The Session was attended by 200 delegates from WHO, FAO, Codex Committee on Food Additives, 54 member countries and one member organization (European Union) and Observers from 27 international organizations. Discussed at the session was the agenda of 18 items including 193 provisions for food additives in ten categories of food in *General Standard for Food Additives* (GSFA), International Numbering System for Food Additives, quality standards for food additives and the priority list of food additives proposed for evaluation by the FAO/WHO Joint Expert Committee on Food Additives (JECFA), provisions for aluminum containing food additives, food additive provision in the standard for infant formulas and the alignment of provisions in Codex Food Standards and GSFA listings, etc. The committee also decided that China should lead the development and maintenance of a database for processing aids, and make the structure of the database and the edition for function display for discussion at the 44th session of Codex Committee on Food Additives.

(Zhao Xuemei)

4. Participating in Work of Codex Alimentarius Commission in 2011

In 2011, the Ministry of Health participated in the electronic working group on aluminum containing food additives, led the formulation of standards for the maximum level of arsenic in rice, led the maintenance of the database for processing aids and vigorously participated in the working groups for the formulation of relevant standards. Information exchange and propaganda of Codex Alimentarius were carried out vigorously, training workshops on Codex Alimentarius were held, *Chinese News Reports on Codex Alimentarius* were published and the propaganda of Codex Alimentarius was intensified via the websites.

(Zhao Xuemei)

5. Progress of Work on National Center for Food Safety Risk Assessment

5-1. National Center for Food Safety Risk Assessment was founded

On October 13, 2011, National Center for Food Safety Risk Assessment was officially founded. The unveiling ceremony was attended by Chen Zhu, Ministry of Health, Zhang Mao, Secretary of the Party Group of MOH, Zhang Yong, Vice Secretary-General of the State Council and Director of Food Safety Office of the State Council, Zhang Chonghe, Vice Director of the State Commission Office for Public Sector Reform, Chen Xiaohong, Director General of the Council of National Center for Food Safety Risk Assessment and Vice Minister of Health, Liu Peizhi, Vice Director General of the Council of National Center for Food Safety Risk Assessment and Vice Director of Food Safety Office of the State Council, responsible officials and leaders of the Ministry of Industry and Information Technology, State Administration for Industry & Commerce, State Food and Drug Administration, State Administration of Grain, as well as directors of the Council of National Center for Food Safety Risk Assessment. The founding of National Center for Food Safety Risk Assessment was an important measure for the Central Committee of CPC and the State Council to enhance food safety and an important base for deeply implementing and practicing *Food Safety Law of the People's Republic of China* and effectively improve the scientific management of food safety in our country. The founding of National Center for Food Safety Risk Assessment filled the gap of professional centers for food safety risk assessment that we didn't have for a long time and the center would play an important role in enhancing the country's food safety research and scientific regulatory capacity, improving food safety quality, protecting public health and strengthening international cooperation and communication.

(Zhao Xuemei)

Chapter V Frontier Health Inspection and Quarantine

Frontier Health Inspection and Quarantine in 2011

In 2011, the whole system of General Administration of Quality Supervision, Inspection and Quarantine (AQSIQ) conducted quarantine inspection on entry/exit persons 343 million person times and 11,848 person times were detected with symptoms of infectious diseases, 6,241 suspected-cases were detected on site with 630 confirmed cases of 14 categories of infectious diseases. Healthcare centers in all the localities conducted physical exams on entry/exit persons 955,213 person times, and 37,037 cases of various infectious diseases were detected. The whole system reported 1,561 events of excessive harmful radioactive factors.

I. Regulating working procedures

Targeting at the different characteristics of work at the ports, General Administration of Quality Supervision, Inspection and Quarantine made corresponding working procedures. At the outbreaks of epidemics, work was conducted from six aspects, i.e. verification of the epidemics, evaluation within the departments, evaluations by the experts, formulation of prevention and control measures, reporting and informing, and coordination with relevant departments to handle the epidemics jointly, etc. Risk assessments were conducted throughout the working procedures, the necessity and effectiveness of work at different stages were assessed while the epidemics were handled and the measures for working were adjusted according to the results of the assessments.

II. Strengthening risk assessment

General Administration of Quality Supervision, Inspection and Quarantine (AQSIQ) applied the concept of risk assessment into every aspect of health inspection and quarantine. Firstly, the mechanism of risk assessment was perfected by the system. The platform of risk pre-warning was established including the retrieval, collection, analysis and evaluation of public health information and the system of pre-warning release, and the working mechanism of risk assessment of public health at ports was further improved. Risk analysis and assessments were conducted on seventeen types of infectious diseases home and abroad including enterohemorrhage E. Coli (EHEC) and poliomyelitis etc. twenty-four announcements and warning -notifications were released and adequate corresponding measures for prevention and control were taken to improve the prevention and control for infectious diseases and work efficiency. Secondly, risk assessment was strengthened in practice. With the occurrence of a series of emergencies, General Administration of Quality Supervision, Inspection and Quarantine (AQSIQ) took timely measures and invited experts to make scientific analysis at the different stages of the emergency occurrence and development, assess the possible impact of the emergencies, research on the responding strategies at ports and scientifically determine the different measures so that steady, orderly and effective response was achieved.

III. Improving the construction of working group mechanism for health quarantine

The framework of working group for health quarantine at ports was further improved. Working groups were established including the working group for management and policy at the healthcare center, the working group for health quarantine and disease monitoring, and the working group for risk analysis of health quarantine and examination for infectious diseases at ports. We gave full play to the role of technical support of the working groups, integrated the resources available and made full use of our professional advantages so that, relying on the technical cooperative group for sanitization, the technical cooperative group for the emergency monitoring on medical vectors and the working group for health quarantine on international cruises etc., we further strengthened the research, analysis and assessment on work related to health quarantine, organized and carried out academic research and educational training etc. to effectively push forward all the work on health quarantine.

IV. Ensuring work quality

Firstly, supervision was made on the inspection of harmful CBRN (chemical, biological, radiological and nuclear) factors at ports. Supervision groups were organized to conduct supervisory inspection on the testing of harmful CBRN and fulfillment of duties at ten ports directly affiliated to AQSIQ in Beijing and Tianjin etc. Secondly, inspections on sanitization were conducted. Self-inspections, sampling inspections and supervisory inspections were made to carry out supervision and inspection on the quality safety of sanitization at ports within the whole system, focusing on the purchase, use, storage and transport of drugs for sanitization etc, to keep abreast of the use of drugs for quarantine handling at ports. Thirdly, inspections on food safety at ports were conducted. On the basis of self-inspections by all the bureaus, an inspection group consisting of relevant professionals made inspection on six ports of four bureaus, i.e. Guizhou Bureau, Yunnan Bureau, Jiangxi Bureau and Anhui Bureau, which further improved the capability of safeguarding food safety at ports. Fourthly, inspections were conducted on the posts of examination at healthcare centers and ports. Special efforts were made to improve the nuclear capability and detection capability of quarantine examination at ports.

(Zhao Xuemei)

Chapter VI Rural Health

1. Work of Rural Health in 2011

I. The new rural cooperative medical system was consolidated and the objectives of the medical and health reform were fulfilled smoothly

According to the requirements of the objectives of the medical and health reform, all the localities and relevant departments put the subsidy into effect, adjusted plans, promoted the reform, enhanced supervisory management and fulfilled all the objectives smoothly. By the end of 2011, 2,637 counties (county-level cities, districts) launched the new rural cooperative medical care; the number of farmers participating in the new rural cooperative medical system amounted to 832 millions with the participating rate of 97.48%, of whom 215 million, 349 million and 268 million were in the eastern, middle and western regions respectively and the participating rate was 98.83%, 97.19% and 96.79% in each region. The funds raised for the new rural cooperative medical care also increased steadily and all-level financial department heightened the subsidiary standard to about 200 RMB Yuan per capita each year and the ratio of personal payment for the new rural cooperative medical care was also raised appropriately. More than 90% of overall-planning areas carried out the overall planning for the new rural cooperative medical care in the outpatient department. The ratio of compensation for policy-related hospitalization expenses in overall-planning areas amounted to about 70% basically and the maximum compensatory limit was increased to 6 times of farmer's per capita net income which was no less than 50 thousand RMB Yuan. The work of the improvement of the level of medical security for leukemia and congenital heart disease was carried out in an all-round way by each province and the pilot work of newly-added diseases was pushed forward smoothly. Instant settlement of medical expenses was realized in most of the overall-planning areas. Reform in the modes of payment for the new rural cooperative medical care such as pre-payment for total amount of expenses in the outpatient department and quota payment for specific diseases was conducted successfully. Such work was promoted steadily as entrusting commercial insurance agencies with participation in administrative services, improvement of overall-planning level of the new rural cooperative medical care and orderly integration of the administrative resources of the basic medical security.

II. The beneficial coverage of the farmers participating in the new rural cooperative medical system was expanded increasingly and farmers' beneficial level improved steadily

All the localities put into effect the subsidy for the new rural cooperative medical care in an all-round way and in 2011, the total sum of funds raised for the new rural cooperative medical care was 204.756 billion RMB Yuan and the actual fund-raising level throughout the country was 246.21 RMB Yuan per capita, which was 89.64 RMB Yuan higher than last year. Per capita funds raised in Shanghai and Beijing were up to 987.04 RMB Yuan and 637.19 RMB Yuan respectively. The average personal payment of farmers participating in the new rural cooperative medical care nationwide was 36.27 RMB Yuan, 53.58 RMB Yuan in the eastern region and 30.24 RMB Yuan in the middle and western regions. In 2011, 1.315 billion person times of farmers reaped the benefit of the system with average 1.58 times for each farmer, of whom 70.3247 million person times enjoyed in-patient compensation; 1.055 billion person times enjoyed the outpatient overall-planning compensation; 112 million person times enjoyed outpatient family-account compensation;4.4243 million person times enjoyed inpatient normal-parturition compensation;10.0648 million person times enjoyed outpatient large-sum compensation for the treatment of special diseases; 24.6564 million person times enjoyed physical-examination compensation; 38.3656 million person times enjoyed other kinds of compensation. In comparison with that in 2010, beneficial person times throughout the country increased by 21.02% and the person times enjoying hospitalization compensation increased by 6.82%.

III. The new rural cooperative medical system was pushed forward steadily and the whole system functioned well

Supervisory management of the funds of the new rural cooperative medical care was further enhanced. In May 2011, the Ministry of Health and Ministry of Finance jointly issued the *Opinions on Strengthening the Fund Management of the New Rural Cooperative Medical Care* which put forward explicit opinions on the issues concerning further enhancement of the management of the participation in the new rural cooperative medical care, regulation of the use of the funds, intensification of the supervisory management of designated medical institutions, promotion of the reform of payment modes, rigorous enforcement of financial and accounting systems, regulation of supervisory and restrictive mechanisms within the administrative organizations, acceleration of informationized construction, strictly enforcement of the three-level regular notification system and serious investigation and punishment of illegal conducts. The Ministry of Health notified fraudulent obtainment of the funds in some regions of Yunnan Province and violations of the laws and disciplines concerning the funds of the new rural cooperative medical care in Guangnan County of Wenshan Prefecture, Yiliang County of Kunming City and Zhenxiong County of Shaotong City. Shandong Province issued the *Measures for Accountability for Violations of Laws and Disciplines of the New Rural Cooperative Medical Care* in the form of a government order which defined exactly the range, principles of disposition, categories, extent of authority and law enforcement entity in the accountability for the violations of the laws and disciplines. Shanxi Province carried out the early warning system for the funds and published yellow and red early warning information according to the indexes of current year's fund balance and previous years' accumulated balance and the degree of safe functioning of the funds. The Department of Health and the Department of Public Security of Henan Province jointly issued the *Notice on Severely Cracking Down on Violations and Crimes of Fraudulent Obtainment of the Funds of the New Rural Cooperative Medical Care* which raised demands for the issues concerning cracking down on the violations and crimes of fraudulent obtainment of the funds and required that personnel and designated medical institutions violating laws and disciplines should be handled seriously in accordance with the law and suspected criminal cases should be transferred to the department of public security.

The work of medical security for rural residents' major serious diseases was actively promoted. In 2011, the Ministry of Health organized and held conferences to promote the pilot work of medical security for rural residents' major serious diseases and newly-added diseases and required all the provinces to carry out the work of medical security for rural children's major serious diseases in an all-round way and by the end of October, all the provinces (cities, autonomous regions) already carried out the work of medical security for rural children's major serious diseases in an all-round way and the pilot of newly-added diseases. According to the statistics, 7,244 children with leukemia were rescued and treated with the total medical expenditure of 144.958 million RMB Yuan, the accumulated sum of compensation of 93.693 million RMB Yuan (including 7.508 million RMB Yuan medical assistance compensation) and the actual compensatory ratio of 65%. 22,692 children with congenital disease were rescued and treated; the total medical expenditure amounted to 577.362 million RMB Yuan; the accumulated sum of compensation was 450.143 million RMB Yuan (including 64.731 million RMB Yuan medical assistance compensation) and the actual compensatory ratio was 78%.

The work of reform in the modes of payment for the new rural cooperative medical care was pushed forward positively. In 2011, the Ministry of Health held four terms of training classes on the reform of modes of payment for the new rural cooperative medical care in Beijing and Shanghai and managerial staff in nearly 400 counties (cities, districts) were trained. Meanwhile, by holding regional meeting and conducting research and supervisory guidance, the Ministry of Health strengthened the guidance on the work of all the localities. All the localities made active exploration and carried out the reform in the payment modes. Jiangsu Province expanded pre-payment for the total amount of expenses in the outpatient department and quota payment for specific diseases to all the overall-planning regions and initiated the reform of mixed payment of combining quota payment for specific diseases with per diem payment in Changshu and Lianyungang. Anhui Province selected 65 groups of diseases for quota payment, carried out clinical pathways and classified diagnosis and treatment and from July 1, the pilot was launched in all the public county-level hospitals of the whole province and every hospital selected no less than 10 groups of diseases for the quota payment.

Participation of commercial insurance agencies in the administrative service work of the new rural cooperative medical care was actively pushed forward. On the basis of investigation and survey made in 2010, the Ministry of Health reported the situation concerning the participation of commercial insurance agencies in the administrative services of the new rural cooperative medical care to the State Council in 2011. With the active promotion of the Ministry of Health, Zhengzhou City started the work that China Life Property & Casualty Insurance Company Limited, Zhengzhou Branch was entrusted with the administrative service work of the new rural cooperative medical care. 6 overall-planning regions in Guangzhou City of Guangdong Province entrusted commercial insurance agencies with the management of affairs of the new rural cooperative medical care. Fujian Provincial Health Department and China Insurance Regulatory Commission Fujian Bureau jointly held on-the-spot symposiums on the participation of commercial insurance agencies in the management of affairs of the new rural cooperative medical care and required all the localities to sum up experience, make innovation and development and do well the work.

The construction of the capacity for the management of the new rural cooperative medical care was enhanced. In 2011, in the light of training on the reform in payment modes, the Ministry of Health added new contents related to the construction of the capacity for the management of the new rural cooperative medical care and held training on report forms of major diseases. At the same time, in the light of the situation that funds of the new rural cooperative medical care were brought into fund budget management of social insurance, training classes for province-level financial personnel were held. By the project of financial transfer payment of the Central Finance, the Ministry of Health continued to support each province to organize and impart training for managerial personnel in all the localities and help them further improve professional level and service capacity. Linyi City of Shandong Province fully carried out county-level vertical management of managerial personnel and county-level managerial organizations dispatched auditors and directors to township managerial organizations.

The informationized construction of the new rural cooperative medical care was accelerated. The Ministry of Health positively pushed forward the construction of the county-level information platforms and all the localities also accelerated the informationized construction of the new rural cooperative medical care in 2011. Information systems were set up in most of the counties (cities, districts) and online verification and reimbursement could be done in some localities. Province-level information platforms began to operate in provinces of Jiangsu, Henan, Hubei, Anhui and Hainan; the construction of the state-level information platform of the new rural cooperative medical care was initiated and the pilot of linking it with information platforms of provinces of Henan, Hainan and so on was launched.

The legislative work of the new rural cooperative medical care was pushed forward energetically. The Ministry of Health led all the localities to make active exploration and promoted the legislative work for the new rural cooperative medical care. Jiangsu Province issued the *Jiangsu Provincial Administrative Regulations on the New Rural Cooperative Medical Care* which put forward normative requirements on administrative systems, fund-raising mechanisms, responsibilities of supervision and management and legal relations.

IV. Reform in the systems and mechanisms of rural grassroots medical and health institutions was deepened.

The comprehensive reform of grassroots medical and health institutions was promoted. The Ministry of Health held seminars and forums on the comprehensive reform of rural grassroots medical and health institutions successively in 2011. 86% of counties (cities, districts) throughout the country carried out the comprehensive reform in grassroots medical and health institutions and all the government-run township health care centers implemented the essential drug system. Fujian Province basically established the multi-channel compensatory mechanism in grassroots medical and health institutions and in 2011, the year-on-year increase in the total subsidiary sum from the three financial levels of province, city and county (including subsidies from the Central Finance) was 46.8%. Zhejiang Province issued the *Opinions on Deepening the Comprehensive Reform of Grassroots Medical and Health Institutions* and proposed to add the establishment of the mechanism of overall-planning distribution of county-level, township and village medical resources and the guarantee mechanisms for the operation of village clinics.

Reform in personnel system was deepened. In May 2011, in cooperation with the State Commission Office for Public Sector Reform, the Ministry of Health issued the *Guiding Opinions on the Standard for the Staffing of Township Health Care Centers* which explicitly provided that staffing standard should be about 1% of the population served. 31 provinces (autonomous regions, cities) and the Xinjiang Production and Construction Corps formulated and issued *the Standard for the Staffing of Township Health Care Centers;* 91.8% of counties re-checked the numbers of the staff in government-run grassroots medical and health institutions; 95.5% of counties finished post establishment and 92.3% finished staff employment. 867 township health care centers in Fujian Province were classified into three groups and the classified management of staffing, financial subsidy and professional management was conducted according to specified standards. Staff members of grassroots medical and health institutions of the whole province competed for post and those succeeding were fully employed.

Mechanisms for performance evaluation were perfected. In March 2011, the Ministry of Health issued the *Opinions on Carrying out Performance Evaluation in Township Health Care Center and Village Clinics* and required all the localities to conduct evaluation on the general management, public health service, basic medical service and degree of satisfaction of township health care centers and village clinics. Governments enhanced the responsibilities for investment by reform and multi-channel compensatory mechanisms were set up initially. 27 provinces issued charging standards for general diagnosis and treatment; 97.2% of counties implemented merit-based salary system in grassroots medical and health institutions and 95.2% of counties conducted comprehensive quantitative performance evaluation in government-run grassroots medical and health institutions. In accordance with the actual realities, all the localities of Zhejiang Province worked out methods for performance evaluation and made active exploration and innovation in evaluation modes. Chongqing City carried out performance evaluation in all the municipal grassroots public medical and health institutions and set up systems of linking evaluation results with financial subsidies, hospital leaders' evaluation results with the evaluation on cadres and the promotion in post and employers' performance evaluation results with their income. Zhangzhou City of Fujian Province appraised and evaluated 64 grassroots medical and health institutions in an all-round way, involving 67 indexes in 10 respects including personnel management, financial management, quality of basic medical services, degree of people's satisfaction and so on and attached importance to performance management, basic public health tasks and quality of basic medical services of grassroots medical and health institutions.

V. Management of rural medical and health institutions was regulated.

In July 2011, the Ministry of Health and the State Development and Reform Commission, the Ministry of Finance, the Ministry of Human Resources and Social Security, the Ministry of Agriculture jointly issued the *Measures for the Administration of Township Health Care Centers (for trial implementation)* which defined the properties, planning for the establishment of organizations, basic functions and the executive, professional, financial and performance administration and promoted the standardized and institutionalized management of township health care centers. Through the activity of "year of management of township health care centers", Hunan Province further regulated the management of township health care centers and improved the medical and health service level. According to the *Measures for the Administration of Township Health Care Centers (for trial implementation)* and local situations, all the localities researched and formulated detailed implementing rules and promoted the standardized and institutionalized management of township health care centers.

VI. On-the-job training for rural health personnel was held

In 2011, the Central Finance invested 257 million RMB Yuan into the on-the-job training for rural health personnel in the middle and western regions and 722 thousand person times and 1.251 million person times from township health care centers and village clinics were trained respectively. The Ministry of Health organized supervisory guidance and inspection on the project of training rural medical and health personnel.

VII. The work of the basic public health service in rural areas was pushed forward

The per capita subsidy for the basic public health service increased from 15 RMB Yuan in 2009 to 25 RMB Yuan in 2011 and service items were expanded to 10 categories, involving 41 items. Basic public health items were fully provided in rural areas and all the task indexes were fulfilled. The rate of the construction of rural residents' standardized electronic health files amounted to 62.6% and the standardization of the files also improved continuously. All the localities discussed and worked out plans for the division of township and village tasks for the basic public health service items and village doctors were required to undertake no less than 40% of the task, which fully aroused village doctors' enthusiasm for participation in the equalization of the basic public health. Some localities attached importance to the play of the role of county-level professional public health institutions and made these institutions participate in training, guidance, inspection and evaluation completely and deeply, which improved the quality and level of the basic public health service items in the grassroots.

(Zhao Yinghong)

2. *Guiding Opinions of the General Office of the State Council on Strengthening the Construction of the Contingent of Village Doctors* Was Issued

In July 2011, in cooperation with the State Council Healthcare Reform Office, the Ministry of Health formulated the *Guiding Opinions of the General Office of the State Council on Strengthening the Construction of the Contingent of Village Doctors* which specified village doctors' responsibilities and staffing standards and the establishment of organizations and construction standards of village clinics, required that the management of village doctors and village clinics should be strengthened and village clinics should also implement the essential drug system and the overall-planning compensation of the out-patient department of the new rural cooperative medical care, meanwhile, demanded explicitly that multi-channel compensatory policies should be perfected. After implementation of the essential drug system in village clinics, village doctors could be compensated by three ways. Firstly, village doctors could be compensated for the offering of the basic public health service, mainly by reasonable subsidies given by governments. In accordance with village doctors' actual work and performance assessment, appropriate percentage of basic public health service funds raised by the state would be allocated to village doctors. Secondly, village doctors could be compensated for the offering of the basic medical service, mainly by personal payment and funds of the new rural cooperative medical care. Thirdly, special subsidies would be allocated to the village clinics that implemented the essential drug system. Subsidiary standards should be made according to the number of served population or checked number of village doctors and village cadres' subsidiary level could be used as a reference for village doctors' subsidiary level. At the same time, localities where conditions permitted were encouraged to heighten the subsidiary level for village practitioners who worked for a long time and for those who worked in remote areas and areas with harsh conditions.

(Zhao Yinghong)

3. The "Project of Promoting Rural Community Health" of the Ministry of Health and the Kadoorie Charitable Foundation (Phase II)

In order to improve the health level of disadvantaged groups in poverty-stricken areas and with support of the Kadoorie Charitable Foundation (Hong Kong), the Ministry of Health continued to carry out the "Project of Promoting Rural Community Health" (Phase II) in provinces of Gansu, Qinghai, Shanxi and Xinjiang Uygur Autonomous Region in 2011. Work concerned was carried out in 2011; equipment was purchased by inviting public bids and houses were built; general evaluation on 4 provinces, 16 counties and 42 towns was conducted and reports on the evaluation were formed; personnel were organized to make external evaluation and evaluation reports were also formed. In May, leaders of the Ministry of Health went to Xinjiang Uygur Autonomous Region with the executive director of the Kadoorie Charitable Foundation to supervise and guide the project and in August, the conference was held to sum up the "Project of Promoting Rural Community Health" of the Ministry of Health and the Kadoorie Charitable Foundation (Phase II). The implementation of the project effectively improved the service capacity of township health care centers and village clinics in the project areas and heightened local residents' health consciousness and health level.

(Zhao Yinghong)

Chapter VII Maternal and Child Health Care and Community Health

1. Work of Maternal and Child Health Care in 2011

In 2011, under the guidance of the 12th Five-Year plan, the *Outline Program for the Development of Chinese Women (2001-2010)* and *the Outline Program for the Development of Chinese Children (2001-2010)*, the work of maternal and child health care closely centered on the key working tasks of deepening the medical and health reform and efforts were made to solve the major issues that affected maternal and child health, deeply promote maternal and child health care service, strengthen the construction of maternal and child health system and push forward the steady development of the work of maternal and child health and positive contribution was made to the improvement of maternal and child health level.

Health level of women and children was improved steadily. In 2011, maternal and child health level was improved unceasingly and the mortality of pregnant and puerperal women, infants and the children under 5 declined continuously, down from 30.0/100000, 13.1‰, 16.4‰ in 2010 to 26.1/100000, 12.1‰, 15.6‰ in 2011 respectively. The morbidity of severe malnutrition for children under 5 fell from 1.55% in 2010 to 1.51% in 2011.

The laws and regulations on maternal and child health were perfected gradually. In 2011, the Ministry of Health stuck to "one law and two programs",(one law referring to *the Law of the People's Republic of China on Maternal and Infant Health Care;* two programs referring to the *Outline Program for the Development of Chinese Women [2001-2010]* and the *Outline Program for the Development of Chinese Children [2001-2010]*) , seriously carried out and implemented *the Law of the People's Republic of China on Maternal and Infant Health Care* and the implementation measures and in cooperation with the State Council Working Committee on Women and Children, fulfilled the summary of the implementation of the two programs (2001-2010) and the issue of the two programs for 2011-2020 and also discussed and worked out plans for the implementation of the two new programs. The Ministry of Health issued the *Administrative Measures for Pregnant and Puerperal Health Care,* the *Working Regulations on Pregnant and Puerperal Health Care* and the *Implementation Plan on Preventing Mother-to-Child Transmission of AIDS, Syphilis and B Hepatitis,* revised and perfected the *Measures for Marketing and Management of Breast-milk Substitutes* and other such normative documents.

The capacity for maternal and child health care service was heightened continuously. Firstly, the Central Finance invested 4.3 billion RMB Yuan in support of the equipment of facilities and the repair of houses for 2,250 county-level maternal and child health care institutions in the middle and western regions, which played a positive role in the improvement of service capacity of grassroots maternal and child health care institutions in the middle and western regions. Secondly, training on numerous special techniques was held to improve the weak capacity of grassroots maternal and child health care institutions. 1,200 professionals in the examination of cervical cancer, 1.256 professionals in breast ultra-sonography and 240 professionals in breast X-ray examination in the grassroots were trained and the teacher training on provincial advanced learning support in obstetrics for 22 provinces (autonomous regions, cities) and Xinjiang Production and Construction Corps was complete. Thirdly, with focus on target regions and groups of people, international cooperative projects were carried out, including pilots of maternal and child health care service for mobile population, adolescents' reproductive health, medical intervention in the women experiencing violence, health care service for pregnant and puerperal women in ethnic minority areas for the promotion of cultural sensitivity, emergency response service of reproductive health, maternal and child health support in Yushu disaster areas, child health care management in China's poverty-stricken areas and integrated maternal and child health and the construction of service capacity at the grassroots levels was strengthened.

The major health problems of women and children were solved constantly. In 2011, for the solution to the major problems that affected maternal and child health, a series of projects concerning major public health service were carried out continuously, such as projects of the reduction of the mortality of pregnant and puerperal women and the elimination of neonatal tetanus (hereinafter referred as project of "reduction and elimination"), hospitalization childbirth subsidies for rural pregnant and puerperal women, the supplement of folic acid for neural tube defect prevention, the examination of "two cancers" for rural women and the prevention of mother-to-child transmission of AIDS. 4 million rural women of childbearing age were screened for cervical cancer, 400 thousand for breast cancer in 2011; as a result, sick women were timely diagnosed and treated. 9.94 million RMB Yuan were subsidized to rural pregnant and puerperal women for hospital childbirth; 8.4 million rural pregnant and puerperal women were offered AIDS consulting service; about 8.7 million had HIV antibody test and compared with that in the period before the implementation of the project, the rate of mother-to-child transmission of AIDS fell from 34.8% to 7.4%. In 2011, rural pregnant and puerperal women's hospital delivery rate was up to 98.1%, which forcefully safeguarded the safety of mothers and infants and difference in the mortality of urban and rural women was basically eliminated;

regional differences were also gradually narrowed and good social benefits were gained. Meanwhile, work of comprehensive prevention and treatment of birth defects was pushed forward steadily. All the localities innovated in working mechanisms and explored modes of providing free premarital physical examination; therefore, the rate of premarital physical examination rose from 31% in 2010 to 41% in 2011. The project of the supplement of folic acid for neutral tube defect prevention was conducted and 10.98 million rural women of childbearing age were supplemented folic acid, which promoted the decline of the incidence of neutral tube defects. The activity of "elimination of infants' anemia" was launched, which improved children's nutrition and health in poverty-stricken areas and popularized knowledge on scientific feeding.

Maternal and child health management was intensified continuously. The Ministry of Health earnestly intensified the routine supervision and management on maternal and infant health care technical service, regulated the management of baby-friendly hospitals, conducted performance assessment on county-level maternal and child health, promoted the rating appraisal on maternal and child health care institutions and the connotation construction of maternal and child health care institutions was strengthened constantly. The information system of maternal and child health was perfected gradually; monitoring on birth defects, death of pregnant and puerperal women and children under 5 was enhanced continuously and in 2011, monitoring on children's nutrition and health was newly added. Annual reports on maternal and child health and monitoring on maternal and child health care institutions were promoted steadily; information on maternal and child health was more comprehensive, accurate and timely and relevant data provided a scientific foundation for the formulation and perfection of health policies, particularly, policies on maternal and child health. In 2011, the Ministry of Health integrated the major projects of maternal and child public health service and the project of "reduction and elimination" with the performance assessment on county-level maternal and child health, organized comprehensive supervision and guidance on maternal and child health work in provinces (autonomous regions) of Heilongjiang, Inner Mongolia, Shaanxi, Anhui, Jiangsu and Qinghai, supervised the work, found out the experience and methods of the projects and forcefully pushed forward the development of maternal and child health work.

(Zhao Yinghong)

2. *Report on the Development of the of Undertaking of China's Maternal and Child Health (2011)* Was Issued

On September 21, 2011, the Ministry of Health issued officially the *Report on the*

Development of the of Undertaking of China's Maternal and Child Health (2011) .It was the first annual report issued by the Ministry of Health on maternal and child health work, which was to fully reflect the development of the undertaking of our country's maternal and child health, lead every part of society and international community to be more concerned about maternal and child health and create a sound environment for the development of the undertaking. In the preface, Chen Zhu, Minister of the Ministry of Health, encouraged all the maternal and child health workers to understand the situation, proceed with confidence, overcome difficulties and make greater efforts to promote the rapid and sound development of the undertaking of maternal and child health.

The report included preface, situations of maternal and child health, situations of maternal and child health care service, development of the undertaking of maternal and child health and conclusion. By deep analysis and comparison, the report fully exhibited the remarkable achievements, objectively analyzed the challenges and opportunities and also briefly introduced the train of thought for the development of the undertaking of maternal and child health in the 12th Five-Year-Plan period. Moreover, in the report, attention was paid to the introduction of a series of major projects beneficial to maternal and child health that were organized and carried out in our country since the start of deepening the medical and health reform and the initial achievements gained.

(Zhao Yinghong)

3. *The Outline Program for the Development of Chinese Women (2011-2020)* and the *Outline Program for the Development of Chinese Children (2011-2020)* Were Issued and Implemented

In July 30, 2011, the State Council officially issued *the Outline Program for the Development of Chinese Women (2011-2020) and the Outline Program for the Development of Chinese Children (2011-2020)*. The two new programs adopted the same framework system of the two programs for 2001-2010 and the two new programs added the part of "guiding ideology and basic principles" respectively. The content concerning "women and social security" was added to *the Outline Program for the Development of Chinese Women (2011-2020)*, while the content of "children and welfare" was supplemented to *the Outline Program for the Development of Chinese Children (2011-2020)*.

The Outline Program for the Development of Chinese Women (2011-2020) covered 7 fields including health, education, economy, participation in government and political affairs, social security, environment and law, 57 objectives being set and 88 strategies and measures being put forward, of which 8 objectives and 11 strategies and measures related to woman health. The main objectives for woman health included: (1) women should enjoy good basic medical and health services in their life time and women's life expectancy should be prolonged; (2) the mortality of pregnant and puerperal women should be controlled below 20/100000.The gap between urban and rural areas should be narrowed gradually and the mortality of mobile pregnant and puerperal women should be reduced; (3) the rate of regular screening of woman common diseases should be more than 80%; the rate of early detection and treatment of cervical cancer and breast cancer should be heightened and mortality should be lowered; (4) female HIV-AIDS infection rate should be under control; (5) the morbidity of severe anemia for pregnant and puerperal women should be reduced; (6) the rate of popularizing the knowledge on woman psychological health and psychiatric disease prevention should be improved; (7) women should be guaranteed the right to know the truth and to choose the ways of birth control ; unwanted pregnancies should be decreased and induced abortion rate should be dropped; (8) the percentage of women doing regular physical exercises should be heightened; more attention should be paid to woman mental and physical health and quality of life and the gap between women in different regions and groups should be narrowed.

The Outline Program for the Development of Chinese Children (2011-2020) covered 5 fields including health, education, welfare, social environment and legal protection, 52 main objectives being set and 67 strategies and measures being put forward, of which 14 objectives and 13 strategies and measures related to children's health. The main objectives for woman health included: (1) the rate of severe multiple-disabled birth defects should fall gradually and disability caused by birth defects should be reduced; (2) the mortality of infants and children under 5 should be controlled below 10‰ and 20‰ respectively and the mortality of mobile infants and children under 5 should be lowered; (3) death and disability caused by injuries should be decreased and injury mortality of children under 18 should be 1/6 less than that in 2010; (4) the incidence rate of children's common diseases and major diseases such as AIDS, syphilis, tuberculosis and B hepatitis should be under control; (5) the rate of vaccination in the National Immunization Program should be more than 95% in each town; (6) the morbidity of neonatal tetanus should be decreased to below 1‰; (7) the incidence rate of low birth weight should be controlled below 4%; (8) the rate of exclusive breastfeeding babies aged 0-6 months should be above 50%; (9) the morbidity of anemia for children under 5 should be controlled below 12% and that for primary and high school students should be 1/3 less than that in 2010; (10) the rate of growth retardation of children under 5 should be controlled below 7% and the rate of low weight should be reduced to below 5%; (11) primary and high school students' qualified rate *for the National Standards for Student Physical Health* should be heightened and the prevalence rate of primary and high school students' poor vision, decayed tooth, overweight/obesity and malnutrition should be under control; (12) the incidence of child psychological and behavioral problems and the morbidity of child psychiatric diseases should be reduced; (13) the rate of popularizing the knowledge on sexual and reproductive health for eligible children should be increased; (14) the harm of environmental pollution to children should be reduced.

(Zhao Yinghong)

4. International and Domestic Cooperative Projects

The project of the seventh period of the Ministry of Health-the United Nations Population Fund was launched and implemented. The Project included 5 subprojects: promotion of the implementation of policies concerning national reproductive health, post-disaster health emergency response service, opposition to violence against women, cultural sensitive health care for pregnant and puerperal women and adolescent sexual and reproductive health. The retrospect reports on China's policies on reproductive health and the indexes of monitoring and assessment on reproductive health and the plans for field investigation and research on the implementation of policies relevant to reproductive health were basically finished; *the Teacher's Manual on the Training of Post-Disaster Emergency Response Service of Reproductive Health* was compiled and training classes were held. Health and education activities suitable to pregnant and puerperal women's healthcare service were carried out in ethnic minority areas and health care out-patient departments for youngsters were set up.

The project of the Ministry of Health-the United Nations Children's Fund (2011-2015) was launched and implemented. The project in this period included: support to the post-disaster reconstruction of maternal and child health, maternal and child health support in Yushu disaster areas, quality improvement of maternal and child information, maternal and child health care service for mobile population and prevention of mother-to-child AIDS transmission. The project of supporting the post-disaster reconstruction of maternal and child health carried out such activities as training of grassroots personnel, communication on health, examination and comment on the critical cases of pregnant and puerperal women and final investigation and on November 24-25, 2011, the conference was held in Chengdu City, Sichuan Province to summarize experience and popularize the achievements. The project of maternal and child health support in Yushu disaster areas organized training and further study for maternal and child health care personnel, provided 463 medical equipment of 12 categories for project areas, adapted Chinese-Tibetan bilingual mother-and-child healthcare materials and distributed them to project areas. The project of maternal and child health care service for mobile population carried out baseline investigation in project areas, worked out plans for health communication and initially established the multi-sector coordinative mechanisms.

The subproject of maternal and child health in the Project of Culture and Development of the Spain Millennium Development Goals Achievement Fund was finished smoothly. From 2009 to 2011, the Ministry of Health, the National Population and Family Planning Commission, the United Nations Population Fund and the World Health Organization jointly conducted the project. 7.18 million RMB Yuan were invested and activities were carried out in 6 ethnic minority counties (cities) of provinces (autonomous regions) of Guizhou, Yunnan, Tibet and Qinghai, including developing the training materials on maternal and child health care which were suitable to local cultural features and holding training classes on cultural sensitivity and technical service of maternal and child health care, which improved the management and service level of maternal and health in ethnic minority areas and promoted the provision and utilization of maternal and child health care service.

In 2011, centering on the main problems that affected maternal and child health, the Ministry of Health also launched the project of the prevention of reproductive tract infection and the project of perinatal nutrition (phase II) and continuously explored the new patterns of maternal and child health care service.

(Zhao Yinghong)

5. Comprehensive Project of Mother and Child Health of the Ministry of Health and the United Nations International Children's Emergency Fund

In order to better the health of pregnant and puerperal women and children aged 0-6 years in the western regions, push forward governments to formulate and implement policies and regulations on maternal and child health, improve service quality of maternal and child health care in the localities and promote the accessibility, availability, equality and sustainability of rural maternal and child health care service, the Ministry of Health and the United Nations International Children's Emergency Fund launched the comprehensive project of mother and child health in 2011. The project was carried out in 35 counties of 7 provinces (autonomous regions) in the middle and western regions of China and women planning to become pregnant, pregnant and puerperal women, children aged 0-6 years and their parents (with attention paid to children under 3 years), medical personnel providing maternal and child health service and relevant governmental personnel in project regions were the target people. In July 2011, the conference was held in Chengdu City of Sichuan Province to launch the project and the conference on the establishment of the state-level expert panel and a seminar were held in Beijing in September. The Ministry of Health organized the expert panel to compile the texts for the project and revise the technical materials of the previous phases such as *the Guidelines for Mother and Child Health Care Service, the Manual on Mother and Child Health* and the *Instruction Manual for Rural Medical Personnel on Mother and Child Health.* In November 2011, training classes for teachers were held in Beijing and 160 maternal and child health care professionals from project regions attended the training.

(Zhao Yinghong)

Chapter VIII Medical Administration

1. Work of Medical Administration in 2011

I. The work related to medical reform progressed smoothly

The management of clinical pathway was pushed forward continuously. Firstly, the compilation and issuing of clinical pathways for some categories of diseases were carried on. In 2011, the clinical pathways for 109 diseases were compiled and issued. From March, 2009 to the end of 2011, the clinical pathways for 331 categories of 22 specialties were completed. Secondly, the pilot of clinical pathway management was further strengthened, which instructed all the localities to organize the pilot of clinical pathway management scientifically and effectively. The coverage of pilot hospitals was expanded. By the end of 2011, 25,503 departments in 3,476 medical institutions nationwide had implemented clinical pathway management. The number of enrolled patients increased. From January to October, 2011, altogether 1,414,543 cases of clinical pathway management were conducted nationwide, with 251,745 cases of variation, the variation rate being 17.8%. 150,723 cases quitted, the completion rate being 89.34%. Thirdly, pilot of the third-party evaluation was carried out. Fourthly, the data reporting platform of www.ch-cp.org.cn was improved, and at present 833 hospitals made on-line real-time reports of data on clinical pathway management. Fifthly, publicity on the clinical pathway management was strengthened.

Pilot of the informationization construction for hospitals was pushed forward with the electronic medical records as the core. Firstly, the coverage of pilot hospitals was further expanded and another 92 hospitals were chosen as the pilot hospitals for electronic medical records in 2011. So far, five cities had been chosen as pilot cities for electronic medical records and 189 hospitals had been chosen as pilot hospitals at the ministerial level nationwide. Secondly, *Measures and Standards for Classified Evaluation on Applying the Function of Electronic Medical Record System (trial)* was formulated to start the classified evaluation on the electronic medical records in hospitals. Thirdly, *Circular on Pushing forward Pilot of Informationization Construction for Hospitals with Electronic Medical Record as the Core* was formulated and issued, which clarified the division of work among the pilot cities and pilot hospitals. Meanwhile, the work conference and the on-site conference on the pilot of electronic medical records were held to make deployments on the pilot work and exchange experience on the pilot work.

The treatment of catastrophic diseases for the residents was further ensured.

Firstly, training on the standardization of peritoneal dialysis was carried out and pilot of peritoneal dialysis at the county-level hospitals and medical institution at the grassroots was started. Thirty-one hospitals were chosen as demonstration centers for peritoneal dialysis and pilot of peritoneal dialysis was carried out in twenty-nine provinces. Secondly, good work was done on providing medical treatment of catastrophic diseases for rural residents. From June 2010 to the end of August 2011, altogether 15,217 kids with congenital heart disease and 3,266 kids with leukemia were treated nationwide. As for the pilot diseases newly added in 2011, altogether 11,819 patients with end-stage renal disease, 8,791 patients with breast cancer, 1,231 patients with cervical cancer, 7,519 patients with holergasia and 7,846 patients with multiple-drug resistance tuberculosis had been granted subsidies for catastrophic diseases by the end of August 2011.Thirdly, the clinical pathways for the catastrophic diseases including the two cancers for women were formulated and issued, which improved the standardized diagnosis and treatment system for catastrophic diseases.

Excellent nursing services were forcefully promoted. In June 2011, the Ministry of Health printed and issued *Guidelines for Clinical Nursing Practice (2011 Edition),* which required to conduct the third-party satisfaction survey as the routine tasks. Performance evaluation was conducted in hospitals carrying out the excellent nursing services nationwide, and 76 hospitals were determined as excellent hospitals, 361 excellent wards and 694 excellent individuals.

The project of Sight Restoration for Millions of Cataract Patients in Poverty was completed. In 2011 500,000 cataract patients in poverty had their vision restored through surgeries. From the time the project was launched to the end of 2011, altogether 1,090,000 cataract patients were operated on to restore sight.

Efforts were made to push forward the mutual recognition of check-up results among medical institutions at the same level. In accordance with the requirements of the Ministry of Health and on the basis of strengthening the informationization construction, all the localities pushed forward the mutual recognition of check-up results among medical institutions at the same level to promote the share of resources and reduce the costs. Relevant guidelines were promulgated successively in Beijing, Guangdong, Hubei, Jiangsu, Liaoning, Guizhou and Shanxi etc. to organize the medical institutions to carry out mutual recognition of check-up results.

II. Strengthening the construction of medical service system and improving the medical service capability

The medical service system wan established and perfected. Firstly, work was done to instruct all the localities to adjust the setting-up of medical institutions and encourage them to leave enough space for the social capitals to run medical institutions. Taking into consideration their respective real conditions, all the localities made plans to adjust the network of medical service. Eight provinces (municipalities) including Shanghai, Jiangsu and Fujian had formulated new *Plan for the Layout of Medical Institutions.* Liaoning Province and Jiangsu Province etc. had set up concentrated clinical laboratories to improve the efficiency of utilizing resources. Secondly, the construction of medical service capability was strengthened. 110 regional medical centers in the mid and west regions were put into use to strengthen the construction of pediatrics departments in the mid and west regions and in the county-level hospitals as well as the construction of children's hospitals at the county level nationwide. Zhejiang Province, Hainan Province and other eight provinces also actively coordinated with relevant departments to strengthen the construction of medical service system.

The construction of the national key clinical departments was carried on. The commission for the management of the national key clinical department projects and the consultant group for the project were established and the work conference for the construction of the national key clinical department was held to clarify the general ideas, basic principles and specific requirements for the construction of the national key clinical departments. Evaluation on the national key clinical department projects in 2011 was completed and 316 construction projects of 20 disciplines including cardiovascular departments were decided on. Surveys on the present situations of clinical discipline at the tertiary hospitals were launched. Guided by the construction of the national key clinical departments, all the provinces (regions, municipalities) also carried out the construction of the provincial key clinical departments. Nineteen provinces (municipalities) including Liaoning Province, Hunan Province, Shanghai Municipality and Jiangsu Province carried out the construction of provincial key clinical departments.

The management of medical institutions was strengthened and social capitals were encouraged to run medical institutions. Ten pieces of opinions were promulgated to promote the development of non-public medical institutions and the pilot of private clinics run by qualified people by law was conducted in Tianjin, Changchun and Kunming etc. *Interim Measures on the Management of Chinese-foreign Joint Venture and Cooperative Medical Institutions* was revised, which devolved the rights of examination and approval of Chinese-foreign joint venture and cooperative medical institutions so that pilots of hospitals wholly owned by Taiwanese, Hong Kongers and Macanese were conducted in some provinces and cities. The standards for the examination and approval of specialized hospitals were delegated and the local health administrative departments were allowed to approve the specialized hospitals for which the Ministry of Health had no standards. By the end of October 2011, there were 671 more private hospitals nationwide. The coverage of the pilot of doctors' multi-sited practices was expanded to all the provinces (regions, municipalities). Special supervisory inspections were conduced on medical cosmetology to regulate the practice of medical institutions.

The construction of health talent team was strengthened to provide talents for deepening the medical and health care reform. *Interim Measures for Administration of Short-term Medical Practice in China by Foreign Doctors* and *Regulations on the Handling of Violations in Qualification Examination of Doctors* were revised. Doctors' qualification examination in 2011 was organized and the pilot of computerized examination was carried out. The coverage of examinations for town-ship registered assistant doctors was expanded to 21 provinces (regions, municipalities) in need and approximately 30,000 examinees passed the examination. The policies for the registration of general practitioners were perfected and training for doctors in weak disciplines was carried out.

Evaluations on training and demonstration sites for opening hospital affairs were conducted and 146 county-level hospitals and township clinics were determined as demonstration sites to guide the county-level hospitals and medical institutions at the grassroots to work well on opening hospital affairs.

Ⅲ. Improving the system of medical quality management and control to ensure medical quality and medical safety

The campaign of "Three Excellent and One Satisfactory" and the campaign of "Long March of Medical Quality" were further carried on. *Circular of the Ministry of Health on Launching the Campaign of "Three Excellent and One Satisfactory" in the Medical* and *Health System Nationwide and Quantitative Index on Division of Tasks for the Campaign of "Three Excellent and One Satisfactory" in the Medical and Health System Nationwide* were issued. Work conferences on the campaign of "Three Excellent and One Satisfactory" were held at regular intervals to push forward the progress of the campaign and provide a platform for communication among regions. Consequently, the campaign progressed well. *Plan for Campaign of "Long March of Medical Quality" in 2011* was formulated and issued to carry on the campaign with the theme of "Continuously Improving Quality and Ensuring Medical Safety". From October to December 2011, the Ministry of Health organized supervisory inspections in 30 provinces (regions, municipalities), with the focus on 113 specialized hospitals in four specialties, i.e. gynecology and obstetrics, pediatrics, oncology and stomatology, which effectively promoted the improvement of management and medical quality in specialized hospitals. Taking advantage of the campaign of "Long March of Medical Quality", we conducted special inspections on the management of hospital infections nationwide and supervisory inspections were conducted on blood safety in 112 blood collecting and supplying institutions in 11 provinces (regions, municipalities) nationwide.

Pharmaceutical administration was strengthened in medical institutions to promote rational clinical medication. Firstly, the special rectification on clinical use of antibacterial agents was conducted nationwide and the special rectification on clinical use of antibacterial agents was determined as an important part of the public hospital reform and the campaign of "Three Excellent and One Satisfactory". From November to December 2011, taking advantage of the campaign of "Long March of Medical Quality", we conducted supervisory inspections on he special rectification on clinical use of antibacterial agents in 30 provincial health administrative departments and 323 medical institutions nationwide. As was revealed by the results of the inspections, periodical achievements were made in the special rectification on clinical use of antibacterial agents, i.e. the number of antibacterial agents conformed to the specific number, the rate of antibacterial agent use by the outpatients and inpatients conformed to the standards, the intensity of antibacterial agent use somewhat declined, the rate of microorganism testing gradually increased and the preventive use of antimicrobial agents for clean operations got regulated. Secondly, relevant rules on pharmaceutical administration were further improved. The Ministry of Health, State Administration of Traditional Chinese Medicine and the Health Bureau of the PLA General Logistics Department jointly formulated and issued *Regulations of Pharmaceutical Administration for Medical Institutions, drafted Measures for the Management of Clinical Use of Antibacterial Agents, and Measures for the Management of Clinical Pharmacists,* and formulated and issued *Guidelines on the Clinical Use of Glucocorticoid.* Research and preparation were made on the legislation of *Pharmacists Law.* Thirdly, efforts were made to strengthen the construction of national monitoring net for clinical use of antibacterial agents and national monitoring net for bacterial drug resistance. Fourthly, training on rational drug use was carried on to improve the capability of microorganism testing and rational use of antibacterial agents at the grassroots medical institutions. Fifthly, experts were organized to draft *National Guidelines on Antimicrobials* and *Chinese National Formulary for Children.* Sixthly, good work was done on the qualification accreditation, verification and examination for institutions of clinical drug trials.

Work was done on medical quality management and control. The construction of provincial medical quality control centers for clinical medicine was vigorously pushed forward. The quality control index for tertiary general hospitals and the second batch of single diseases were formulated and issued and the quality control index for the tertiary specialized hospitals and key laboratories were drafted to guide the health administrative departments and hospitals to work on medical quality control. Besides, the national information system for the quality control of single diseases was established and quality control for single diseases was conducted. The examination and admission of the third type of medical technology was pushed forward steadily, and the administration of interventional therapies, endoscopic therapies and blood purification was strengthened. Standardized diagnosis and treatment for catastrophic diseases was conducted, including cardiovascular diseases, strokes, chronic renal failure and cancers etc. Norms for the diagnosis and treatment of six common carcinomas were researched on and formulated, i.e. primary lung carcinoma, primary hepatic carcinoma, pancreatic carcinoma, breast carcinoma, gastric carcinoma, colorectal carcinoma, the national information system for cases of common carcinomas was being gradually established and training for the medical staff was carried out.

The management of hospital infection and first aid was strengthened to work well on the treatment of emergencies. Technical norms including *Technical Guidelines on Prevention and Control of Hospital Infection of Multi-drug Resistant Bacteria (trial)* were printed and issued and *Catalogue of Medical Waste Classification* was revised. The information reporting system for the outbreaks of hospital infection was established and improved and training was conducted for the management of hospital infection at the grassroots. *Management Measures for Pre-hospital First Aid* was drafted to standardize pre-hospital first aid.

IV. Further pushing forward blood donation and management of blood safety

Blood donation was further pushed forward. In 2011, approximately 12,320,000 people donated about 4,164 tons of blood, the number of donors and the amount of blood donated increased by 3.71% and 5.18% respectively as compared with those in the year 2010. Hence, the blood donation rate reached 9.2 per thousand people. Centering round the goal of "continuously establishing and improving the long-term working mechanism for blood donation which is guided by the government, collaborated by multi-departments and participated by the whole society", we focused on the following key work:

Efforts were made to implement the requirements of the State Council. *Circular on Further Strengthening AIDS Prevention and Control* issued by the State Council required that blood donation should be effectively pushed forward, publicity of non-commercial ads for blood donation should be carried out widely and volunteer organizations for blood donation should be set up vigorously. In order to implement the requirements of the State Council and strengthen the organization and leadership for blood donation, the Ministry of Health, Health Bureau of the PLA General Logistics Department and Red Cross Society of China jointly issued *Circular on Further Strengthening Work on Blood Donation,* requiring all the localities to fully understand the importance and urgency of blood donation, improve the long-term mechanism for blood donation which is guided by the government, collaborated by multi-departments and participated by the whole society, carry on the publicity, lead the whole society to participate and promote the work on blood donation together.

Awards for blood donation were granted. In February 2011, the Ministry of Health held the national awarding conference for blood donation, to which the Vice Premier Li Keqiang sent a congratulatory message. Han Qide, Vice Chairman of the Standing Committee of NPC attended the conference and took photos with the winners. The conference granted awards to 112,347 individuals with the title of "Contribution Award for Blood Donation", 80 units and 13 individuals with the title of "Promotion Award for Blood Donation", 9 provinces and 240 cities (districts) with the titles of "Advanced Province (City) for Blood Donation", 18 military units with the title of "Advanced Military Units for Blood Donation" and 616 individuals with the title of "Contribution Award for Donating Hematopoietic Stem Cell".

Publicity on blood donation was strengthened. Publicity on June 14 World Blood Donor Day was carried out. Non-commercial ads and information on relevant work were played and released via the media including CCTV and all the localities were required to make publicity to create the atmosphere for blood donation. The campaign of blood donor month was conducted. *Circular on Launching Campaign of Blood Donor Month in 2011* was issued jointly with the Ministry of Education, Central Committee of Youth League, State Administration of Radio, Film and Television, Health Bureau of PLA Logistics Department and Red Cross Society of China, which determined December 2011 as the blood donor month and "donating renewable blood to save non-renewable lives" as the theme of the campaign. Aiming at the hot issues in the society, we held media briefings and press conferences to publicize information concerning blood donation and work on blood so as to gain understanding and support on blood donation from the society. Work on blood donation was publicized. Comparison was made on the amounts of blood collected and the numbers of donors between the same period in 2010 and 2011. The results of the comparison were publicized, which helped all the localities to strengthen the service of collecting and supplying blood more specifically and thus ensured the blood supply and the safety of blood using.

Blood safety was intensified. *Technical Operation Procedures for Plasma Collection Station (2011 Edition)* was formulated and issued and other normative documents were formulated including *Health Examination Criteria for Blood Donors* and *Quality Standards for Whole Blood and Blood Components* etc. 2011 work conference on nucleic acid testing and blood safety for blood stations was held and the pilot of nucleic acid testing was expanded. The supervisory inspections on blood safety of the campaign for 2011 Long March of Medical Quality were conducted and over 100 experts on blood management made supervisory inspections at 98 blood stations and 14 plasma collection stations in 11 provinces (regions, municipalities) i.e. Liaoning, Heilongjiang, Zhejiang, Anhui, Henan, Hebei, Hubei, Guangdong, Hainan, Sichuan, and Qinghai. A fund of 77.12 billion RMB Yuan for central finance projects was arranged to support the management of blood quality in all the localities and hold training workshops for the technicians from blood collecting and supplying institutions at the prefectural level.

Rational clinical blood use was pushed forward. *Measures for the Management of Clinical Blood Use at Medical Institutions (2011 edition, Draft for Soliciting Opinions)* was revised. Training on clinical blood use was conducted to popularize the experience from some hospitals on the management of clinical blood use and the on blood conservation techniques.

The construction of standardization for blood management information was strengthened. The reporting indexes for the current blood collecting and supplying information system were adjusted, and *Ministry of Health Statistic Indexes for Blood Collecting and Supplying Information (for Blood Stations, 2011 Edition)* was formulated. Consequently, the functions of data were improved and the national unified statistic information for blood collection and supply was adopted on the basis of the pilot.

Partner assistance was provided well. Firstly, the capability construction of blood collection and supply in Tibet was strengthened. *Circular on Providing Partner Assistance for Blood Collection and Supply to Tibet and Tibetan Areas in Yunnan, Gansu, Qinghai and Sichuan* was issued, which defined that Shanghai, Jiangsu, Zhejiang, Anhui, Fujian, Chongqing, Shanxi and Institute of Blood Transfusion, Chinese Academy of Medical Sciences provided partner assistance to Tibet and collaborated and deployed the assistance for blood collection and supply in Tibet. Secondly, vigorous efforts were made to aid Xinjiang in blood supply. While vaccinating poliomyelitis vaccines in South Xinjiang, we organized Hebei, Jiangsu, Zhejiang, Shandong and Sichuan to aid Xinjiang in blood supply and effectively ensured the blood supply in Xinjiang.

Assistance was provided in preparing for researching on the implementation of *Law on Blood Donation* and revising it. The diagnosis and treatment of hemophilia and its management were carried on to coordinate manufactures of blood products to increase the production of prothrombin complex. The management of the bank of umbilical cord blood hematopoietic stem cells was standardized.

V. Nursing care was strengthened comprehensively

Regulations on Nurses was implemented and practiced to strengthen the construction of nurse team. In 2011, there were over 190,000 new nurses nationwide, so that the total number of nurses had amounted to 2,240,000 nationwide. *Interim Management Measures for Hospital Nurses and Measures for Foreign Nurses Practicing in China* were drafted and *Management Measures for Clinical Practice of Nursing Education* was formulated. By the end of 2011, over a thousand nurses had been trained specializing in intensive care, emergency first-aid treatment and hemopurification etc. In 2011, eight nurses in China were awarded 43rd Nightingale Medal and it was the fifth time that General Secretary of CPC Central Committee and President of China, Hu Jintao, had granted the award to the winner nurses. *The Outline for Developing Nursing Care in China (2011-2015)* was formulated and issued. *Basic Standards of Nursing Home (2011 Edition)* was issued and relevant research on the long-term nursing care was conducted. Pilot was conducted in some cities to formulate and improve policies and measures for long-term nursing care. Communication with and guidance on hospitals with the national clinical key specialized nursing projects were strengthened and working plans for the projects of nursing in hospitals were formulated.

VI. Pushing forward the management of rehabilitation, blindness prevention and treatment and the management of drug rehabilitation

Pilot of establishing and improving the rehabilitation medicine system was launched in 14 provinces (regions, municipalities) nationwide. *Outline for Developing Rehabilitation Medicine in China (2011-2015)* was formulated. *Operation Procedures of Common Rehabilitation Techniques* was drafted and special work was organized on the rehabilitation for the disabled. National training was conducted for the management of rehabilitation and the management of blindness prevention and treatment. Phrase Ⅲ of the project of Vision First-China in Action was launched. Laws and regulations were implemented including *Narcotics Control Law* and *Regulation on Drug Rehabilitation* and training was conducted for 141 drug rehabilitation institutions nationwide. *Agreement on Voluntary Drug Rehabilitation* and *Record of Drug Rehabilitation in Hospital* were formulated to strengthen the management of drug rehabilitation nationwide by law.

(Zhao Xuemei)

2. The Rights of Examination and Approval for Chinese-foreign Joint Ventures and Cooperative Medical Institutions Was Delegated to Provincial Health Administrative Departments

In order to implement the essence of *Circular of the General Office of the State Council on Transmitting and Issuing the Opinions of National Development and Reform Commission, the Ministry of Heath and Other Departments on Encouraging and Leading Social Capitals to Run Medical Institutions* and simplify and regulate the examination and approval procedures for foreign capital to run medical institutions, the Ministry of Health issued *Circular of the Ministry of Health on Adjusting Examination and Approval Rights for Chinese-foreign Joint Ventures and Cooperative Medical Institutions* in January 2011, which adjusted the examination and approval rights for Chinese-foreign joint ventures and cooperative medical institutions. *The Circular* clarified that the examination and approval rights for the layout and changing of Chinese-foreign joint ventures and cooperative medical institutions would be delegated to the provincial health administrative departments. In accordance with the essence of *the Circular,* the layout of Chinese-foreign joint ventures and cooperative medical institutions should, after being examined by the municipal health administrative departments where the medical institutions were located, be reported to the provincial health administrative departments for examination and approval. The applicants could run both profitable and non-profitable medical institutions. The applicants should submit application to relevant commercial departments in charge in accordance with relevant laws and regulations for the layout, changing and ending of Chinese-foreign joint ventures and cooperative medical institutions after being approved by the provincial health administrative departments.

(Zhao Xuemei)

3. *The Outline for Developing Nursing Care in China (2011-2015)* Was Issued

According to the general plan on developing health care and deepening reform of the medical and health care system during the 12th Five-Year Plan period and *Long-Term Development Plan for Medical Professionals (2011-2020),* the Ministry of Health issued *The Outline for Developing Nursing Care in China (2011-2015)* to promote the development of nursing care in China.

The Outline summarized and analyzed the achievements and experience of nursing care in China during the 11th Five-Year Plan period. The 11th Five-Year Plan period was a truly extraordinary time in the course of healthcare development, which had made remarkable achievements. Particularly, with the deepening of medical and healthcare institutional reform, great progress had been achieved in nursing care, which had been reflected by the growing number of nurses. By the end of the 11th Five-Year Plan period, the total number of registered nurses in China had amounted to 2.05 million, an increase of 52% as compared with that in 2005, which meant the structure where the number of nurses substantially outweighs the number of physicians was changed gradually. The number of nurses who had received college education accounted for 51.3% of the total. All the localities vigorously carried out standardized training on specialist nurses. As a result, the professional skills of nurses had been continuously improved. During the course of public hospital reforms, hospitals at all levels promoted quality nursing service by reforming nursing service mode and carrying out an integrated and accountability-based nursing care. Consequently, clinical nursing service was greatly improved. Service gradually extended to families and communities and played an active role in elderly care, chronic disease care and hospice care.

The Outline pointed out the main objectives of developing nursing care during the 12th Five-Year Plan period as the followings: improving nursing service and quality, enriching nursing content and broadening service scope were the key points; strengthening nurse team construction and service mode reform were the starting points; with promoting excellent nursing service and long-term caring for the elderly, chronic patients and hospice patients as entry points, nursing capability and professional skills would be continuously enhanced and comprehensive, coordinated, and sustainable development of nursing care would thus be promoted. The main tasks included: *the Regulation on Nurses* should be further implemented; the construction of nurse team should be strengthened; clinical nursing care should be improved; nursing management at public hospitals should be deepened; training system for specialized nursing care jobs and training system for nursing management should be established; and long-term nursing care service system should be explored and established.

Apart from what were mentioned above, the *Outline* also deployed work on accelerating the reform and development of nursing care, forcefully promoting TCM nursing care and strengthening cooperation and communication with international counterparts as well as those in Hong Kong, Macao and Taiwan.

(Zhao Xuemei)

Chapter IX Medical Service Supervision and Management

1. Work on Medical Service Supervision and Management in 2011

I. Pushing forward pilot projects for public hospital reform

Documents on the pilot projects for public hospital reform in 2011 were formulated to push forward work vigorously. On the basis of thoroughly summarizing work and widely soliciting opinions, *Arrangements for Public Hospital Pilot Reform in China in 2011* (herein after referred to as *Arrangements)* was drafted, revised and improved and issued by the General Office of the State Council on February 28, 2011. The Ministry of Health and the leading group for medical and healthcare reform of the State Council held the work conference on the pilot projects for public hospital reform in Beijing on March 19 to implement the essence of the national work conference on the pilot for deepening medical and healthcare system reform and the *Arrangements* and accelerate the pilot for public hospital reform. In April, a conference was held in Xiamen to deploy the major tasks in 2011 for the national level pilot cities for public hospital reform; in June, the 28th session of the ministerial leading group office for medical reform and the 21st session of the ministerial leading group for medical reform were held to further research and discuss *Working Plan for the Pilot Projects of Comprehensive Reform of County-level Hospitals* and *Guiding Opinions on Establishing the Mechanism of Division of Responsibility and Coordination between Public Hospitals and Urban and Rural Medical and Healthcare Institutions at the Grassroots-level;* on September 2, experience exchanging conference was held in Changchun on the pilot of public hospital reform; in September and November, communication conferences for the pilot of public hospital reform in the North and South were held respectively in Beijing and Shanghai.

Investigations and instruction on the pilot cities as well as the summarizing and spreading of experience were strengthened. In April 2011, the Ministry of Health listened to the report on the implementation plans on the major tasks of medical reform by seven pilot cities, i.e. Zhenjiang, Weifang, Shenzhen, Wuhu, Luoyang, Zhuzhou and Baoji and discussed on propelling all the tasks of reforming public hospital systems and mechanism in 2011. Investigations and instruction were organized to keep abreast of the progress of the pilot in all the localities, summarize beneficial experience and find out difficulties and deficiencies. The system of accredited contacts for national level pilot cities for public hospital reform and the system of coordination group for the pilot of public hospital reform were established.

The system of information reporting for pilot cities was established and 26 issues of *Dynamic on Public Hospital Reform and Management* were compiled and published as well as 133 issues of *Briefing on Pilot of Public Hospital Reform.*

Specialized and professional trainings for public hospitals were conducted. In order to research on and establish the specialized and professional system and training system for the directors of public hospitals and cultivate a group of directors of public hospitals with thorough understanding of policies, open mind, abundant knowledge and excellent capability of management, the launching ceremony for the training program for specialized and professional public hospitals & seminar was held in Beijing on May 26, 2011. Vice Minister of the Ministry of Health, Mao Xiaowei, attended the ceremony, delivered an address and granted letters of appoints to the member of the expert committee of the program.

The comprehensive reform of county-level hospitals was effectively pushed forward. In accordance with the deployments of the State Council, priority was given to developing county-level hospitals and the comprehensive reform of county-level hospitals as the breakthrough to push forward the reform of public hospitals. CPC Central Committee planed to select 300 county-level hospitals to push forward the pilot of public hospital reform. On the basis of making wide investigations and research and soliciting opinions, we formulated *Working Plan for the Pilot Projects of Comprehensive Reform of County-level Hospitals* and *Guiding Opinions on Establishing the Mechanism of Division of Responsibility and Coordination between Public Hospitals and Urban and Rural Medical and Healthcare Institutions at the Grassroots-level.* Selection on pilot counties and pilot provinces for comprehensive reform of public hospitals kicked off and 21 provinces (regions, municipalities) submitted application documents. The seminar was held in March 2011 to discuss the working plan for the pilot projects of comprehensive reform of county-level hospitals and the symposium was jointly held with the Office of Medical Reform of the State Council on the pilot projects of the comprehensive reform of county-level hospitals to solicit opinions from the local governments, relevant experts and experts on *Working Plan for the Pilot Projects of Comprehensive Reform of County-level Hospitals.*

Measures for providing convenient and beneficial service were pushed forward. *Circular on Further Pushing forward Clinic Appointment Service* was drafted and issued, and an introduction on the progress of providing clinic appointment service in public hospitals nationwide was made via the press conference. The national video and teleconference on clinic appointment service was held, at which achievements were summarized on the clinic appointment service obtained in the previous two years, the experience gained in Beijing, Zhejiang and some hospitals such as Affiliated Hospital to Xiamen University was spread and deployments were made on the future work.

By the end of 2011, 1,125 tertiary hospitals nationwide and some qualified secondary hospitals had provided clinic appointment service.

II. The construction of county-level hospitals was pushed forward

The Project of Ten Thousand Doctors Supporting Rural Health was carried on, and inter-provincial partner assistance between the eastern and western regions was conducted. Work on the Project of Ten Thousand Doctors Supporting Rural Health in 2011 was deployed to enhance the management of the project and improve the use of evaluation results. Experts were organized to make supervisory inspections on the Project of Ten Thousand Doctors Supporting Rural Health and random inspections were made via telephones on the attendance of supporting doctors, the results of which were reported nationwide. The information management system for partner assistance between the urban and rural hospitals was established to grasp the real-time situations of work in all the localities. In 2011, over 1,100 tertiary hospitals sent approximately ten thousand medical workers to 2,139 supported county-level hospitals, over 3.5 million person times county-level medical workers were trained, members of the medical teams sent treated over 1.65 million person times of patients and applied new techniques and conducted new business approximately 6,200 times. Free diagnosis and treatment, health checkups and tour medical services were provided and the medical devices and other things in great need were donated. The national work conference on partner assistance between urban and rural hospitals was held in Yunnan Province to summarize and spread the experience from Shanghai providing partner assistance to the county-level hospitals in Yunnan Province. The summary conference on inter-provincial partner assistance between the eastern and western regions was held to make timely summary of experience, find out the deficiency and promote our work. The summary conference on hospitals affiliated to the Ministry of Health (administrated by the Ministry of Health) assisting rural health in the western regions was held to exchange experience and praise those with excellent performance in 2011. Peking Union Medical College Hospital, Zhongshan Hospital affiliated to Fudan University and the First Hospital Affiliated to Zhongshan University were entrusted to found the national medical team, which provided tour medical services to the former revolutionary base areas, areas inhabited by ethnic groups, remote and border areas and poverty-stricken areas in eighteen provinces (regions, municipalities). Thus the excellent medical resources were given full play to.

Communication with the key contact hospitals at the county level was strengthened. In January, March and August 2011, the Ministry of Health held conferences respectively in Hainan, Shanghai and Jilin for the directors of the key contact hospitals at the county level and the officials in charge of the medical administrative departments from the provincial (regional, municipal) health bureaus. At the conferences, discussions were made on working mechanism and working mode of the key contact hospitals at the county level, the problems confronted by the reform and development of the county-level hospitals and the criteria of examination and evaluation of county-level general hospitals. From late March on, the Ministry of Health dispatched personnel to conduct on-site investigations and research in the key contact hospitals at the county level in Hebei Province, Ningxia Province, Henan Province, Hubei Province, Anhui Province and Yunnan Province etc. to keep abreast of the work at the county-level hospitals on medical service, management, the construction of talent team and partner assistance etc. Surveys were conducted on the basic situations in the key contact hospitals at the county level to provide the first-hand information about the pilot of the comprehensive reform of county-level hospitals.

Training programs for the key doctors were carried on. The symposium on the training programs for the key doctors at the county-level hospitals was held in Xinjiang to exchange and summarize experience on carrying out the programs in 2010 and deploy work in 2011. *Management Measures for Training Key Doctors at County-level Hospitals (Draft for Soliciting Opinions)* was formulated to solicit opinions from all the localities and relevant units. Meanwhile, the program of Getting to the West for training health talents was carried on with 32 training workshops held in Guangxi, Hunan, Guizhou, Jiangxi and Yunnan etc. training 3,622 medical personnel and management personnel for hospitals.

The establishment of distance diagnostic system was pushed forward. With the help of the central finance, the Ministry of Health proceeded with the project of establishing the distance diagnostic system for the middle and west regions in 22 provinces (areas, municipalities) in the middle and west regions including Hebei, Shanxi, Inner Mongolia and Xinjiang Production and Construction Corps. On the basis of summarizing the work in 2010, *Plan for Establishing Distance Diagnostic System in 2011* was printed and issued to deploy work on the construction of distance diagnostic system in the middle and west regions. Work conference on distance diagnostic was held. Experts were organized to instruct and inspect 22 provinces (regions, municipalities) with the program and Xinjiang Production and Construction Corps as well as 12 hospitals affiliated to (administrated by) the Ministry of Health to urge all the localities to work well on the program.

Ⅲ. Supervision and management on medical quality and safety was strengthened

Firstly, *Measures for Supervision and Management of Medical Service (Draft for Soliciting Opinions)* was drafted, which defined the institutional system of supervision and management on medical service, the contents and requirement for supervision and management, supervision and management personnel and their duties and punishment etc. Secondly, norms for medical service were established. Experts were organized to draft *China's Guidance for Pilot of Grading Emergency Patients* to push forward the normalization for emergency departments. In order to improve diagnosis and treatment at the medical institutions at the grassroots level, the normalized diagnosis and treatment were started for 20 types of common diseases and the drafts of diagnosis norms for eight types of diseases were completed, i.e. bronchopneumonia, acute upper respiratory infection, chronic obstructive pulmonary disease, nodular goiter, inguinal hernia, acute appendicitis, acute pancreatitis, urinary calculus. Thirdly, guidance on medical conducts was strengthened. Focusing on normalized diagnosis and treatment of tumors, the Ministry of Health held the national work conference on the pilot of normalized diagnosis and treatment of common tumors at the county-level hospitals in Beijing on March 22, 2011, at which 23 hospitals in 15 national contact pilot cities for public hospital reform were selected to conduct pilot of normalized diagnosis and treatment of eight types of common tumors, i.e. lung cancer, liver cancer, gastric cancer, esophageal cancer, colorectal cancer, pancreatic cancer, breast cancer and cervical cancer. The assessment on the application of consultation specialists at the pilot hospitals and provincial consultation centers for distance consultation of tumor pathology was conducted and examination was organized for the 70 candidates of the pilot hospitals for the distance consultation of tumor pathology in late July, which meant the pilot of distance consultation of tumor pathology was formally launched. In mid October, work conference on the supervision and evaluation of pathology quality was held. Fourthly, methods for service supervision and management were perfected. *Interim Regulations on Reporting Events of Medical Quality and Safety* was formulated and promulgated. From May 1 on, the health administrative departments at various levels and various medical institutions at various levels nationwide started the on-line direct reporting system for events of medical quality and safety. Consequently, supervision and management on medical quality and safety were strengthened. Joint efforts were made with the industrial and commercial administrative departments to strengthen supervision and management on medical advertisements. Statistics were collected at regular intervals on the examination & certification of medical advertisements, surveillance on them and the punishment of illegal medical advertisements in all the localities. All the problems found were thoroughly investigated and the medical institutions that released fraud and illegal medical advertisements were punished by law.

The campaign of Safe Hospital was carried out and efforts were made to create harmonious doctor-patient relationship. The health system vigorously assisted the rectification on the violation and crimes of disturbing the security order at the medical institutions with remarkable achievements. The establishment of medical liability insurance was promoted throughout the nation as an important working mechanism for the construction of Safe Hospital and investigations and supervisory inspections on the medical liability insurance were made in Beijing and Zhenjiang in May and August 2011 respectively. In December, the Ministry of Health, the Office of CPC Comprehensive Administration Commission for Social Order, the Ministry of Public Security, the Ministry of Justice and China Insurance Regulatory Commission jointly held the national experience exchanging conference on handling medical disputes in Jingdezhen, Jiangxi Province.

IV. Examination, evaluation and supervision on hospitals were pushed forward

Examination and evaluation system was established. *Examination Criteria for Tertiary General Hospitals (2011 Edition), Examination Criteria for Tertiary Cardiovascular Hospitals, Children's Hospitals, Tumor Hospitals, Maternity Hospitals and Eye Hospitals (2011 Edition)* were compiled and issued together with the supportive document *Detailed Rules on Implementing Examination Criteria for Tertiary Comprehensive Hospitals (2011 Edition). Interim Measures for Hospital Examination* and *Measures for Administration of Expert Bank for Hospital Examining (trial edition)* were compiled and issued. Various measures were explored to evaluate hospitals, including the application of Patient-Oriented tracer methodology in hospital evaluation, spreading the use of DRGs to strengthen routine supervision and evaluation of hospitals and establish the long-term working mechanism of conducting patient satisfaction surveys by the third party. On the basis of hospital examination and evaluation, efforts were made to gradually push forward the construction of hospitals.

Inspections were made on large hospitals. By means of listening to reports and making on-site inspections, the first stage of inspections was made in eleven hospitals administrated by the Ministry of Health including Xiangya Hospital Central-South University, and Qilu Hospital Shandong University, etc. from the aspects of the public welfare of public hospitals, the development and construction of hospitals, medical service and hospital safety etc.

Supervision and administration on organ transplant techniques were strengthened.

Conferences were held to research and discuss human organs transplantation and the pilot of human organ donation at present. Vigorous efforts were made to coordinate the Legislative Affair Office of the State Council and other relevant departments to push forward the revision of *Regulations on Human Organ Transplantation.* Efforts were made to assist the China Red Cross Society to push forward human organ donation and communication conference on the pilot of human organ donation was jointly held. Training workshops were held on Chinese system of human organ distribution and share. Organ Donation Committee and Organ Procurement Organization were established. *Circular on Launching Pilot of Organ Transplant Deceased after Cardiac Death* was issued to further improve the working mechanism, plans and procedures of pilot of human organ donation and gradually establish the Chinese system of human organ donation. A special rectification was launched to severely crack down on the illegal human organ transplant by the non-organ-transplant medical institutions to intensify the detection of the non-organ-transplant hospital and the medial institutions at the grassroots level. National teleconference on the supervision and administration of human organ transplant was held to deploy relevant work and clarify that grading accountability would be carried out if illegal transplant occurred.

(Zhao Xuemei)

2. Pilot of Public Hospital Reform in 2011

Reform on major systems and mechanism were effectively pushed forward in the pilot cities. Separated supervision and operation were conducted in thirteen cities among the seventeen national contact pilot cities. The administration of the government on public hospitals was strengthened in all the localities by signing entrusted administration contracts or responsibility documents of comprehensive target administration, establishing the performance evaluation system with the orientation of public interests and establishing the corporate governance structure with the board of directors as the core. Four methods of separating medical service from medicine markups were explored and formed, i.e. reforming way of payments, lowering or canceling medicine markups by increasing financial investment or adjusting prices for medical services, practicing separate management on revenue and expenditure and establishing management centers for medicines independent from hospitals, and meanwhile policies for government funding were being improved gradually. Identification standards and administration system for the operation nature of medical institutions were perfected to attach more importance to developing qualified private medical institutions and strengthen the supervision and administration on them.

Measures providing convenience and benefits to people were widely adopted throughout the nation. All the localities endeavored to improve patients' medical experience by establishing the system of appointment service and the system of time-interval controlled appointment, providing excellent nursing care, adopting real time settlement of basic medical insurance, and pushing forward the campaign of Three Excellent and One Satisfaction (excellent service, excellent quality, excellent medical ethics, satisfaction from the patients). The problem of expensive medical service was alleviated by conducting the management of clinical pathways and mutual recognition of inspection results, launching the special rectification on antibacterial drugs and adopting comprehensive measures to rectify the soaring medical expenses. Compared with the same period in 2010, the outpatient expenses at the secondary and above public hospitals rose by 5.8% in comparative prices and 0.3% in current prices; the inpatient expenses rose by 5.3% in comparative prices and decreased by 0.1% in current prices. Therefore, the patient satisfaction improved significantly and they really benefited from the medical reform.

The adoption of the measures providing convenience and benefits to people also promoted the comprehensive reform of system and mechanism. In Shanghai, the prices of over 4,000 medical services were adjusted, which helped to rationalize the system of prices; in provinces like Anhui and Zhejiang, the provincial pricing departments delegated the authority of price adjustment. Among the 338 cities, 261 cities had established the performance evaluation system for hospitals, 185 cities had established the system for the selection and management of directors, and 152 cities had established the incentive and restraint mechanism for directors; 156 cities explored DRGs-based payment system, 94 cities explored capitation payment system, and 134 cities explored global budget payment system (some cities explored the co-existence of multiple payment systems).

The service system of public hospitals was improved. All the localities took measures such as building, removing, restoring and enlarging and integrating public hospitals to strengthen the capability construction in the weak areas and weak fields. The capability construction for regional medical centers was strengthened by constructing the key specialties, the development of county-level hospitals was given priority to by means of partner assistance and training for key doctors, and the service of urban and rural medical system was improved with the regional medical centers and county-level hospitals playing the leading role. Within the medical service system, the mechanism of division of labor between public hospitals and medical institutions at the grassroots level was established by means of establishing medical groups and medical complex, trusteeship, operation by the hospital and administrated by the hospital and technical collaboration etc.

The system of personnel management was reformed to motivate the medical personnel. The performance evaluation system was improved to various degrees in all the localities, the salaries were paid in accordance with the results of the evaluation and the payments of the clinical staff were increased; in cities like Wuhu and Zhenjiang etc, personnel posts were increased for public hospitals on the basis of rational calculation; special documents were promulgated on the normative training for resident doctors in eight pilot cities, among which Shanghai made it clear that normative training is indispensable for doctors to practice medicine; and multi-site practice by licensed practitioners was conducted to promote the rational turnover of medical personnel.

The pilot of comprehensive reform of county-level hospitals was pushed forward in all aspects. In 2011, deployments were made in 29 provinces (regions, municipalities) on pushing forward the pilot of comprehensive reform of county-level hospitals and the pilot had been officially launched in 18 provinces including Shanxi, Jiangsu and Zhejiang etc. with 561 pilot hospitals. In the majority of the pilot counties, the focus was on reforming compensation mechanism, strengthening capability construction and establishing the mechanism of division of labor and coordination.

(Zhao Xuemei)

3. Sino-French Communication and Cooperation on Public Hospital Reform

Sino-French cooperation on public hospital reform was pushed forward. The Ministry of Health, relevant officials from Talent Exchanging Center of the Ministry of Health (the Sino-French Collaborating Center for Health Professional Training) and the counselor of social affairs from the French Embassy and her entourage held a talk in Beijing to discuss the working plan in 2011 on Sino-French cooperation on public hospital reform. Two jobs were started after the meeting: Firstly, to assist the Ministry of Health in preparing for the Sino-French forum on public hospital reform to be held in April. Secondly, to decide on the Chinese cooperative hospitals for Sino-French Cooperation on Public Hospital Reform to select some public hospitals in the 16 national contact pilot cities to cooperate with the counterpart hospitals in France.

The seminar on Sino-French public hospital reform was jointly held by the Ministry of Health and France Ministry of Labor, Ministry of Employment and Ministry of Health. On April 19, 2011, the seminar on Sino-French public hospital reform was jointly held by the Ministry of Health and France Ministry of Labor, Ministry of Employment and Ministry of Health in Beijing. Ma Xiaowei, Vice Minister of Health, and Ms Nora Berra, French Health Secretary of the State, attended and addressed the seminar. The seminar was jointly hosted by Talent Exchanging Center of the Ministry of Health (the Sino-French Collaborating Center for Health Professional Training) and the Social Affairs Department from French Embassy. Communication and discussion were focused on topics like the programming of medical service, the governance and supervision on public hospitals, safety and quality of medical service and doctor-patient relationship and the payment system for medical service etc.

Cooperative partnership was established between 18 public hospitals in 16 pilot cities and 17 French hospitals. On April 19, 2011, program for the partnership of Sino-French public hospitals and the name list for the cooperative hospitals were announced at the seminar on Sino-French public hospital reform. Work was done to instruct the pilot cities to cooperate with relevant hospitals in France in conducting investigations, communication and discussion on the quality of medical service, promoting the progress in medical technology and promoting training of talents, etc.

(Zhao Xuemei)

4. Pilot of Human Organ Donation

Pilot of donated organ transplant deceased after cardiac death was launched. On April 26, 2011, the Ministry of Health launched the pilot of donated organ transplant decreased after cardiac death in accordance with the essence of the 8th session of Organ Transplant Committee of the Ministry of Health (herein after referred to as OTC). It was clearly demanded that qualified tertiary hospitals should obtain the qualification for undertaking transplant of donated organs deceased after cardiac death after being examined by OTC if they undertook a certain number of organ donations and accomplished correspondent transplant from May 2011 to May 2012. If the hospitals with the qualification failed to undertake transplant of donated organs deceased after cardiac death in the two years after the pilot ended, their qualifications for undertaking transplant would be canceled.

The national communication conference on the pilot of human organ donation was held. On March 10 and 11, 2011, the Ministry of Health and Red Cross Society of China jointly held the national communication conference on the pilot of human organ donation to further promote the pilot of human organ donation in our country and summarize and exchange experience in the past year since the pilot of human organ donation was launched. At the conference, we conscientiously summarized the experience of human organ donation from all the localities, analyzed the difficulties faced by the present work and made deployments on the work in the next stage.

The national training workshop for coordinators of human organ donation was held. From August 8 to 11, 2011, the Ministry of Health and Red Cross Society of China jointly held the national training workshop for coordinators of human organ donation in accordance with relevant requirements of the working plan for the pilot of human organ donation. Over 110 people attended the workshop including people in charge of Red Cross branches and the pilot hospitals for organ transplant and coordinators from 16 pilot provinces and cities for organ donation. Special investigations were made on the pilot work of human organ donation in Shandong and Shanghai etc.

China Organ Transplant Response System was put into use. In order to push forward the pilot of human organ donation actively and steadily, the Ministry of Health commissioned China Liver Transplant Registration Center to, on the basis of conducting research into international standards and relevant policies, formulate China Basic Principles for Human Organ Transplant Response and Policies for Liver, Kidney Transplant Response, in line of which China Organ Transplant Response System was developed. From April 6, 2011 when the response system was put into use till December 2, 2011, 51 organ donators of cardiac death were registered from 10 provinces nationwide (22 cases from Guangdong, 9 cases from Zhejiang, 7 cases from Guangxi, 6 cases from Jiangsu, 2 cases from Liaoning, 1 case from Hunan, 1 case from Shandong, 1 case from Sichuan, 1 case from Inner Mongolia, 1 case from Chongqing). 41 DCD livers and 66 DCD kidneys were allocated through the system.

The coverage of human organ donation pilot was expanded. In May 2011, the Ministry of Health and Red Cross Society of China jointly expanded the coverage of human organ donation pilot from some cities in Jiangsu, Fujian and Hubei to all the cities in these provinces and added Inner Mongolia, Jilin, Henan, Guangxi and Shanxi as new pilot provinces. Hence, there had been 16 pilot provinces for the pilot of human organ donation. By December 20, 158 cases of donation were achieved through the pilot of human organ donation (among which 46 cases were from Guangdong, 16 cases from Tianjin, 15 cases from Hunan, 13 cases from Zhejiang, 10 cases from Hubei, 10 cases from Liaoning, 11 cases from Guangxi, 6 cases from Shandong, 10 cases from Jiangsu, 8 cases from Jilin, 4 cases from Henan, 3 cases from Jiangxi, and 2 cases from Fujian), with 409 donations of large organs (among which 129 were livers, 272 kidneys, 4 hearts and 3 lungs).

Investigation and evaluation on the pilot of human organ donation were conducted. In late November 2011, the Ministry of Health and Red Cross Society of China jointly conducted investigation and evaluation on the pilot of human organ donation in the provinces (regions, municipalities) of Fujian, Zhejiang, Hunan, Tianjin, Liaoning, Jilin, Shandong, Jiangxi, Hubei, Jiangsu, Guangdong and Guangxi etc, to summarize the experience from the pilot and find out the problems. Consequently, the working modes for donation had primarily come into being, which laid a foundation for spreading organ donation throughout the whole country.

(Zhao Xuemei)

5. Revision of Regulation on Human Organ Transplant

With the progress of human organ donation, some clauses of *Regulation on Human Organ Transplant* (herein after referred to as *Regulation*) could no longer meet the need of present work. So in September 2010, the Ministry of Health started the revision of *Regulation.* After soliciting opinions from relevant departments and some experts on transplant and law, *Regulation on Human Organ Transplant (Amendment)(draft)* was formulated. The draft had been submitted to Legislative Affairs Office of the State Council. The draft clearly defined the duties of Red Cross Society for human organ donation, relevant requirements on the transplant of living organs and the legal responsibilities taken by the main officials of the hospital undertaking transplant. The draft provided legal protection for regulating human organ transplant and donation.

(Zhao Xuemei)

Chapter X Medical Education

1. Work of Medical Education in 2011

I. With focus on general practitioners, the work of standardized training for resident doctors was pushed forward

In cooperation with the Healthcare Reform Office of the State Council, the Ministry of Health formulated and issued *the Guiding Opinions of the State Council on the Establishment of the System of General Practitioner,* drafted and worked out the *Standards for Standardized Cultivation of General Practitioners* and jointly with the Degree Administration Office of the State Council, drafted and formulated *the Trial Measures for Master's Degree in Clinical Medicine (General Practice Medicine)* and made feasible schemes for linking resident doctors' standardized training with the system of master's degree in clinical medicine. Efforts were also made to assist the selection and construction of general practitioners' training bases.

The Ministry of Health organized the formulation of such documents as *the Guiding Opinions on the Establishment of the Training System for Resident Doctors, the Administrative Measures for Resident Doctors' Standardized Training* and the *Administrative Measures for the Assessment on Resident Doctors' Standardized Training* and perfected the training system, which laid a foundation for the implementation of the standardized training for resident doctors throughout the country. Work was also done to organize and work out project programs for resident doctors' standardized training.

II. Job-transfer training for general practitioners was organized and carried out.

Job-transfer training for general practitioners was promoted and *the Notice on Effectively Carrying out the Work of Job-Transfer Training for General Practitioners in 2011* was issued. The Central Finance invested 128.05 million RMB Yuan in the training and by the end of 2011, 18 thousand general practitioners were trained in all the localities.

III. Ordered, directional and free cultivation for rural medical students was organized and implemented

The Notice on Effectively Performing the Work of Ordered, Directional and Free Cultivation of Rural Medical Students in the Middle and Western Regions was issued and the work of compilation of plans for the requirement, enrollment and admission of free medical students and the signature of employment agreement was guided in all the localities so as to ensure the effective implementation of the cultivation task. 5,315 free medical students were admitted and cultivated in 2011 (including 1000 students majoring in traditional Chinese medicine)

IV. Management on continuing medical education was further regulated and strengthened

The Ministry of Health organized and worked out *the 12th Five-Year Plan for Continuing Medical Education and the Education Planning for Village Doctors (2011-2020),* organized experts to conduct re-evaluation on the development situations of the 11th Five-Year Plan for continuing medical education throughout the country and also organized experts to carry out examination and evaluation on the 6,831 state-level continuing medical education projects of 2012. The compilation of annual progress reports of continuing medical education on general practice medicine, tumor, imageology and cardio-angiology was organized.

V. Training for health personnel and relevant work were pushed forward comprehensively

In the light of the working mode of "integration of overall planning with classified management", the Ministry of Health took the lead in the overall planning of the Central Government's transfer payment for the project of training the personnel of the medical and health reform. 10 projects were set up for the training of health personnel in 2011 and the Central Finance invested 945 million RMB Yuan, about 1.5 million persons being trained. The Office of Teaching Materials of the Ministry of Health was organized and established.

VI. The National Conference on the Reform of Medical Education was held

The Ministry of Education and the Ministry of Health jointly held the National Working Conference on the Reform of Medical Education. Liu Yandong, State Councilor, made special instructions; Han Qi-de, Vice-Chairman of the Standing Committee of the National People's Congress attended the conference and delivered a speech and principal leaders of the Ministry of Education and the Ministry of Health made deployment for the work concerning how to promote medical education to better adapt to the medical and health reform and development.

(Zhao Yinghong)

2. Science and Technology Major Project of "Prevention and Treatment of AIDS, Viral Hepatitis and Other Major Serious Infectious Diseases" Was Organized and Implemented

The year 2011was a crucial year in which the 11th Five-Year Plan for science and technology major projects was summarized in an all-round way and the 12th Five-Year Plan was to be initiated and implemented. The Science and Technology Major Project of "Prevention and Treatment of AIDS, Viral Hepatitis and Other Major Serious Infectious Diseases" (hereinafter referred to as Project of Infectious Diseases) focused on key targets of lowering the morbidity and mortality of AIDS, viral hepatitis and tuberculosis and improving the capacity for emergency response and comprehensive prevention and control of newly-emerging and emergent infectious diseases, intensified top-level designs, paid attention to systemic integration, made efforts to innovate mechanisms and enhanced process management so as to enable the work in various respects to develop smoothly.

I. The formulation of the 12th Five-Year implementation plan was fulfilled.

In accordance with the comprehensive balance suggestions of the Ministry of Science and Technology and the National Development and Reform Commission, experts were organized to compile and revise the 12th Five-Year implementation plan for the project. The objectives of the 12th Five-Year implementation plan for the project were: firstly, to offer scientific and technologic support to the effective control of the epidemics of AIDA, viral hepatitis and tuberculosis and secondly, to heighten the capacity and level of the prevention, diagnosis, treatment and control of infectious diseases in an all-round way so as to do contribution for improvement of people's health level and guarantee of' the security of our country , the harmony and stability of the society and the sustainable development of the economy. Key tasks were to explore the patterns and mechanisms of the prevention and control of infectious diseases that were suitable to the situations of our country, obtain some breakthroughs and products in key technology, solve some bottleneck problems in the prevention and control of infectious diseases and in the development of relevant industries, promote the transformation and application of achievements of scientific research and cultivate a rationally structured and high-level researcher contingent.

II. The summary and evaluation on the 11th Five-Year planning tasks were accomplished.

According to the *Measures for the Administration of the Inspection and Acceptance of National Science and Technology Major Projects* and the principle of "being scientific, objective, open and impartial; relying on experts and conducting classified evaluation", the summary and evaluation schemes and classified evaluation standards were worked out. 188 subjects of the 11th Five-Year planning tasks were summarized and evaluated from the end of May to the middle of June, 2011 by three stages of the summary of research groups, the evaluation of experts in charge and the examination and approval of the group in charge of the project. Except 2 research subjects, the remaining 186 research subjects passed the evaluation. In general, the 11th Five-Year plan for the project was conducted well, key tasks in every respect being carried out smoothly and phased objective being realized basically.

III. Key tasks of the 12th-Five-Year-plan were arranged.

In the light of the 12th Five-Year plan for the project, the Ministry of Health attached more importance to the focal work, strengthened mechanic innovation and systemic integration, initiated the implementation of 6 subjects set up in 2011 and arranged 113 million RMB Yuan of funds for them. On the basis of the summary and evaluation of the 11th Five-Year plan and with focus on the landmark achievements, the Ministry of Health adopted the modes of ceaseless optimum selection, adjustment selection and top-down entrustment, held more than 40 conferences of the expert group, 4 conferences of the standing committee and 3 conferences of all the members of the group in charge of the project successively; 70 suggestions on the establishment of projects of 2012 were put forward and nearly 2.6 billion RMB Yuan of funds by the Central Finance were expected to arrange.

IV. Organizational management, systemic construction and process management were strengthened.

The Ministry of Health further perfected all-level executive and technologic managerial systems for the project, intensified the coordination of leading implementing sectors, set up and optimized internal coordinative mechanisms and unceasingly enhanced the construction of managerial contingents and the construction of systems for the project.

Management by objectives was enhanced. According the objectives and roadmap of the project, the Ministry of Health decomposed research tasks and key objectives in the management, clarified the timing, phased objectives and persons and institutions in charge and drew diagrams to show decomposed tasks and based on which the examination, supervisory guidance and evaluation were conducted.

Supervision and assessment were intensified. In accordance with the characteristics of different tasks of special research, technical platforms, demonstrative regions and product researches and development, classified management was carried out and supervisory guidance and assessment were conducted at regular intervals. The assessment and practice of online labs of emergency testing and monitoring of infectious diseases were strengthened and the introduction of the third-part independent assessment mechanisms was explored. The construction of security systems such as bio-safety, medical ethics, genetic resources and research integrity was enhanced and the system of "one-vote veto" was carried out. The management of demonstrative regions was taken as an important component of the co-construction of the Ministry of Health and each province and the results were closely connected with the assessment on relevant local health executive performances.

Innovation was also made in the modes of the organization of the key tasks. By open collection and the establishment of project bank, top-down planning for the project which was closely centering on key tasks was organized. By several rounds of experts' demonstration, implementation plans were perfected. Supporting resources and policies were coordinated to offer support and dynamic adjustment was carried out according to the development of the project.

V. Cooperative mechanisms for tackling key problems were perfected and transformation and application of scientific achievements were promoted.

Aiming at key tasks such as the construction of demonstrative regions, mechanisms were put forward to promote the achievements in scientific research to be timely applied in the demonstrative regions that intensified the coordination of the central and local governments, the organic linking between scientific researches and demonstrative regions and the evaluation on the demonstrative regions. Personnel of the group in charge of the project, the expert group responsible for demonstrative regions and administrative offices went to key demonstrative regions in provinces of Sichuan and Yunnan several times to do research and supervisory guidance, coordinated and solved problems. Schemes of unified clinical diagnosis, treatment and research of AIDS and other diseases in the demonstrative regions were revised; achievements suitable to be popularized were selected and the linking between the demonstrative regions and other research subjects was enhanced. Coordinative mechanisms were set up and concerted operation between tasks such as research on the prevention and treatment of infectious diseases and research and development of medicines was enhanced. For fulfilling the clinical research task of the morbidity and mortality from AIDS, hepatitis B and tuberculosis, unified research standards and technical regulations were formulated and research on the controlled treatment with traditional Chinese medicine and western medicine was particularly intensified, which further promoted the integrated level, relational degree and concertedness of various kinds of tasks with the integral multi-centered research pattern.

The exhibition tour of the national major achievements in scientific research in the 11th Five-Year-Plan period was organized and finished and on December 1, 2011, the 24th World AIDS Day, the progress and achievements in the scientific research of AIDS prevention and treatment were reported to Premier Wen Jiabao. Party and state leaders and the society spoke highly of and widely accepted the achievements gained in the 11th Five-Year plan for the project.

(Zhao Yinghong)

3. Entry-Exit Examination of Special Medical Articles in 2011

In January 2011, the Department of Medical Science, Technology and Education of the Ministry of Health organized the personnel concerned in key regions to hold the Symposium on the Entry-Exit Administration of Special Medical Articles, at which experience in different localities was exchanged and it was proposed that technical examination of special medical articles should be further regulated. In October, in response to the application of some enterprises in Shanghai for the entry-exit of special medical articles and after consultation with the State Administration of Quality Supervision, Inspection and Quarantine, the Ministry of Health issued *the Reply on the Relevant Issues Regarding the Transitional Measures on Enterprises' Application for the Entry-Exit Certificate of Special Medical Articles* which required, before submitted to the Ministry of Health for examination and verification, enterprises' entry-exit of special medical articles should be examined by provincial administrative departments in charge of the enterprises and health administrative departments and for the detailed requirements, the entry-exit administration of special medical articles could be consulted, but special application forms must be used. In December, on the basis of the extensive solicitation of opinions, the Ministry of Health revised the previous *Application Form for the Entry-Exit of Special Medical Articles and issued the Notice of the General Office of the Ministry of Health on Starting to Use the Application Form for the Entry-Exit of Special Medical Articles.* According to the statistics, the exit of 51 batches and the entry of 432 batches of special medical articles and 71 scientific and technologic cooperative projects of genetic resources conducted by the institutions affiliated to the Ministry of Health were examined all together in 2011.

(Zhao Yinghong)

4. Working Progress of the Personnel Exchange Center of the Ministry of Health

4-1. Project of Tobacco Control of the China Medical Board

In April 2011, the Personnel Exchange Center of the Ministry of Health (hereinafter referred to as the Personnel Center) applied to the China Medical Board for the training project of smoking control for health administrative cadres in four provinces (autonomous regions of China) which was approved. Under the guidance of the Ministry of Health, the Personnel Center organized the experts from the Chinese Center for Disease Control and Prevention, the China Health Education Center (the News and Publicity Center of the Ministry of Health), the Collaborating Centre for Tobacco Control of the World Health Organization, the Chinese Association on Tobacco Control and other organizations to design the training courses systematically and held a series of training courses in Shandong Province, Henan Province, Tibet Autonomous Region and Xinjiang Uygur Autonomous Region. Most trainees were leaders of the health department of these provinces (autonomous regions), members of the leading groups of prefectures, counties and districts and leaders of the health bureau and up to 1,200 persons participated in the training courses. The training contents included the framework and development of the conventions on tobacco control, the interpretation of policies on tobacco control, the implementation of the construction of smoke-free medical institutions and the exchange of the experience. By participating in the training, the administrative cadres of health sectors in these four provinces (autonomous regions) deepened their understanding of our country's policies on tobacco control, improved the capacity for the execution and management and accumulated the experience for the creation of a sound environment for carrying out the long-term work of tobacco control at the grassroots level.

(Zhao Yinghong)

4-2. China-Australia Training Project of the Essential Drug System

In order to further keep abreast of the construction of international medical and health service systems, the foreign health systems and the formulation of drug policies, the Personnel Exchange Center of the Ministry of Health undertook the China-Australia Training Project of the Essential Drug System and in December 2011, finished the organization of the training in Australia for drug administrators, 23 directors of drug administrative department from provinces (autonomous regions, cities) of Hunan, Hubei, Xinjiang, Gansu, Liaoning, Shandong and so on participating in all the training courses.

The University of Sydney, Australia, engaged high-quality teachers and from the perspectives of politics, economy, society and management and by means of introduction to theories, comparative studies, case analyses, site inspection and classroom interaction, teachers and trainees analyzed and discussed key and difficult issues in Australian medical treatment, health and security. They were also arranged to go to numerous drug stores and hospitals for inspection and study and also communicated with the governmental health administrative personnel of the Department of Health and Ageing, staff of the Australia Medical Association and other agencies on the formulation and enforcement of drug policies and other issues concerned. The *Pharmaceutical Benefits Scheme of Australia* written by the training class to introduce the advanced system of the Australian pharmaceutical benefits scheme was published in the *Trends of Deepening the Reform of the Medical and Health System (Journal 188),* which offered reference to our country's reform in the medical and health system.

(Zhao Yinghong)

Chapter XI Medical Science and Technology

1. 2011 Work on Medical Science and Technology

I. The organization and implementation of major scientific projects were pushed forward

The summary and evaluation of the subject of the 11th Five-Year Plan of major S&T special projects were carried out. In accordance with the tasks and targets of the 11th Five-Year Plan of two major scientific projects, experts were organized to perform summary and evaluation for infectious diseases and new drugs. Overall, these two special projects were carried out better, with each key task going well and stage targets basically achieved. In the special project of infectious diseases, the scientific support system with the characteristic of new-type whole-nation system was initially established. A number of key techniques and products were obtained to provide support for effective reduction of "three diseases, two rates". With remarkable improvement in the emergency capacity of emerging, emergent infectious diseases, the organization implementation mechanism suitable for the characteristics of the special projects was initially established. In the special project of new drugs, a number of innovative drugs were studied and developed with quantity targets overfulfilled and the quality of some types considerably enhanced. The innovative system of drugs of our country was initially established while the innovative capacity of enterprise technique was improved. A number of key technical breakthroughs were obtained. A set of new-type management mechanism was initially established.

The 12th Five-Year Plan for the special projects was worked out and launched. In accordance with the latest trend of science and technology in related fields at home and abroad, and the implementation plan of two special projects, the implementation plan for the special projects in the period of the 12th Five-Year Plan was worked out and was approved by the leader's group of the two special projects and three departments. According to the work thinking of the implementation plan, the focal points were highlighted further. With the mechanism innovation and system integration strengthened, the implementation of 2011 projects approved and initiated was completed, so was the organization of 2012 projects approved and initiated.

The coordination and system construction were strengthened. Administrative systems and technical management systems at all levels for two special projects were further improved. With the coordination of implementation departments strengthened, the internal coordination mechanisms of the Ministry of Health were improved. Full-time deputy directors were appointed for the two special projects and special branches were set up. Professional staff of implementation management office was reaffirmed. The ministerial coordination group and work group for the demonstration area were established for the special project of infectious diseases. The combination with disease control and prevention was strengthened. The implementation of technical management responsibility for the special project of new drugs was strengthened. The team construction of responsible experts was intensified. Aimed at candidate drugs and technical innovation, the corresponding public relation coordination group was established according to drug category, disease type and direction of key techniques. As a result, researches on different technical routes were conducted in a collaborative way under the unified deployment. The implementation management office of two special projects constantly strengthened and improved the system construction of special project system. *Administrative Measures for Major Special Projects and Administrative Measures for the Subjects of Major Special Projects* were revised. Such supportive documents as the implementing rules for the management of major special intellectual property were improved. To raise the level of standardized management, such internal management documents as *Service Regulations of Office* was formulated. Based on the characteristics of different tasks, the indexes of examination and evaluation as well as the examination panel point were set. *An Administrative Manual of Subject Process* was worked out.

Funds management was strengthened. The first was to conduct trainings for budgeting and financial management to further improve the quality of budgeting. The second was to accelerate the report and appropriation of funds use plan. The subject organizations were guided to improve the system of financial management and perfect the internal control system and supervision mechanism. The third was to coordinate the department of financial management to complete the funds reimbursement and funds approval for duty-free imports. We also coordinated with the State Auditing Administration to carry out the key audit to strengthen constantly the funds regulation. Meanwhile, aiming at the problems found in the process management, we coordinated with the issue of *A Circular of the General Office of the Ministry of Health on Further Strengthening the Funds Management of Major Scientific Special Projects* to further perfect the regulatory mechanism of funds. *An Outline of State Mid and Long-Term Talent Development* was carried out. As a result, the Thousand Person Plan implemented for two special projects attracted dozens of overseas high-level talents. Meanwhile with the special task as the carrier, needed talents were introduced through other channels and ways.

II. Revolving around the industry needs, the planning guide and project implementation were strengthened

The 12th Five-Year Plan for the development of medical science and technology was worked out and issued. We worked out and issued *The 12th Five-Year Plan for the Development of Medical Science and Technology* with the Ministry of Science and Technology and nine other ministries, which made clear the guiding ideology, basic principle, strategic targets and key tasks for the next five years' development of medical science. Besides six key tasks were put forward, based on which *The Development Plan for Health Science in the Period of the 12th Five-Year Plan was drawn up.*

The special project of scientific research for health industry was carried out. The policy of industry needs was adhered to with the orientation of research and development, integration, transformation, transfer, promotion and application of mid- and lower-level technique. Top-level design and overall planning were highlighted. Therefore the organization and operating mode of close contact needs, effective integration of resources and open to combination. In 2011, the project bank was established based on the key tasks and need of medical reform, and experts were organized to conduct research for demonstration with 24 projects put forward.

The acceptance and implementation of scientific support project were completed. In 2011, the acceptance and summary of 15 projects including "key techniques of food safety" were completed. The research findings of some of the projects played an important supporting role in health work. For example, the project of "prevention, early diagnosis and comprehensive treatment and study of common malignant tumors" provided technical support for the gradual turning of health resources to preventive interventions and early diagnosis and early treatment. The project of "key techniques and product development of major digital medical equipment holds greater realistic significance to the development of independent intellectual property products, the promotion of development of domestic medical devices industry and turning around the situation of medical equipment dependent on imports. In accordance with the *12th Five-Year Plan for the Development of Medical Science and Technology,* in three areas of "population health, public safety and modern service industry", 15 projects of sci-tech support plan for the 12th Five-Year Plan were demonstrated, including malignant transformation and comprehensive research of prevention and control, and researches on the new techniques and new approaches of malignancy diagnosis and treatment, and researches on key technique of the prevention and control of major mental diseases. Besides the report, feasibility demonstration and implementation plan of these projects were completed, and so was the compilation of project budget book with the funds from the central treasury of approximately 0.9 billion RMB Yuan.

The organization of other scientific research project was completed. According to related requirements of the Ministry of Science and Technology, the proposals, reports, approval and process management of such subjects as "973" plan, "863" plan, special scientific project of scientific research institutions, project of soft science and special project of basic scientific research. Especially for close contact with the construction of medical reform informationization, 17 subjects were organized and implemented, like "the project of development of digital medical engineering technique" under "863" plan. We positively coordinated with and organized related scientific research power of health system to conduct the organization of the systemic subject of health application in the civil part of major special project of high resolution earth observation. The assessment and organization of scientific research fund subject of the Ministry of Health conducted jointly by the Ministry of Health, Zhejiang and Henan, which promoted the improvement of the capacity of local scientific research and development.

III. Technical management and popularization went smoothly and related system construction was strengthened

The first was to explore new management mode of clinical research of medical high technology. On the basis of extensive survey and research and soliciting opinions from all sides, we organized and worked out *Guiding Principles for Clinical Research Management of Medical High Technology (Exposure Draft)*, which standardized the conduct of clinical research of medical high technology. Studying and discussing the problems and countermeasures in the assessment study of health technique of our country, we worked out *A Guide to Health Technique Assessment (First Draft).* Coordinating with related departments, we drafted *A Plan for Clinical Research on Stem Cells and Application Specification Rectification* and took the lead in carrying it out. In addition, we issued *A Circular on Self-examination and Self-correction for Clinical Research and Application of Stem Cells* and started relevant work. The second was to explore the establishment of effective mechanism for appropriate popularization of health technique. With appropriate popularization mechanism of health technique and related policy researches completed, we issued the compilation of research data to related organizations and personnel in various localities for reference. With the popularization of appropriate health technique held positively, training workshops for technique popularization of emergent first-aid, screening tests for cervical cancer and breast cancer and basic diagnosis of cardiovascular disease were held in Jiangxi, Guizhou and Sichuan. The third was to push forward the regulation of intellectual property. We took the lead in working out the plan for special operation of cracking down on infringing, fake and low-quality commodities in health industry, and we coordinated with related departments to push forward the implementation of every task. We also carried out publicity, popularization and training of The National Intellectual Property Strategy Compendium, and studied and worked out the guiding opinions on the management of intellectual property of health field. The communication class of ethics board under medical institutions was held to promote capacity and system constructions of the ethics boards of various institutions. The fourth was to strengthen the examination and approval of exit and entry of medical special items. In coordination with General Administration of Quality Supervision, Inspection and Quarantine, we made clear the verification procedure of exit and entry of biological products declared by enterprises, which facilitated the enterprises' declaration while strengthening the regulation.

IV. The management of laboratory biosafety and base construction were strengthened

The first was to carry out the prevention and control of imported poliomyelitis in Xinjiang Uygur Autonomous Region and the management of laboratory biosafety related to Shenzhen Universiade and Xi'an Garden Expo. The second was to preserve bacterial and viral strains of pathogenic microorganism and draw up *A Planning for Preservation Organizations.* The third was to organize and conduct trainings, supervision and inspections a number of times for laboratory biosafety. The review and reevaluation for the qualification of class III biosafety laboratories were conducted as prescribed. The fourth was to commission Chinese Academy of Medical Sciences (CAMS) to complete the evaluation for 65 key laboratories of the Ministry of Health. The fifth was to establish two national key laboratories approved by the Ministry of Science and Education, and national engineering laboratory for digital stomatology approved by National Development and Reform Commission (NDRC). The sixth was to conduct regulation for qualification authentication and examination accreditation. *Teaching Material for Quality Management and Safety of Health Testing Laboratories and A Work Guideline for Qualification Authentication of Food Inspection Agencies* were compiled. With trainings for quality management of laboratories conducted many times, the review panel of health industry completed field review and examination for qualification authentication of laboratories of 23 health testing agencies in 2011.

(Shan Yongxiang)

2. The Progress of Implementation for Major Scientific Project of "Major New Drugs Development"

The year 2011 was the first year for comprehensive summary of the achievements of major scientific projects in the "Twelfth Five-year Plan" period. The leading departments of major scientific project of "major new drugs development", namely the Ministry of Health and Health Bureau of PLA General Logistics Department, seriously carried out the guiding spirits of the leaders of the State Council on strengthening the combination of special projects with medical reform to form fighting capability of large troop formation. According to the strengthening of strategic study and clarification of key task orientation put forward by the supervision and evaluation group, they centered on the targets of livelihood guarantee and medicine industry promotion. Priority was given to the cultivation of major products, met needs of importance and resolve of key problems. Besides the implementation mechanism was innovated, top-level design was paid attention to and system integration was intensified. The purpose was to further centralize national targets and highlight further the key tasks.

I. The implementation plan for the 12th Five-Year Plan was revised and perfected

Based on the comprehensively balanced opinions of National Development and Reform Commission (NDRC) and the Ministry of Science and Technology, we organized experts to centralize targets and highlight the key points for the completion of the compilation and revision of the implementation plan of the special projects for the 12th Five-Year Plan. For the overall targets of the special projects for the 12th Five-Year Plan, the first was to provide support for the safeguard and improvement of livelihood. The second was to promote effectively the rapid development of pharmaceutical industry, speed up the transformation of our country's pharmaceutical science and technology from copying to creation, and push forward the transformation of our country's pharmaceutical industry from big country of pharmaceutical industry to great power of pharmaceuticals. Key tasks were: through the establishment and perfection of the country's innovative system of drugs, the construction of a number of development platforms and industrialization bases was strengthened; key techniques of new drug development and industrialization were mastered; and the species of major drugs with a promoting effect on livelihood safeguard and promotion of industry development were created. The special project for the 12th Five-Year Plan will be deployed in five areas based on the implementation plan: research and development of innovative drugs, technical transformation for major species, construction of technical platform, enterprise incubators and key techniques.

II. Summary and evaluation were conducted to sort out symbolic achievements

As required by *Administrative Measures for National Acceptance of Special Scientific Projects,* we studied and worked out the summary and evaluation plan and clarified the classified assessment indexes. In June, 2011, summary and evaluation were conducted for 631 subjects of the task for the 11th Five-Year Plan approved in 2008 and 2009. Through this work, the progress of the special project for the 11th Five-Year Plan was further understood and symbolic achievements were sorted out, which laid a good foundation for 2012 subject establishment of the 12th Five-Year Plan.

III. 2012 subject establishment was organized, and 2012 implementation plan for the special projects was compiled and examined

The organization of 2012 subject establishment was carried out in three ways. The first was to organize experts for top-level design. They present solutions, integrated power; with full demonstration, they entrusted directionally major innovative subjects from the bottom-up. The second was to selectively support some subjects which were carried out better. The third was to publicize the guide and selectively choose some newly added subjects. Accordingly 2012 implementation plan for the special project was compiled and examined. In accordance with the opinions of the office of leaders' group for the special project of new drugs, coordination group for major special projects and, the joint conference of the first administrators and technical leaders, we revised many times the implementation plan which passed the examination of the leaders' group meeting for the special projects.

IV. The top-level and classified management of subjects were strengthened to promote collaborative innovation

Based on the principle of "highlighting focal points and system integration", with major innovative species as the principal line and according to "major products", "important needs" and "key problems", we further strengthened top-level design and promoted system integration.

To further highlight the key points, we made clear such key tasks as major innovative species, the construction of public resources platform and the construction of comprehensive platform, on the basis of original five major tasks of the special projects. Exploring the whole-nation system of new type, we held the symposium on the implementation of key tasks for the 12th Five-Year Plan, the meeting on the demonstration of major species, symposium on the platform of public resources and discussion on experts' demonstration. We held the meeting on such subjects as bio-medical park, platform of laboratory animals, which promoted the implementation of subjects. We also coordinated the industry-university-research alliance of the special project of new drugs to connect with the comprehensive platform, which provided support and coordination for holding the achievement fair, and effectively promoted the transformation and the combination of industry-university-research of the achievements of special projects.

(Shan Yongxiang)

Chapter XII Food and Drug Supervision & Administration

1. Food and Drug Supervision & Administration in 2011

I. Good working was done on the major special work concerning the overall situation.

Firstly, active efforts were made to include the contents of "safeguarding food and drug safety" into the outlines of national general plan, which provided solid basis for the subsequent work. We took lead in compiling *National Program for Drug Safety (2011-2015)*, which had been discussed and approved by the State Council executive meeting. We participated in compiling more than ten relevant plans including *National Program for Basic Public Service System (2011-2015), National Program for Supervision & administration System of Food Safety (2011-2015), and Program for Construction of Vaccine Supply System*, which reflected the contents concerning food and drug supervision & administration from multiple aspects. More than 20 provinces (regions, municipalities) also succeeded in including food and drug safety into the special plans of the governments. Secondly, supervision & administration on the quality of essential drugs were implemented. The rise and promulgation of standards for essential drugs were fulfilled. Sampling-inspections covering all types of drugs were implemented. Electronic supervision & administration were conducted on all the essential drugs taking part in the bidding. The construction of monitoring system for adverse drug reaction at the prefectural level was completed. Full coverage of supervision and inspection was implemented on the manufacturers and distributors of essential drugs. Thirdly, special rectifications on food and drug safety were conducted. The violations of laws and regulations to illegally add and abuse food additives were severely cracked down on and special rectifications on school canteens and clenbuterol hydrochloride, with 7,133 cases meted out administrative penalties. We participated in the comprehensive rectifications on Recycled Gutter Oil, Plasticizer and alcohol etc. so that the food safety orders of catering service were further regulated. The two-year-long special rectification on drug safety was accomplished, during which special actions were taken to intensively crack down on infringing intellectual rights and producing and selling fake and counterfeit commodities. Cooperating with the departments of industry and information, public security, supervision, finance, commerce, health, customs, industry and commerce and traditional Chinese medicine etc. we cracked down on the production and sale of fake drugs, which effectively purified food and drug markets.

II. Routine supervision & administration on food and drug were strengthened.

The supervision & inspection and investigation & evaluation on the key sites and key types of products were strengthened and 86,000 sampling inspections were fulfilled. The demonstration projects of food safety for catering services were launched and 117 provincial demonstration counties were selected. Supervision & administration on health food products and cosmetics were strengthened. The management systems of examining the material suppliers etc. were implemented, focusing on the supervision & administration on materials of propolis, donkey-hide gelatin and pear powder etc. The pilot of qualified person for manufacturers was carried out. Special exanimations on formula technique were organized. Illegal labeling was rectified. Besides, surveillance on safety risks was carried out. Remarkable progress was made in the construction of demonstration counties for drug safety. The implementation of the newly revised GMP was pushed forward effectively and 154 drug manufacturers had passed the certification examination. Supervision & administration on the high risk products such as vaccines were strengthened. Special examinations on narcotic drugs and psychotropic drugs were made to standardize the production and management of compound preparations of ephedrine. Illegal advertisements were rectified, with the sales of illegal products suspended 994 times and 61 approval numbers for advertisement canceled or recalled. *Good Manufacturing Practice for Medical Devices (GMP)* was implemented for the manufacturers of sterile and implantable medical devices and the special inspections were conducted on the management system of production and quality of products such as dialysis products, intravascular stents and allergenic bones etc. The action plan for popularizing knowledge on food and drug safety was implemented. Safeguarding food and drug safety was successfully provided for the major events such as Universiade, World Horticultural Exposition, China-Eurasia Expo, China ASEAN Expo and National Games for Ethnic Minorities etc. as well as the major holidays and festivals.

III. Food and drug supervision & administration were improved.

Firstly, the construction of legislation was further strengthened. Regulations and normative documents were formulated and revised such as *Good Manufacturing Practice for Drugs, Provisions for Medical Device Recall, Provisions for Adverse Drug Reaction Reporting and Monitoring, Measures for Drug Supervision and Administration in Medical Institutions (for trial implementation), Examination Standards for License of Central Kitchen, Operating Standards for Food Safety in Catering Services and Requirements for Record Keeping of Domestic Non-Special* Cosmetics etc, which legally ensured supervision & administration. Secondly, the construction of responsibility system was accelerated. The pilot of evaluating the responsibility system for drug safety was implemented, which covered 15 provinces (regions, municipalities), 385 counties, to explore and establish a set of comparatively complete index system of evaluation. Performance evaluations on food safety supervision in catering services were conducted. Valuable experience was accumulated on motivating the local governments and ensuring supervisory resources at the grassroots etc. Thirdly, the construction of technical support system was strengthened. The examination and approval capabilities for health food, cosmetics, drugs and medical devices were improved and the team construction for examination experts was strengthened. Primary achievements were made in the division of authority for the supplementary application for drug registration, the evaluation of drug packaging materials and the lot release for biological products. The compilation of *Chinese Pharmacopoeia (2015 edition)* progressed smoothly, with the approval of scientific research projects and the selection of pharmaceutical products accomplished. The formulation and revision of standards for 150 medical devices were conducted. The program of equipping testing devices and equipment for catering services, health food and cosmetics was implemented, which meant the further improvement of inspection and testing system. The capabilities of supervisory evaluation and risk pre-warning were improved. The construction of risk control system and adverse response monitoring system was accelerated. Fourthly, the process of internationalization for supervision & administration was pushed forward. For the first time, on-site inspections were conducted on drug production by manufacturers abroad. Drug supervision officials were sent abroad to implement relevant bilateral cooperation agreements. International communication and cooperation were carried out vigorously and China-ASEAN Drug Safety Forum & Conference for Commissioners of Drug Administration was held successfully. We successfully got WHO approval for vaccine regulatory system, which was a historic achievement for the internationalization of our drug supervision & administration.

IV. Construction of supervisory & administrative system was strengthened.

Firstly, the campaign of Excelling in Work and Safeguarding Food and Drug Safety was carried on and the effectiveness and cohesiveness of the party groups at the grassroots level were further enhanced, embodied by a large number of advanced groups and individuals represented by Shi Junqin, and Gao Liqin etc. Secondly, the team construction was intensified. The transition of the functions for food safety supervision in catering services was finished by food and drug administrations in

28 provinces (regions, municipalities) and the transition of functions for supervision on health food and cosmetics was finished in 31 provinces (regions, municipalities). Thirdly, *National Medium and Long-term Plan for Development of Food and Drug Supervision & Administration Talents (2010-2020)* was formulated. Reform of personnel system for cadres was deepened, and public selection and taking up a job through competition were intensified so that more attention was paid to selecting cadres from the grassroots. Training Program for Top Leaders at Grassroots was carried out, i.e. rotational training was implemented for the members of the leading bodies of the provincial food and drug administrations, the chief officials of administrative supervisory organs at the prefectural and county levels and the chief officials of technical supervisory organs at the provincial and prefectural levels. The construction of licensed pharmacist team was strengthened. Fourthly, the construction of the system for punishing and preventing corruption was promoted with great efforts. Supervision and inspection on leaders'clean practice in work were strengthened, integrity risk control was conducted and the construction of the system of combating corruption and building a clean government was strengthened. Consequently, a number of cases violating laws and disciplines were severely punished, which provided political safeguard for food and drug supervision & administration.

(Zhao Xuemei)

2. A State Council Executive Meeting Approved *National Program for Drug Safety (2011-2015)*

On December 7, Premier Wen Jiabao chaired a State Council executive meeting, at which *National Program for Drug Safety (2011-2015)* was discussed and approved. *The Program* clarified the overall objectives and key tasks for drug safety in the Twelfth Five-Year Plan period. By 2015, all drug manufacturing should meet the requirements of the newly revised *Good Manufacturing Practice for Drugs*, drug safety would improve greatly and people would be more satisfied with drug safety. The main tasks are: (1) National standards should be improved. Efforts should be made so that the national standards for pharmaceutical chemicals and biological products conform to the international standards and the national standards for Chinese traditional medicines take lead in formulating the international standards. (2) Drug control system should be completed. The construction of national drug control institutions should be strengthened, the labs of provincial and prefectural drug control institutions should be improved and the capability of rapid testing should be enhanced at the county-level institutions. (3) Total quality control should be strengthened on drugs and medical devices. Standards for drug research should be perfected so as to conform to the international standards. The coverage of on-site supervision and inspection on clinical trials should be improved. The tracing system for the circulation of Chinese traditional medicinal materials should be established to promote the standard production of common Chinese traditional medicinal materials. The construction of informationization for supervision & administration should be sped up, i.e. coding management should be conducted on all the drugs approved of entering the market and electronic supervision & administration should cover all types of drugs. (4) Safety monitoring and pre-warning should be strengthened. The monitoring system for adverse drug reaction and drug abuse should be improved, and the post market re-evaluation system for drugs should be completed, with the focus on monitoring and evaluating the safety of new drugs, TCM injections and high-risk drugs. Emergency pre-plans should be improved to ensure the timely and efficient supply of emergency drugs. (5) The manufacturing and supplying of national essential drugs should be improved to ensure their quality, safety, equity and availability. (6) The long-term mechanism for the supervision & administration of drug safety should be established. The pricing mechanism of drugs, the policies for concentrated procurement and the mechanism of drug sampling should be improved and the mechanism of recalling drugs with problems or drugs driven off the market should be completed. The evaluation of credit rating for drug enterprises should be conducted and the integrity files for enterprises should be established to deprive those who violate rules or discredit themselves of the access to the industry. Sales of counterfeit and substandard drugs should be severely cracked down on by law. (7) Reform should be deepened and legislation should be improved. Reform on the administrative approval system for drugs should be deepened to adopt stricter standards and regulate procedures. The system and mechanism of drug law enforcement should be innovated to enhance supervision on law enforcement. The circulation orders of drugs should be regulated and the circulation links should be deduced. The formulation and revision of laws and regulations concerning drug administration should be accelerated.

(Zhao Xuemei)

Chapter XIII Management of the Undertaking of Traditional Chinese Medical Science and Medicines

1.Work of Traditional Chinese Medical Science and Medicines in 2011

I. The position of the traditional Chinese medical science and medicines in economic and social development was heightened

Support to the development of the traditional Chinese medical science and medicines was listed out as a separated chapter in the *Outline of the 12th Five-Year Plan for National Economic and Social Development of the People's Republic of China (hereinafter referred to as the National Outline of the 12th Five-Year Plan)*and it was one of the six key tasks in "the perfection of the basic medical and health system"; meanwhile, the traditional Chinese medical science and medicines was also included in the part of "optimization of the structure of foreign trade" and "maintenance of Hong Kong's long-term prosperity and stability". The traditional Chinese medical science and medicines was taken as an important component of the energetic enhancement of science and technology for people's livelihood in both *the National 12th Five-Year Plan for Scientific and Technologic Development and the 12th Five-Year Plan for the Development of Medical Science and Technology* and the talent engineering of inheritance and innovation was regarded as one of five major ones in *the Medium- and Long-Term Program for the Development of Medical and Health Talents* (2011-2020). Formulation of the *Five-Year Plan for the Development of the Undertaking of the Traditional Chinese Medical Science and Medicines* was fulfilled and organization of the implementation was started and some key projects such as the construction of service capacity of hospitals of traditional Chinese medicine and ethnic minority medicine were carried out also. Special programs on the informationization, standardization, innovation in science and technology, cultural construction and foreign exchange and cooperation were fulfilled or being worked out. Formulation and implementation of the 12th Five-Year Plan for the development of the traditional Chinese medical science and medicines were promoted smoothly in all the localities; level of the formulation was heightened in considerable number of localities and support to the development of the traditional Chinese medical science and medicines was increased greatly; for example, Shanghai and some other localities listed the program on development of the traditional Chinese medical science and medicines into provincial or municipal special programs for the first time; Inner Mongolian Autonomous Region listed the infrastructure construction of the hospitals of traditional Chinese medicine and Mongolian medicine in all the cities and counties into the 12th Five-Year plan of the autonomous region;

Liaoning Province allocated 45 million RMB Yuan of special funds to the support of the development of the traditional Chinese medical science and medicines in 2011 and planned continuous investment in the 12th Five-Year-Plan period and Hubei Province strengthened the infrastructure construction of the hospitals of traditional Chinese medicine in all the localities.

II. The role of the traditional Chinese medical science and medicines in the medical and health reform was brought into play

In 2011, the Ministry of Health and the State Administration of Traditional Chinese Medicine jointly issued *the Opinions on further Play the Role of Traditional Chinese Medicine in Deepening the Reform of Medical and Health System (hereinafter referred to as the Opinion)* which made comprehensive deployment on how to play the role of the traditional Chinese medical science and medicines and strengthen the talent cultivation in the five key tasks of the in-depth reform of the medical and health system.

In the construction of the basic medical security system, more attention was paid to the encouragement of the provision and use of the service of the traditional Chinese medical science and medicines. Increase in the compensatory percentage required by the new rural cooperative medical system further mobilized farmers' enthusiasm for the use of the traditional Chinese medical science and medicines and enabled them to reap the benefits. Henan Province issued *the Circular on Relevant Issues concerning the Guidance and Encouragement of the Use of Traditional Chinese Medical Service in the Basic Urban Medical Insurance.* The number of the service items of traditional Chinese medicine and the categories and numbers of traditional Chinese medicines that was brought into the coverage of payment by the medical insurance were increased unceasingly and most provinces (autonomous regions, cities) explicitly defined that Chinese herbal preparations were brought into the range of payment.

In the construction of the essential drug system, the principle of putting equal stress on traditional Chinese medicine and western medicine was adhered to and importance was attached to encouraging the use of traditional Chinese medicines. 102 kinds of Chinese patent drugs and the Chinese traditional medical herbal pieces with promulgated national standards were listed into *the National Essential Drug List (for provision and use of grassroots medical and health institutions).* All the localities actively promoted the supplement of the kinds of traditional Chinese medicines to the additional essential drug lists and a great number of localities added more kinds of traditional Chinese medicines than western medicines; the addition accounted for nearly 62% in Guizhou Province and the added drugs were mainly ethnic drugs in

Tibet and other ethnic minority regions.

In the work of the equalization of public health service, application of preventive and healthcare techniques and methods of traditional Chinese medicine was actively pushed forward. *The National Basic Public Health Service Norms (2010)* newly added the requirements of traditional Chinese medical service for child health care, specified the demands for the health management of the patients with hypertension and type 2 diabetes, formulated technical regulations on the health management of children, pregnant and puerperal women, old people and patients with hypertension and diabetes, meanwhile, initiated the pilot project of the basic public health service of traditional Chinese medicine. Gansu Province set up the department of traditional Chinese medicine in all the institutions of disease prevention and control, took "preventive treatment of diseases" of traditional Chinese medicine as a basic public health service item and required that the contents concerning traditional Chinese medicine should be no less than 20% and 10% respectively in residents' health records and health education. A special fund of 10 RMB Yuan per capita was allocated to TCM identification of constitution for old people over the age of 55 in Qingdao City of Shandong Province; Shijiazhuang City of Hebei Province required that no less than 10% of the funds of public health service projects should be allocated to the traditional Chinese medical science and medicines and in Gongshu District of Hangzhou City, Zhejiang Province, 10 RMB Yuan of the total 25 RMB Yuan of public health funds was specially for each person's payment of TCM service items.

In the construction of urban and rural grassroots medical and health service systems, attention was paid to the improvement of the accessibility to traditional Chinese medical service. 382 county-level TCM hospitals were reconstructed and standardization was promoted in the construction of the department of traditional Chinese medicine and the dispensary of traditional Chinese medicines in a great number of township and community health care centers. 13 prefecture-level and above cities including Beijing, Shanghai, Tianjin, Hangzhou, etc. and 139 counties (cities, districts) won the honorary title of "national grassroots (rural, community) advanced unit in the work of the traditional Chinese medical science and medicines". Achievements were gained in the exploration of unified management of county-level, township and village rural work of the traditional Chinese medicine and medicines (ethnic minority medical science and medicines) in provinces of Anhui and Heilongjiang and autonomous regions of Guangxi and Inner Mongolia; Yunnan Province allocated 12.3 million RMB Yuan to the provision of medical equipment for 4,100 village clinics; all the township health care centers in Hubei Province conducted the construction of *"san tang yi shi"("san tang":guo yi tang:*place for national honored great TCM masters practicing medicine; *ming yi tang:* place for famous TCM doctors practicing medicine; *yang sheng tang:* place for people to consult on health preservation; *yi shi:* office of famous TCM doctors); the construction of *"guo yi tang"* was pushed forward comprehensively in community and township health care service centers and exploration was made in the patterns of comprehensive service of TCM general practice in Tianjin City and for the treatment of 4 common diseases at the grassroots level, 10 prescriptions of Chinese traditional medical herbal pieces and 10 appropriate techniques were formulated and popularized in Ningxia Autonomous Region.

In the pilot of the reform of public TCM hospitals, attention was paid to the play of the characteristics and superiorities. Efforts were made to explore investment and compensation mechanisms beneficial to full play of the characteristics and superiorities of the traditional Chinese medical science and medicines. Fully-budgeted management was conducted for the salary of the staff in public hospitals of traditional Chinese medicine (ethnic minority medicine) in the provinces (autonomous regions, cities) such as Beijing, Inner Mongolia, Shaanxi and so on.; patients going to the outpatient department and inpatient department of government-run TCM hospitals were compensated 8 RMB Yuan each time and 15 RMB Yuan each day respectively in Ningbo City of Zhejiang Province and exploration in compensatory mechanisms for the service of the traditional Chinese medical science and medicines in public TCM hospitals was carried out in Jining City of Shandong Province and Pingxiang City of Jiangxi Province. A great number of TCM hospitals continuously perfected performance evaluation systems and made active exploration in the incentive mechanisms that encouraged the application of techniques and methods of the traditional Chinese medical science and medicines. The pilot work of comprehensive reform in county-level TCM hospitals was pushed forward in an orderly way and the pilot of the formulation and implementation of clinical pathways of traditional Chinese medicine developed gradually, the total number of the clinical pathways being up to 210. The activity of TCM hospital management year with the theme of "taking patients as the center, play of the characteristics and superiorities of the traditional Chinese medical science and medicines as the focus" was carried out; measures beneficial to the masses were put into effect; process of medical care was optimized and conducts were regulated. The engineering that promoted the application of TCM medical equipment was carried out; small packages of Chinese traditional medical herbal pieces were popularized and used; guidance on the construction and management of clinical departments were intensified and the construction of key specialties was promoted orderly; the connotation construction of TCM hospitals was strengthened and the maintenance and play of the characteristics and superiorities were pushed forward. Evaluation and acceptance inspection on 9 units of the key construction project of the combination of traditional Chinese medicine and Western medicine were complete and working guidelines for hospitals of traditional Chinese medicine and Western medicine were formulated. The acceptance inspection on 10 units of the key construction project of the hospitals of ethnic minority medicine was finished and the investigation on the standards of the medical qualification examination for the doctors of ethnic minority medicine was conducted. 93 general hospitals were constructed into the exemplary units of traditional Chinese medical work. The State Administration of Traditional Chinese Medicine issued opinions on the intensification of the work of folk medicine in order to further promote the exploration in it.

Ⅲ. Policies of the State Council on supporting and developing the undertaking of the traditional Chinese medical science and medicines were implemented

Greater efforts were made to carry through and implemented the State Council's *Several Opinions of the State Council on Supporting and Promoting the Development of TCM Undertaking* (hereinafter referred to as *Several Opinions*). All-level committees and governments strengthened the organization and leadership on the traditional Chinese medical work, gave more policy support and financial input and adopted measures to promote the solution to difficulties and problems in the development, which forcefully pushed forward the development of the undertaking in all the localities. In 2011, provinces of Liaoning, Heilongjiang, Hunan, Shaanxi and Hebei issued the implementation opinions on supporting and promoting the development of the traditional Chinese medical science and medicines or the action plans on accelerating the development; Guangxi Zhuang Autonomous Region, in particularly, issued the decision on accelerating the development of traditional Chinese medical science and medicines and the development of ethnic minority medical science and medicines, the plans for the vitalization of Zhuang and Yao medical science and medicines and the implementation schemes on 10 key projects concerning the development of the traditional Chinese medical science and medicines and ethnic minority medical science and medicines; Sichuan Province and Xinjiang Uygur Autonomous Region fulfilled the draft of the implementation opinions on carrying out the State Nations' *Several Opinions*. Provinces of Jilin, Shaanxi, Hebei, Guizhou and Hunan held conferences on the development of the traditional Chinese medical science and medicines and the industry of traditional Chinese medicines in the name of provincial government and Tibet Autonomous Region and some other regions sped up the preparation for the conferences. Moreover, principal Party and governmental leaders of numerous provinces (autonomous regions, cities) such as Hebei, Shanxi, Jilin, etc. gave instructions and put forward requirements on the acceleration of the development of the traditional Chinese medical science and medicines. Since the issue of the *Several Opinion*, 19 provinces (autonomous regions, cities) issued special documents on the implementation opinions on carrying through and implementing the *Several Opinions* or on the support and promotion of the development of the undertaking of the traditional Chinese medical science and medicines and 11 provinces (autonomous regions, cities) held conferences on the traditional Chinese medical science and medicines and the ethnic minority medical science and medicines.

Joint action of all-level administrations of traditional Chinese medicine was strengthened and innovation was made in the working mechanisms for the scientific development of the undertaking of the traditional Chinese medical science and medicines. The State Administration of Traditional Chinese Medicine signed the agreement with Gansu Provincial Government on the construction of the demonstrative province of the pilot of comprehensive reform in the development of the traditional Chinese medical science and medicines, the cooperative agreement with Hainan Provincial Government on the promotion of the development of the traditional Chinese medical science and medicines, the cooperative agreement with Chongqing Municipal Government on the promotion of overall-planning urban and rural development of the undertaking of the traditional Chinese medical science and medicines and issued the specific opinions on support to the development of the undertaking of Tibetan medical science and medicines in Tibet Autonomous Region and the rapid development of Xinjiang Production and Construction Corps. The State Administration of Traditional Chinese Medicine incorporated "promotion of the development of the traditional Chinese medical science and medicines" into the agreement signed by the Ministry of Health and Shanghai Municipal Government on further deepening ministerial-municipal cooperation, signed agreements with Jiangsu Provincial Government and Henan Provincial Government respectively on the joint construction of Nanjing University of Chinese Medicine and Henan University of Traditional Chinese Medicine and supported the China Academy of Chinese Medical Sciences and Qinghai Tibetan Medicine Research Institute to sign the agreement on the cooperative promotion of the researches on the inheritance and innovation of Tibetan medical science and medicines.

Active efforts were made to obtain support and more funds were invested in the development of the traditional Chinese medical science and medicines. In 2011, the Central Finance invested nearly 6 billion RMB Yuan, of which 4.212 billion RMB Yuan were invested in the construction of service capacity of 1,814 county-level hospitals of traditional Chinese medicine (hospitals of ethnic minority medicine), 58 prefecture-level and city-level hospitals of ethnic minority and 88 prefecture-level and city-level hospitals of traditional Chinese medicine in the western regions; 1.014

billion RMB Yuan were allocated to the support of the construction of 70 county-level hospitals of traditional Chinese medicine; 300 million yun of newly-added funds were invested in the construction of 88 specialties of traditional Chinese medicine in the national construction project of key clinical specialties and 412 million RMB Yuan were allocated to the support of projects such as the construction of offices for inheritance of national veteran TCM doctors' experience and so on. Meanwhile, all-level governments also increased input in the development substantially.

Communication and coordination were further enhanced and policy measures on the support and promotion of the development of the traditional Chinese medical science and medicines were made further specific; for example, the *Guiding Opinions of the State Council on the Establishment of the System of General Practitioners* included the contents of the traditional Chinese medical science and medicines, which provided a policy guarantee for TCM general practitioners' standardized training, admittance and employment; the *Guiding Opinions of the General Office of the State Council on further Strengthening the Construction of the Contingent of Village Doctors* clarified the responsibilities and requirements for village doctors' treatment of rural residents with common diseases and frequently-encountered diseases with traditional Chinese medical science and medicines. 1,093 college students majoring in traditional Chinese medicine were to be enrolled in the 2011 plan for directional and free cultivation of rural medical students. The pilot of the reform in the modes of cultivation of TCM clinical talents combining college education with master-disciple education was launched and reform in education and teaching of TCM colleges and universities was promoted. The first selection of "National Honored Great Master of Traditional Chinese Medicine" was conducted; methods for the evaluation of TCM medical staff's titles of professional technical posts were adjusted and exploration was made in the establishment of incentive mechanisms for TCM talents. The construction of the systems of clinical research on the prevention and treatment of infectious diseases with the traditional Chinese medical science and medicines and the special projects or subjects concerning the traditional Chinese medical science and medicines were set up in 973 Program (Key Project of Chinese National Programs for Fundamental Research and Development), the National Science and Technology Support Program, the special science and technology projects of public-welfare industries and the major special science and technology projects of the prevention and treatment of infectious diseases and the creation and preparation of new medicines. The registration system for traditional Chinese medicines was perfected and opinions on the management of Chinese herbal preparations in medical institutions were discussed and worked out. Measures on the intensification of the work of TCM intellectual property were put forward and policies on the promotion of the development of service trade were clarified. Implementation schemes for recent prior work in ethnic minority medical science and medicines were issued to accelerate the promotion of the development. In close cooperation with the Health Bureau of the PLA Logistic Department, the integration of military-civil resources of the traditional Chinese medical science and medicines was actively promoted.

IV. Work of the legislation of the Law of Traditional Chinese Medicine and the standardization and informatization of the traditional Chinese medical science and medicines

The Law of the People's Republic of China on Traditional Chinese Medicine (Draft)(hereinafter referred to as *Draft*) was adopted after examination and approval by the conference of the Ministry of Health and was reported to the State Council by the end of 2011. The general train of thought of the *Draft* included following points: the first was to focus on the legislative purpose of protection, support and promotion of the development of the traditional Chinese medical science and medicines; the second was to obey laws of the development, embody the characteristics, attach importance to institutional innovation and strive to make breakthroughs; the third was to take traditional Chinese medical service as a foundation, highlight the characteristics superiorities and satisfy people's needs for the service of the traditional Chinese medical science and medicines; the fourth was to highlight focal points, make overall plans and take all factors into consideration and promote the comprehensive, coordinative and sustainable development of the traditional Chinese medical science and medicines. *The Draft* made institutional arrangements for attaching importance to highlighting the characteristics, playing the role of the traditional Chinese medical science and medicines, strengthening the inheritance, encouraging the innovation and promoting the coordinative development of the traditional Chinese medical science and medicines.

The standardization of the traditional Chinese medical science and medicines was pushed forward in an all-round way. Guangdong Province took the lead in setting up the standardization technical committee of traditional Chinese medical science and the standardization technical committee of traditional Chinese medicines and Shenzhen City also promoted local construction of the standardization. The informationized construction of TCM hospitals was accelerated and the website construction of TCM administrations was intensified. Supervision on the traditional Chinese medical science and medicines was further enhanced and great efforts were made to monitor and punish false and illegal TCM medical advertisements.

V. The cultural construction of the traditional Chinese medical science and medicines

The State Administration of Traditional Chinese Medicine held the National Working Conference on the Cultural Construction of Traditional Chinese Medicine which comprehensively reviewed the experience and achievements made in the cultural construction carried out by the whole system of the traditional Chinese medical science and medicines, put forward objectives and tasks for the development of the culture and formulated measures on the acceleration of the cultural construction. The first was to energetically propagandize the core values of the traditional Chinese medical science and medicines and by organizing a series of activities such as Zhang Zhongjing Cultural Festival of Medical Science and Technology, Li Shizhen Medical Festival and Sun Simiao Cultural Festival of *Traditional Chinese Medicine,* do researches on the cultural essence and connotation and the core value system of the traditional Chinese medical science and medicines, develop and expand the value of "great masters' super skill and absolute sincerity", inherit the cultural spirit, set up good medical ethics and promote harmonious doctor-patient relationship. The second was to make greater efforts to publicize the popular science of the traditional Chinese medical science and medicines with more diversified forms, rich contents and extensive platforms. The activity of "the Traditional Chinese Medical Science and Medicines in China•Entering Villages, Communities, Families" was popular with the masses; programs on health care with the traditional Chinese medical science and medicines organized by some media developed into brands; the full-length documentary film, *Traditional Chinese Medicine,* produced jointly with the CCTV began shooting and the lectures on the popular science knowledge of health care with the traditional Chinese medical science and medicines held for diplomatic envoys to China also created a positive stir. The third was to make active exploration in the mechanisms that integrated the cultural construction with health protection. Provinces and cities such as Beijing, Guangdong, etc. launched TCM cultural and healthcare tourist demonstrative bases and the culture and health care of the traditional Chinese medical science and medicines were incorporated into the construction of the international tourist island in Hainan Province. The construction of publicity and education bases of the culture of the traditional Chinese medical science and medicines was strengthened continuously and cultural construction of TCM hospitals was pushed forward unceasingly. The work of news propaganda for the traditional Chinese medical science and medicines was further intensified.

VI. The inheritance and innovation of the traditional Chinese medical science and medicines

In September 2011, Tu Youyou, a researcher from China Academy of Chinese Medical Sciences, won the 2011 Lasker DeBakey Clinical Medical Research Award for the discovery of artemisinin, a drug therapy for malaria. The scientific and technologic work of the traditional Chinese medical science and medicines focused on the acceleration of the construction of national clinical research bases and strengthened the construction of clinical scientific and technologic systems. The train of thought was put forward that the research on the key diseases should be taken as the foundation of the professional construction of the bases, the construction of the sharing system of the information on clinical scientific research as the principal part and the regulation of clinical scientific research and the training of backbone talents as the "both wings" and the guidelines for the construction of the information sharing system and the guiding opinions on the regulation of clinical scientific research were worked out. The training for the backbone of scientific research of the bases was strengthened and the cooperative mechanism with research alliances as the main body was basically set up.

Systematic researches were conducted in theories, clinical treatment and medication for influenza and other exogenous diseases and positive progress was made, of which the comparative study on the effectiveness of oseltamivir and the Chinese traditional prescription of "ma xing shi gan" (4 kinds of traditional Chinese medicines) and Lonicerae and Forsythiae Powder on Influenza A (H1N1) proved the effect of the traditional Chinese medical science and medicines and release of the research result drew an extensive concern of the world.

The inheritance research on the traditional Chinese medical science and medicines was enhanced; new achievements were gained in research-based inheritance of the famous veteran experts in traditional Chinese medicine and the achievements such as "the comprehensive service platform of famous veteran TCM experts' clinical experience and academic ideology" and "prescription analysis system of traditional Chinese medicine" acted as means of improvement in the efficiency of inheritance research. The collation of the third batch of 400 ancient books went on smoothly and the formulation and implementation of working guidelines for the collation of literature on ethnical minority medical science and medicines and the selection of the projects of the popularization of TCM appropriate techniques regulated the collation and selection.

The transformation and application of the research achievements in the prevention and treatment of major complicated and difficult diseases and common diseases, the characteristic acupuncture and moxibustion therapy, technical standards, key technology in traditional Chinese medicines in the 11th Five-Year-Plan period were strengthened, which provided scientific and technologic support for the medical service, construction of the essential drug system, popularization of appropriate techniques and training of grassroots talents.

According to the unified technical standards and task requirements, the pilot of survey on natural resources of Chinese medicinal materials was conducted orderly and forcefully in 6 provinces (autonomous regions), including Anhui, Sichuan, Xinjiang and so on. The State Administration of Traditional Chinese Medicine seriously implemented Vice Premier Li Keqiang's instruction, investigated the causes for the rise in the prices of Chinese medicinal materials and reported countermeasures and suggestions to the State Council.

VII. The construction of talent contingents of the traditional Chinese medical science and medicines

The State Administration of Traditional Chinese Medicine earnestly carried through and implemented Vice-Premier Li Keqiang's and State Councilor Liu Yandong's instructions on the education work of the traditional Chinese medical science and medicines and in accordance with the requirements of *the Medium- and Long-Term Development Program on Medical and Health Talents(2011-2020),* launched the project of "talent engineering of inheritance and innovation of the traditional Chinese medical science and medicines". The first was, for the purpose of the cultivation of high-level talents, to steadily promote the projects concerning the inheritance of the academic experience of veteran experts in the traditional Chinese medical science and medicines, the further study of excellent TCM clinical talents, the cultivation of the academic pacemakers and so on, strengthen the management on the link between master-disciple education and professional degrees, establish 226 offices for the inheritance of the academic experience of the national famous veteran experts in the traditional Chinese medical science and medicines and explore the "classes of great masters of traditional Chinese medicine" for the experience of the cultivation of high-level talents. The second was to enhance the cultivation of grassroots talents and train 2,375 county-level clinical technical backbone of traditional Chinese medicine. Cultivation of general practitioners of traditional Chinese medicine and standardized training for resident doctors were forcefully pushed forward. Job-transfer training for general practitioners of traditional Chinese medicine was launched and more than 2,200 TCM personnel from grassroots medical and health institutions took part in the training. The construction of training bases of TCM general practitioners was carried out and the pilot of standardized training for TCM resident doctors was launched. The third was, by the joint construction of the State Administration of Traditional Chinese Medicine and each province, to strive to push forward the connotation construction of colleges and universities of traditional Chinese medicine; meanwhile promote the reform in education and teaching. The construction of key disciplines was pushed forward actively and construction programs on 323 key disciplines were made. The fourth was to accelerate the development of the occupational education. The National TCM Occupational Education and Teaching Committee was set up and the First National Skill Competition of Occupational Education was organized. Training for teachers evaluating professional skills of 5 types of jobs peculiar to the industry of the traditional Chinese medical science and medicines including pharmacists of traditional Chinese medicines and the appraise on 3 kinds of professional technical personnel including *gua sha shi* (doctors treating patients' illness by scraping the patient's neck, chest or back) were initiated. The fifth was to intensify the continuing education and play the role of the continuing education bases of the superior disciplines and the urban community and rural demonstrative training bases of knowledge and skills on the traditional Chinese medical science and medicines. Therefore, the quality and coverage of the continuing education were improved greatly.

VIII. The foreign exchange and cooperation of the traditional Chinese medical science and medicines

The National Working Conference on Foreign Exchange and Cooperation of the Traditional Chinese Medical Science and Medicines was held which defined the guiding thought and basic principles and proposed the key tasks and specific measures for promoting the traditional Chinese medical science and medicines to have more extensive influence on the world. Multilateral platforms were made good use of and the role of a big country in traditional medicine was well played. Efforts were made to further implement *the Resolution of Traditional Medicine* adopted in the 62nd World Health Assembly, take an active part in the formulation of the part of the traditional medicine for ICD of WHO (International Classification of Diseases of the World Health Organization), positively promote WHO Western Pacific Region to formulate and carry out *the Regional Strategy for Traditional Medicine in the Western Pacific Region (2011-2020)* and manage to establish 5 working groups at the second conference of ISO Technical Committee of Traditional Chinese Medicine (tentative name) with Chinese experts being the organizers of 3 groups. Moreover, after examination and approval of the UNESCO, two ancient books of Huang Di Nei Jing (Emperor's Inner Canon) and Ben Cao Gang Mu (Compendium of Materia Medica) were selected into the Asia-Pacific Memory of the World Register. The State

Administration of Traditional Chinese Medicine timely pushed forward China and the European Union to establish mechanisms that promoted the registration of traditional Chinese medicines and further promoted the construction of the high-level China-ASEAN cooperation platform. Bilateral cooperation was consolidated and developed and with focus on carrying out inter-governmental agreements, fields of cooperation were further expanded. Abundant achievements were gained in the Sino-America Seminar on Traditional Chinese Medicine, the Sino-Russia First Meeting of the Working Group of Traditional Chinese Medicine and the Sino-Korean Cooperation and Coordination Committee for Traditional Medicine and cooperation with Malaysia, Vietnam, New Zealand and Australia was enhanced. Provinces (Autonomous regions) of Heilongjiang, Fujian, Guangxi, Yunnan, etc. brought regional advantages into play and the service trade of traditional Chinese medical science and medicines developed positively. The Administration of Traditional Chinese Medicine and Xiamen Municipal Government jointly held the Cross-Strait Forum on Traditional Chinese Medicine and some prominent figures in the field of traditional Chinese medical science and medicines, including some academicians and national honored great masters, went to Taiwan to attend the Third Cross-Strait Forum on Cooperation and Technologic Exchange in Chinese Herbal Medicines and other such activities.

IX. The activity of striving to excel in the performances

The State Administration of Traditional Chinese Medicine earnestly studied and carried through the spirits of the General Secretary Hu Jintao's important speech on July 1, deeply carried out the activity of striving to excel in the performance in the course of deepening the medical and health reform and a great number of advanced collectives and excellent Party members sprang up, including Guang'anmen Hospital, China Academy of Chinese Medical Sciences, Guangdong Hospital of Traditional Chinese Medicine, Chongqing Hospital of Traditional Chinese Medicine and Zhang Boli from Tianjin City, Chen Xiangyi from Jilin Province, Lu Youqiang from Shaanxi Province and so on, which created a good atmosphere that every Party member competed in study, work and devotion and also learned from and caught up with each other and tried to be the advanced; therefore, Party members' and cadres' capacity and level of putting people first and governing for the people were greatly improved. Hospitals of traditional Chinese medicine combined "three good and one satisfaction" (good service, good quality, good medical ethics; masses' satisfaction) with the activity of striving to excel in the performances, cultural construction, connotation construction and the construction of mechanisms that promoted the play of the characteristics and superiorities of the traditional Chinese medical science and medicines and created a series of advanced working experience. The Affiliated Hospital of Shanxi Provincial Hospital of Traditional Chinese Medicine put forward "whether patients were rich or poor, saved their life first"; Yanzhou Municipal Hospital of Traditional Chinese Medicine of Shandong Province raised the mode of "rescuing and treating patients before their payment and enabling everyone to get access to green life passage"; Jingde Municipal Hospital of Traditional Chinese Medicine of Jiangxi Province resolved doctor-patient conflicts and constructed harmonious doctor-patient relationship and service vehicles of traditional Chinese medicine of Fangshan Hospital of Traditional Chinese Medicine travelled through all the villages of Fangshan District of Beijing City.

(Zhao Yinghong)

2. Selection of the Top Ten News Events on Traditional Chinese Medicine in 2011

On January 16, 2012, results of the selection of the top ten news events on traditional Chinese medicine in 2011 that was jointly organized by the Information Office of the State Administration of Traditional Chinese Medicine and the China News of Traditional Chinese Medicine were published. Results were as follows:

I. Traditional Chinese medicine was listed out as a separated chapter in the *Outline of National 12th Five-Year Plan* for the first time and the Central Finance invested 5.9 billion RMB Yuan in support of the development of traditional Chinese medical science and medicines at the beginning of the 12th Five-Year-Plan period

Development of the traditional Chinese medical science and medicines was listed out as a separated chapter in the *Outline of the 12th Five-Year Plan for National Economic and Social Development of the People's Republic of China* for the first time and also taken as one of the six key tasks of "perfection of the basic medical and health system". At the beginning of the 12th Five-Year-Plan period, the Central Finance allocated 5.9 billion RMB Yuan of special funds to offering greater support to the development of the undertaking of the traditional Chinese medical science and medicines.

II. Tu Youyou won the 2011 Lasker DeBakey Clinical Medical Research Award

Tu Youyou, a researcher from China Academy of Chinese Medical Sciences, won the 2011 Lasker Award (Lasker DeBakey Clinical Medical Research Award) for her outstanding contribution to the research on the artemisinin. Enlightened by the curative effect of sweet wormwood *(Artemisia annua)* for malaria described in the classic books on traditional Chinese medicine, she discovered for the first time that the lower-temperature ether extraction was an effective drug therapy for malaria, which was of vital importance for the research and development of the effective preparation of sweet wormwood *(Artemisia annua)*. Artemisinin, an effective drug therapy for malaria, saved millions of lives across the globe.

III. Huang Di Nei Jing (Emperor's Inner Canon) and Ben Cao Gang Mu (Compendium of Materia Medica) were accepted for inscription on the Memory of the World Register

At the 10th International Advisory Committee (IAC) Meeting held in Manchester, England, from May 23-26, 2011, *Huang Di Nei Jing* (Emperor's Inner Canon) and *Ben Cao Gang Mu* (Compendium of Materia Medica) were accepted for inscription on the UNESCO Memory of the World Register, which symbolized the identification of the international community to Chinese cultural values.

IV. Traditional Chinese medical science and medicines played an active role in deepening the medical and health reform and the policies concerned were put into effect

The Ministry of Health and the State Administration of Traditional Chinese Medicine issued *the Opinions on further Playing the Role of Traditional Chinese Medical Science and Medicines in Deepening the Reform of Medical and Health System* and the traditional Chinese medical science and medicines played an important role in the fulfillment of the five key tasks in deepening the medical and health reform. Polices and measures defined by *the Several Opinions of the State Council on Supporting and Promoting the Development of TCM Undertaking* were put into effect by central and local governments in an all-round way.

V. A new prospect was opened up in the cultural construction of the traditional Chinese medical science and medicines and the popular science knowledge was popular with people

The State Administration of Traditional Chinese Medicine held the National Working Conference on the Cultural Construction of Traditional Chinese Medical Science and Medicines for the first time and issued the guiding opinions on strengthening the cultural construction of the traditional Chinese medical science and medicines. The activity to recommend national excellent popular science books on the traditional Chinese medical science and medicines was organized for the first time and the order of publishing books on health protection was regulated. Some programs on health care with the traditional Chinese medical science and medicines organized by some media developed into brands and activities of "the Traditional Chinese Medical Science and Medicines in China•Entering Villages, Communities, Families" and "Tour of Lectures on Popular Science Knowledge on the Traditional Chinese Medical Science and Medicines" were carried out deeply.

VI. The report of the survey on the basic status quo of traditional Chinese medicine publicized for the first time that there were 900 million visits to doctors of traditional Chinese medicine each year

The publication of *the Report of the Survey on the Basic Status Quo of Traditional Chinese Medicine in 2009* provided a scientific basis for the development of the undertaking of the traditional Chinese medical science and medicines. The report showed that the total number of visits to the outpatient and emergency departments of traditional Chinese medicine was 907 million annually throughout the country; 59.6% medical institutions could provide traditional Chinese medical service and there were 3.06 doctors of traditional Chinese medicine for every ten thousand persons.

VII. Joint working mechanisms of the State Administration of Traditional Chinese Medicine and each province were established and first demonstrative province for the comprehensive reform of the traditional Chinese medical science and medicines was constructed in Gansu Province

The State Administration of Traditional Chinese Medicine and Gansu Provincial Government signed an agreement on the construction of the demonstrative province for the pilot of the comprehensive reform in the development of the traditional Chinese medical science and medicines and Gansu Province adhered to the principle of putting equal stress on traditional Chinese medicine and Western medicine, opened up a new prospect of reform in conformity with the actual situations of the province and played an exemplary role for the whole country. The State Administration of Traditional Chinese Medicine also signed cooperation agreements with provincial governments of Hainan, Jiangsu and Henan for the joint promotion of the development of the undertaking of the traditional Chinese medical science and medicines.

VIII. Rise in the prices of traditional Chinese medicinal materials caused great social concern and measures to stabilize the rising prices gained results

Prices of traditional Chinese medicinal materials rose irrationally and for the solution to this problem, relevant departments conducted a comprehensive survey, rectified the order of circulation, investigated and punished the conducts of hoarding for speculation according to the law; as a result, the momentum was suppressed and the prices gradually fell. Of the 500 kinds of traditional Chinese medicinal materials inspected, more than half dropped in prices and more than 100 kinds decreased by 21%~50%.

IX. Folk traditional Chinese medical work was strengthened

For solution to difficult problems in the development of folk medical science and medicines, the State Administration of Traditional Chinese Medicine issued the *Opinions on Strengthening Folk Medical Work*, intensified the exploitation and collation of folk medical science and medicines and did a good job in the management of medical qualification. All the localities adopted the measure of "discovering treasures in apricot grove" (apricot grove was used in ancient time to refer to the field of traditional Chinese medicine) and other measures to find out more folk medical techniques and methods and helped folk doctors with special skills obtain the qualification for practicing medicine legally and offering services of prevention and health protection of traditional Chinese medicine.

X. The mode of "rescuing and treating patients before their payment and enabling everyone to get access to green life passage" put forward by Yanzhou Municipal Hospital of Traditional Chinese Medicine of Shandong Province and the ideology that "whether patients were rich or poor, saved their life first" raised by the Affiliated Hospital of Shanxi Provincial Hospital of Traditional Chinese Medicine created a positive stir in the system of traditional Chinese medicine and the whole society

In the in-depth medical and health reform and the activities of "striving to excel in the performances" and "three good and one satisfaction", the two hospitals put people first, made bold innovation in service modes and ideology, improved service quality, promoted harmonious doctor-patient relationship, created new experience and made the highlights in the reform and development of the traditional Chinese medical science and medicines and even the whole medical and health system.

(Zhao Yinghong)

3. National Working Conference on Foreign Exchange and Cooperation of Traditional Chinese Medicine Was Held

On February 22, 2011, the National Working Conference on Foreign Exchange and Cooperation of Traditional Chinese Medicine and the inaugural meeting of the Advisory Committee of Experts on Foreign Exchange and Cooperation were held in Nanjing.

Wang Guoqiang, Vice Minister of the Ministry of Health and concurrently Chief of the State Administration of Traditional Chinese Medicine reviewed the new achievements gained in recent years' foreign exchange and cooperation, analyzed opportunities and challenges on the road to the world and deployed key working tasks for the next stage in his speech.

The Advisory Committee of Experts on Foreign Exchange and Cooperation was established during the conference and the first working meeting was convened. Wang Guoqiang awarded letters of appointment to representatives of committee members, encouraged them to fully play the role and provide advice, opinions and suggestions to the work of foreign exchange and cooperation.

Relevant leaders of the Foreign Trade Department of the Ministry of Commerce and the International Cooperation Department of the Ministry of Science and Technology made reports respectively entitled *the Policy Research and Development Prospect for the Service Trade of Traditional Chinese Medicine and the International TCM Scientific and Technologic Cooperation Promotes Traditional Chinese Medicine to Move towards the World.*

Group discussions about Wang Guoqiang's report and *the Medium- and Long-Term Program for TCM Foreign Exchange and Cooperation* were organized and opinions and suggestions on future ten years' working principles, development objectives and key tasks were solicited extensively.

Leaders of health department (bureau) responsible for traditional Chinese medical work of all provinces (autonomous regions, cities) throughout the country, leaders of departments, offices and the subordinate units of the State Administration of Traditional Chinese Medicine, representatives of relevant departments of the Central Party Committee and the state organs and members of the Advisory Committee of Experts on Foreign Exchange and Cooperation attended the conference. 12 units, including the China Academy of Chinese Medical Sciences, exchanged experience at the conference.

(Zhao Yinghong)

4. The State Administration of Traditional Chinese Medicine and the Ministry of Health of Malaysia signed the Memorandum of Understanding on the Cooperation in the Field of Traditional Medicine

On November 7, 2011, Wang Guoqiang, Vice Minister of the Ministry of Health and concurrently Chief of the State Administration of Traditional Chinese Medicine met with Liao Zhonglai, Minister of the Ministry of Health of Malaysia and his delegation.

Two sides exchanged and communicated fully about the cooperation in the field of traditional medicine and the establishment of the "Center of Excellence for Traditional Medicine". After the talk, Wang Guoqiang and Liao Zhonglai signed *the Memorandum of Understanding of the Government of the People's Republic of China and the Malaysian Government on Cooperation in the Field of Traditional Medicine* on behalf of the two countries respectively. The memorandum covered policies and regulations, education and training, scientific research and development, information exchange and so on in the communication of traditional medicine, which laid foundation for the establishment of long-term mechanisms of cooperation in traditional medicine of two countries.

(Zhao Yinghong)

Chapter XIV Management of Pharmaceutical Industry

Production and Operation of the Pharmaceutical Industry in 2011

In 2011, the production of the pharmaceutical industry grew steadily but with slower speed; compared with last year, growth of total profits and sales profit ratio reduced; situations for the deficit of pharmaceutical enterprises were not good; foreign trade increased slowly and there were still unstable factors in export.

I. Production

In 2011, the accumulated gross output value of the pharmaceutical industry reached 1,570.77 billion RMB Yuan, a year-on-year increase of 28.5%. Viewed from the accumulated gross output value of the pharmaceutical industry in each quarter, the trend was better than that of last year.

Of the total, growth of Chinese medical herbal pieces processing industry, Chinese patent medicine manufacturing industry, health materials and medical supplies manufacturing industry was higher than the average of the pharmaceutical industry.

Table-1 Total accumulated gross output value of the pharmaceutical industry in 2011

Sub-industry	Accumulated gross output value (100 million RMB Yuan)	Year-on-year increase (%)
chemical material medicine manufacturing industry	3081.9	25.0
chemical medicine preparation manufacturing industry	4231.3	24.1
Chinese medical herbal pieces processing industry	880.9	51.2
Chinese patent medicine manufacturing industry	3499.8	33.7
biological and biochemical product manufacturing industry	1592.1	23.5
health materials and medical supplies manufacturing industry	942.9	37.5
medical equipment, device & machine manufacturing industry	1398.5	27.1
pharmaceutical machinery manufacturing industry	80.2	11.5
pharmaceutical industry	15707.7	28.5

From January to December 2011, the year-on-year increase in the added value of the pharmaceutical industry was 17.8%, higher than the average of the whole national industry (13.8%).

II. Sales

In 2011, the accumulated sales value of the pharmaceutical industry reached 1,502.51 billion RMB Yuan, a year-on-year increase of 29.3%. The increase of 2010 continued to the first half of 2011 and the rise of the sales value kept the same pace with that of the gross output value, but the speed was slower in the fourth quarter.

Of the total sales value, the increase amplitude of the three sub-industries of Chinese medical herbal pieces processing industry, health materials and medical supplies manufacturing industry, Chinese patent medicine manufacturing industry was higher than that of the average of the pharmaceutical industry, particularly, the rise of Chinese medical herbal pieces processing industry was 25.5% higher than the average, while that of chemical medicine preparation manufacturing industry was 4.1% lower than the average.

Table-2 Total finished sales value of the pharmaceutical industry in 2011

Sub-industry	Accumulated gross sales value (100million RMB Yuan)	Year-on-year increase(%)
chemical material medicine manufacturing industry	2922.9	24.5
chemical medicine preparation manufacturing industry	4044.7	25.2
Chinese medical herbal pieces processing industry	873.5	54.8
Chinese patent medicine manufacturing industry	3305.2	34.1
biological and biochemical product manufacturing industry	1529.7	25.5
health materials and medical supplies manufacturing industry	918.2	38.4
medical equipment, device & machine manufacturing industry	1354.1	27.5
pharmaceutical machinery manufacturing industry	76.7	12.6
pharmaceutical industry	15025.1	29.3

III. Production and Sales Ratio

In 2011, the total production and sales ratio of the pharmaceutical industry was 95.7%. The production and sales ratio returned to normal in the first half year after a rise in the first quarter and then showed a rebounding tendency in the next half year. Generally speaking, the production and sales of the pharmaceutical industry were in a stable and coordinative state.

Of the total, the production and sales ratio of the three sub-industries of chemical material medicine manufacturing industry, chemical medicine preparation manufacturing industry and Chinese patent medicine manufacturing industry was lower than the average of the pharmaceutical industry.

Compared with the same period of 2010, except chemical material medicine manufacturing industry, all the sub-industries increased the production and sales ratio of to a certain extent, of which Chinese medical herbal pieces processing industry increased mostly, the increase percentage being 2.4 .

Table-3 Production and sales ratio of the pharmaceutical industry in 2011

Sub-industry	Production and sales ratio (%)	Year-on-year increase (%)
chemical material medicine manufacturing industry	94.8	−0.4
chemical medicine preparation manufacturing industry	95.6	0.9
Chinese medical herbal pieces processing industry	99.2	2.4
Chinese patent medicine manufacturing industry	94.4	0.3
biological and biochemical product manufacturing industry	96.1	1.6
health materials and medical supplies manufacturing industry	97.4	0.7
medical equipment, device & machine manufacturing industry	96.8	0.3
pharmaceutical machinery manufacturing industry	95.7	−1.4
pharmaceutical industry	95.7	0.6

IV. Steady and slow increase in foreign trade

(1) Export delivery value

Viewed from the accumulated export delivery value of all the sub-industries in 2011, the increase amplitude of chemical material medicine manufacturing industry that accounted for a considerable large proportion of the whole was lower than the average of the pharmaceutical industry, which lowered the growth level of the pharmaceutical industry. Negative growth of Chinese medical herbal pieces processing industry in the first half year (-9.1%) turned to positive growth (18.9%) and the increase amplitude was higher than the average of the pharmaceutical industry. The year-on-year increase of health materials and medical supplies manufacturing industry was 34%.

Table-4 Finished export delivery value of the pharmaceutical industry in 2011

Sub-industry	Export delivery value (100 million RMB Yuan)	Year-on-year increase (%)
chemical material medicine manufacturing industry	528.2	12.2
chemical medicine preparation manufacturing industry	123.3	15.6
Chinese medical herbal pieces processing industry	21.0	18.9
Chinese patent medicine manufacturing industry	51.6	20.3
biological and biochemical product manufacturing industry	190.2	20.4
health materials and medical supplies manufacturing industry	114.5	34.0
medical equipment, device & machine manufacturing industry	405.6	17.8
pharmaceutical machinery manufacturing industry	5.2	5.5
pharmaceutical industry	1439.5	17.0

(2) Import and export surplus

Customs data showed that the total accumulated import-export amount of pharmaceuticals reached $73.28 billion, a year-on-year increase of 39.1% and compared with the year-on-year increase of 24.6% in 2010, it increased sharply. The export value was $44.52 billion, a year-on-year increase of 34.9% and an increase of nearly 10% compared with 24.9% of 2010, while the import value was $28.77 billion, a year-on-year increase of 46.1% and an increase of 22.1% compared with 24% of 2010. The trade surplus was $15.75 billion, increased by 18.3% and decreased by 7.5% compared with 25.8% of 2010. The import and export of the pharmaceutical industry showed a steady rising trend with the import relatively active, slow speed of the export in the fourth quarter and declining increase amplitude of the trade surplus.

Viewed from the three major categories, medical equipment and devices ranked first in the year-on-year increase of the total import-export amount and traditional Chinese medicines came next. Medical equipment and devices and traditional Chinese medicines ranked first in the year-on-year increase of the total export amount, whereas medical equipment and devices and Western medicines ranked first in the year-on-year increase of the total import amount. The need of our country's pharmaceutical market for the import of chemical medicines and biochemical medicines and transnational enterprises' seizure of our country's market were increasing.

Table-5 Import and export of pharmaceuticals from January to November 2011

	Amount of export (100 million dollar)	Year-on-year increase (%)	Percentage (%)	Amount of import (100 million dollar)	Year-on-year increase (%)	Percentage (%)
Chinese medicines(including health care products, plant extracts,、Chinese patent medicines 、Chinese herbal medicines and Chinese medical herbal pieces)	23.3	36.5	5.2	7.2	29.1	2.5
Western medicines(including raw materials, preparations and bio-chemical products)	264.7	25.7	59.5	171.7	41.4	59.7
medical equipment and devices (including dressing, disposable medical supplies, products of hospital diagnosis and treatment, health protection and rehabilitation, dental equipment and materials)	157.1	53.6	35.3	108.9	55.6	37.8
total	445.2	34.9	100	287.7	46.1	100

V. Economic benefits

(1) Main business income

In 2011, the accumulated main business income reached 1,525.48 billion RMB Yuan, a year-on-year increase of 28.8%.

The main business income grew steadily throughout the year but slower in the fourth quarter.

Table-6 Finished main business income of the pharmaceutical industry in 2011

Sub-industry	Main business income (100 million RMB Yuan)	Year-on-year increase (%)
chemical material medicine manufacturing industry	3050.2	22.6
chemical medicine preparation manufacturing industry	4105.0	24.0

Continued

Sub-industry	Main business income (100 million RMB Yuan)	Year-on-year increase (%)
Chinese medical herbal pieces processing industry	853.7	56.1
Chinese patent medicine manufacturing industry	3378.7	34.8
biological and biochemical product manufacturing industry	1515.5	26.7
health materials and medical supplies manufacturing industry	920.9	39.4
medical equipment, device & machine manufacturing industry	1354.3	26.6
pharmaceutical machinery manufacturing industry	76.6	9.8
pharmaceutical industry	15254.8	28.8

(2) Growth of the total profits rebounded

The accumulated total profits finished from January to November 2011 amounted to 157.69 billion RMB Yuan, a year-on-year increase of 23.2%.

The increase in the quarterly total profits of the pharmaceutical industry showed that the first quarter had the least increase which was 19.7% and then it rose gradually and rebounded to 23.2% in the fourth quarter.

Table-7 Total finished profits of the pharmaceutical industry in 2011

Sub-industry	Total profits (100 million RMB Yuan)	Year-on-year increase (%)
chemical material medicine manufacturing industry	247.9	20.1
chemical medicine preparation manufacturing industry	442.3	12.8
Chinese medical herbal pieces processing industry	64.4	65.3
Chinese patent medicine manufacturing industry	372.4	40.4
biological and biochemical product manufacturing industry	206.7	6.5
health materials and medical supplies manufacturing industry	89.4	41.6
medical equipment, device & machine manufacturing industry	146.2	26.7

Continued

Sub-industry	Total profits (100 million RMB Yuan)	Year-on-year increase (%)
pharmaceutical machinery manufacturing industry	5.6	33.2
pharmaceutical industry	1576.9	23.2

(3) Sales profit ratio

In 2011, the sales profit ratio of the pharmaceutical industry reached 10.3% and drop in the sales profits indicated that the profitability of the pharmaceutical industry declined.

VI. Asset growth

(1) Investment in the fixed assets

In 2011, the total accumulated fixed asset investment of the pharmaceutical industry reached 295.05 billion RMB Yuan, a year-on-year increase of 46.2%.

Of all the sub-industries, Chinese medical herbal pieces processing industry ranked first in the increase of the investment (increased by 59.4%) and chemical material medicine manufacturing industry and medical equipment, device & machine manufacturing industry came next (increased by 56.8% and 51.8% respectively). Viewed from the scale of the sub-industries, biological and biochemical product manufacturing industry invested most in the fixed assets; health materials and medical supplies manufacturing industry came next and chemical material medicine manufacturing industry, chemical medicine preparation manufacturing industry and Chinese medical herbal pieces processing industry all invested considerable numbers of funds in the fixed assets.

Table-8 Finished fixed asset investment of the pharmaceutical industry in 2011

Sub-industry	Fixed asset investment (100 million RMB Yuan)	Year-on-year increase (%)
chemical material medicine manufacturing industry	510.5	56.8
chemical medicine preparation manufacturing industry	489.4	32.7
Chinese medical herbal pieces processing industry	281.5	59.9
Chinese patent medicine manufacturing industry	471.2	44.1

Continued

Sub-industry	Fixed asset investment (100 million RMB Yuan)	Year-on-year increase (%)
biological and biochemical product manufacturing industry	485.3	43.2
health materials and medical supplies manufacturing industry	247.2	49.9
medical equipment, device & machine manufacturing industry	335.2	51.8
pharmaceutical industry	2950.5	46.2

(2) Total assets

In 2011, the total assets of the pharmaceutical industry amounted to 1,376.17 billion RMB Yuan, a year-on-year increase of 23%.

Table-9 Total assets of the pharmaceutical industry in 2011

Sub-industry	Total assets (100 million RMB Yuan)	Year-on-year increase (%)
chemical material medicine manufacturing industry	2810.7	18.4
chemical medicine preparation manufacturing industry	4017.5	24.4
Chinese medical herbal pieces processing industry	516.4	40.6
Chinese patent medicine manufacturing industry	3105.8	24.1
biological and biochemical product manufacturing industry	1571.2	18.9
health materials and medical supplies manufacturing industry	561.0	30.3
medical equipment, device & machine manufacturing industry	1115.5	21.7
pharmaceutical machinery manufacturing industry	63.6	30.0
pharmaceutical industry	13761.7	23.0

Ⅶ. Deficit

In 2011, there were 615 enterprises in deficit, a year-on-year drop of 40.5%. Deficit enterprises accounted for 10% and the accumulated losses reached 4.02 billion RMB Yuan, a year-on-year increase of 39.2%.

Table-10 Deficit of the pharmaceutical industry

Sub-industry	Deficit enterprise (companies)	Amount of losses (100 million RMB Yuan)	Year-on-year increase (%)
chemical material medicine manufacturing industry	140	10.4	66.8
chemical medicine preparation manufacturing industry	134	11.3	19.3
Chinese medical herbal pieces processing industry	28	0.7	5.6
Chinese patent medicine manufacturing industry	135	5.7	2.7
biological and biochemical product manufacturing industry	47	5.5	126.9
health materials and medical supplies manufacturing industry	36	0.8	-2.9
medical equipment, device & machine manufacturing industry	91	5.6	57.3
pharmaceutical machinery manufacturing industry	4	0.1	21.3
pharmaceutical industry	615	40.2	39.2

(Zhao Yinghong)

Chapter XV Basic Medical Insurance System

1. Urban Basic Medical Insurance in 2010

I. The coverage of urban basic medical insurance was continuously expanded.

Firstly, the problem of medical insurance for retirees from closed and bankrupt state-owned enterprises and retirees from enterprises with financial difficulties was properly solved. The Ministry of Finance and the Ministry of Human Resources and Social Security jointly decided on the plan to allocate the incentive and subsidizing funds from the central finance to solve the problem of medical insurance for retirees from closed and bankrupt state-owned enterprises. In October 2011, an incentive and subsidizing fund of 7.6 billion RMB Yuan was allocated and all the localities were required to solve the problem of medical insurance for retirees from closed and bankrupt collective-owned enterprises and retirees from enterprises with financial difficulties. Heretofore, 50.9 billion RMB Yuan of central finance subsidies had all been allocated. By the end of 2010, according to statistics, altogether 5.96 million retirees from closed and bankrupt state-owned enterprises were covered by medical insurance for employees and meanwhile the problem of basic medical insurance for over 2 million retirees from other closed and bankrupt enterprises and enterprises with financial difficulties was properly solved. Secondly, *Social Insurance Law of the People's Republic of China* was implemented and practiced and policies on the unemployed enrolling in the medical insurance were researched on and promulgated. In June 2011, the Ministry of Human Resources and Social Security and the Ministry of Finance jointly issued *Circular on Relevant Problems concerning People Living on Unemployment Pension Enrolling in Basic Medical Insurance for Employees (Ministry of Human Resources and Social Security [2011] No. 77)* to properly solve the problem of people enrolling in basic medical insurance for employees while living on unemployment pension, work well on the transfer of basic medical insurance accounts and ensure rational medical treatment. Thirdly, the coverage of medical insurance for urban residents was further expanded. Efforts were made to instruct the local governments to give full play of the role of communities and schools, with the focus on the enrolling in insurance of the migrant population, new pupils and newly-born babies, etc. so as to cover all the residents with medical insurances. By the end of 2011, a total of 473.43 million people had enrolled in the basic medical insurance for urban residents, exceeding the goal of 440 million people set by the State Council, outnumbering that at the end of 2009 by 40.8 million. Among the total, 252.27 million people enrolled in the basic medical insurance for urban employees, 22.116 million people enrolled in the basic medical insurance for non-working urban residents and 46.41 million migrant workers enrolled in the medical insurance.

II. Fund-raising standards and benefit levels were improved steadily.

In 2011, governments at all levels raised government subsidies on basic medical insurance for non-working urban residents to no less than 200 RMB Yuan per person per year, and appropriately increased rates for individual contributions. On such basis, the benefits of medical insurance also steadily improved. In 2011, the maximum amount payable by the medical insurance for urban employees and the medical insurance for urban residents in the great majority of places was increased to about six times of the annual average salary of local employees and disposable income of residents respectively, with the maximum amount of no less than 50,000 RMB Yuan paid by the medical insurance. The proportion of inpatient medical expenses for urban employees paid out of the medical insurance fund within the scope of policies reached over 75% and the proportion for non-working residents while treated in medical institutions beneath secondary institutions within the scope of policies reached around 70%. Secondly, efforts were made to push forward the risk pooling of outpatient services for residents. In May 2011, the Ministry of Human Resources and Social Security issued *Opinions on Popularizing Risk pooling of Outpatient Services for Urban Residents (Ministry of Human Resource and Social Security [2011] No.59)*, requiring all the localities to popularize risk pooling of outpatient services for residents with the focus on insuring the frequently-encountered diseases and chronic diseases for outpatients, rely on the medical and health resources at the grassroots to keep the cost of medical services under strict control and improve the usage effectiveness of funds.

III. The reform on payment methods was further pushed forward

In June 2011, the Ministry of Human Resources and Social Security issued *Opinions on Further Pushing forward Reform on Payment Methods (Ministry of Human Resource and Social Security [2011] No.63)*, which definitely suggested that, in combination with the budget management of fund to strengthen the control of total expenses, global budget should be explored, on the basis of which capitation should be explored in combination with outpatient medical insurance and DRG should be explored in combination with the insurance for inpatient diseases and outpatient catastrophic diseases. Firstly, the working system of key contact for the reform of payment methods was established. All the provinces (regions, municipalities) were organized to select 103 key contact cities, on the basis of which 40 cities were determined as the ministerial key contact cities. Payment reform was conducted in all the localities, where plans for reform were formulated seriously and the compound payment method with the combination of multiple methods was pushed forward. Secondly, training was strengthened. In September 2011, the training workshop was held on the payment reform for medical insurance. Over 300 people attended the workshop, including officials in charge from the provincial bureaus, institutions of basic medical insurance system and the key contact cities.

IV. The management of medical insurance was further improved.

Firstly, the management of funds was regulated so that municipal pooling was mostly achieved. In line with the requirements of deepening the reform on medical and healthcare system, the reference standards for the municipal pooling were proposed, which proposed 14 requirements from the aspects of fund management, system and policies, settlement of medical expense account, service by the institutions of basic medical insurance system and information system etc. to instruct all the localities to vigorously strive for the municipal pooling. By the end of 2011, municipal pooling had been basically achieved. In Beijing, Tianjin, Shanghai and Tibet Autonomous Region, the provincial pooling was practiced. In 2011, the premium for urban basic medical insurance nationwide was 553.9 billion RMB Yuan, and the expenditure 443.1 billion RMB Yuan, which meant the balance of revenue and expenditure and smooth operation. Secondly, supervision on medial insurance was strengthened and working modes for supervision and administration of medical services were innovated. The agreement management was further improved to push forward the hierarchical management of designated medical institutions; modern information techniques were made full use of to establish a complete monitoring system for medical insurance, and insurance frauds were cracked down on even more severely by law.

V. Service quality for medical insurance was further improved.

Firstly, real-time settlement of medical expenses was pushed forward. By the end of 2011, 99% of the regions with fund-pooling of medical insurance for employees and 98% of the regions with fund-pooling of medical insurance for non-working residents had practiced real-time settlement of medical expenses within the regions with fund-pooling. Secondly, the management of site-off settlement of medical insurance was strengthened. 29 provinces (excluding Beijing, Tianjin and Shanghai) had made arrangements on site-off settlement within the province, among which 15 provinces practiced real-time settlement for site-off medical service within the province. Meanwhile, all the localities vigorously pushed forward the cooperation on the management of cross-province site-off medical service, for instance, the cooperation framework agreement on the management of site-off medical services among north-western provinces was signed in the northwest. 25 provincial and municipal institutions of basic medical insurance system signed the cooperation agreements to practice cross-province real-time settlement.

IV. The unification of urban and rural medical insurance was pushed forward with primary achievements.

As was required by *Opinions of the CPC Central Committee and the State Council on Deepening the Health Care System Reform([2009] No. 6),* efforts should be made to further improve the basic medical insurance management system ; The central government unitarily should formulate the framework and policies of the basic medical insurance system, while local governments should take the responsibility of organizing the implementation and management, create conditions for gradually uplifting the level of fund-pooling; Efforts should be made to effectively integrate the resources handling the basic medical insurance, and progressively achieve unified administration of urban and rural basic medical insurance. Acting on these requirements, we instructed the local governments to push forward the unification of urban and rural medical insurance and some regions have explored actively on the system to ensure the unification of urban and rural medical insurance. At present, unification of urban and rural medical insurance was practiced in 5 provincial administrative regions, i.e. Tianjin, Chongqing, Qinghai, Ningxia Hui Autonomous Region and Xinjiang Production and Construction Corps, over 40 big or medium cities and over 160 counties. Most localities started by regulating management system, unifying information standards and integrating the institution resources to gradually unify the urban and rural medical insurance systems. The unification of urban and rural medical insurance met the needs of the mobility of population to the urban areas, increased the insurance benefits for the rural residents, avoided repetitive insurance to a certain extent, decreased repetitive payment of premium, improved the management efficiency and service quality and brought convenience to the participants.

(Zhao Xuemei)

2. Work on New Rural Cooperative Medical Care System (NRCMS) in 2011 Was Deployed

In order to implement the work plan on the five key tasks of health care reform in 2011, the Ministry of Heath and the Ministry of Finance jointly issued *Circular on Working Well on New Rural Cooperative Medical Care System (NRCMS) in 2011*, in which detailed requirements were proposed for all the localities: Firstly, to improve fund raising for NRCMS, and raise the government subsidy to 200 RMB Yuan per person per year. Secondly, to optimize the compensation plan from the pooling fund, improve benefits, increase the reimbursement rate for hospitalization within the scope of policies to around 70%, raise the ceiling line of the pooling fund to six times of the rural per capita net income and no less than 50,000 RMB Yuan, and spread risk pooling of outpatient service. Thirdly, to expand the pilot for catastrophic diseases, improve benefits for children's leukemia and congenital heart disease within the respective province (region, municipality), and gradually expand the pilot scope of diseases. Fourthly, to accelerate the reform of payment methods and keep the irrational increase of medical expenses under control. Fifthly, to strengthen the supervision of fund, and ensure the steady operation of the fund. Sixthly, to assist the implementation of national essential drug system and promote the reform of operation mechanism for the rural grassroots medical institutions. Seventhly, to accelerate the informationization construction for NRCMS and carry out the pilot of All-in-One Card. Eighthly, to strengthen the capability construction of management and handling, innovate the handling modes, strengthen the connection between supplementary medical insurance and basic medical insurance, and better the construction of rural medical security system.

(Zhao Xuemei)

Chapter XVI The Management of Planning and Finance

1. The 2011 Management of Health Planning and Finance

In 2011, centering on the work plan of "one central point, highlighting six focal points and achieving four breakthroughs, the management of health planning and finance constantly intensified the responsibilities of "planning", "security", "regulation" and "resource allocation". As a result, significant achievements were made in all work.

I. The medical and health system reform was pushed forward greatly.

(1) Scientific planning and guidance for medical reform. *Suggestions of the Ministry of Health on Deepening Medical and Health System Reform in the Period of the 12th Five-Year Plan* was studied and put forward. We got involved in the revision of *Planning and Implementation Plan for Deepening Medical and Health System Reform in the Period of the 12th Five-Year Plan (2012-2015)* of Medical Reform Office of the State Council. *A Study Report on Medical Reform of Finance for Health Planning of the 12th Five-Year Plan* was completed, which made clear the guiding ideology, main tasks, major measures, key projects and main action plan for the medical reform planning of the 12th Five-Year Plan of the Ministry of Health.

(2) Funds were put to use and medical reform was guranteed. The year 2011 witnessed an input of 161.1 billion RMB Yuan of the central treasury for health services, with an increase of 52.4 billion RMB Yuan and growth rate of 48% compared with 2010. It was a year in which the central treasury put in the greatest investment in health services.

(3) Policies were made and medical reform was deepened. Centering on the reform of system and mechanism, we got involved in studying and worked out guiding opinions on multiple work and conducted prospective studies on various major policies. We also studied and issued related provisions for the connection of new and old accounting systems.

(4) Regulation was intensified and medical reform was safeguarded. With the construction of the platform for fund regulation of medical reform, we pushed forward the surveillance for total expenditure on health and government's investment for medical reform, and achieve basically complete coverage of various localities. The comprehensive supervision and inspection for special funds for medical reform were organized. And local authorities were asked to report in time how the tasks for

medical reform were under way.

(5) Investigations and instructions were conducted and medical reform was pushed forward. The were mainly as follows: comprehensive investigations for medical reform, supervision and investigations for pilot reform of public hospitals, investigations for regional health planning, criteria for health resource allocation, and layout and structure adjustment of public hospitals, investigations for the control of medical expenditure and investigations for comprehensive reform of county-level hospitals. These investigations played an important role in finding solutions to medical reform.

(6) Theoretical research was conducted to serve medical reform. The bidding for 10 subjects was organized, like the relationship of government health investment and the control of medical expenditure, which provided theoretical support for making health and economical policies of medical reform. Related experts were organized to conduct comparative study on health systems of China and Italy. Based on the study results, the experts put forward eight policy proposals suitable for the conditions of our country, which gave advice and suggestions to deepening medical reform. The revision of final report on "Healthy China 2020" was carried out seriously.

II. The task for health planning and finance was completed

(1) Planning related to health work was worked out in a scientific way. The first was to study and put forward *Basic Thinking for the 12th Five-Year Plan of Health Services and An Outline of the 12th Five-Year Plan for the Development of Health Services (Manuscript)*. The second was to carry out regional health planning actively and steadily, and guide and push forward various localities to carry out regional health planning. In addition, *Guiding Opinions on Strengthening Regional Health Planning* was revised. The third was to study and revise *The Construction and Planning for Health Supervision System*. Beside the following plans were studied and drawn up: *A Construction Plan for Rural First-Aid System, A Construction Plan for Clinical Training Base of General Practitioners, A Construction Plan for the Project of Medical and Health Management at the Primary Level, A Construction Plan for Rural Circuit Hospital Cars in Central and Western Regions* and related guiding opinions on constructions. The fourth was to guide organizations affiliated to the Ministries to conduct compilation and implementation of total construction and planning of development. Organizations affiliated to the Ministry were asked to compile first the development planning of services before compiling total construction planning of development to determine construction projects.

(2) The budget management was strengthened to accelerate budget

implementation. The first was that big issues in budget management must be settled by the working committee of budget management under the Ministry of Health after centralized study and examination. The second was to study and develop "ten measures" which accelerated budget implementation, including intensifying the management responsibility of the main of budget implementation body. As a result, the budget implementation schedule of the Ministry of Health was enhanced more significantly than previous years. The third was to take the initiative to make public the departmental budget, and final accounts, which would be subject to public supervision. The fourth was to compile scientifically 2011 departmental budget of the Ministry of Health and coordinated with the Ministry of Finance to guarantee the need of key funds. The fifth was to boost the performance appraisal for the expenditure of medical reform at the level of the Ministry and carry out the pilot work for performance appraisal of project expenditure.

(3) Targeted inspection was conducted in an in-depth way. The first was to complete the specific rectification of "unit-owned exchequer" and issued *A Circular of the Ministry of Health on Establishing and Perfecting a Long-Term Mechanism for Prevention and Control of "Unit-Owned Exchequer"*. The second was to push forward special rectification of prominent problems in the area of engineering construction in health system. A spot test was performed, focusing on twenty organizations affiliated to the Ministry and health construction projects of 100 counties. The third was to conduct supervision and inspection of budget funds. Through strict management of budget examination and approval, and conducting self-exams of budget enforcement, we guaranteed the safety of budget fund use. The fourth was to organize the compilation of *An Operator's Guide to Internal Audit in Health System*, which boosted the standardization of internal audit in health system. The fifth was to push forward the construction of general accountant system. The sixth was to conduct the audit of economic responsibility and financial revenues and expenditures to ensure safe and effective use of funds. *Provisions for the Economic Responsibility Audit of Principal Leading Cadres of Organizations Directly Under the Ministry of Health* was studied and worked out.

(4) Work was done for providing health aid for Xinjiang and Tibet, and for poverty alleviation by health and post-disaster reconstruction. The first was to continue to carry out and implement the spirit of Central Conference on Xinjiang Work, and held special sessions, such as 2011 Coordination Meeting of National Health System on Partner Assistance for Xinjiang. The second was to continue to carry out and implement the spirit of the 5th Central Conference on Tibet Work, and held special sessions, such as the work conference of six provinces (cities) on partner assistance for the Tibetan areas in Qinghai, and the work meeting of national health system on partner assistance for Tibet. The third was to hold the meeting on

poverty alleviation by health and coordinated with organizations affiliated to the Ministry to raise designated funds and determined poverty relief projects in 2011. The collaborative agreement was signed by the Ministry of Health and Guizhou Provincial People's Government to support the leapfrog development of health services in Bijie experimental area. The work thought of regional development and poverty alleviation in Luliang Mountain area was studied. The fourth was to complete all the tasks of post-disaster reconstruction. The summary meeting of health system on post-disaster reconstruction of Wenchuan earthquake was held to sum up experiences comprehensively, and specific requirements were put forward. The post-disaster reconstruction projects of Yushu and Zhouqu were carried out as scheduled. The fifth was to conduct health emergency security. A special fund of 97.28 million RMB Yuan was provided for the emergency disposal of imported wild poliovirus in Xinjiang, which effectively guaranteed the prevention and control of the epidemic situation. Meanwhile we kept an eye on earthquakes, typhoons and floods in various localities, contacted the affected provinces and actively applied for relief funds.

(5) The centralized procurement of drugs, large medical equipments and high-value consumables was pushed forward. The first was to conduct studies on special topics like drug evaluation system and quantity procurement. Also "the data base for bidden price inquiry of national centralized procurement of drugs" was developed. The second was to complete the procurement of surgical robot, TOMO and PET-CT, and reduced the price of equipment procurement greatly. The third was to establish the price information bank for high-value medical consumables for data collection, classification and aggregation. Besides work rules for centralized procurement of high-value medical consumables were drawn up.

(6) The management of capital construction was strengthened. The first was to strengthen the management of capital construction of organizations affiliated to the Ministry and revise *Administrative Measures for the Capital Construction of Organizations Affiliated to the Ministry of Health*. The second was to study and worked out *Distribution Measures for the Base Parts of the Departments of Central Budgetary Investments*. Nine different factor indexes were transformed into weight coefficients, which made fund distribution more scientific and transparent. The third was to compile and printed *An Atlas of the Construction of Health Supervision Institutions* and started the compilation of *Construction Standards for Children's Hospitals*. The fourth was to strengthen energy conservation and emission reduction of medical and health institutions to push forward the scientific, standard and informative management of energy conservation.

III. A new breakthrough in the management of health planning and finance was made

(1) The breakthrough in the control and management of health planning and finance was made. *A Project Specification for National Medical Service Price* was completed, while *Interim Provisions on Strengthening the Internal Price Management of Medical Institutions* was issued. With the pilot work for single-diagnosed disease fee system done, we issued jointly with National Development and Reform Commission (NDRC) *A Circular on Issues Related to Pilot Reform of Diagnostic Related Groupings.* With national inspection for health service price conducted, we gave guidance to correct definition of price violation in various localities. We also conducted surveillance of the cost of medical service prices, which provided bases for strengthening cost accounting. With financial analysis, we formed special analysis report on An Analysis of Economic Operation of Hospitals Affiliated to the Ministry in the Period of the 11th Five-Year Plan.

(2) The breakthrough was made in the adjustment of health resource allocation. *Guiding opinions on Layout and Structure Adjustment of Public Hospitals in Pilot Cities, 2011-2015 National Configuration Planning of Positron Emission Tomography-computed Tomography (PET-CT), National Configuration Planning of Group B Large Medical Equipments and Administrative Measures for Medical Equipment of Medical and Health Institutions* were issued and printed. Prospective management measures for Positron Emission Tomography-Magnetic Resonance (PET-MR) and *Administrative Provisions for the Configuration of New Large Medical Equipments (Exposure Draft)* were studied and put forward.

(3) The breakthrough was made in the regulation measures of funds. The first was to strengthen the construction of regulation platform of medical reform fund, further understand the capital arrangement and appropriation in various localities, urge local governments at all levels to perform responsibilities for investment and accelerate the capital enforcement of medical reform. The second was to push forward total expenditure on health and surveillance of government investment in medical reform, design special software, combine site submission with cyber submission and achieve basically full coverage in various localities. The third was to initially establish the financial database for central treasury subsidy of major special projects for medical reform since 2011 to conduct data collection analysis and provide data support for leadership decisions.

(4) The breakthrough was made in formation mechanism of major public health projects. The first was to study and set up the formation mechanism of major special projects for medical reform, in which the professional department put forward needs,

experts were organized to demonstrate, planning and financial department organized the examination and approval, and the budget board of the Ministry of Health centered on the discussion. The second was to set up project libraries for special projects of the 12th Five-Year Plan of medical reform and conduct rolling management. Currently fifty-four projects have been included in project libraries with a project fund of 884 billion RMB Yuan. The third was to reform issuing ways. Departments at the central level only issued task load and assessment requirements while departments at the provincial level just refined implementation requirements of projects. The fourth was to establish the special information reporting system for funds of medical reform, which made local authorities make overall arrangements for funds and develop measures combining with local actual realities.

IV. The overall level of health planning and finance was improved

(1) The informationization construction of health planning and finance was pushed forward. The first was to establish the information communication platform for health planning and finance, which was open to the health planning and financial departments in various localities as well as the financial departments of organizations affiliated to the Ministry. The second was to conduct the construction of surveillance platform for medical reform investment, which included the medical reform investment of governments at all levels in the range of surveillance, and urged governments at all levels to establish and perfect the investment mechanism, and carry out the government responsibilities for investment. The third was to strengthen the construction of regulation for medical reform funds, establish the system of periodic report and step up the enforcement of medical reform funds. The fourth was to push forward the information system construction for budget management of the Ministry of Health. The interconnection and real-time monitoring were initially achieved between the Ministry of Health and various budget organizations affiliated to the Ministry. The purpose was to improve the efficiency of budget management. The fifth was to establish the information management system of national large medical equipments, and set up the cyber platform of examination and approval for the configuration of Group A large medical equipments.

(2) The safety and integrity of state-owned assets were safeguarded. The transition of publishing houses was pushed forward. The special fund for the development of culture industry was reported. *The 3rd Suggestion for Bid List of Health GPA Accession and The Influence of GPA Accession on China's Health and Report on Countermeasure Study were completed.*

(Shan Yongxiang)

2. The Study on Health Accession to GPA of WTO

Based on the work arrangements and work focus of the Ministry of Finance and the Ministry of Commerce concerning the accession to GPA of WHO, the Ministry of Health organized experts to make a serious study. Proceeding from the procurement object, they analyzed the influence of GPA accession on medical equipment industry, procurement system of essential drugs, health services (including TCM services) and the central health entity as well as the countermeasures. On the basis of above study, *The 3rd Suggestion for Bid List of Health GPA Accession and The Influence of GPA Accession on China's Health* and *2010 Report on Health Accession to GPA of WHO* were completed and reported to the Ministry of Finance and the Ministry of Commerce.

(Shan Yongxiang)

Chapter XVII Health Education, News and Publication

1. 2011 Work on Health Promotion and Health Education

In 2011, health promotion and health education centered on the central task of medical reform and main health issues. Health promotion and health education of medical reform were actively carried out. The comprehensive coordination and overall planning of health promotion and health education were strengthened, which achieved stage progress. The main tasks were as follows:

I. The comprehensive coordination and overall planning of health promotion and health education were strengthened. In March, 2011, National Conference on Health Promotion and Health Education was held, which comprehensively summed up the job performance of health promotion and health education in the period of the 11th Five-Year Plan. The situation and challenge facing health promotion and health education in the period of the 11th Five-Year Plan were analyzed. In addition, priorities areas of work on health promotion and health education in the period of the 12th Five-Year Plan were arranged. Also experience changes and site visits were under way. Commendations were conducted for the exemplary organizations carrying out *A Planning Outline for National Health Promotion and Health Education (2005-2010)*. Besides the exemplary organizations in the establishment of smoke-free medical and health system were praised. The 12th Five-Year Plan for health promotion and tobacco control was studied and related contents were brought into the 12th Five-Year Plan for health.

II. The publicity and surveillance of residents' health literacy. Based on 2008 and 2009 surveillance results of health literacy, the evaluation index system of health literacy was revised and perfected, which laid a foundation for further surveillance of health literacy evaluation. The network testing and study system of health literacy was developed to explore and conduct network learning and self-assessment for health literacy. Knowledge and skills of residents' health literacy were popularized through network. In pushing forward the promotion action of health literacy of the whole nation, Jiangsu and Jilin pushed forward local health promotion and health education with the provincial surveillance of health literacy as the grasp.

III. *Measures for Performance Assessment of Health Education Institutions* was issued and printed. In August, 2011, *Measures for Performance Assessment of Health*

Education Institutions was issued. Health education institutions at all levels were given instructions in conducting performance assessment for technical consulting and policy proposals, professional guidance and training, summary and popularization of appropriate technology, information management and publishing, enforcement of surveillance and evaluation, and work effectiveness. Moreover performance pay system in health education institutions was studied and explored. Health administrative departments at all levels were responsible for the performance assessment of health education institutions in their jurisdictions. In all localities (especially at the prefecture level and county level), proper adjustment might be made for index weight and scoring criteria in accordance with local actual conditions. In principle performance assessment was conducted once a year. Health education institutions at all levels were responsible for technical support for performance assessment and accepted assessment. Based on the result of performance assessment in the previous year, health administrative departments at all levels checked and ratified the total performance pay of organizations examined for the present year. The result of performance assessment was taken as the important basis for financial subsidy, commendation and reward as well as examination and appointment of leading cadres. The result of performance assessment should be recorded in the files of performance assessment.

IV. The education health project of national basic public health services was pushed forward and carried out. We coordinated with the formulation of the specifications for 2011 health education project of basic public health services. We also gave guidance to primary-level medical and health institutions in carrying out health education project. Furthermore we strengthened the coordination and distribution of responsibilities of health education institutions and primary-level health institutions. Finally we conducted experience exchanges and carried out the medical reform task. In Ningxia Hui Autonomous Region, "health for all people of Ningxia" was held. The local health education institutions gave full play to support and guidance. They carried out health promotions toward primary-level organizations, gave publicity to health knowledge, and improved residents' health and living quality.

V. Implementation measures for tobacco control of health departments were pushed forward. The establishment of smoke-free medical and health system was pushed forward. Cross-supervision was conducted for the establishment of smoke-free medical and health system. Trainings on tobacco control were conducted for health administrators, and publicity and education for the implementation measures for tobacco control were also carried out. In combination with World No-Tobacco Day, publicity materials were given out. *2011 Report on China Tobacco Control* was issued while the theme publicity for national smoke-free day was given. We got involved in the work of the leaders' group of ministerial coordination for the implementation of tobacco control, and the writing of the 2nd implementation report of our country. *A Planning for China Tobacco Control (2011-2015)* was drawn up. As the international exchanges and cooperation for tobacco control implementation were strengthened, we learned from international experience to boost tobacco control implementation of our country.

(Shan Yongxiang)

2. Mass Communication Activity for China Tobacco Control

2011 mass communication activity for China tobacco control centered on such work as carpet tobacco control in medical and health institutions. A wider range of media campaign was launched with greater development of form and coverage, which exerted a more far-reaching social influence. Work was carried out in the following areas:

I. The annual commendation and kick-off meeting was held. On November 23, 2011, the Ministry of Health held 2010-2011 summary commendation and 2011-2012 kick-off meeting on mass communication activity of China tobacco control in Beijing. Over one hundred and forty people attended the meeting, including the officials of members of the leaders' group for tobacco control implementation of national health institutions, leaders of organizers and related supporting organizations, international organizations and domestic tobacco control experts, award-winning organizations and individuals, and reporters from over 20 domestic media. At the meeting, 2008-2009 award-winning agencies and individuals received commendation and awards. The activity for the current year was started.

II. Special web page for the activity and official m-blog were launched. On May 26, 2011, when the 24th World No-Tobacco Day was coming, a special web page was opened at Sina.com themed with In Tobacco Control Action I Support Smoke-Free Environment. Meanwhile official m-blog was launched. Voices from media, experts and netizens were aggregated, and dynamic information and hot topics in tobacco control area were released in time. With m-blog platform, "snapshots" for tobacco control focused on smoking in medical and health system, and netizens were asked to expose smoking. By December 31, 2011, there had been 25,865 fans of official m-blog, and 47,630 m-blog fans for snapshot of tobacco control.

III. Media training for tobacco control was conducted and business communications was held. Training courses for coverage of media from Central China area and Southwestern area were held. Directors, producers and reporters of related media from 16 provinces (regions, cities) were invited to the courses. Centering on the implementation process of China tobacco control, hot issues in tobacco control, and responsibility for media supervision by public opinions on tobacco control, tobacco control experts and media representatives held exchanges and communications. Jointly hosting the salon news conference of health page editors of media with the economic society department of People's Daily and people.com.cn, we discussed the integration of media resources of health and the expansion of media coverage results of tobacco control.

IV. 2010 top ten news stories on China tobacco control were chosen through public appraisal and released. Experts were organized to conduct preliminary screening for 2010 major news stories in domestic tobacco control. After netizens and media reporters voted, 2010 top ten news stories on tobacco control were chosen through public appraisal, including "tobacco control becoming a hot issue among deputies to the two Conferences drew attention".

V. Media works collection and selection. Words, television and radio related to tobacco control and published from July 1, 2010 to June 30, 2011 were retrieved. And experts were organized for the appraisal and selection. After more than 20,000 pieces of works were collected, repeated news stories and brief news stories were rejected through preliminary screening. At last there remained over 2,700 text category of works, 41 television category of works and 10 radio category of works, covering over 400 media organizations. After experts' preliminary assessment and final assessment, 36 pieces of works for three categories were selected.

(Shan Yongxiang)

3. Health Communication of Prevention and Control for HIV/AIDS, Hepatitis, Tuberculosis and Other Major Infectious Diseases

In 2011, Chinese Center for Health Education organized the theme campaign for 12.1 World AIDS Day. Anti-AIDS documentary With was put on display for awards winning and promotion at Berlin International Film Festival, Hong Kong International Film Festival, Beijing International Film Festival and Golden Rooster & Hundred Flowers Film Festival. The documentary won excellent documentary award at Beijing International Film Festival. The collaborative project for Youth Ambassador of love for

AIDS Prevention of the United Nations Children's Fund was carried out. *A Collection of Pictures for the Achievements of China-UK HIV/AIDS Strategy Support Project was published. And A Reader of HIV/AIDS Prevention and Control for Cadres* was revised.

A series of campaigns for the prevention of hepatitis were launched. Public-service ads and feature films were produced and broadcasted, and propaganda posters were printed and issued. We worked with News Probe of CCTV on shooting the feature film to launch a probe and discussion on hepatitis B discrimination and vaccination. A national campaign was launched for health consultation moving station of hepatitis C. The sunshine project for hepatitis B was started for patients' health education.

A campaign for World TB Day was launched and the feature film *TB—A New Threat to Age-Old Infectious Diseases.* An educational campaign of "vaccination publicity week" for parents was launched. Children's parents' education class was held for China Health Babies Plan. A series of spreading materials were produced: flash animation for popularization of SciTech for malaria, poster for National Vaccination Day, poster for Iodine Deficiency Disorders Day, education material for dental care, pumps, influenza and bacillary dysentery.

(Shan Yongxiang)

4. The Meeting on the Compilation of the 3rd Edition of English-Chinese Glossary of Medical Terms

On August 12, 2011, the meeting on the compilation of the 3rd edition of English-Chinese Glossary of Medical Terms was held at Tongji Hospital affiliated to Tongji Medical College of Huazhong University of Science and Technology in Wuhan. Over 80 people attended the meeting, including Professor Chen Anmin, Member of the Standing Committee of the CPC of Huazhong University of Science and Technology in Wuhan and Director of Tongji Hospital, Editor-in-Chief and professor Lu Zaiying, advisers, editor-in-chief, associate editors and editorial board members. Du Xian, Associate Editor and Deputy Director of People's Medical Publishing House Co., Ltd and related personnel from Medical Education Publishing Center also attended the meeting. At the meeting, the compilation contract of the 3rd edition of English-Chinese Glossary of Medical Terms was signed. The list of advisers, editors-in-chief, associate editors and editorial board members was announced, and letters of appointment were awarded to the advisers, editors-in-chief and associate editors.

(Shan Yongxiang)

Chapter XVIII International Cooperation and Foreign Exchange

International Cooperation and Exchange in 2011

I. Participating Actively in High-rank Talks and Global Health Issues to facilitate the nation's diplomatic activities.

The high-rank talks attended included the China-US Strategic and Economic Dialogue,the Sino-German Government Consultations, the China-Russia Committee on Humanities Cooperation and etc.. Active actions were conducted and resulted in the 10 national level strategic cooperation documents and foreign visit outcomes ,including the incorporation of health issues into SCO (Shanghai Cooperation Organization) . Apart from this, 4 cooperation documents were signed by our visiting state leaders with the coordination of the health departs. All of the above mentioned lent great support to the realization of our country's general goals in foreign affairs.

The meetings of our state leaders with Margaret Chan Fung Fu-chun, Director-General of the World Health Organization (WHO) and Michel Sidibe, Executive Director of UNAIDS were proposed and arranged. On behalf of China, the leaders of the Health Ministry attended the High-Level Meeting on Noncommunicable Diseases (NCDs) and the High-Level Meeting on AIDS of the UN General Assembly. They stated our country's concepts in health work and raised the proposals for the active global cooperation in the health issues. They conveyed our country's attention to our people's livelihood issues and health, the concepts in the reform and development of the medical and pharmaceutical systems and the ideas of prevention first in China's disease control work.

First BRICS Health Ministers' Meeting was successfully held and passed the outcome documents, which deepened the cooperation relationship between our nation and Brazil, India, Russia and South Africa and laid a basis for the cooperative mechanisms among the emerging powers in the international health issues.

II. Centering on the Medical Reform and Actively Carrying out International Cooperation and Exchange

Centering on the medical reform, the visits of the ministerial leaders were carefully arranged. They went to visit the medical and health institutions, held relevant symposiums, observed and studied the foreign medical systems, investigated the measures and experience of the visited countries in their development of the health undertaking. These efforts provided reference for our country's medical reform. At the same time, in order to boost our country's medical reform and exchange the experience in the reform, we made full use of the bilateral and multilateral cooperation platforms. Hong Kong was invited to introduce the basic drug system. The international symposiums between China and US, Canada, Australia, ASEAN and other entities were held and they were symposiums centering on medical reform, which greatly promoted the development of policies and the cooperation among different organizations. And for the first time, the famous international experts were invited to conduct independent evaluation on China's medical reform via WHO and they gave constructive opinions on China's medical reform.

In response to the 2011 world health theme "noncommunicable disease control", the ministerial leaders led delegations to attend the World Conference on Social Determinants of Health in Brazil and the First Global Ministerial Conference on Healthy Lifestyles and Noncommunicable Disease Control in Russia. By the cooperation mechanisms of BRICS, China-ASEAN and so on, we promoted the discussion and study on the chronic diseases, raised constructive suggestions to the prevention and control of chronic diseases and made our nation reach broad consensus on the issue of chronic disease control.

The international cooperation projects were taken as the breakthrough points and provided opportunities of policy and personnel training for the grassroots institutions. The cooperation projects on the public hospital reform with France, Switzerland and other countries and the policy research projects with US were conducted. The cooperation programs in general practice medicine, health emergency response, emerging infectious diseases, control of AIDS, tuberculosis and malaria and so on were carried out as well. The Sixth Experience Sharing Conference of International AIDS Projects was held and 3 foreign experts who made great contribution to the prevention and control of AIDS in China were awarded the certificates of honor.

III. Cooperating with WHO and Other International Organizations and Boosting Our Country's Health Undertaking.

We attended the important international conferences, like the World Health Assemble, the WHO Western Pacific Committee Meeting, the meeting of the WHO Executive Board, the Board Meeting of the Global Fund to Fight AIDS, Tuberculosis and Malaria, the meeting of UNAIDS Program Coordinating Board and so on. We successfully organized the Board Meeting of Roll Back Malaria Partnership, pushed forward the reform of WHO and the Global Fund and lent support to Margaret Chan for running for reelection as Director-General of WHO.

Close cooperation was maintained with WHO and timely response was made to the emergencies like the polio outbreak in Xinjiang, the nuclear radiation and pollution from Japan, the E coli outbreak in Germany and so on. WHO was encouraged to give inclination to the west region of our country to support the reform and development of the health work in that area. We also cooperated with the Chinese State Food and Drug Administration and the succeeded in passing the evaluation of WHO on our nation's inspection and supervision system of the vaccines, which was the premise for our country's vaccine manufacturers to develop the international market.

Proper response was made to the suspension of fund allocation from the Global Fund and the inspection and supervision of the projects were strengthened. Cooperation was maintained with UNAIDS, UNICEF, UNFPA (the United Nations Population Fund), APEC. The annual working plans and memorandums were signed with UNICEF and UNFPA. The implementation of projects for the UN Millennium Development Goals was organized and coordinated. Assistance was given to the World Bank in issuing *the Report on Chronic Diseases in China.*

IV. Increasing the Bilateral Exchange in the Health Field and Advancing the Cooperation with Neighboring Regions.

Attention was given to the realization of the outcomes of the visits by our state and ministerial leaders and the cooperation with the developing countries in South Africa and Southeast Europe was conducted as the priority. The South-South Cooperation in the health field was deepened by the cooperation in disease control, traditional Chinese medicine, food safety and so on. The bilateral high-rank communication with the developed countries in Europe and America was maintained and deepened and the range of cooperation was widened. The exchange was enhanced in the aspects of medical system, hospital management, disease control, biosafety, traditional medicine, food safety, health emergency response, telemedicine, translational medicine, health techniques, personnel training and so on.

Emphasis was laid on strengthening the cooperation with the neighboring countries in Asia and other continents. We held the tripartite health ministers' meeting of China, Japan and South Korea and attended about 20 international conferences on the themes of hospital management, disease control and prevention and so on. After Japan was struck by the tsunami and the nuclear leakage, the ministers wrote to express their sympathy and solicitude and invited Japanese experts to attend the symposium on the health response to the emergency of nuclear leakage. The new-round application for Japan-China Sasakawa Medical Fellowship was started. Visits were paid to the North Korea and free medical service was provided. In addition, medicines and medical devices were donated to the North Korea. The prevention and control programs on AIDS, malaria and dengue in the bordering regions with Vietnam, Laos and Burma were conscientiously continued and a lab for the primary screening of AIDS was donated to Laos. The negotiations over the standards of bird's nest with Malaysia and Indonesia were conducted. *The Regional Health Cooperation of China(2003-2010)* was compiled and published.

V. Pursuing Excellence in Performance and Doing Well the Work of the Foreign Medical Aiding Teams.

The communication with the African countries was maintained. With the visits of the high-rank officials, the bilateral cooperation was pushed forward, the achievements and experience in our country's medical reform was demonstrated and the Chinese enterprises were aided to enter the African markets.

The dispatch of foreign-aiding medical teams was continued. Within the year, 24 batches, 365 teams, and totally 1072 medical worker were sent to work in 48 countries. 23 inter-governmental agreements on the dispatch of medical teams were signed and another 16 were under discussion. The aiding medical team to the south Sudan was sent. We assisted the evacuation of Chinese overseas from Libya and arranged the emergent withdrawal and re-station of the medical teams during war. We lent support to the hospital construction in Africa and organized the African experts of key medical disciplines to receive clinical training in China. New foreign-aiding patterns were created. Our oculists went to Yemen, Botswana and Algeria to carry out cataract operations for the local people and an ophthalmic center was donated to Yemen. All of these efforts helped to set up a good image of our nation among the African people.

The activity of pursuing excellence in performance was carried out in all the medical teams. The preparations for the observation of the 50th anniversary of the initiation of the foreign-aiding medical teams were conducted. We coordinated the relevant departments, enhance the investigation of the foreign-aiding medical teams and solved the problem they met. The information network construction of the foreign-aiding work and the annual assessment of the team members were pushed forward. And thus, the management of the medical teams was improved.

VI. Implementing the Agreements on Health Cooperation and Maintaining the Stability and Prosperity of Hong Kong, Macao and Taiwan.

The Cross-strait Food Security Protocol and the Cross-strait Medical and Healthcare Cooperation Agreement and the medical and healthcare section of the ECFA (Economic Cooperation Framework Agreement) were firmly implemented. The exchange among the professionals with Hong Kong, Macao and Taiwan was intensified. The exchange and cooperation with Hong Kong and Macao in the fields of health emergency response, control of influenza and Health of the elderly were conducted and more convenience was provided for the Hong Kong and Macao residents to practice medicine or open up medical institutions. The Mainland and Hong/Macao informed each other of the epidemics 127 times and the epidemic reporting mechanisms were well maintained. The video conferences on the control of influenza A(H1N1) were held and the communication of the information on the epidemic situation was strengthened. The Lifeline Express carried out 9464 cataract operations in 10 regions of 7 provinces. The programs like the one of Hong Kong Huaxia Foundation achieved positive results and beneficial experience in the training for community nurses, rural community health promotion and vaccination of hepatitis B among adults.

The cross-strait conferences and symposiums on food safety, healthcare investment and so on were held. According to the annual plan, about 70 students from 7 Taiwan universities were invited to Beijing, Chengdu and other places to attend the summer camp, which greatly influenced the medical students in Taiwan and great increased their sense of identity of the Chinese nation and their interests in the historical origins.

VII. Establishing the Multi-department Meeting Mechanism on Going Abroad on Business.

The name of the Working Group on Forbidding the Travel out of China with Public Funds was changed to the Multi-department Meeting Mechanism on Going Abroad on Business of the Health Ministry. A long-lasting mechanism on forbidding the travel out of China with public funds was set up. The multiple departments made concerted efforts in the administration from different aspects. The members of the multi-department meeting mechanism carried out inspection and supervision in China's CDC, the Beijing Hospital, the Chinese Medical Association, Chinese Academy of Medical Sciences and so on. The inspection was conducted over the working norms of foreign affairs, administration of visas, the approval of the application for going abroad and the management of expenses for going abroad. They also lectured on the relevant policies and regulations of going abroad.

The departments and bureaus of the Health Ministry publicized the detailed accounts of the visits to foreign countries on the internal network according to actual needs of daily management and requirement for the report of statistics of going abroad on business. The reports of going abroad were shared and publicized. The quality and transparency of the visits to foreign countries were elevated and it was easy for the supervision of the public.

(Qu Yang)

Section 1 Important Visits to Foreign Countries

1. Zhang Mao, Party Group Secretary and Vice Minister of Ministry of Health, Paid a Visit to India and Yemen

During January 10th—19th, 2011, Zhang Mao, Party Group Secretary and Vice Minister of Ministry of Health, paid a visit to India and Yemen with the delegation of the Health Ministry headed by him. During his visit to India, Zhang Mao with the delegation paid visits to the medical institutions, observed the healthcare system of India and attended the China-India Symposium on Reform of the Medical and Pharmaceutical Systems. During his visit to Yemen, Zhang Mao met with Premier of Yemen and attended the ceremony for the donation of ophthalmic equipment to Yemen and the opening ceremony of China-Yemen Ophthalmic Center. In addition, Zhang Mao went to visit the Chinese foreign aiding medical team in Yemen and expressed his solicitude .

(Qu Yang)

2. Chen Zhu, Minister of Ministry of Health, Led a Delegation to Visit France and Morocco

During March 26th—April 4th, 2011, Health Minister Chen Zhu, heading a delegation, visited France and Morocco on invitation of these two countries' health ministries. During his visit to France, Chen Zhu met with some high-rank French officials. He also attended the Seventh Session of BIOVISION-the World Life Sciences Forum and the Sixth Meeting of the Steering Committee of the Sino-French Cooperation on Prevention Program against Emerging Infectious Diseases. During his visit to Morocco, Chen Zhu met with Moroccan Minister of Foreign Affairs and Cooperation Taieb Fassi Fihri and Health Minister Yasmina Baddou. He also paid visits to Moroccan medical institutions and went to express his solicitude to the Chinese foreign aiding medical teams in Morocco.

(Qu Yang)

3. Shao Mingli, Vice Minister of Ministry of Health Paid a Visit to the Seychelles and Kuwait

During April 12th—21st, 2011, Shao Mingli, Vice Minister of Ministry of Health and Commissioner of the State Food and Drug Administration, paid a visit to the Seychelles and Kuwait on invitation of their health ministries and went to see the Chinese medical teams in these two countries. During his visit to the Seychelles, Shao Mingli had a courtesy meeting with Danny Faure, Vice President of the Seychelles and Deputy Secretary of the Seychelles People's Progressive Front. He also had a meeting with Erna Athanasius, Minister of Health of the Seychelles. He inspected the Victoria Hospital where the Chinese medical team worked and visited the Chinese foreign aiding health workers. The national TV station of the Seychelles interviewed Shao Mingli and gave coverage to the cooperation between China and the Seychelles. During his visit to Kuwait, Shao Mingli had a talk with Ibrahim Alabdulhadi, the Under Secretary for the Ministry of Health of Kuwait and observed the drug administration bureau and the national medicine storehouse of Kuwait. In addition, Shao Mingli paid a visit to the traditional Chinese medicine clinic in Al Sabah Hospital where the Chinese aiding medical team worked.

(Qu Yang)

4. Vice Minister of Health Ma Xiaowei Paid a Visit to Hungary and Montenegro

During April 20th—29th, 2011, Vice Minister of Health Ma Xiaowei, heading the Chinese delegation, paid a visit to Hungary and Montenegro on invitation of the Hungarian National Resource Department and the Ministry of Health of Montenegro. During his visit to Hungary, Ma Xiaowei had a talk with Miklós Szócska,Minister of State for Health at the Ministry of National Resources of the Republic of Hungary and signed *The Executive Plan of China-Hungary for the Cooperation in Health Issues and Medical Science (2011-2013)*. The two sides exchanged opinions over the further cooperation within the framework of bilateral agreement in the health field in the aspects of reform of the medical system, control of infectious and chronic diseases, hospital management, evaluation of the quality of medical service, etc.. The Chinese delegation visited the Semmelweis University, its affiliated ophthalmic, pathologic and cardiovascular departments and other medical institutions.

During his visit to Montenegro, Ma Xiaowei had a talk with Gorica Savović, Vice Health Minister of Montenegro and signed *the Memorandum of Understanding on Medical and Health Cooperation between China and Montenegro*. The two sides exchange opinions over the further cooperation within the framework of *The Understanding*

Memo in the fields of medical reform, control of diseases, traditional medicine and so on. The delegation visited the Medical Center of Montenegro, the Medical Institute of Montenegro and other medical institutions.

(Qu Yang)

5. Vice Minister of Health Huang Jiefu Attended the First Global Ministerial Conference on Healthy Lifestyles and Noncommunicable Disease Control and Visited Austria

During April 26th—May 5th, 2011, Vice Minister of Health Huang Jiefu, heading the Chinese delegation, attended the First Global Ministerial Conference on Healthy Lifestyles and Noncommunicable Disease Control and visited Austria.

Huang Jiefu with the delegation attended the conference and delivered a speech. He pointed out that China, as a major developing country, was confronted with the challenge of the prevention and control of noncommunicable diseases and the solution to this problem was of great importance to the health of the Chinese people and the social and economic development. The Chinese government was highly concerned about the chronic diseases and the governments at different levels all issued relevant policies and formulated relevant measure to counter the problem. The prevention and control of chronic diseases was integrated into the overall social and economic development plan of the local governments. The coordinating mechanism among different departments was established and the whole society was mobilized to participate in the control of chronic diseases. The funding was actively carried out and the sufficient investment was guaranteed. The monitoring and evaluation were enhanced and the level of scientific control was elevated. Huang Jiefu called on all the countries to consider the control of noncommunicable diseases as important as the development of economy and cooperate together to tackle this global health issue.

During April 30th—May 4th, Huang Jiefu and the delegation visited Austria and investigated the medical and healthcare system, the hospital management and the management organ transplantation in Austria. On May 2nd, Huang Jiefu had a bilateral talk with Austrian Health Minister Alios Stoeger. Huang Jiefu pointed out that his visit took place during the 40th anniversary of the establishment of diplomatic relations between China and Austria and the bilateral cooperation in the health field developed steadily. He expressed satisfaction with the bilateral cooperation in the aspects of medical system, traditional Chinese medicine, hospital management and so on. Stoeger spoke highly of the sound development trend of the bilateral health cooperation promoted by the health departments of two countries. Both sides agreed to expand the range of cooperation in the health field and actively guide and coordinate the institutions at different levels to participate in the cooperation. The

Austrian side gave a relatively comprehensive introduction to the development of the Austrian medical system, including the policies and measures of Austria and EU for the administration of organ transplantation. The delegation visited the Vienna General Hospital and other medical institutions.

(Qu Yang)

6. Vice Minister of Health Yin Li Attended the Third Round of China-US Strategic and Economic Dialogue

During May 9th—10th, 2011, the third round of China-US Strategic and Economic Dialogue was held in Washington, USA. The Chinese delegation, headed by Vice Premier Wang Qishan and State Councilor Dai Bingguo, who were special representatives of Chinese President Hu Jintao, attended and chaired the dialogue held in US. As a companion, Vice Minister of Health Yin Li was presented at the meeting.

The main goal of the dialogue was to implement the important agreement struck between the presidents of two countries during Chinese President Hu Jintao's visit to the USA and to boost the construction of the overall reciprocal economic partnership. The two sides had in-depth discussions on the comprehensive, strategic and long-term issues and achieved many win-win outcomes. Vice Premier Wang Qishan and US Treasury Secretary Timothy Geithner signed *The China- U.S. Comprehensive Framework for Promoting Strong, Sustainable and Balanced Growth and Economic Cooperation,*which required that the two countries carry out expanded, closer, and more extensive economic cooperation.

On the morning of May 10th, Vice Premier Wang Qishan chaired the session of the Economic Track. During the third debate Promoting the Structural Adjustment and the Change of Development Style at the Economic Track, Chinese Vice Health Minister Yin Li made a speech to introduce the main contents and development of the reform of medical and pharmaceutical systems in China. Yin Li exerted that both China and the USA were under the medical reform and the two sides should strengthen and expand the cooperation. Both sides should learn from each other, try to advance the medical reform and bring benefits to the people in the two countries.

During the dialogue, Yin Li met with Howard Koh, the assistant secretary for Health for the U.S. Department of Health and Human Services (HHS), on May 9th. They exchanged opinions over the issues like medical reform, control of infectious and chronic diseases, health promotion and so on. Both of them agreed to deepen the cooperation between the health departments of the two nations.

(Qu Yang)

7. Chen Zhu, Minister of Health Attended the 64th World Health Assembly (WHA)

During May 16th—24th, 2011, the 64th World Health Assembly (WHA) was held in Geneva, Switzerland. The Chinese delegation headed by Minister of Health Chen Zhu attended the assembly. The delegation consisted of representatives from Ministry of Health, Ministry of Foreign Affairs, Ministry of Finance and other relevant departments.

During the general debate session, Chen Zhu made a key-note speech—*High Time to Control Noncommunicable Diseases*. He called on the international society to increase their sense of mission and urgency, firmly carry out the global strategy over the control of noncommunicable diseases, integrate the control of noncommunicable diseases into the core index measuring the level of a nation's social and economic development and further strengthen the construction of the medical and healthcare system.

Prior to the assembly, Chen Zhu met with Margaret Chan Fung Fu-chun, Director-General of WHO and Dr. Christos Patsalides, President of the 64th World Health Assembly and Health Minister of Cyprus. During the assembly, Chen Zhu met with the ministers from different countries and the chiefs from the international organizations like UNAIDS, IAMP and the Global Fund to Fight AIDS, Tuberculosis and Malaria. They exchanged opinions over the bilateral of multilateral cooperation. Chen Zhu also attended the preparation meeting for the BRICS Health Ministers' Meeting to give publicity of the oncoming ministers' meeting in July and to implement the outcomes on the health cooperation achieved during the third summit of the leaders of the Brics.

The Chinese delegation participated actively in the discussion of the different issues, especially the issues like noncommunicable disease control, HIV/AIDS control and elimination of smallpox. They stated the concerns of our country, safeguarded our nation's interest and successful completed their mission.

(Qu Yang)

8. Vice Minister of Health Yin Li Attended the 2011 UN General Assembly High Level Meeting on AIDS

During June 8th—10th, 2011, the Sixty-fifth UN General Assembly High Level Meeting on AIDS was held at the HQs of UN in New York. The Chinese delegation, headed by Vice Minister of Health Yin Li, attended the meeting.

During the discussion of the general assembly, Yin Li gave a key-note speech—"Action,Cooperation,Realization of the New Goals". Yin Li pointed out that, every nation, organization and individual should take action, further the cooperation, clarify their responsibility and set up the mechanism of joint prevention. The prevention and control of HIV/AIDS in China was an important part of the global action. The Chinese government would continue its efforts and establish the working mechanism in which the leadership of the government would be strengthened, the different departments would cooperate and the whole society would get engaged. And meanwhile, China would further the cooperation and exchange with the international society and face the new challenges together.

The Chinese delegates, coming from the Department of International Cooperation of Ministry of Health, the Disease Control Bureau of Ministry of Health, China CDC, Chinese civil societies, and the China's permanent mission to the United Nations, attended the meeting.

(Qu Yang)

9. Li Xi, the Discipline Inspection Team Leader to Ministry of Health Paid a Visit to Venezuela and Ecuador

During June 15th—24th, 2011, the Chinese health delegation, headed by Li Xi, the Discipline Inspection Team Leader to Ministry of Health, visited Venezuela and Ecuador.

During his visit to Venezuela, Li Xi met with Venezuelan Health Minister Eugenia Sader and they signed *The Memorandum of Understanding on Cooperation in Health Issues between the Chinese Ministry of Health and the Venezuelan Ministry of Health.* Li Xi pointed out that it was of great importance to sign *The Memorandum of Understanding* for both countries and he believed that his visit would advance the cooperation between the two nation's ministries of health and bring benefits to the people in both countries. Sader noted that the relationship between Venezuela and China was very close and the two countries cooperated in many fields. In addition, Venezuela was in need of China's support in the aspects of medicine, medical devices and so on. The medicine distribution center was under construction with the cooperation of Chinese enterprises. What's more, China's aid was an indispensable factor for the development of the health undertaking of Venezuela and *The Memorandum of Understanding* would guarantee the smooth development of the bilateral health cooperation. The Chinese delegation went to the medicine bidding and purchasing fair organized by the Venezuelan Ministry and paid a visit to the Pediatric Heart Center.

During his visit to Ecuador, Li Xi had talks with Onal, the Vice Health Minister of Ecuador and other relevant officials and they sighed *The Agreement on Health Cooperation between the Chinese Ministry of Health and the Ecuadoran Ministry of Public*

Health. Li Xi noted that his visit and the signature of the agreement were milestones in the bilateral health cooperation. At present, China was well under the reform of the medical and pharmaceutical systems and needed to learn the experience of other countries. The Chinese Ministry of Health would strengthen the exchange in control of infectious diseases, basic medical service, medical reform and traditional medicine within the framework of the agreement. Onal extended a warm welcome to the visit of the first ministerial delegation of China's Health Ministry. Ecuador was making efforts to intensify the construction of a sound medical service network to promote the health of the mass people. And Onal wished that the two sides would carry out pragmatic cooperation in the health field after signing the agreement.

The delegation had a discussion with the Ecuadoran health officials over the topics like medical and healthcare system, medicine purchasing regulations, hospital management, telemedicine and so on. The delegation also visited the Public Hospital, the Pediatric Hospital of Ecuador and other medical institutions.

(Qu Yang)

10. Vice Minister of Health Chen Xiaohong Paid a Visit to Italy and Albania

During June 22nd—July 1st, 2011, Vice Minister of Health Chen Xiaohong paid a visit to Italy and Albania on invitation of the two nations' ministries of health.

During his visit to Italy, Chen Xiaohong had a talk with Ferruccio Fazio, Italian Health Minister and they signed *The Executive Plan for the Memorandum of Understanding on Cooperation in Health and Medical Science between Chinese Ministry of Health and Italian Ministry of Health (2011-2014)* and witnessed the signing of *The Memorandum of Understanding on Research and Academic Cooperation in the Medical and Health Field between the National Health Development Research Center of Chinese Ministry of Health and the Italian Higher Institute of Health.* They had in-depth exchange over the further cooperation within the framework of *The Memorandum of Understanding* in the fields like reform of the medical and health system, food safety, health information network and telemedicine and prevention and control of infectious diseases. The delegation also met with He Changchui, the Assistant Director-General of Food and Agriculture Organization of the United Nations and visited the Italian Higher Institute of Health, the Ospedale Spallanzani Hospital and other medical institutions.

During his visit to Albania, Chen Xiaohong met with Sali Ram Berisha, the Prime Minister of Albania and Edmond Haxhinasto, the Deputy Prime Minister and Minister of Foreign Affairs. In addition, Chen Xiaohong had a talk with Albania's Minister of Health Petrit Vasili and they signed *The Executive Plan for Health Cooperation between Chinese Ministry of Health and Albanian Ministry of Health (2011-2015).* The two sides had in-depth exchange over the opinions on the future cooperation in the fields like reform of the medical and health system, construction of the medical institutions, exchange and training of medial staff, medicine production and so on. The delegation visited the Albania's Public Health Institute, the Mother Theresa Medical Center and other medical institutions.

(Qu Yang)

11. Zhang Mao, Party Group Secretary and Vice Minister of Ministry of Health, Attended the Sino-German Government Consultations

During June 26th—29th, 2011, Zhang Mao, Party Group Secretary and Vice Minister of Ministry of Health, with 5 colleagues attended the first round of the Sino-German Government Consultations held in Berlin, Germany. On June 28th, Chinese Premier Wen Jiabao and German Chancellor Angela Merkel co-chaired the first round of Sino-German Government Consultations. The delegation of Chinese Ministry of Health had counterpart consultations with Germany Federal Ministry of Health. Zhang Mao met with Daniel Bahr, Germany Federal Minister of Health, attended the symposium on hospital management chaired by Annette Widmann-Mauz, Parliamentary State Secretary at the Federal Ministry of Health and inked with Annette *The Joint Declaration on the Establishment of Partnership on the Hospital Management between Chinese Ministry of Health and Germany Federal Ministry of Health.* Zhang Mao listened to the introduction of Federal Ministry of Health over the response to the epidemic situation of E coli and went to visit some medical institutions in Berlin.

(Qu Yang)

12. Vice Health Minister Huang Jiefu Paid a Visit to Azerbaijan and Israel

During August 23rd—September 1st, 2011, Vice Health Minister Huang Jiefu, heading the Chinese delegation, visited Azerbaijan and Israel on invitation of the two nations' ministries of health.

During his visit to Azerbaijan, Huang Jiefu met with Abid Sharifov, the Vice Premier of Azerbaijan and Oktay Shiraliyev, Azerbaijani Health Minister. Huang Jiefu pointed out that since the establishment of the diplomatic relationship between China and Azerbaijan in 1992, the relation between the two nations had developed steadily. Both sides trusted each other politically, the cooperation in the fields of economy, trade expanded continuously and the exchange in the humanistic aspects like the medical and health field achieved remarkable outcomes. China was the second largest country that carried out organ transplantation and the medical devices made in China were of high quality and relatively low prices. Azerbaijan had full coverage of the medical security network and provided many kinds of service for diabetes, cancer, maternal and child healthcare. This yielded good results and set good examples for China to follow. Huang wished that the Azerbaijani would approve the agreement on health cooperation between the two nations and deepen the bilateral health cooperation. Huang Jiefu visited the largest surgical center in Azerbaijan and had talks with the relevant medical experts.

During his visit to Israel, Huang Jiefu had a talk with Israeli Deputy Minister of Health Yakov Litzman and signed *The Plan for the Cooperation in Health Issues and Medical Science between Chinese Ministry of Health and Israeli Ministry of Health (2011-2015)*. The two sides exchanged in-depth opinions over the bilateral cooperation in the fields like prevention of infectious diseases, reform and management of hospitals and so on. In addition, the Chinese delegation visited the largest Israeli medical center—Sheba Medical Center and investigated the development of organ transplantation in Israel.

(Qu Yang)

13. She Jing, Chairperson of World Federation of Chinese Medicine Societies Paid a Visit to the UK and Italy

During August 31st—September 9th, 2011, She Jing, chairperson of World Federation of Chinese Medicine Societies visited the UK and Italy. She Jing addressed the opening ceremony of the 8th World Congress of Chinese Medicine (WCCM) held in London, took part in the discussion in a sub-session of the meeting and communicated with the international organizations over the inhibition of using animals as drugs. During this period of time, She Jing chaired the election session of World Federation of Chinese Medicine Societies and its third conference of the representatives and had discussion with the Association of Traditional Chinese Medicine and Acupuncture UK over the legislation of the traditional Chinese medicine.

She Jing made a key-note speech on the strategy for the globalization of the standards of traditional Chinese medicine at the European Symposium of International TCM Standards held in Italy. She also attended a series of academic activities in Italy and investigated the clinics and hospitals of TCM in Rome and Venice, which brought about the cooperation among the medical institutions of China and Italy.

(Qu Yang)

14. Chen Zhu, Minister of Ministry of Health, Attended the 2011 UN General Assembly High-level Meeting on Non-communicable Diseases and the Third Meeting of Sino- Canadian Policy Dialogue on Health

During September 26th—28th, 2011, Chen Zhu, Minister of Ministry of Health, visited Canada with the delegation headed by him. He attended the third meeting of Sino- Canadian Policy Dialogue on Health held in Toronto and co-signed *The Executive Plan of China-Canada for the Cooperation in Health Issues(2011-2014)* with Leona Aglukkaq, the Canadian Minister of Health.

During this round of dialogue, the two sides had in-depth exchanges over the concerns of the both nations in the aspects of the financing for healthcare in rural and remote areas, the medical human resources in rural areas and the medical information network in rural areas. Both sides agreed that they were confronted with the same challenge in solving the problems of availability of medical service and financing for healthcare in the rural areas. The training and medical service based on the telemedicine, cultivation of appropriate medical talents and proper approaches to the problems in the work and life of the local health workers were the effective solutions to the challenge. In addition, both sides agreed to put emphasis on the cooperation in strengthening the evaluation of health policies, training of general practitioners, reform of public hospitals, construction of basic drug system, construction of health information network, control of chronic diseases and scientific research of traditional Chinese medicine and biomedicine.

Chen Zhu visited the Toronto Pediatric Hospital and investigated the medical and health information network of Canada. In the Chinese embassy in Toronto, Chen Zhu delivered a speech on China's deepening the reform of medical and pharmaceutical systems and had discussions with the Chinese biomedicine experts living in Canada.

(Qu Yang)

15. Vice Minister of Health Liu Qian Paid a Visit to Romania and Armenia

During October 12th—21st, 2011, the Chinese delegation headed by Vice Minister of Health Liu Qian, visited Romania and Armenia to observe and study their work in medical system, maternal and child healthcare and rural health.

During the visit to Romania, Li Qian met with Rodica Nassar, Chairman of the Health Committee in the Parliament of Romania and had a talk with Ladislau Ritli, Health Minister of Romania. They spoke to each other about the reform and development in the health field. Both sides expressed their willingness to deepen the bilateral cooperation in health policies and traditional medicine on the basis of the close cooperation over more than six decades since the establishment of diplomatic relationship between the two countries. The delegation visited the biggest pediatric hospital in Romania, the county pediatric hospitals and the family doctor's clinic.

During his visit to Armenia, Liu Qian had a meeting with Health Minister of Armenia Harutyun Kushkyan and they co-signatured *The Executive Plan for the Cooperation in Health Issues and Medical Sciences between Ministry of Health of China and Ministry of Health of Armenia (2010-2015).* The two sides exchanged in-depth opinions over deepening the cooperation in the fields like traditional Chinese medicine within the framework of the bilateral health cooperation agreement. The delegation also paid visits to the medical centers and maternal and child healthcare institutions at different levels.

(Qu Yang)

16. Zhang Mao, Party Group Secretary and Vice Minister of Ministry of Health Went to Brazil to Attend the World Conference on Social Determinants of Health

During October 19th—21st, 2011, the World Conference on Social Determinants of Health co-sponsored by WHO and the Brazilian Ministry of Health was held in Rio de Janeiro, Brazil. Zhang Mao, Party Group Secretary and Vice Minister of Ministry of Health, heading the Chinese delegation, attended the conference. Approximately 1,200 people participated in the meeting and they were the ministers from over 60 countries, the representatives from over 120 member nations and the representatives and experts from the UN special agencies, academic societies, and non-governmental organizations.

During the conference, Zhang Mao had a bilateral talk with Alexandre Padilha, the Brazilian Minister of Health and signed *The Executive Plan for the Joint Health Action of China and Brazil (2011-2014).*

(Qu Yang)

17. Vice Minister of Health Liu Qian Paid a Visit to Uzbekistan and Hong Kong

During November 25th—December 2nd, 2011, the Chinese delegation, headed by Vice Minister of Health Liu Qian, went respectively to Uzbekistan and Hong Kong on the invitation of the Health Minister of Uzbekistan and the Hong Kong government. The delegation attended the Uzbekistan International Symposium on Maternal and Child Healthcare and investigated the development of Hong Kong's medicine industry and medical technology.

During the visit to Uzbekistan, Liu Qian attended the Uzbekistan International

Symposium on Maternal and Child Healthcare. The symposium was co-sponsored by WHO and the Uzbekistan government, aiming to share the international experience on maternal and child healthcare. Uzbekistan's president, Islam Karimov and WHO Director-General, Margaret Chan attended and addressed the opening ceremony. The health officials and experts on maternal and child healthcare from 36 countries took part in the symposium. During the meeting, Liu Qian met with the Uzbekistan's Health Minister and Deputy Health Minister and had a talk with them. They spoke to each other about the reform and development in the health field. Both sides expressed their willingness to deepen the bilateral cooperation in E-medicine, immunization planning and training of medical workers.

During the visit to Hong Kong, Liu Qian visited the laboratories of the Medicine Research Department and the Biology Institute of Hong Kong University, the central laboratory of the Molecular Science and Technology Research Institute of the Chinese University of Hong Kong (CUHK), the Biomedicine Institute of CUHK and other medical facilities in Hong Kong. The delegation investigated the management models, the research orientations, the research outcomes and the cooperation programs with the mainland in the laboratories at different levels. They also observed the educational system of general practitioners and the community basic medical service network in Hong Kong and had discussions with the relevant departments over the cooperation on medicine research and development and training of general practitioners.

On November 30th, Liu Qian attended the evening gala hosted by Hong Kong AIDS Foundation and he spoke about the challenges the Ministry of Health confronted in the prevention and control of AIDS in recent years and the relevant policies formulated by the ministry.

(Qu Yang)

Section 2 Important Visits from Other Countries

1. Shin Young-soo, WHO's Regional Director for the Western Pacific, Paid Three Visits to China

On invitation of the Chinese Ministry of Health, Shin Young-soo, WHO's Regional Director for the Western Pacific, paid three visits to China respectively on March 14th, August 18th and August 28th—30th, 2011.

On March 14th, the Chinese National Influenza Center held the opening ceremony of the WHO influenza reference and research cooperation center in Beijing. Chinese Health Minister Chen Zhu and Doctor Shin Young-soo jointly held the key and opened the red door of the center, which symbolized China's entry into the family of WHO influenza reference and research cooperation center. Later the key was given to Shu Yuelong, director of the Chinese National Influenza Center. Shin Young-soo with his colleagues visited China's CDC and left an inscription.

On August 18th, Minister Chen Zhu met with Shin Young-soo in Beijing and they exchanged opinions over the future cooperation. Chen Zhu appraised the long-term support from WHO and especially the support from the Western Pacific office to the reform and development of the medical industry in China. Chen also thanked Shin Young-soo for his presence at the China Health Forum. Shin Young-soo congratulated China on the fast and overall development in the public health. He pointed out that in the future cooperation, the priority should be given to the development of the medical service network in the western regions of China. Chen Zhu and Shin Young-soo exchanged opinions over the issues like the control of chronic diseases, the role of the WHO Collaborating Center and so on. When attending the China Health Forum, Shin Young-soo made a key-note speech at the round tables and he exerted that equality, accessibility and affordability were the main goals of the development of medical system in all the countries. During August 28th—30th, Shin Young-soo visited Shanghai. He investigated the development in the construction of healthy city and medical system and attended the opening ceremony of The WHO Health City Cooperation Center. He said that Shanghai had a great deal of experience in building a healthy city, which would provide a model for other countries in the western pacific region to follow. The cooperation center could also help Shanghai share the experience with others. On August 29th, the opening ceremony of The WHO Health City Cooperation Center was held. Dr. Shin, Deputy Mayor of Shanghai Shen Xiaoming and the representatives from the relevant departments like the Department of International Cooperation of Ministry of Health, Shanghai Health Bureau and Shanghai Health Promotion Committee attended the opening ceremony.

(Qu Yang)

2. Nicola Roxon, Australian Minister for Health and Ageing, Attended the First Meeting of Sino-Australian Policy Dialogue on Health

On April 18th, 2011, the First Meeting of Sino-Australian Policy Dialogue on Health was held in Beijing. This meeting was co-sponsored by Chinese Ministry of Health and the Australian Ministry for Health and Ageing and supported by the Chinese Ministry of Commerce and the Australian Agency for International Development. Chinese Health Minister Chen Zhu and Australian Minister for Health and Ageing Nicola Roxon attended the meeting and they made key-note speeches on the reform of the medical system. Deputy Head of Mission to China Graeme Meehan attended the meeting and addressed the opening ceremony.

Chen Zhu stated that the bilateral health cooperation brought huge benefits to the people in both countries and contributed greatly to the global stability and development. He hoped that the mutual understanding and trust would be strengthened and the cooperation between the organizations in the two countries would be further pushed forward. Nicola Roxon pointed out that this meeting was an opportunity for both sides to know the new concepts and approaches of the medical and health system and for both sides to cooperate to improve the medical and health system.

The health policy makers and experts of China and Australia had discussions on the topics like control of chronic diseases, psychological health, prevention and control of emerging and re-emerging diseases and health emergency response. They also discussed the possible collaborating fields that both sides were interested in. Over 120 representatives from the Chinese Ministry of Health, the Chinese Ministry of Commerce, the Australian Ministry for Health and Ageing, the Australian Agency for International Development and the executive departments of the China-Australia Health and HIV/AIDS Facility attended the meeting.

Prior to the meeting Chen Zhu and Nicola Roxon had a bilateral talk, exchanged opinions over issues like tobacco control and noncommunicable disease control and co-signatured *The Executive Plan of China-Australia for the Health Cooperation (2011-2014).*

Nicola Roxon was invited by the Chinese Ministry of Health. During her stay in Beijing, she visited the China CDC, the Beijing Jishuitan Hospital and the community health center of Desheng Community.

(Qu Yang)

3. Didier Burkhalter, the Swiss Interior Minister, Paid a Visit to China

On April 25th, 2011, Chinese Health Minister Chen Zhu met with the visiting Swiss Federal Councilor and Interior Minister Didier Burkhalter.

Chen Zhu explained the new development in China's deepening of the medical reform, hospital management, tobacco control, noncommunicable disease control and other aspects. And he gave positive response to Didier Burkhalter' suggestions on cooperation. He also expressed willingness to strengthen the cooperation in the fields like the payment system, training of resident doctors, construction of health information network, chronic disease control, tobacco control, traditional Chinese medicine, global health issues and so on. Burkhalter also expressed willingness to share the experience and information with China and he also wished to learn the working experience of China in health issues. The two sides agreed to issue a joint declaration on the bilateral health cooperation between the two nations' health ministries and launched the cooperation partnership among 4 pairs of cities of the two nations in health policies and public hospital reform.

Burkhalter was invited to China by the Chinese Ministry of Science and Technology. The Swiss Ambassador to China and the relevant officials from the State Administration of Traditional Chinese Medicine and the Department of International Cooperation and the Department of Medical Administration of the Chinese Ministry of Health attended the meeting.

(Qu Yang)

4. Michel Sidibe, Executive Director of UNAIDS, Paid Two Visits to China

On invitation of the Chinese Ministry of Health, Michel Sidibe, Under-Secretary-General of the United Nations and Executive Director of UNAIDS paid two visits to China respectively during July 7th—13th and November 30th—December 2nd, 2011.

During his visit in July, Sidibe attended the First BRICS Health Ministers' Meeting in Beijing, met with Vice Premier Li Keqiang and the WHO Goodwill Ambassador for Tuberculosis and HIV/AIDS Peng Li Yuan, had discussions with the relevant officials from the Chinese Ministry of Health and the Chinese Ministry of Civil Affairs and went to Chengdu to investigate the prevention and control of HIV/AIDS in China.

During his meeting with Li Keqiang, Sidibe and Li exchanged opinions over the 4 issues of China' s strategy for HIV/AIDS Control, China's participation in the international cooperation on HIV/AIDS Control, promotion of the accessibility to medicine and further cooperation between China and Africa.

During November 30th—December 2nd, Sidibe met with the Chinese Health Minister Chen Zhu and was invited to the work conference on control of HIV/AIDS chaired by the Chinese Premier Wen Jiabao. He also attended charity activity for 2011 World AIDS Day held in the Great Hall of the People. At the work conference chaired by Premier Wen, Sidibe pointed out in his speech that the conference demonstrated Premier Wen's political commitment to the control of HIV/AIDS. And he thought that the Global Fund shouldn't slash the program funds of China and China should focus on the reduction of discrimination in the control of HIV/AIDS and provide antivirus drugs with less side effects.

(Qu Yang)

5. Margaret Chan Fung Fu-chun, Director-General of the World Health Organization (WHO) Paid a Visit to China

During July $9^{th}-16^{th}$, 2011, on invitation of the Chinese Ministry of Health, Margaret Chan Fung Fu-chun, Director-General of the World Health Organization (WHO) visited China. During her stay in China, Margaret Chan met with Premier Wen Jiabao, attended the First BRICS Health Ministers' Meeting, had talks with the officials of Ministry of Health and Ministry of Foreign Affair and went to visit Yan'an and Shanghai.

During the meeting with Premier Wen Jiabao, they exchanged opinions mainly over the issues of the development of biomedicine, the deepening of the medical and health reform and Margaret Chan's running for next term of office. Premier Wen noted that though the biomedicine industry in China started relatively late, in recent years, breakthroughs had been made in the establishment of basic drug system and the research and development of vaccines. In addition, more impetus would be given to the development of the biomedicine industry. When came to the ongoing reform of the medical and pharmaceutical systems, Premier Wen pointed out that the reform went well and was in the "deep water zone". The keys were to establish the basic drug system, push forward the system of general practitioners, make good preparations for the reform of public hospitals and make the public health service accessible to everyone. Premier Wen also hoped that by ways of change and training, WHO would continue its participation and support to China's medical and health reform. Premier Wen also spoke highly of Margaret Chan for her outstanding organizing and coordinating capacity during her term in WHO and stated clearly that the Chinese government would support Margaret Chan to run for next term of office.

During her meeting with Minister Chen Zhu, Margaret Chan praised China's achievements in the medical reform and she hoped that China would share the experience with the international society. Chen Zhu thanked WHO and Margaret Chan for the support to the reform and development of China's medical system and appreciated the long-term and practical cooperation of China and WHO in the health field.

In Yan'an, Margaret Chan went to visit the three-tier medical institutions of the county, township and village in Zichang County. She talked with the local medical workers and patients and investigated the development of the reform of the medical and health system.

In Shanghai, Margaret Chan visited the Pharmaceutical Engineering Center of the China State Institute of Pharmaceutical Industry, attended the China Symposium on Pharmaceutical Industry hosted by the Chinese Ministry of Health, inspected the

National Institute of Parasitic Diseases of China CDC and had a talk with director of WHO collaborating center.

(Qu Yang)

6. Mexican Secretariat of Health José Angel Córdova Villalobos Paid a Visit to China

On invitation of the Chinese Ministry of Health, Mexican Secretariat of Health José Angel Córdova Villalobos visited China during August $17^{th}-19^{th}$, 2011. José Angel Córdova Villalobos attended the Second China Health Forum, had a talk the Chinese Health Minister Chen Zhu and met with the relevant chiefs from the General Administration of Quality Supervision, Inspection and Quarantine of China and other departments.

On August 18th, 2011, the Chinese Health Minister Chen Zhu met with José Angel Córdova Villalobos and the delegation headed by him. They had a meeting over the bilateral health exchange and the reform of the two nations' medical system.

Chen Zhu spoke highly of the achievements in the bilateral health cooperation between China and Mexico and thanked Mexico for the support to the Second China Health Forum. He stated that the measures and successful experience of Mexico in the overall coverage of basic medical service and the equality in getting medical service were worth studying and he hoped that the two sides would enhance the exchange and cooperation in traditional medicine, health system reform and so on.

José Angel Córdova Villalobos congratulated China on the success in holding the Second China Health Forum. He stated that he would push forward the bilateral health cooperation in the fields like traditional medicine and reform of the medical and healthcare system. The two sides also had in-depth exchange over the reform of healthcare system, reform of WHO, food safety standards and so on.

The chiefs from the Department of International Cooperation and the Department of Health Law Enforcement and Supervision of Chinese Ministry of Health and the Mexican ambassador to China attended the meeting.

(Qu Yang)

7. French Minister of Labour, Employment and Health Xavier Bertrand Paid a Visit to China

On the morning of August 18th, 2011, the French Minister of Labour, Employment and Health Xavier Bertrand attended the Second China Health Forum and made a key-note speech on the French medical system and the reform of the medical system.

Bertrand explained the general situation of the French medical system and the reform of it, including the measures in medical insurance, health information network, hospital management and so on. He noted that the main goal of the medical reform in France was to increase the quality and accessibility of the medical service and boost the healthy development of the medical industry. He also spoke highly of the ongoing bilateral cooperation in the fields like personnel training and prevention and control of infectious diseases. He hoped that the cooperation could be expanded into more fields like medical science research, first aid and control of chronic diseases in the future.

(Qu Yang)

8. Ghanaian Minister of Health Joseph Yieleh Chireh Paid a Visit to China

During September 26th—October 1st, 2011, Ghanaian Minister of Health Joseph Yieleh Chireh with the delegation headed by him visited China. Zhang Mao, Party Group Secretary and Vice Minister of Ministry of Health met with the delegation and co-signatured with Joseph Yieleh Chireh the agreement on China's sending new aiding medical teams to Ghana. The delegation visited the first affiliated hospital to Zhengzhou University where they observed the internal information network and the remote video consultation system of the hospital. The delegation also visited the Guangdong Provincial People's Hospital. In addition, they had a talk with the Health Department of Guangdong province and met with the second batch of aiding medical workers who would leave for Ghana in the near future.

(Qu Yang)

9. Ferruccio Fazio, Italian Health Minister, Paid a Visit to China

On October 10th, 2011, Chinese Health Minister Chen Zhu met with the visiting Italian Health Minister Ferruccio Fazio and they exchanged opinions on strengthening the bilateral health cooperation. Chen Zhu briefly introduced the achievements and challenges in China's health work and the development in the new round of medical reform. He hoped that the two sides would have more high-rank dialogues and give encouragement to the direct cooperation between the two nations' organizations. In addition, the two nations should expand the range of cooperation within the framework of the bilateral cooperation agreement and strengthened the exchange and collaboration in the fields like medical reform, research of health policies, food safety, promotion of healthy lifestyle and traditional Chinese medicine. Fazio praised China for the remarkable achievements China made in the health work and he was impressed with the Chinese government's concepts and measures that prioritize the health of the mass people. Fazio introduced the healthcare system and the disease prevention system in Italy and expressed willingness to further the cooperation with China. Both sides agreed to first strengthen the cooperation in health policies and training of medical personnel.

(Qu Yang)

10. Miograg Radunovic, Health Minister of Montenegro, Paid a Visit to China

On the morning of October 24th, 2011, the Chinese Minister of Health Chen Zhu met with Health Minister of Montenegro Miograg Radunovic. They exchanged opinions on pushing forward the bilateral health cooperation. Minister Chen Zhu gave a brief introduction to the development in China's medical and pharmaceutical systems, prevention and control of chronic diseases, hospital management and hospital information network. He expressed his appreciation over the memorandum of understanding between the two nation signed in April and the active cooperation conducted within the framework of the memorandum. Radunovic said that Montenegro cherished the friendship with China and wished to deepen the health cooperation in different fields. The two sides had in-depth exchange over the issues like the reform of the medical and pharmaceutical systems, the reform of public hospitals, traditional medicine, health information network and so on. Both sides agreed that the cooperation and exchange in medical human resource, health information network, supervision of the quality of medical service and etc. should be strengthened.

(Qu Yang)

11. Anne Milton, the UK Parliamentary Under Secretary of State for Public Health, Paid a Visit to China

On the afternoon of November 8th, 2011, Huang Jiefu, the Vice Chinese Health Minister met with Anne Milton, the UK Parliamentary Under-Secretary of State for Public Health and had a talk over strengthening the bilateral health cooperation.

Huang Jiefu stated that the bilateral health cooperation between China and the UK had a long history and was of great achievements. China would like to learn the successful experience of the UK in the healthcare system to promote the reform and development of China's medical and health system. Milton said that the cooperation between the two nations' ministries of health went well and both sides benefited from the cooperation. She hoped that the cooperation would be furthered to bring benefits to both nations. The two sides exchanged opinions over the issues like food safety, noncommunicable disease control and training of general practitioners. They agreed that the cooperation at different levels, including the cooperation at provincial level and between the organizations should be strengthened to push forward the extended, practical and effective cooperation.

The relevant officials from the Department of International Cooperation and the Department of Medical Science, Technology and Education of the Ministry of Health attended the meeting.

(Qu Yang)

12. Kondi Charles AGBA, Health Minister of Togo, Paid a Visit to China

During November 15th—24th, 2011, on invitation of the Chinese Ministry of Health, Health Minister of Togo Kondi Charles AGBA with the delegation headed by him visited China and attended the board meeting of Roll Back Malaria Partnership held in Wuxi city of Jiangsu province. The Chinese Health Minister Chen Zhu had a meeting with the delegation. Chen Zhu spoke highly of the bilateral health cooperation between China and Togo. Kondi Charles AGBA thanked China for the selfless support from China in the health field. The two sides unanimously agreed to strengthen the bilateral cooperation in strengthening the medical personnel training for Togo. Vice Chinese Health Minister Huang Jiefu had a talk with Minister AGBA. Huang Jiefu gave a high appraisal to the bilateral relationship and the achievements in the health cooperation. AGBA thanked China for the long-term efforts in sending aiding medical teams to Togo, constructing hospital for Togo and safeguarding the health of the people of Togo. The two sides had in-depth exchange of opinions over the cooperation in aiding medical teams, training of medical personnel, assistance in the hospital construction and medical supplies and so on. The delegation also visited Shanghai city and Shanxi province.

(Qu Yang)

13. Maria Larsson, Swedish Minister for Children and the Elderly, Paid a Visit to China

On the afternoon of November 22nd, 2011, the Chinese Health Minister Chen Zhu met with the Swedish Minister for Children and the Elderly, Maria Larsson and they had a talk over strengthening the bilateral health cooperation.

Chen Zhu made a brief review of the bilateral health cooperation and gave a high appraisal to it. He said that after signing the executive plan for the bilateral health cooperation, the collaboration in many fields was actively conducted on the basis of mutual respect and friendship. Larsson stated that the Swedish Ministry of Health attached great importance to the cooperation with China and she had paid four visits to China within the past four years. The two countries had a lot in common in health and healthcare for the elderly. The two sides exchanges opinions and reached broad consensus over the cooperation on issues like collaborating mechanism, healthcare for the elderly, health information network, training of medical personnel and traditional Chinese medicine. Chen Zhu answered the question about the development in the reform of the medical and pharmaceutical systems. Larsson said that China was a nation with a large population and a vast area and it was a great challenge for such a nation to carry out a large-scale medical and health reform. She congratulated China on the great achievements China had made within the last 3 years.

The relevant officials from the Department of International Cooperation, the Department of Maternal and Child Health Care and Community Health, the Department of Medical Administration and the Department of Medical Science, Technology and Education of the Chinese Ministry of Health attended the meeting.

(Qu Yang)

Section 3 Important International Conferences

1. The Chinese Delegations Attended the 128th Session and the 129th Session of the Executive Board of WHO

The 128th Session and the 129th Session of the Executive Board of WHO were held in Geneva respectively during January 17th—24th and on May 25th, 2011. About several hundred people from 34 member states, relevant observers and international organizations attended the meeting. The Chinese delegation headed by Ren Minghui, director of the international cooperation department of the Ministry of Health attended the meetings as a member of the Executive Board. The Chinese delegation actively participated in the discussion of different issues, the revision of resolutions and the consultations outside the meeting session.

The 129th Session of the Executive Board of WHO was chaired by R.El Makkoui, the Secretary-General of the Ministry of Health of Morocco. During this session, the outcomes of the 64th World Health Assembly were reported. The administrative and financial issues like the specific steps of the reform of WHO, the implementation policies on publication of WHO and the working procedures of the executive board were discussed. In addition, the constitution of the sub-committees under the executive board was determined.

(Qu Yang)

2. The 43rd Session of the Codex Committee on Food Additives (CCFA) Was Held in Xiamen, China

The 43rd Session of the Codex Committee on Food Additives (CCFA) was held in Xiamen, China during March 14th—18th, 2011. This session was attended by 200 delegates from 54 Codex Member Countries, one member organization (the European Union), 27 international observer organizations, and FAO and WHO Secretariat staff. Professor Chen Junshi from the Chinese Ministry of Health Communicable Disease Center chaired this session.

The 43rd session proceeded with an agenda of 11 items and the discussion was mainly focused on the Codex General Standard for Food Additives (GSFA), maximum levels for aluminum containing food additives, food additive provisions for infant formula and formulas for special medical purposes and so on.

The Chinese delegation with 17 delegates from Ministry of Health, Ministry of Agriculture, Ministry of Commerce and other departments attended the 43rd session. Over 30 representatives from the regional food safety supervisory departments, trade association and food manufacturing enterprises sat in at this session. The 43rd CCFA session was the fifth session chaired by China since China was elected as the host country.

(Qu Yang)

3. The Ministry of Health Attended the APEC Conference

The First APEC Health Working Group (HWG) meeting of 2011 was held in Washington DC, US during March 6th—7th, 2011. Representatives of 15 APEC economies attended the meeting.

The main goals of the 2011 APEC conference were as the following: strengthening regional economic integration and expanding trade by advancing "next-generation" trade and investment issues, promoting green growth and fostering job creation in green industries and expanding regulatory cooperation and advancing regulatory convergence. The meeting proposed that the Health Working Group should carry out dialogues with LSIF and strengthen the cooperation between them. The cooperation should mainly cover the issues like study of risky behaviors, noncommunicable diseases, ageing, health planning and health information technology. China proposed the project "containing the highly infectious avian influenza via safety of food trade", which was seconded by Tailand and Chinese Taipei.

At the meeting 7 projects of five APEC economies were suggested. The project of Shanghai CDC of China "training for public health emergency response" was seconded by Sigapore and the South Korea and the project of the General Administration of Quality Supervision, Inspection and Quarantine of China "containing the highly infectious avian influenza via safety of food trade" was seconded by Thailand and Chinese Taipei. The meeting determined that the next Health Working Group (HWG) meeting be held in Russia in February and June. As the host country, Russia mainly pushed forward the issues like noncommunicable diseases, healthy lifestyle, maternal and child healthcare and so on.

The policy dialogue of the Health Working Group would was held on September 15th. It continued with the topic of ageing from last dialogue and the theme of this round was "ageing, health and innovation: idea to action". The attending parties reached consensus on the following principles: Firstly, the government should view the ageing of population as investment instead of consumption. Secondly, the cooperation between public organizations and private organizations should be strengthened and the public policy should be integrated with the innovation of the private organizations. Thirdly, the learning at different stages of life could elevate the productivity. The high-rank dialogue on innovation in the health system was held during September 16th—17th. The dialogue, centering on innovation of the health system, put emphasis on global challenge of noncommunicable diseases and economic burden brought by the diseases. It encouraged the innovation in the healthcare system and used the outcomes of studies to prove that investment in the innovation in the healthcare system could yield substantial economic return.

(Qu Yang)

4. Sino-French Forum on Public Hospital Reform Was Held in Beijing

During April 19th—20th, 2011, the Sino-French Forum on Public Hospital Reform, co-sponsored by the Chinese Ministry of Health and the French Ministry of Labour, Employment and Health, was held in Beijing. Vice Chinese Health Minister Ma Xiaowei and French Federal Secretary for the Ministry of Labour, Employment and Health Norah Béla attended and addressed the opening ceremony. Ren Minghui, director of the Department of International Cooperation of the Chinese Ministry of Health hosted the opening ceremony.

Ma Xiaowei spoke highly of the long-term health cooperation between China and France. He briefly introduced the background and contents of deepening the reform of the medical and pharmaceutical systems in China and laid emphasis on the development and working plans in the pilot work of public hospital reform. He pointed out that the reform of the public hospital was a long and complicated task that needed the experience accumulated from the pilot work and the mature measures learned from the international societies. France was rich in experience in the planning and administration of public hospitals and could provide guidance for China. Norah affirmed China's active collaboration with France in the reform of the public hospitals and she believed that the bilateral health cooperation was rich in contents. In the future, the cooperation could extend to the provincial or municipal level instead of being limited to the national level.

During the forum, the two sides had extensive and in-depth exchange over the issues like the basic situation of the public hospital system, planning of medical service, management and supervision of public hospitals, and so on. The participants of the forum thought there were common grounds between China and France in the principles and goals of public hospital reform. Both countries laid emphasis on the responsibility of the government, the accessibility to medical service and the mobilization of the medical workers to provide safe, effective, convenient and inexpensive medical service to the mass people. In the formulation of the specific policies, the two countries shared many commonplaces in establishing the socialized medical expense coverage system, emphasizing the function of the community medical institution and pushing forward the reform of payment models. The Chinese representatives thought that super-ministry system in France helped to integrate the medical resources, ensured the coordination and consistency of the medical service and laid a solid foundation for the improvement of the performance in the hospitals. The hospital presidents were appointed by the government and given the status as public servants and the performance of the hospitals was assessed by the government as well. Thus, the management of the hospitals was strengthened. The salaries of the medical workers in the public hospitals were fixed and the performance assessment of them was enhanced. As a result, the behavior of the medical workers was regulated. The expenses for medical service were controlled by reform of the payment models and the highly developed health information network facilitated the management and supervision of the hospitals. In order to deepen the bilateral cooperation in the reform of the public hospitals, the two nations formulated the partnership hospital projects. The forum publicized the list of the 17 French hospitals and 18 Chinese hospitals in 16 pilot cities. The forum was organized by the Human Resource Exchange Center of the Chinese Ministry of Health and the French embassy to China.

(Qu Yang)

5. Ministry of Health Attended the 20th Session of Roll Back Malaria Partnership

During May 11th—13th, 2011, the 20th Session of Roll Back Malaria Partnership (hereinafter referred to as RBM) was held in Geneva, Switzerland. Approximately

80 people, including the ministers and high-rank representatives from the afflicted countries like Angola and South Africa, the representatives from the donor countries like France and USA and the representatives from WHO, UNICEF, academic and research institutions, non-government organizations, private organizations, attended the session. Chinese director of the International Cooperation Department of the Ministry of Health, Ren Minghui, on behalf of Vice Health Minister Huang Jiefu, attended the meeting as the board member of the Asian-Pacific countries afflicted with malaria.

At the meeting, the representatives discussed the report of the executive director, the implementation of the GMAP and the goals, priorities and quotas of RBM in 2011-2015. The meeting decided to continue the exploration of the flexibility of innovative financing. Victor Makwenge Kaput, health minister of the Democratic Republic of Congo was voted as the next chair of the board of RBM by secret ballot at the meeting.

(Qu Yang)

6. Ministry of Health Attended the 23rd, 24th and 25th Board Meetings of the Global Fund

The 23rd and 24th board meetings the Global Fund to Fight AIDS, Tuberculosis and Malaria were held in Geneva, Switzerland respectively during May 10th—12th and September 26th, 2011. The 25th board meeting was held during November 21st—22nd in Accra, Ghana. The Chinese Ministry of Health attended the meetings as the board member of the Western Pacific Region.

At the 23rd board session, the key issues of the Global Fund like the 5-year strategy framework, the plan for the reform of the Global Fund and the financial auditing were discussed and the board also approved the preliminary framework of reform and the establishment of a High-level Independent Review Panel. The delegation of the Western Pacific Region consisted of delegates from the International Cooperation Department and the Disease Control Department of the Chinese Ministry of Health, the non-government organizations in China and the island countries of the West Pacific Region like Vietnam and Samoa. The board approved the decisions on the policy of eligibility criteria, the prioritization of proposals for funding and the counterpart financing requirements. In addition, the new country coordinating mechanisms, the 2010 annual report and financial report of the Global Fund were also approved. The board discussed the report and suggestions of the General Inspector and elected Martin Dinham, Director General of the UK Department for International Development, as chair of the board and Mphu Ramatlapeng, Health Minister of the

Kingdom of Lesotho as vice chair.

At the 24th board session, the report of the High-level Independent Review Panel was discussed. The board was co-hosted by Simon Bland, chair of the board and Mphu Ramatlapeng, vice chair of the board. The representatives from China CDC sent by the Chinese Ministry of Health and the reprehensive from New Caledonia, the South Pacific island country attended the board meeting as the board member of the Western Pacific Region. The board accepted the report of the High-level Independent Review Panel and the analysis and proposals of it. In order to implement the proposals in the report, the board needed to formulate a detailed plan based on the best practice and the past experience. The new plan would integrate the ongoing reform plan to form a working scheme for implementation.

The 25th Board Meeting approved the Global Fund Strategy 2012-2016 Framework, the Consolidated Transformation Plan, the Charter for each new standing Committees of the Board, the appointment of chairs and vice chairs for the committees and the 2012 Operating Expenses Budget of the Secretariat. The board endorsed the Consolidated Transformation Plan which aimed to transform the following elements: resource allocation, investment, results management and evaluation; risk management; grant management; Secretariat organization, management and culture; board governance; and resource mobilization to turn the Global Fund into an effective and efficient organization. Taking the international economic condition and the funding of the Global Fund into consideration, the board restated that priority would be given to the projects of the low-income countries and measures would be taken to cut down the grants to middle or high-income countries.

(Qu Yang)

7. Ministry of Health Attended the Meetings of UNAIDS Programme Coordinating Board

The twenty-eighth and the twenty-ninth meetings of UNAIDS Programme Coordinating Board (PCB) were held in Geneva, Switzerland respectively during June 21st—23rd and December 13th—25th, 2011. Over 150 representatives from the 22 members of PCB, the non-government organizations of Asia-Pacific, North America, Europe, Africa and Latin America and the cosponsors like WHO and World Bank attended the two meetings. The Chinese delegation consisting of representative from the International Cooperation Department and the Disease Control Department of Ministry of Health attended the meeting.

At the 28th meeting, UNAIDS Executive Director Michel Sidibé pointed out in his report that now it was a critical stage for the prevention and control of AIDS and the international societies should act on the new strategy of UNAIDS and make efforts to follow the roadmap to realize the vision of "zero new AIDS infections, zero discrimination and zero AIDS-related deaths". The sustainable funding approaches should be explored, the efficiency of the funds should be elevated and the operating cost should be reduced. The new emerging economies like the Brics should pay a more important role in the global control of AIDS. The issues of nutrition, food safety and AIDS were discussed during the meeting. The meeting determined that UNAIDS should help the relevant nations formulate policies that required the different departments to participate in the improvement of the food supply and nutrition for the people affected by HIV/AIDS. The board listened to the report of the Secretariat on the drafting of the 2012-2015 Unified Budget, Results and Accountability Framework (UNAIDS) and had discussion over contents within the framework.

At the 29th board meeting, Sidibé pointed out that in order to realize the vision of "zero new AIDS infections, zero discrimination and zero AIDS-related deaths" , the models for the global control of AIDS and the fund-raising should be innovated. The board listened to and reviewed the following issues: the report of the 28th board meeting, the report of the Executive Director, the report of NGO representatives, follow-up to the 2011 UN General Assembly High Level Meeting on AIDS, progress report on the global plan toward the elimination of new HIV infections among children by 2015 and keep their mothers alive, second independent evaluation of UNAIDS, UNAIDS results, accountability and budget matrix, UNAIDS technical support, next programme coordinating board meetings and election of officers. During the thematic segment: the theme of HIV and Enabling Legal Environments was discussed. The participating countries exchanged experience over the following three components of legal environment: access to justice, law enforcement and law and regulations.

(Qu Yang)

8. Sino-German Forum on Hospital Management Was Held in Germany

The Sino-German Forum on Hospital Management chaired by Annette Widmann-Mauz, Parliamentary State Secretary at the Federal Ministry of Health of Germany, was held in Berlin on the morning of June 28th. The Germany representative introduced the work done by the Sino-German Medical Association on the hospital management, which included the regular annual conference, personnel training and mutual visits and exchange.

In addition, the Germany representative gave a brief introduction to medicare reimbursement model of Diagnosis Related Group (DRG) and suggested that the implementation of DRG payment system should take a nation's specific situation into consideration and should be based on the advanced record of medical cases and well-developed information network.

(Qu Yang)

9. The First BRICS Health Ministers' Meeting Was Held in Beijing

On July 11th, 2011, the First BRICS Health Ministers' Meeting was held in Beijing. The meeting was hosted by Chen Zhu, Chinese Minister of Health. Delegations from the other four countries led by Alexandre Padilha, Minister of Health of Brazil, Tatyana Golikova, Minister of Healthcare and Social Development of the Russian Federation, Ghulam Nabi Azad, Minister of Health and Family Welfare of India, and Aaron Motsoaledi, Minister of Health of South Africa, attended the meeting. Margaret Chan, Director General of World Health Organization, and Michel Sidibé, Executive Director of UNAIDS attended the meeting as observers.

The First BRICS Health Ministers' Meeting was consistent with the mandate of the Sanya Declaration of the BRICS Leaders Meeting held in Sanya on 14th April, 2011. The theme of this meeting was "Global Health- Access to Medicine". Discussions were carried out on several topics. *The First BRICS Health Ministers' Meeting Beijing Declaration* was issued. It pointed out that public health was an essential element for social and economic development and should be reflected accordingly in national and international policies.

In light of the theme of the meeting "Global Health-Access to Medicine", which aimed to promote innovation and access to affordable medicines, vaccines and other health technologies of assured quality, in support of reaching MDGs 4, 5, 6 and 8 and other public health challenges, the following priority areas were identified:

1) Collaboration to strengthen health systems and overcome barriers to access to affordable, quality, efficacious, safe medical products, vaccines and other health technologies for HIV/AIDS, tuberculosis, viral hepatitis, malaria and other infectious diseases and non-communicable diseases.

2) Collaboration to explore and promote, where feasible, effective transfer of technology to strengthen innovation capacity to benefit public health in developing countries.

3) Collaboration with and support of international organizations, including WHO and UNAIDS, the Global Fund to Fight AIDS, Tuberculosis and Malaria and the GAVI alliance, to increase access to affordable, quality, efficacious and safe medicines, vaccines and other medical products that serve public health needs.

(Qu Yang)

10. The Third Experts' Meeting on Sino-South Korean Food Standards Was Held in Beijing

On July 21st, 2011, the Third Experts' Meeting on Sino-South Korean Food Standards was held in Beijing. The two sides had exchange over the food standard issues like the health standard for non-sterilized fermented food, the health standard for copper in cocoa products, flavored laver, white sugar, the standards for bacteria in ready-to-eat-food, the standard for iron and nitrite in ablactational food, the application of the standard for composite food and the administrative policies and the formulation of the regulations of food additives. The Chinese representatives for the Department of Health Law Enforcement and Supervision, the Department of International Cooperation and the Department of Disease Control of Ministry of Health and the South Korean representatives from South Korean Ministry of Food and Drug Safety (MFDS) attended the meeting.

(Qu Yang)

11. The First Senior Officials' Meetings on Health Development of ASEAN plus China, Japan and South Korea (10+3) and ASEAN plus China (10+1) Were Held in Burma

The first Senior Officials' Meetings on Health Development of ASEAN plus China, Japan and South Korea (10+3) and ASEAN plus China (10+1) were held in Naypyitaw, Burma during July 26th—29th, 2011. Wang Liji, Deputy Director of the International Cooperation Department of Chinese Ministry of Health, attended the meetings. At the ASEAN+3 Senior Officials Meeting on Health Development, the ASEAN Secretariat reported the cooperative activities carried out after the 4th ASEAN+3 Health Ministers Meeting held in Singapore in July and the contents of *the ASEAN Strategic Framework on Health Development (2010 -2015)*. The Chinese representative introduced the ASEAN+3 Symposium on Non-communicable Diseases to be held in Qingdao in November and issued invitation to ASEAN, Japan, South Korea, WHO and etc.. The meeting approved that the second Senior Officials Meetings on Health Development of ASEAN Plus China, Japan and South Korea (10+3) and ASEAN Plus China (10+1) would be held in Cebu, Philippines and the 5th ASEAN+3 Health Ministers Meeting would be held in Phuket Island, Thailand. At the Senior Officials Meeting on Health Development of ASEAN plus China, the Chinese delegation reported the 10+1 health collaboration carried out by China and the 5 projects China planned to cooperate with ASEAN in 2011 and the first half of 2012. The representatives had a discussion over the draft of *the Memorandum of Understanding between the Member States of ASEAN and the Government of the People's Republic of China on Health Cooperation* and they reached a consensus over the contents of the draft. The meeting also approved that the 4th China-ASEAN Health Ministers Meeting would be held in Phuket Island, Thailand in July of 2012.

(Qu Yang)

12. Ministry of Health Attended the 62nd Session of the World Health Organization (WHO) Regional Committee for the Western Pacific Region

During October 10th—13th, 2011, the 62nd Session of WHO Regional Committee for the Western Pacific Region was held in Manila, Republic of the Philippines. The Chinese delegation, consisting of representatives from the International Cooperation Department of Ministry of Health (MOH) , the Health Law Enforcement and Supervision Department of MOH, the Medical Administration Department of MOH, the Disease Control Department of MOH, the Chinese State Food and Drug Administration and the State Administration of Traditional Chinese Medicine attended the meeting.

Adanan Yusof, head of the Brunei delegation and Brunei Health Minister, was elected as chair of the 62nd session and Ren Minghui, Director of the International Cooperation Department of the Chinese Ministry of Health elected as vice chair. Liow Tiong Lai, chair of the 61st session and the Health Minister of Malaysia, Margaret Chan Fung Fu-chun, Director-General of WHO and Shin Young-soo, WHO's Regional Director for the Western Pacific attended the meeting and addressed the opening ceremony.

The committee reviewed the mid-term report on the operation of Western Pacific Regional Strategy (2011-2012) and passed 5 resolutions on proposed programme budget (2012-2013), non-communicable disease control, antibiotic resistance, regional strategy for traditional medicine, Western Pacific regional strategy for food safety (2011-2015). At this session, the topics like regional strategy for the elimination of malaria, control of dengue, mental health, essential medicines and planned immunization were discussed. The Chinese representatives fully participated in the discussion. In addition, they proactively gave an overall introduction to the imported case of polio in Xinjiang of China and the response to this emergency, which was unanimously acknowledged by WHO and the member states of the Western Pacific Region.

(Qu Yang)

13. Vice Minister of Health Huang Jiefu Attended the 11th and 12th Session of China-Russia Committee on Humanities Cooperation

On October 11th, 2011, Liu Yandong, State Councilor and Chair of the China-Russia Committee on Humanities Cooperation on the Chinese side, met with Zhukov, Deputy Russian Prime Minister and Chair of the China- Russia Committee on Humanities Cooperation on the Russian side, in Beijing. Both sides co-chaired the 12th session of the China-Russia Committee on Humanities Cooperation. Vice Chinese Health Minister and Chair of the Sub-committee on Health of China-Russia Committee on Humanities Cooperation Huang Jiefu attended the session.

The two sides fully summarized the achievements and experience in the bilateral humanities cooperation and came up with the plans and proposals for the next stage. In addition, they planned to strengthen the cooperation and exchange in the aspects like traditional medicine and prevention and control of infectious disease.

(Qu Yang)

14. China-Japan-South Korea Forum on Health Response to the Fukushima Nuclear Disaster Was Held in Beijing

On October 18th, 2011, the China-Japan-South Korea Forum on Health Response to the Fukushima Nuclear Disaster co-sponsored by the Chinese Ministry of Health, the Japan Ministry of Health, Labour and Welfare and the South Korean Ministry of Health and Welfare was held in Beijing. The Japanese experts introduced the Japan's medical response to the earthquake-and-tsunami-induced Fukushima Nuclear Disaster in March, 2011 and laid emphasis on the food safety measures. The Chinese and Korean representatives respectively introduced their work in public health, risk assessment and risk communication in response to the Fukushima Nuclear Disaster. The representatives from the relevant Japanese, Chinese and South Korean departments attended the forum. The Japanese representatives were from the Department of Health Crisis Management of the Japan National Institute of Health Sciences (NIHS) and the Department of Food Safety of the Pharmaceutical and Food Safety Bureau of the Japan Ministry of Health, Labour and Welfare. The South Korean representatives were from the South Korean Ministry of Health and Welfare, the South Korean National Center for Nuclear Emergency Response. And the Chinese representatives were from the International Cooperation Department of Ministry of Health (MHO), the Office of Health Emergency of MHO, the Department of Food Safety Standards, Monitoring and Assessment of MHO, National Institute for Radiological Protection of China CDC and other departments.

(Qu Yang)

15. The 5th Tripartite Health Ministers' Meeting between China, Japan and South Korea Was Held in Qingdao

On November 13th, 2011, The 5th Tripartite Health Ministers' Meeting between China, Japan and South Korea was held in Qingdao. Chinese Health Minister Chen Zhu, Japan Minister of Health, Labour and Welfare Yoko Komiyama and Korean Minister of Health and Welfare Rin Che Min attended the meeting with the delegations headed by them. Shin Young-soo, WHO's Regional Director for the Western Pacific Region attended the meeting as an observer. At the meeting, the three sides reviewed the health cooperation among the three countries, had discussion on the collaborating issues like noncommunicable disease control and issued a joint declaration. Prior to the meeting the three health ministries met respectively with the Office of the WHO Western Pacific Region and exchanged opinions. After the meeting, the representatives from the health ministries of China, Japan and South Korea and the representatives from the ministries of ASEAN countries attended the ASEAN+3 Symposium on Noncommunicable Disease Control hosted by China.

(Qu Yang)

16. The 21st Board Meeting of Roll Back Malaria Partnership Was Held in Jiangsu

During November 16th—18th, 2011, the 21st Board Meeting of Roll Back Malaria Partnership was held in Wuxi, Jiangsu, China. Vice Chinese Health Minister Huang Jiefu, as member of the RBM Partnership Board, attended the meeting and delivered a speech at the opening ceremony.

Huang Jiefu pointed out that as a global concern, the control of malaria was listed within the UN Millennium Development Goals. The Chinese government attached great importance to the prevention and control of malaria. In recent years, China had made great achievements in controlling malaria. In order to further safeguard the health of the people, China promulgated *the National Operating Plan for Elimination of Malaria (2010-2020).* He stated that as a major developing country, China was actively participating in the international cooperation and giving support to the neighboring nations and other developing countries in their efforts to fight malaria. By hosting this meeting, China wished to play a more active role in the global control of malaria, push forward the exchange in policies and technology and enable the early realization of the goal for elimination of malaria.

The RBM Partnership was launched in 1998, in an effort to provide a coordinated global response to the disease and put an end to it. The Board of RBM was the decision-making body and the 21st Board Meeting was the first board meeting ever hosted in China. Over 80 representatives and observers from the malaria endemic countries, donors, WHO, the World Bank, foundations, the private sector, and research and academic institutions attended the meeting.

(Qu Yang)

17. The 11th Meeting of the Health Sub-committee of the China-Russia Committee on Humanities Cooperation Was Held in Beijing

On December 13th, 2011, The 11th Meeting of the Health Sub-committee of the China-Russia Committee on Humanities Cooperation was held in Beijing. Chair on the Chinese side and Vice Health Minister Huang Jiefu, and Chair on Russian side and Vice Minister of Ministry of Health and Social Development of the Russian Federation Veronika I.Skvortsova co-hosted the meeting.

The two sides reviewed the achievements and process in the bilateral and multilateral health cooperation between China and Russia and had discussions over the issues like prevention and control of infectious diseases, rehabilitation medicine, traditional medicine, pharmaceutical supervision and disaster medicine. Both sides agreed to deepen the effective cooperation on the basis of mutual trust and benefits. They would proactively push forward the construction of the bilateral emergency response mechanism, strengthen the joint prevention and control of infectious diseases along the bordering regions and the academic exchange of medical sciences, start the construction of China-Russia rehabilitation center in Hainan, build traditional Chinese medicine medical centers in Russia and take measures to realize other cooperative intentions.

The Health Sub-committee was one of the sub-committees of the China-Russia Committee on Humanities Cooperation and the sub-committee meeting was held annually in China and Russia alternately. The Chinese representatives from Ministry of Health, State Food and Drug Administration, State Administration of Traditional Chinese Medicine, Health Department of Heilongjiang Province and Health Department of Hainan Province, and the Russian representatives from Ministry of Health and Social Development of the Russian Federation attended the meeting.

(Qu Yang)

Section 4 International Cooperation Projects

1. Chinese Short-term Expert Team Carried out Free Cataract Operations in Botswana

On the 30th anniversary of the initiation of Chinese medical aiding teams to

Botswana and in order to strengthen the health cooperation between China and Botswana, the Chinese Ministry of Health sent a short-term expert team to carry out free cataract operations in Botswana. The Chinese oculists conducted over 200 cataract operations in the capital of Botswana and trained the local medical workers. In order to extend the influence of this action, the Chinese Ministry of Health donated ophthalmic equipment and consumables worth 1.35 million RMB Yuan to Princess Marina Hospital where the Chinese aiding medical team worked. The Chinese officials from Chinese embassy to Botswana and the Economic and Commercial Councilor's Office, the Botswana officials from the national government, Ministry of Health and Ministry of Foreign affairs, the relevant experts of Botswana and the representatives of Botswana media attended the celebration of the 30th anniversary and donation of the ophthalmic equipment.

(Qu Yang)

2. China/WHO Cooperation Projects of the Annual Budget Planning (2010-2011)

The China/WHO Cooperation Projects of the Annual Budget Planning (2010-2011) were completed. The total budget was 5.2 million dollars, which was less than that of last year. There were 73 biannual projects, which covered the fields like prevention and control of infectious diseases, epidemic monitoring and response, noncommunicable disease control, maternal and child healthcare, construction of rural health, reform of the medical system, development of traditional Chinese medicine and safety of food and drugs. 69 organizations were involved in the projects, 14 of which were subordinates of the Chinese Ministry of Health. The projects distributed in 22 provinces/municipalities, 10 of which were in the west region. The projects were centered on China's key fields of the health development as well as on the priorities of WHO global strategy. They facilitated the China's deepening the reform of medical and pharmaceutical systems. And at the same time, they covered the fields like traditional medicine and control of chronic diseases that were less involved in the international cooperation.

(Qu Yang)

3. China-US Cooperation—Global AIDS Program

In 2011, the China-US Cooperation—Global AIDS Program(GAP) went well. Based on the existing management framework of GAP, the two sides established the highest management body— the Program Management Committee and held the 3rd committee meeting on October 28th, 2011. The committee reviewed the work report of

GAP (2010-2011), the operating plans for GAP (2011-2012), the revision of the strategy of GAP and *the GAP Management Handbook (the 4th edition).*

(Qu Yang)

4. China-US Collaborative Program on Emerging and Re-emerging Infectious Diseases

The China-US Collaborative Program on Emerging and Re-emerging Infectious Diseases went well in 2011. The program mainly focused on the following fields and tasks: continuing the efforts in monitoring and quick-response capability to check the spread of H5N1, supporting China's training programs on field epidemiology and capacity construction of health communication, strengthening the monitoring and quick-response capability of the provincial laboratories of foodborne diseases, strengthening the construction of the management and collaborating platform for emerging and re-emerging infectious diseases, enhancing the study on the public health implication of newly isolated arboviruses and infectious fevers, enhancing the capacity construction in public health information and intensifying the control of the infection of tuberculosis. Meanwhile, projects in new fields were carried out and they were the projects on the emergency preparedness and response capacity, and testing capacity building for laboratories of congenital cytomegalovirus infection. The provincial projects on control of nosocomial infection, the diagnosis and treatment of infectious diarrhea, respiratory diseases and meningitis, study on epidemiology of pediatric influenza and burden of disease were strengthened. The periodic goals of the research projects were achieved. The study on the characteristics of hand-food-and-mouth disease deceased cases and the virus-carrying ratio among healthy people and cases of close contacts was conducted. In addition, the academic researches on canine leishmaniasis in western China, optimization of inhibitors of influenza virus A membrane fusion and other subjects were carried out.

(Qu Yang)

5. The Progress of China-Australia Health and HIV/AIDS Facility

Initiated in August of 2007, the China-Australia Health and HIV/AIDS Facility (CAHHF) was jointly overseen by China's Ministry of Health, Australia's Department of Health and Ageing, China's Ministry of Commerce and the Australian Agency for International Development (AusAID), which also funds the Facility. CAHHF was a partnership between the Government of the People's Republic of China and the Australian Government. CAHHF was a 5-year project with a total budget of 25 million

Australian dollars. The Facility used expertise from both Chinese and Australian health institutions to support the Chinese Government's health reform priorities. The Facility acknowledged the mutual national interests of China and Australia. It was a new form of development partnership that was flexible and responsive.

Since the commencement of this initiative in 2007, CAHHF had approved a total of 53 research and development activities. These were being led by 29 Chinese organizations, working in partnership with 26 Australian partner institutions. 36 of activities supported the five key priorities of China's health care reform and 4 of these activities directly supported China's public hospital reform. 3 activities lent support to the food safety in China. By the end of December of 2011, 19,410,000 Australian dollars had been allocated and the actual disbursement rate was as high as 80%.

(Qu Yang)

6. The Progress of the China-Australia HIV/AIDS Asia Regional Program (HAARP)

The China-Australia HIV/AIDS Asia Regional Program (HAARP) went well in 2011. According to the annual plan, the estimated budget for 2011 was 9,947,000 RMB Yuan. The fund execution rate was 99.5%. Progress was made in the multi-department cooperation. Many multi-department cooperation activities at the provincial and county levels were carried out. At the county level, HAARP mainly focused on the reduction of the harm of drug abuse and advocated the multi-department collaboration. At present, in the 31 projects counties in Yunnan Province and Guangxi Autonomous Region, 45 needle exchange centers provided service for harm reduction like clean needle exchange and referral.

In 2011, the national program office and the program offices of Yunnan Province and Guangxi Autonomous Region organized a series of activities and achieved desired results. The activities mainly included: (1) With the financial and technical support of the AusAID, Yunnan Police Officer Academy carried out training on how to reduce drug-related harms for the senior anti-narcotics police officers from the Southeast Asian Countries like Vietnam, Burma, Laos and Cambodia.(2) Within the majority of the project counties, the local public security departments agreed not to arrest the drug users in the needle exchange centers and the methadone clinics, which increased the accessibility of the relevant service to the target groups. (3) The web and data management system developed by HAARP was adopted by Yunnan Provincial AIDS Prevention Bureau and was applied in the information management of the drug users in Yunnan. (4) The grounds for policy advocacy were laid. The Yunnan province program office gave financial and technical support to Yundi-Harm Reduction Network(YDHR)for its policy advocacy for the benefits of the targeted groups. Based on the previous survey and research, *the Flexibility Report on Deleting EX-drug Users from the Dynamic Surveillance System* was submitted to the National Anti-narcotics Commission and it provided the relevant suggestion for further improvement of the management and control system. On June 26th, 2011, the new version of *Detoxification Ordinance* came into force and it prescribed that the ex-drug users who hadn't had contact with drug for over 3 years would be deleted from the Dynamic Surveillance System of Drug Users. The promulgation of *Detoxification Ordinance* demonstrated that the advocacy had reached the legal level and great progress had been made in advocacy.

(Qu Yang)

7. Progress of the AIDS Prevention and Treatment Program of Bill & Melinda Gates Foundation (BMGF)

In 2011, the AIDS Prevention and Treatment Program of MOH & State Council AIDS Working Committee Office with Bill & Melinda Gates Foundation went well. The management of the program, as well as the quality control and utilization of the statistics, was strengthened. In order to realize the goals and strategy of the program, new ways were explored. More social organizations and medical institutions were involved in the AIDS control and the performance of the disease prevention and control centers improved greatly. The cooperation among social organizations, disease prevention and control centers and medical institutions was enhanced, the service chain connecting intervention, mobilization, screening, consultation, treatment and care was formed and the 3-demontional intervention model was established. In 2011, 3,024 new cases of HIV positive were detected among MSM and that made a total of 7,704 new cases. 253,553 persons/times were mobilized or intervened. 76,628 persons/times accepted the screening of HIV and syphilis antibody and 4.563 cases of HIV positive were detected.

(Qu Yang)

8. Progress of AIDS Prevention and Treatment Program between the Ministry of Health and the Clinton Foundation

In order to review the work and achievements since the initiation of the program in 2004 and to exchange the experience and popularize the best practice, the end-cycle project appraisal meeting was held in Beijing Friendship Hotel on October 31st, 2011. The meeting maintained that the Clinton Foundation had given great support to the Chinese government in the issues like the standardized antivirus treatment for children, training of rural doctors on antivirus treatment and laboratory diagnostic techniques. All of these facilitated the smooth development of the relevant fields. In the past 6 years, the Clinton Foundation, as the first international NGO that cooperated with the Chinese government, fully exercised its advantage in setting up projects according to the actual needs and integrated itself closely with Chinese tasks in AIDS prevention and control and the international collaborating programs. The AIDS Prevention and Treatment Program between the Ministry of Health and the Clinton Foundation was an important part and supplement to China's prevention and control of AIDS.

(Qu Yang)

9. China-MSD HIV/AIDS Partnership

In 2010, the management and implementation organizations of the program carried out activities according to the plans in the following 6 areas: (1) health education, (2) effective interventions to change the high risk behaviors, (3) screening and treatment of HIV/AIDS patients, (4) care and fight against discrimination (5) support to ability construction and (6) supervision and assessment. Priority was given to the following tasks: strengthening the discovery of HIV/AIDS patients, increasing the coverage of the antiretroviral treatment, and enhancing the ability construction, human resource support and plans for public advocacy.

In 2010, two meetings of the Oversight Committee for the China-MSD HIV/AIDS Partnership (hereinafter referred to as C-MAP) were held and the key proposals approved by the committee were implemented. The key events and activities of the program included the Business Summit on HIV/AIDS Control, the Summing-up Meeting of the Project (2008-2009), the forum of the MSD top management, the project mid-term evaluation, the initiation of national bidding and entrustment, the financial management training and hearings, the provision of technical supports for the AIDS prevention in Liangshan prefecture in collaboration with HIV/AIDS prevention centers, 2011 Annual Plan Initiative, 2011 framework and integrated plans for the overall AIDS prevention in Liangshan prefecture of Sichuan province and so on.

30 indexes out of the 33 project indexes in 35 project counties of Sichuan province and 10 project cities with MSM groups were accomplished by 100%, which constituted 90% of all the indexes. 81 among the 90 indexes in 17 project counties/county-level cities in Liangshan prefecture were accomplished by 100%, which constituted 81% of all the indexes. By the end of December 2010, the budget for Level-3 programs was 71,734,606 RMB Yuan and the actual expenditure was 59,884,800 RMB Yuan, with an executive rate of 83%.

(Qu Yang)

10. Progress of the Advanced International Courses of Health Development and Reform

The Advanced International Courses of Health Development and Reform were held in September of 2011 in Tsinghua University and Harvard University. 25 trainees from the State Council, Ministry of Health, Ministry of Finance, National Development and Reform Commission, China Health Education Center and provincial/municipal Health Bureaus took part in the courses. The training combined the theories with practice, the international experience with China's basic conditions, widening of horizons with solutions to problems and training with discussion. The courses were highly appraised by the trainees.

Based on the China Senior Health Executive Education Program (2005-2010), Ministry of Health and Harvard University signed the memorandum of understanding on cooperation and launch a new 3-year cooperation program which aimed to improve ability of Chinese senior health executives in policy formulation, implementation and evaluation, and upgrade them with latest concepts and experiences on health management.

(Qu Yang)

11. Progress of Smile Train—the Cleft Lip and Palate Repair Program

In 2011, the Smile Train—the Cleft Lip and Palate Repair Program carried out 27,464 free operations in 397 project hospitals in China. The Smile Train donated over 90 million RMB Yuan for the operations and held training courses in Xinjiang, Liaoning, Yunnan, Hebei, Shandong and Shenzhen. All together 433 persons/times of surgeons and anesthetists were trained and 85 persons/times of the surgeons and anesthetists received the further advanced training for 1-2months. The program compiled *the Phonetic Training Course for the Cleft Lip and Palate Patients* and organized a training camp during November 9th-14th, 2011 in Wuhan city of Hubei province, where 40 phonetic doctors and therapists from all over the country were trained.

On July 25th, 2011, the third meeting of steering committee of the Smile Train—the Cleft Lip and Palate Repair Program was held in Beijing. Huang Jiefu Deputy Health Minister and Director of the Steering Committee attended and addressed the meeting. Special Advisor of the Program and Standing Committee Member of CPPCC Zhang Wenkang delivered a speech at the meeting. The representatives from Ministry of Health, the China Charity Federation, Chinese Stomatological Association, USA Smile Train took part in the meeting. Huang Jiefu pointed out that the Smile Train program made great contribution to relieving the pain of the cleft lip and palate patients, increasing their life quality and lessening the burden of their family and the society. He thanked USA Smile Train, the China Charity Federation, and Chinese Stomatological Association for their support to the program. And he stated that Ministry of Health would mobilize and organize the health system and the relevant institutions and individuals to support and participate in the program to ensure the successful implementation of the program.

The meeting listened to the work report from January of 2009 to June of 2011, passed *the Management Handbook of the Smile Train—the Cleft Lip and Palate Repair Program (2011)*and reached consensus on the key missions in the future. The meeting required that the publicity of the program should be enhanced to make more patients have accessibility to the free operations and to ensure the medical service quality of the project hospitals.

The Smile Train—the Cleft Lip and Palate Repair Program was an joint initiative of Ministry of Health, the China Charity Federation, Chinese Stomatological Association, USA Smile Train launched in 2007. It gave free operations to the cleft lip and palate patients and provided professional training for the medical staff in the project hospitals. From January of 2009 to June of 2011, 69,000 operations were conducted within the 397 project hospitals.

(Qu Yang)

12. Rehabilitation Program of Project Hope

In 2011, Rehabilitation Program of Project Hope compiled the program textbook *the Series for Rehabilitative Education* and revised *the Service Guidance for Community Rehabilitation Therapists: Injuries of Joints.* The program also organized the third and fourth therapist-to-therapist training courses respectively on osteoarthrosis and the treatment of pain of cervical vertebra and lumbar vertebra. In addition, the refreshing training courses for grassroots rehabilitation therapists were carried out. All of these activities elevated the rehabilitative service ability in Dujiangyan of Sichuan. In May of 2011, the program launched the pilot work of two-way transfer of rehabilitative patients between Sichuan Provincial People's Hospital and Dujiangyan Orthopedic Hospital. In July, the education activity of the program was conducted in the communities. And in September, a return visit was paid and the on-the-spot teaching activities were conducted by the program. These efforts all achieved desired results.

(Qu Yang)

13. China-USA Senior Health Executive Education Program

The first cycle of China Senior Health Executive Education Program was carried out in the Central Party School of the Communist Party of China and Stanford University of USA form May 22nd-June 11th. 23 trainees from the Central Party School of the Communist Party of China, State Development and Reform Commission, Ministry of Finance, Ministry of Human Resources and Social Security, Ministry of Health and provincial health departments participated in the program. The major objective of the program was to help China produce a critical mass of well-informed, open-minded, and highly responsible leaders and executives at the national and provincial levels who can effectively develop and implement sound policies while dealing with local issues. Given the public health challenges that have accompanied China's rapid economic development, there was an urgent need for such progressive and resourceful leaders.

The China-USA Senior Health Executive Education Program was a cooperative initiative between the Chinese Ministry of Health and GlaxoSmithKline (GSK) China. The program aimed to develop the participants' comprehensive understanding of the major global, national, and regional health development and health system reform issues and sharpen the participants' problem-solving, strategic planning, and leadership skills to help them design, introduce, and sustain major policy and institutional actions directly related to their own environment. Lasting for 3 years, the program would hold annual training courses in the Central Party School of the Communist Party of China and Stanford University of USA for 4 weeks. About 25 trainees would be training each time and the contents would cover the issues like administration, health economy, policy formulation, ethnics and case study of international medical reform.

(Qu Yang)

14. Strategic Partnership between Chinese Ministry of Health and Dartmouth College

On October 17th, 2011, the Ministry of Health of the People's Republic of China (PRC) and Dartmouth College signed the agreement to enter into a five-year strategic partnership that aimed to serve the efforts of the Chinese government to reform health services and medical education. Following the official signing of the five-year agreement, Professor Al Mulley, Director of The Dartmouth Center for Health Care Delivery Science (TDC), led a faculty delegation in delivering two symposia in the Chinese cities of Shanghai and Suzhou that identified potential areas of collaboration between Dartmouth and the PRC government. The first steering committee meeting would be held in April of 2011 in Dartmouth College.

(Qu Yang)

15. The Progress of the Sino-French Cooperation on Prevention Program against Emerging Infectious Diseases

On March 30th, 2011, the sixth meeting of the steering committee of the Sino-French Cooperation on Prevention Program against Emerging Infectious Diseases was held in Paris. Health Minister Chen Zhu and President of Mérieux Foundation Alain Mérieux co-chaired the meeting and made speeches. 23 Chinese representatives from Ministry of Health, Ministry of Science and Technology, Standardization Administration of China, Certification and Accreditation Administration of China, Chinese Academy of Sciences and the Chinese Embassy to France and over 20 French representatives and experts from Ministry of Foreign Affairs, Ministry of Higher Education and Research, French Agency for the Safety of Health Products (AFFSAPS)and Association Française de Normalisation (AFNOR) attended the meeting. The meeting fully reviewed the development in the cooperation in the fields like training of the medical professionals, scientific research and development, laws and regulations of biosafety, normalization and construction of laboratories. On June 30th, 2011, the commencement ceremony of the core laboratory of P4 project was held. The representatives from the Chinese government, the French Government and the relevant local departments attended the ceremony. The construction was started in September and according to the plan, the civil engineering would be finished in March of 2012. In terms of laws and regulations, the two sides passed the study report on biosafety and biological security. As for the standards, in February of 2011, the Chinese working group on the standards was set up. When it came to the project management, the steering committee held a meeting in April of 2011 and made plans for the final period and the popularization of the project.

On November 24th, 2011, the seventh meeting of the secretariat of the Sino-French Cooperation on Prevention Program against Emerging Infectious Diseases was held in Beijing. The Chinese chief mediator of the project and Director of the Department of International Cooperation Ren Minghui and the French chief mediator of the project Jean-Michel Hubert co-chaired the meeting. The meeting fully reviewed the bilateral cooperation in the fields like training of the medical professionals, scientific research and development, laws and regulations of biosafety, normalization and construction of laboratories, and discussed and passed the meeting minutes of the sixth meeting of the Secretariat and the executive handbook of the project. The meeting stressed that the civil engineering quality and the safety of the P4 lab was of crucial significance. The two sides should communicate closely to inform each other of the relevant situation. The two sides clarified the future cooperation plan and agreed to prioritize the biomedicine and emerging infectious diseases in the bilateral cooperation. In addition, the connection between the relevant organizations and working groups should be strengthened and the construction of the laboratory and the development of the project should be accelerated. The meeting resolved that the eighth meeting of the Secretariat and the seventh meeting of the steering committee be held in Shanghai, China in the first half of 2012.

(Qu Yang)

16. The Progress of the Belgian Damien Foundation Project on Tuberculosis/Leprosy Prevention and Treatment in China

The Belgian Damien Foundation Project on Tuberculosis/Leprosy Prevention and Treatment in China went well in 2011. The project was the cooperation project between the Department of International Cooperation of Chinese Ministry of Health and the Belgian Damien Foundation. The foundation sponsored the prevention and treatment of tuberculosis and leprosy in Tibet, Inner Mongolia, Qinghai, Ningxia and Guizhou.

The project participated in the national reference lab system and carried out pilot work of LED fluorescence microscopy in Xining City of Qinghai Province.

The project sponsored the training courses on the prevention and control of leprosy-induced deformity held by the Leprosy Control Center of China CDC in Wenshan County of Yunnan Province and about 30 trainees were trained. In June and December of 2011, the foundation conducted training on control of TB infection for the clinical medical workers at the provincial, municipal and county level in Qinghai and Ningxia.

The project provinces accomplished the goals set by the Damien Foundation in 2011. The total budget for the project on tuberculosis prevention and treatment was 3,150,000 RMB Yuan and the total allocation was about 3,150,000 RMB Yuan. All the reimbursement was spent. The budget for the prevention and control of leprosy was 280,000 RMB Yuan and the actual executive rate reached 95%.

(Qu Yang)

17. Programs of the Global Fund to Fight against AIDS, TB and Malaria

In 2011, due to the suspension of the reimbursement from the Global Fund to Fight against AIDS, TB and Malaria, the routine work of the programs basically stopped. Apart from lifesaving prevention and treatment services, an overhaul was launched by the Chinese side in late June in a bid to strengthen the management and supervision of grants from the Global Fund and address the concerns that caused it to withhold its money. A detailed plan was worked out to address the issues like self-examination of the programs, working plans, program budgets to allow Global Fund to lift its suspension of funding. In November and December, the Office of the Inspector General of the Global Fund conducted diagnostic evaluation on China's programs. The negotiation for the tenth round of the malaria program with the Secretariat of the Global Fund was completed and the agreement was signed. The funds would be 5,080,000 dollars to the maximum for the first two years and the program would be started from January 2012. All together 78,425,700 dollars were allocated to the Chinese programs.

(Qu Yang)

18. Program on "Improving Nutrition, Food Safety and Food Security for China's Most Vulnerable Women and Children" of the UN-Spain Millennium Development Goals Achievement Fund (UN-Spain MDG-Fund)

After its commencement on June 11th, 2010, the Program on "Improving Nutrition, Food Safety and Food Security for China's Most Vulnerable Women and Children" of the UN-Spain MDG-Fund (hereinafter referred to as the Program of the UN-Spain MDG-Fund), the baseline surveys over the food supply, nutrition of women and children and food safety in the 6 rural project counties were completed and the 89 outcomes were timely shared with the governments and provided reference for the development of policies. The textbooks on nutrition of women and children and food safety were compiled and the ability of the workers in the fields of health, education, quality inspection, nutrition of children and food safety was strengthened. In addition, the construction of the system in safety of food production was enhanced. The Program of the UN-Spain MDG-Fund also supported the relevant the study and popularization of laws on food safety in various ways.

On December 7th, 2011, the meeting of the executive committee of the Program of the UN-Spain MDG-Fund was held at Chinese Ministry of Health. The people present at the meeting were Director of the Department of International Cooperation of Chinese Ministry of Health Ren Minghui, WHO Representative in China Dr. Michael O'Leary, representatives from 7 UN agencies in China, and the personnel from the 21 program implementation departments and research institutions.

The meeting reviewed the implementation of the program of the second year and approved the working plans for the third year. The meeting required that on the basis of the previous two years, all the project departments and institutions should carefully study the opinions for improvement suggested by the external mid-term evaluation. In addition, they should increase the efficiency in implementing the program and timely sum up the experience of success. Moreover they should give support to the key work of *China National Program for Woman Development* and *China National Program for Child Development* to improve the nutrition and food safety condition of the poor women and children in the rural areas.

Lasting for 3 years the Program of the UN-Spain MDG-Fund aimed to explorer an comprehensive way to improve the condition of China's most vulnerable women and children in nutrition, food safety and security status. The UN agencies participating in the program included WHO, FAO, WFP, UNICEF, UNESCO, ILO, UNDP and UNIDO. The Chinese organizations engaged in the program includes Ministry of Commerce, Ministry of Agriculture, Ministry of Education, Ministry of Health, the General Administration of Quality Supervision, Inspection and Quarantine, the State Administration of Work Safety, the State Administration of Radio, Film and Television (SARFT), ALL China Women's Federation, All China Federation of Trade Unions, and China Law Society. The Program of the UN-Spain MDG-Fund piloted a comprehensive approach in six of the poorest counties in Yunnan province, Shaanxi province and Guizhou province.

(Qu Yang)

19. China/UNFPA Cooperation Program

In July of 2011, Ministry of Commerce and UNFPA signed *the China/UNFPA Seventh Country Programme.* As the project executive department, Ministry of Health signed the relevant working plans with UNFPA which covered the issues like reproductive health, prevention and response to domestic violence in China and culture sensitivity and promotion of reproductive health in ethnic regions. The goal of China/UNFPA Seventh Country Programme was to combine HIV/AIDS prevention and control with reproductive health. With the approval of the UNFPA representative to China, Guizhou province, Hainan province and Jiangxi province were determined as the project provinces. The programme would last from August of 2011 to December of 2015, aiming to increase the utility and availability of the service in reproductive health and AIDS prevention for the illicit sex workers in the project provinces and increase the people's awareness on AIDS prevention and control and reproductive rights.

(Qu Yang)

Section 5 Other Important Foreign Affairs

1. Vice Minister of Health Liu Qian Met with the Health Delegation of Slovenia

Vice Minister of Health Liu Qian met with the health delegation of Slovenia headed by Director of the Department of Public Health of the Slovenian Ministry of Health. Ambassador of the Republic of Slovenia to China Marija Adanja attended the meeting.

Liu Qian gave a brief introduction to China's rural healthcare system and medical security system. He expressed that Ministry of Health was willing to strengthen the connection between the counterpart collaborating institutions and carry out sustainable exchanges within the existing framework of bilateral health cooperation. The two sides also exchanged opinions over the cooperation in the fields like public health challenges, infectious disease control, hospital management, health education and training of medical talents for the grassroots institutions. During their stay in Beijing, the delegates attended the meeting held by the National Health Development Research Center of Chinese Ministry of Health on the rural health and the construction of the grassroots healthcare system. In addition, they visited the medical institutions in Beijing like the Shunyi district hospital, the Renhe township hospital and Henancun community health service center.

(Qu Yang)

2. Vice Minister of Health Huang Jiefu Met with President of China Medical Board of USA. Lincoln C.Chen

On January 18th, 2011, Vice Minister of Health Huang Jiefu met with President of China Medical Board of USA. Lincoln C.Chen and they exchanged opinions on deepening the bilateral cooperation. Huang Jiefu thanked the board for its support to China's health undertaking and proposed that the two sides should continue the collaboration in the fields like medical education, organ transplantation, tobacco control, personnel training. He also encouraged the board to carry out concrete collaboration with the specialized Chinese health institutions and give further support to the reform of China's medical and pharmaceutical systems. The relevant officials from the Department of International Cooperation and the Department of Maternal and Child Health Care and Community Health of Chinese Ministry of Health attended the meeting.

(Qu Yang)

3. Minister of Health Chen Zhu Met with Former Italian Prime Minister Romano Prodi

On January 20th, 2011, Minister of Health Chen Zhu met with the visiting former Italian Prime Minister and former President of the European Commission Romano Prodi and they exchanged opinions over the Sino-Italian health cooperation. Chen Zhu spoke highly of the fruitful bilateral health cooperation and thanked Prodi for his active role in pushing forward the health cooperation between China and the European Commission and the health cooperation between China and Italy. Chen Zhu also introduced the development and challenges in China's deepening the reform of the medical and pharmaceutical systems. Prodi stated that the Sino-Italian health cooperation featured a strong compatibility and great potential. The two sides agreed to enhance the high-rank exchange in the aspects of health policies, training of medical professionals, information network management in the hospitals and telemedicine.

(Qu Yang)

4. Minister of Health Chen Zhu Met with the Delegation of Russian Medical Society

On January 24th, 2011, Minister of Health and President of Chinese Medical Association Chen Zhu met with the Delegation of Russian Medical Society.

Chen Zhu spoke highly of the Sino-Russian health cooperation. The high-rank officials of the two sides maintained steady and sound collaborating mechanism and the academic societies in both countries also carried out close and pragmatic cooperation. He encouraged Russian Medical Society to continue its frank exchange with the relevant Chinese institutions like Chinese Medical Association and expand the cooperation in the fields like health policies, training of medical professional and academic research.

(Qu Yang)

5. Vice Minister of Health Liu Qian Met with Dean of the University of Pittsburgh School of Medicine Arthur S.Levine

On February 24th, 2011, Vice Minister of Health Liu Qian met with Dean for the University of Pittsburgh School of Medicine Arthur S.Levine. Liu Qian gave a brief introduction to the priorities in China's reform of the medical and pharmaceutical systems and he hoped that the University of Pittsburgh School of Medicine would carry out cooperation projects with its Chinese partners in the fields like scientific research, education and medical treatment and give support to the development of

China's health undertaking. The relevant persons in charge from the Department of International Cooperation of Ministry of Health and Chinese Academy of Sciences attended the meeting.

(Qu Yang)

6. Minister of Health Chen Zhu Met with US Ambassador to China Jon Huntsman

On February 15th, 2011, Minister of Health Chen Zhu met with US Ambassador to China Jon Huntsman.

Chen Zhu spoke highly of the long-lasting, in-depth and pragmatic bilateral cooperation in health. He introduced the new rural cooperative medical scheme and the relevant policies, characteristics and challenge about the scheme. He proposed that China and USA should strengthen the bilateral health cooperation in the fields like health policies, biomedicine, translational medicine, education of general practitioners and geriatric nursing to push forward the comprehensive development of the bilateral relationship.

Jon Huntsman expressed that health was the field which was critical to the livelihood of the people in both countries and the bilateral cooperation in health conformed to the two nations' strategic goals and mutual interests. He hoped that the two sides would cooperate closely and make contribution to the welfare of the people in both countries and the people all over the world.

(Qu Yang)

7. Vice Health Minister Liu Qian Met With the President of the Milstein Medical Asian American Partnership Foundation (MMAAP)

On December 29th, 2011, Vice Minister Liu Qian met with Dr. Gerald Lazarus, the President of the Milstein Medical Asian American Partnership Foundation, MMAAP, and his colleagues at the Ministry of Health to discuss cooperation in health.

Liu Qian thanked Mr. Milstein, the founder of the MMAAP Foundation, for his interest in China's healthcare and his willingness to develop cooperation with China. The two parties exchanged ideas about the model and priorities of the cooperation between the Foundation and China. They also agreed on developing and strengthening the relationships between the Foundation and Chinese medical institutions with initial cooperative areas being skin research and geriatric medicine.

(Qu Yang)

8. China's Inspection and Supervision System of Vaccines Was Accredited by WHO

On March 1st, 2011, WHO declared in Beijing that China's inspection and supervision system of vaccines was accredited by WHO. The accreditation was a performance evaluation on a nation's supervisory organizations and system on vaccines. Passing the certification meant that China's supervisory ability on vaccines was greatly improved and it also laid the foundation for our country's vaccine manufacturers to develop the international market. Passing the evaluation on the supervisory organizations and system on vaccines was the premise for the nation's vaccine manufacturers to apply for the WHO's accreditation and participate in the international bidding and purchase. Since China's inspection and supervision system of vaccines was accredited, it would be the platform for China's vaccines' entry into the international market and China would provide safe and reliable vaccines for the world.

(Qu Yang)

9. Minister of Health Chen Zhu Met with Sylvie-Agnès Bermann, French Ambassador to China

On March 25th, 2011, Minister of Health Chen Zhu met with French Ambassador to China Sylvie-Agnès Bermann and they exchanged opinions over the bilateral health cooperation and China's reform of the medical and pharmaceutical systems. Chen Zhu congratulated Bermann on becoming the first female French ambassador since the two countries established the diplomatic relationship. He spoke highly of the Sino-French comprehensive strategic partnership and the long-term close bilateral cooperation in the health field. He thanked the French side for the efforts to promote the bilateral health cooperation. Chen Zhu gave a brief introduction to the development of the bilateral health cooperation in public health reform and prevention and control of emerging infectious diseases. On request of Bermann, Chen Zhu also introduced the work on food safety and prevention and control of noncommunicable diseases. Bermann spoke highly of the Sino-French relationship and she expressed that during her tenure, she would proactively push forward the bilateral health cooperation and give support to the cooperation in the fields like medical system, management of public hospitals and food safety.

(Qu Yang)

10. Vice Health Minister Chen Xiaohong Met with Peter Berman, Health Economist of the World Bank

On March 28th, 2011, Vice Health Minister Chen Xiaohong met with Peter Berman, Health Economist of the World Bank. Chen Xiaohong thanked Berman for his support to China's study on health economy. He stated it was a critical stage for China's reform of the medial and pharmaceutical systems and he hoped that Berman could use his rich experience in global health study and policy analysis to provide valuable suggestions for China. Berman thanked the Chinese side for trusting him and he expressed that as the countries of the world gave more attention to health economy and China was having the in-depth study in health economy, he would strengthen the exchange with the relevant organizations in China and. carry out activities in study and exchange.

After the meeting, Chen Xiaohong attended the inauguration ceremony of Berman as the chief financing expert for the National Health Development Research Center of Ministry of Health. The relevant officials from the Department of International Cooperation and the National Health Development Research Center attended the meeting.

(Qu Yang)

11. World Health Day 2011 Was Observed in China

The theme of World Health Day 2011 was "Antibiotic resistance: No action today, no cure tomorrow". In order to observe the World Health Day, Ministry of Health and WHO held the kick-off ceremony for the first Conference on Rational Medication and the activity for World Health Day 2011. Vice Health Minister Ma Xiaowei and WHO Representative in China Dr. Michael O'Leary attended the meeting. WHO Director-General Dr Margaret Chan addressed the ceremony via a video.

Ma Xiaowei stated in his speech that antibiotic resistance was a global health concern. With the extensive application of antibiotics in medical industry, agriculture, animal husbandry and other fields, the bacteria became more resistant to antibiotics. Ministry of Health would take measures to strengthen the administration over the clinical usage of antibiotics, regulate the behavior of the medical workers in the usage of medicines and promote the rational use of antimicrobial drugs. At the same time, he pointed out that it was the joint responsibility of the health administrative departments, medical institutions, pharmaceutical enterprises, academic societies and even the whole society to act on the calling of WHO, push forward the rational usage of antibiotics, and control the resistance to antibiotic drugs.

Dr. Michael O'Leary said that WHO, centering on the theme of World Health Day 2011, introduced a six-point policy package to combat the spread of antimicrobial resistance. He called on all the social sectors to make efforts to solve this problem.

At the kick-off ceremony, the advisory committee for rational medication of Ministry of Health advocated that the medical professionals like doctors, pharmacists and nurses and the mass public should get rid of the misconceptions in medication, promote rational use of medicines and actively combat the abuse of antibiotics.

(Qu Yang)

12. Ms Peng Li Yuan Was Appointed Goodwill Ambassador for Tuberculosis (TB) and HIV/AIDS by WHO

On June 3rd, 2011, WHO Director-General Dr. Margaret Chan appointed the famous Chinese soprano Peng Li Yuan as WHO Goodwill Ambassador for Tuberculosis and HIV/AIDS at WHO headquarters in Geneva. Vice Health Minister Yin Li, Ambassador of Chinese mission in Geneva He Yafei and the senior officials of WHO attended the inauguration ceremony.

In her speech Dr. Margaret Chan stated that every year tuberculosis and HIV/AIDS were responsible for the deaths of more than 3.5 million people all over the world. They posed a threat to people's health and were a great burden to the social and economic development. She was delighted that Ms Peng Li Yuan agreed to represent the WHO as a Goodwill Ambassador for Tuberculosis and HIV/AIDS and her appointment would have a lasting impact in bringing awareness to two of the world's deadliest infectious diseases and the recent advances that had been made in the areas of prevention and treatment of TB and HIV. Ms Peng had captured the attention of millions of fans through her compelling performances. Through her increased profile on a global platform, she would reinforce international commitments to achieving the health-related Millennium Development Goals, set for 2015. Ms Peng said at the inauguration ceremony that it was a great honor for to be given this important role by WHO and she hoped that she would make a significant contribution to the great work of WHO in saving lives from TB and HIV/AIDS, and that her involvement would benefit those who were at most risk.

Goodwill Ambassadors of WHO were usually acclaimed artists or sportsmen who were engaged in the publicity of WHO's strategies, goals and major missions. They communicated the relevant information to the public to elevate the awareness of them.

(Qu Yang)

13. Vice Minister of Health Huang Jiefu Attended the Signature Ceremony of Bill & Melinda Gates Foundation (BMGF) and Baidu Foundation

On June 11th, 2011, Vice Minister of Health Huang Jiefu attended the signature ceremony of BMGF and Baidu Foundation on the agreement to establish strategic charity alliance, promote public health and advocate a smokeless environment. Chair of BMGF Bill Gates and Chair of Baidu Foundation Li Yanhong co-signatured the agreement on the establishment of strategic charity alliance centering on the theme "abide by the smoking ban and say no to passive smoking". The alliance would arouse the passive smokers' awareness of health so they could stand up for their own rights. The alliance would also popularize the scientific methods for quitting smoking to help the smokers.

Huang Jiefu stated in his speech that the Chinese government paid great attention to tobacco control. Since WHO Framework Convention on Tobacco Control (hereinafter referred to as FCTC) came into force in 2005, China had made great progress in honoring the convention. For example, a series of departmental and regional laws and regulations on tobacco control were formulated and relevant activities were conducted. In addition, the goals of a smokeless Olympic Games in 2008 and a smokeless World Expo in 2010 were achieved and according to the 12th Five-Year Plan (2011-2015), the smoking in public places would be totally banned. Huang Jiefu pointed out that it was a long way for China to accomplish the task of tobacco control . Therefore, relying only on the government was far from enough and the support from all sectors of the society was needed for the completion of the task. He hoped that on the basis of the agreement Bill & Melinda Gates Foundation (BMGF) and Baidu Foundation would carry out relevant activities to push forward the tobacco control in China. He also hoped that more and more enterprises and foundations would join the strategic charity alliance and thus, the social environment in which the whole society participated in tobacco control would be created.

The relevant officials from the Department of International Cooperation took part in the signature.

(Qu Yang)

14. Minister of Health Chen Zhu Met with Arnold Munnich, Scientific Adviser for Medical Research and Health to the French President

On June 15th, 2011, Chen Zhu, Chinese Minister of Health met with Arnold Munnich, Scientific Adviser for Medical Research and Health to the French President and they exchanges opinions over the cooperation on the reform of the medical and pharmaceutical systems in both countries and the medical research. Chen Zhu spoke highly of the Sino-French comprehensive strategic partnership and the long-term close bilateral cooperation in the health field. He thanked the French side for the efforts to promote the bilateral health cooperation. Chen Zhu gave a brief introduction to the development of the bilateral health cooperation in public health reform and prevention and control of emerging infectious diseases and he hoped that the high-level strategic collaboration among the two countries medical research institutions and universities could be established. Munnich introduced the ongoing and upcoming reform measures of the French government in the medical and health field, especially in the medical scientific research. The measures included the structural adjustment of the hospital, the improvement of hospital management, the enlargement of the investment in medical research and so on. He also stated that he would proactively support the future bilateral exchange and cooperation in medical research and hospital management.

(Qu Yang)

15. Minister of Health Chen Zhu Met with UNICEF's Representative to China Gillian Mellsop

On June 16th, 2011, Minister of Health Chen Zhu Met with UNICEF's Representative to China Gillian Mellsop and her colleagues. The two sides exchanged opinions over the issues like maternal and child health, nutrition of children, pediatric disease control and immunization. Chen Zhu congratulated Gillian Mellsop on her assuming the office and thanked UNICEF for the long-term support to China's health undertaking, especially for the support to development of the maternal and child health. Chen Zhu stated that there were a lot of challenges for the development of China's health undertaking and he hoped that the international organizations like UNICEF would continue their support to China's health undertaking. China would strengthen the cooperation with UNICEF over the issues like improvement of the nutritional condition of women and children, breast feeding, lowering the cesarean delivery rate, immunization and increasing the average life expectancy. Gillian congratulated China on the achievements in improving the health condition of women and children and on the deepening the reform of the medical and pharmaceutical systems. The two sides agreed to establish an annual consultation mechanism to elevate the effectiveness of the cooperation. The relevant officials from the Department of International Cooperation and Department of Maternal and Child Health Care and Community Health of Chinese Ministry of Health attended the meeting.

(Qu Yang)

16. Vice Minister of Health Huang Jiefu Met with Veronika I.Skvortsova, Vice Minister of Ministry of Health and Social Development of the Russian Federation

On July 12th, 2011, Vice Minister of Health Huang Jiefu met with Vice Minister of Ministry of Health and Social Development of the Russian Federation Veronika I.Skvortsova and the delegation headed by her. The two sides had a talk over the bilateral exchange and cooperation in the health field.

Huang Jiefu stated that in recent years, the China-Russia health cooperation went well and the range of cooperation was continuously expanded. In addition, within the framework of SOC and Sino-Russian-Indian Cooperation Agreement, the health cooperation between China and Russia was further strengthened. The First BRICS Health Ministers' Meeting was successfully held in Beijing and *the Beijing Declaration* was passed as the outcome of the meeting which provided a new mechanism for the China-Russia health cooperation. Huang Jiefu also gave a brief introduction to the development in China's reform of the medical and pharmaceutical systems. He hoped that with the cooperative mechanisms like the Health Sub-Committee of the China-Russia Committee on Humanities Cooperation and the Brics Health Ministers' Meeting, the bilateral cooperation could be further strengthened.

Skvortsova congratulated China on the success in holding the First BRICS Health Ministers' Meeting and she hoped that the multilateral cooperation concerning China, Russia, WHO and other organizations could be enhanced and the practical bilateral health cooperation could be strengthened. In addition, she was looking forward to the 11th Meeting of the Health Sub-Committee to be held in Beijing. The two sides exchanged opinions over the issues like reform of the medical system and construction of the Sino-Russian rehabilitation centers. The Russian delegation was invited by Chinese Ministry of Health to attend the First BRICS Health Ministers' Meeting.

(Qu Yang)

17. Minister of Health Chen Zhu Met with Carlos Miguel Pereira, Cuban Ambassador to China

On July 14th, 2011, Minister of Health Chen Zhu met with Carlos Miguel Pereira, the leaving Cuban Ambassador. The two sides spoke highly of the bilateral cooperation and exchange in health field and exchanged opinions over the future cooperation.

Chen Zhu thanked Pereira for his contribution to the Sino-Cuban health cooperation during his tenure as ambassador to China. He stated that China could learn from Cuba for the experience in providing full coverage of medical service. He hoped that the two sides could strengthen the exchange over the issues like training of general practitioners and training of the grassroots medical workers. Pereira gave a positive review over the bilateral health cooperation in recent years, especially over the cooperation in ophthalmology. He noted that Cuba would further strengthen the cooperation with China in various forms and fields. The two sides also exchanged in-depth opinions over the specific contents and forms of the bilateral health cooperation.

The relevant official from the Department of International Cooperation of Ministry of Health attended the meeting. Pereira's tenure as ambassador to China began from November 2006 and would end in August 2011.

(Qu Yang)

18. The Third Training Course on Global Health Diplomacy Was Held in Beijing

On July 25th, 2011, the commencement of the 2011 Training Course on Global Health Diplomacy was held in the Medical College of Beijing University. Deputy Health Minister Huang Jiefu attended the commencement ceremony and made a speech. He pointed out that with the economic globalization in the 21st century, the concept of health diplomacy came into being, but it was quite challenging to put it into practice. How to construct the new global health partnership was topping the agenda of the reform of international organizations. Huang Jiefu hoped that the international societies could view the global health cooperation from the health perspective as well as from the diplomatic perspective in order to deal with the increasingly complicated global situation and health issues.

The course had been held for 3 successive years. The experts from Switzerland, Brazil, Thailand and China gave instructions to the trainees. The course covered contents like the concept of global health, key issues and challenges of global health, the concept and acting bodies of the global health management, the relationship between health and diplomacy, global health diplomacy, global health negotiation and so on.

(Qu Yang)

19. Minister of Health Chen Zhu Met with Carel Ijsselmuiden, Executive Director of the COHRED Group

On September 13th, 2011, Minister of Health Chen Zhu Met with Carel Ijsselmuiden, Executive Director of the Council on Health Research and Development Group and they exchanged opinions over the issues like innovations in the medical research, development of health technology and experience of China's medical reform. Chen Zhu stated that China's medical reform was a process of evidence-based decision-making, and the innovations in medical research and the development in medical technology would boost the change of the medical system. Chen Zhu hoped that the cooperation with the Development Group would be further continued. China would actively use the view points of the Global Forum for Health Research for reference and make efforts to promote the development of the global health research. Carel IjsselmuidenJ stated that the Council on Health Research and Development Group would commit itself to the development and innovation in the health research field and strengthen its cooperation with the low-income or middle-income countries to adjust to the changing path of health development. The Council on Health Research and Development Group was found in 2011 on the basis of the former Council on Health for Development Group and the Global Forum for Health Research.

(Qu Yang)

20. Minister of Health Chen Zhu Met with Gordon Brown, Former British Prime Minister and Advisor of the World Economic Forum

On September 15th, 2011, Minister of Health Chen Zhu met with Gordon Brown, Former British Prime Minister and Advisor of the World Economic Forum and they exchanged opinions over the global health cooperation.

With the globalization of economy, the health issues were also increasingly internationalized and had become a major global concern. The two sides agreed to promote the information exchange and experience sharing of the global health, optimize the public health policies, increase the accessibility to medical service and make new medicines and treatments available to more people and more countries.

The relevant officials from the Department of International Cooperation, the Department of Health Policy and Regulation, the Department of Disease Control of the Chinese Ministry of Health attended the meeting.

(Qu Yang)

21. Vice Minister of Health Yin Li Met with Chris Wilson, Director of Discovery in the Global Health Program of the Bill & Melinda Gates Foundation

On September 20th, 2011, Vice Minister of Health Yin Li had a meeting with Chris Wilson, Director of Discovery in the Global Health Program of the Bill & Melinda Gates Foundation and the delegation headed by him. And they had discussion on furthering the bilateral cooperation.

Yin Li affirmed the achievements of the cooperation between Chinese Ministry of Health and the Bill & Melinda Gates Foundation in the programs on AIDS and tuberculosis control and he thanked the Bill & Melinda Gates Foundation for its active involvement in China's tobacco control and its advocacy for a smokeless environment. Yin Li gave a brief introduction to the imported case of polio in Xinjiang of China and hoped that the two sides could collaborate in the field of planned immunization. Chris Wilson stated that the Bill & Melinda Gates Foundation was willing to strengthen the cooperation with China and make contribution to China's health undertaking and the health of the mankind.

The relevant officials from the Department of Disease Control, the Department of Medical Science, Technology and Education and the Department of International Cooperation of the Chinese Ministry of Health attended the meeting.

(Qu Yang)

22. Vice Minister of Health Chen Xiaohong Met with the Italian Minister of Health Ferruccio Fazio

On October 10th, 2011, Vice Minister of Health Chen Xiaohong met with the Italian Minister of Health Ferruccio Fazio and the delegation headed by him in Beijing. The two sides exchanged opinions over the bilateral health cooperation. Chen Xiaohong spoke highly of the existing health cooperation between the two countries and briefly introduced the situation of China's reform of the medical and pharmaceutical systems and the development of the medical information technology. Chen hoped that the two sides would proactively carry out the executive plan for the bilateral health cooperation and expand the range of collaboration. He also hoped that the exchange and cooperation in the key fields like medical reform, training of medical professionals, noncommunicable disease control and food safety. Ferruccio Fazio introduced the healthcare system and the disease prevention and control in Italy and he expressed willingness to cooperate with the Chinese side over the issues like health policies, training of medical professional, e-medicine and telemedicine.

(Qu Yang)

23. Minister of Health Chen Zhu Met with the U.S. Ambassador to China Gary Locke

On November 11th, 2011, Minister of Health Chen Zhu had a meeting with the U.S. Ambassador to China Gary Locke.

Chen Zhu gave a positive review over the outstanding achievements in the bilateral health cooperation. He pointed out that the health cooperation between China and USA had a long history and covered a great variety of fields. He suggested that in addition to the collaboration over the prevention and control of infectious diseases, the two sides should strengthen the cooperation in the control of noncommunicable diseases like cancer, cardiovascular diseases and diabetes. At the meantime, China and USA were both reforming the medical and pharmaceutical systems. Even though the actual situation in the two countries was different, the exchange and cooperation in health policies could provide reference for each other. The bilateral collaboration was beneficial to both nations.

Gary Locke stated that the health cooperation was always an important part in the development of Sino-US relationship. He seconded Chen Zhu's opinion on the bilateral health cooperation and he hoped that more private sectors would participate in the health cooperation to contribute to people's health in both countries.

(Qu Yang)

24. Vice Health Minister Huang Jiefu Attended the Signature of the Cooperation Agreement with Dartmouth College

On October 17th, 2011, Vice Health Minister Huang Jiefu met with the Dartmouth College delegation headed by Dartmouth Provost Carol Folt and Dean of the Geisel School of Medicine at Dartmouth Wiley Souba.

Huang Jiefu gave a positive review over the academic achievements of Dartmouth in fields like public health and medical education. Huang also thanked Dartmouth for its support to the reform and development of the medical system in China and its close collaboration with the medical institutions in China. Huang Jiefu pointed out that China was still confronted with great challenges in the medical reform and he suggested that the two sides should strengthen the cooperation in construction of a medical talent contingent, especially in the training of general practitioners.

After the meeting, Huang Jiefu witnessed the signature of the cooperation agreement between Dartmouth College, and the International Cooperation Department and the Exchange Center of Health Professionals of the Chinese Ministry of Health. According to the agreement, the two sides would carry out collaboration over the issues like healthcare service, training of medical professionals and academic exchanges.

(Qu Yang)

25. Minister of Health Chen Zhu Met with Alice Dautry, the Director General of the Pasteur Institute

On October 19th, 2011, Chinese health minister Chen Zhu met with Alice Dautry,

Director General of the Pasteur Institute and they exchanged views on strengthening bilateral cooperation in medical research.

Chen Zhu briefly introduced the situation of infectious disease prevention and control in china. He thanked the Pasteur Institute in France for supporting the establishment and development of the Institute Pasteur of Shanghai. He stated that the Institute Pasteur of Shanghai made great contribution to China's public health and set a good example of the Sino-French cooperation in health. Chen Zhu hoped that the Pasteur Institute and the research institutions in China would carry out closer cooperation in the research of vaccines, diagnostic agents and medicines for infectious diseases like hand-foot-and-mouth disease and hepatitis C. Dautry expressed that the Pasteur Institute would strengthen the cooperation with China in medical research and strive to improve the health of people in China and other developing countries.

(Qu Yang)

26. Vice Health Minister Huang Jiefu Was Given an Honorary Professorship by the University of Sydney

On October 20th, 2011, Deputy Minister of Health of People's Republic of China, Mr. Huang Jiefu met with Governor of NSW Australia and Chancellor of the University of Sydney, Professor Marie Bashir and the delegation at the Ministry of Health. Mr. Huang was appointed as the Honorary Professor of the University of Sydney in this meeting.

Mr. Huang Jiefu expressed his appreciation to the University of Sydney for appointing him as the honorary professor, and he said that the appointment was not only the affirmation to his personal achievement, but also the affirmation to the achievement of Chinese public health and the affirmation to the achievement of Chinese-Australian cooperation and communications in health area. Mr. Huang exerted that he would continuously promote the cooperation and mutual communications between China and Australia in health sector, especially the cooperation with the University of Sydney, so as to benefit the people of both countries.

Professor Bashir congratulated Mr. Huang on his achievement in liver transplantation surgery and expressed her appreciation to him on his great contribution to the Chinese-Australian cooperation and communications in public health.

They also exchanged the information on further cooperation in the education of general practice, nursing, dentistry and pharmacy.

(Qu Yang)

27. Health Minister Chen Zhu Met with Honorary President of French Academy of Engineering Francois Guinot

Health Minister Chen Zhu met with Professor Francois Guinot, Honorary President of French Academy of Engineering & French President of Sino-French TCM Cooperation Committee in the Ministry of Health on October 26, 2011 and exchanged views on cooperation on TCM and the 5th conference of Sino-French TCM Cooperation Committee. Highly commending Sino-French cooperation on health, Chen Zhu said China and France have always kept close contact in the health field with multi-level and multi-channel cooperation pattern already formed. The four conferences of Sino-French TCM Cooperation Committee made fruitful achievements. He said he understood that the fifth conference which was scheduled to be convened in Paris in this September was postponed and hoped that both sides could overcome difficulties by enhancing communications in order to promote the development of TCM in both France and China to benefit peoples of both countries. Professor Francois Guinot agreed with Chen Zhu and suggested that a Sino-French joint working group be set up to further push forward their cooperation.

(Shan Yongxiang)

28. Health Minister Chen Zhu Met with Alberto Jesus Silva, the new Cuban Ambassador Extraordinary and Plenipotentiary to China

Health Minister Chen Zhu met with Alberto Jesus Silva, the new Cuban Ambassador Extraordinary and Plenipotentiary to China on October 27, 2011. Both sides reviewed and spoke highly of China-Cuba cooperation and communication in health and exchanged views concerning the next-step cooperation.

Chen Zhu pointed out that Cuba was the first Latin American country to establish diplomatic ties with China and the people of both countries have maintained a brotherly friendship. Similarly, China-Cuba health cooperation is time-honored and wide-ranging. He encouraged both sides to further strengthen the co-operations and exchanges in the training of general practitioners and health workers at the primary level as well as the cooperation and exchange in medical research and bio-technique. Alberto Jesus Silva positively evaluated China-Cuba friendly and cooperative relations and appreciated the achievements made in China's health development. He also said that Cuba would further enhance health cooperation with China in various areas and in manifold forms. Both side exchanged opinions regarding health workers' training and cooperation in bio-technique of two countries.

Officials from the Department of Medical Science, Technology and Education and the Department of International Co-operation under the Ministry of Health attended the meeting.

(Shan Yongxiang)

29. Deputy Health Minister Yin Li Attended the Summary Meeting on China AIDS Roadmap Tactical Support Project(CHARTS project)

On October 30, 2011, Deputy Health Minister Yin Li attended and addressed the Summary Meeting on China AIDS Roadmap Tactical Support Project (CHARTS project) held in Beijing.

Yin Li pointed out in his address that AIDS, as a major public health issue and a social issue, was highly emphasized by international community and governments around the world. By and large, AIDS epidemic in China was in low prevalence with high prevalence in some areas and among specific population. Attaching greater importance to AIDS prevention and control, as a strategic issue involving economic development, social stability, national security and national rise and fall, the Chinese government integrated them into the important agenda of government work.

Yin Li stressed that China would fulfill its commitment to reinforce AIDS prevention and control. Getting involved in international co-operations, China would introduce international advanced concepts and techniques in the comprehensive AIDS prevention and control, In addition, China would use and absorb the experiences of prevention and control from other countries to promote the development of China's AIDS prevention and control. Meanwhile, China would make due contributions for the realization of UN Millennium Development Goals and curbing the global spread of AIDS together with international community.

Deputy Ambassador of the British Embassy to China Chris Wood, Deputy Ambassador of the Australian Embassy to China Graeme Meehan and UNAIDS Country Coordinator Mark Stirling attended and addressed the Meeting. Representatives from social organizations of the project provinces and project support gave speeches. About 200 people attended the Meeting, who were from the Ministry of Commerce, the Ministry of Public Security, the Propaganda Department of the Central Committee of the CPC and 17 other ministries and commissions, 19 project provinces (autonomous regions) including Yunnan and Xinjiang, embassies of some countries to China, international organizations, scientific research institutes, and representatives from non-governmental organizations.

(Shan Yongxiang)

30. The 6th Experience Exchange Conference of International Cooperation Programs on HIV/AIDS in China Was Held in Beijing

On October 31st, 2011, the 6th Experience Exchange Conference of International Cooperation Programs on HIV/AIDS in China was held in Beijing. Health Minister Chen Zhu addressed the Conference. Chen Zhu said that the Chinese government attaches great importance to the leadership and coordination over the prevention and control of HIV/AIDS. After many years of hard work, the mechanism of "leading-governmental organizations, departments' responsibility and community-wide participation" had initially taken shape. And the policy of "four frees and one care" was fully carried out. Chen Zhu stressed that China, as a responsible world power, would fulfill its solemn commitment of containing and reverse the prevalence of HIV/AIDS by 2015" to make due contributions for the realization of global millennium development goals and curbing the spread of HIV/AIDS.

Nearly 500 people attended the Conference. They were representatives from members of the State Council AIDS Working Committee, WHO, international organizations including UNAIDS and international non-governmental organizations, neighboring countries like Viet Nam, Laos, Myanmar and Cambodia, representatives from individual provinces (autonomous regions and municipalities) and Xinjiang Production and Construction Corps, front-line staff from the regions of international cooperation programs and workers of community organizations.

(Shan Yongxiang)

31. Health Minister Chen Zhu Attended Harvard Forum on Translational Medicine in Shanghai

On November 7, 2011, Health Minister Chen Zhu attended Harvard Forum on Translational Medicine in Shanghai. In his keynote address, Chen Zhu pointed out that promoting the development of translational medicine and meeting health challenge were line with the inherent objective law. He also stressed that, through the construction of two-way channel for laboratory to clinic or vice verse, the complete development of translational medicine should be linked with a deeper understanding of pathogenesis and development mechanism of disease as well as the mechanisms of health protection and promotion. And new disease control strategy should be explored. The results of scientific research should be converted into specific means, technique and plans of diagnoses or interventions, which are practical to clinic and public health as well as cost effective and facilitate popularization. The conversion of medical results should go into system arrangement through evidence-based decision and become an organic component of health policy, health service and security system. That would benefit the vast majority of clinical patients and ordinary people in a sustainable way and push forward the development of medical sciences. The Ministry of Health would try hard to promote and support medical institutions and research institutes at all levels in conducting clinical and translational medicine researches and international co-operations.

Before the Forum, Chen Zhu held talks with related responsible persons from Harvard Medical School, Shanghai Jiao Tong University School of Medicine and Chinese Academy of Medical Sciences. They reached an agreement on the establishment of China-Harvard Medical School Translational Medicine Consortium.

The Forum was hosted by Harvard Medical School and sponsored by Shanghai Jiao Tong University School of Medicine. Officials from the Department of Medical Science, Technology and Education and the Department of International Co-operation under the Ministry of Health attended the above-mentioned activity.

(Shan Yongxiang)

32. Deputy Health Minister Huang Jiefu Met with Dr. Jenny Amery, Chief Professional Officer of Health and Education, UK DFID

On November 15, 2011, Deputy Health Minister Huang Jiefu met with Dr. Jenny Amery, Chief Professional Officer of Health and Education, the UK's DFID at the Ministry of Health. They held talks on strengthening health cooperation between China and UK.

Huang Jiefu said that, over the past 10 years, China's Ministry of Health and UK DFID conducted pragmatic, effective co-operations in the prevention and control of HIV/AIDS and tuberculosis, community health and researches on health policies, which introduced advanced management philosophy and technique into China for sustainable development. The Chinese side expressed appreciation for that and wished to proceed with co-operations with UK in a wider range of areas and share the experiences of health work with international community, particularly other developing countries. He stressed that it had not been the task of certain department or certain country to develop health services; rather, it required multiple departments and countries all over the world to coordinate the response.

Amery said that the British side would like to go on with close communication with China's Ministry of Health, further deepen the cooperative relations of both countries and make contributions for global health through collaborations in global health. Both sides agreed to conduct active consultations for jointly promoting the realization of UN Health-Related Millennium Development Goals and the future development framework of global health to serve the health of the world's people.

Officials from the Department of International Co-operation under the Ministry of Health attended the meeting.

(Shan Yongxiang)

33. Health Minister Chen Zhu Met with Chief Executive of UK Medical Research Council (MRC)

On November 28, 2011, Health Minister Chen Zhu met with Chief Executive of UK Medical Research Council (MRC) Sir John Savill.

Upon request Chen Zhu told about how the deepening of medical and health system reform was under way in China. He stressed that the Chinese government attached importance to the prevention and control of chronic diseases and adopt appropriate technique for basic medical care and health services. Chen Zhu also hoped that the UK would strengthen its support to medical research institutions including Chinese Academy of Medical Sciences (CAMS) and deepen the cooperation between both countries in the research and talent training for chronic diseases and translational medicine. Besides, both sides communicated with each other on diabetes management and health education for chronic diseases.

Officials from the Department of International Co-operation, the Bureau of Disease Control, the Department of Medical Science, Technology and Education under the Ministry of Health as well as Chinese Academy of Medical Sciences (CAMS) attended the meeting.

(Shan Yongxiang)

34. Health Minister Chen Zhu Met with Former Chairman of Cancer Research UK Sir David Newbigging

On November 28, 2011, Health Minister Chen Zhu met with former Chairman of Cancer Research UK Sir David Newbigging.

Chen Zhu extended thanks to Cancer Research UK for its long-term support to China's health services and medical research. He hoped that UK side would go ahead with the close contact with the National Center for Cancer Research under Chinese Academy of Medical Sciences (CAMS). In addition, it was hoped that the cooperation between both countries in cancer research and medical talent training would be deepened. Both sides conducted communications concerning fund-raising for medical researches and the management of research fund operations.

Officials from the Department of International Co-operation under the Ministry of

Health and Chinese Academy of Medical Sciences (CAMS) attended the meeting.

(Shan Yongxiang)

35. Health Minister Chen Zhu Met with President of the University of California, San Francisco (UCSF)

On November 29, 2011, Health Minister Chen Zhu met with President of the University of California, San Francisco (UCSF) Susan Desmond Hellman and her delegation. They communicated with each other on co-training top health talents.

Chen Zhu spoke highly of the achievements made by UCSF in bio-medicine, medical education and voiced support for its conception of establishing long-term cooperative relationship with China's Medical Universities and the conception of the project for training medical students. He hoped that Chinese Academy of Medical Sciences (CAMS), Peking Union Medical College and UCSF, on the basis of existing co-operations, would further strengthen communications and co-operations in scientific research and education, cultivate high-level health talents, and promote the development of translational medicine and bio-medicine.

Officials from the Department of International Co-operation, the Department of Medical Science, Technology and Education under the Ministry of Health, Chinese Academy of Medical Sciences (CAMS) and Peking Union Medical College attended the meeting.

(Shan Yongxiang)

36. Health Minister Chen Zhu Met with Former French Prime Minister Dominique de Villepin

On December 6, Health Minister Chen Zhu met with former French Prime Minister Dominique de Villepin and both sides conducted exchanges on cooperation in health. Chen Zhu positively evaluated the bilateral comprehensive strategic partnership of cooperation and the long-term friendly cooperation in health. And he extended his thanks to Dominique de Villepin for his pushing forward China-France health cooperation during his term of office. Upon request Chen Zhu told about the latest progress of China's medical system reform, the new rural cooperative medical system (NCMS) and the 12th Five-Year Plan for health services development. Dominique de Villepin spoke highly of the achievements made in China's medical reform in recent years and the long-term co-operations in health care between China and France. Both sides agreed to push forward further exchanges and co-operations in health between two countries.

(Shan Yongxiang)

37. Health Minister Chen Zhu Met with Secretary of National Security and Defense Council of Ukraine Raisa Bogatyrova

On December 7, 2011, Health Minister Chen Zhu met with Secretary of National Security and Defense Council of Ukraine Raisa Bogatyrova. Both sides exchanged views on strengthening China-Ukraine health exchanges and co-operations. Chen Zhu said that China and Ukraine shared traditional friendship, and worked extensively and deeply with each other. In particular, in April of 2011, both countries established the intergovernmental cooperation committee and sub-committee of health cooperation under this framework, which started a new chapter of bilateral exchanges and co-operations. Bogatyrova spoke highly of China-Ukraine friendly cooperation and expressed readiness to further conduct health co-operations in various forms and areas. Both sides agreed to strengthen bilateral co-operations and exchanges in disease prevention and control, bio-technique, drug safety and Traditional Chinese Medicine.

(Shan Yongxiang)

38. Deputy Health Minister Yin Li Attended the Opening Ceremony of High-Level Communication Meeting for White Ribbon Alliance in China

On December 13, 2011, the High-Level Communication Meeting for White Ribbon Alliance for Safe Motherhood in China was held in Beijing. Deputy Health Minister Yin Li attended and addressed the Opening Ceremony.

Yin Li pointed out that in recent years the Chinese government took multiple measures to improve the equity and accessibility of maternal and child health services. As a result, the health of women and children was greatly improved. In 2010, the national infant mortality was 13.1‰ and the mortality of children under 5 was 16‰, which achieved UN Millennium Development Goals ahead of schedule. The national maternal mortality was 30/100,000, falling by 66% from 1990. Currently, China's maternal and child health is facing not only the challenge of unbalanced development among urban-rural areas, various regions and various populations, but rare development opportunities. *The Outline of the 12th Five-Year Plan for Economic and Social Development* includes the main health indicators of women and children in the economic and social development planning, which will surely promote the development of China's maternal and child health care.

The Meeting was hosted by Health News. Vice-Chairperson of All-China Women's Federation Zhen Yan and Global Patron of the White Ribbon Alliance for Safe Motherhood addressed the Meeting respectively. Approximately 80 related experts and managers from nearly 20 Provinces (autonomous regions, municipalities) attended the Meeting.

White Ribbon Alliance for Safe Motherhood is an international non-governmental organization committed to promoting maternal and child health. Since its establishment in 1990, its memberships have covered over 152 countries. The current focus of the Alliance is on calling for governments and organizations around the world to pay attention to lowering maternal mortality.

(Shan Yongxiang)

39. The National Conference on Foreign Affairs in Health Was Held

On December 22-23, 2011, the National Conference on Foreign Affairs in Health was held in Shenzhen, Guangdong. Health Minister Chen Zhu presented the work report at the Conference. He affirmed the achievements made in foreign exchanges and co-operations of national health. In addition, Chen Zhu pointed out that profound changes are taking place in domestic and international situations. And situations and tasks set higher requirements on health and foreign affairs. During the period of the 12th Five-Year Plan, foreign exchanges and co-operations of health should be strengthened. We should get deeply involved in collaborations with international organizations including WHO. Practical exchanges and co-operations of health in border regions will be pushed forward. In addition, we will continue to tap potential in health collaborations with developed countries. The management and innovation of medical teams for aiding foreign countries will be reinforced. And the agreements and mechanisms of health collaborations with Hong Kong and Macao and on both sides of the Taiwan Straits. In accordance with the principle of medical reform, foreign collaborations should promote the development of medical sciences and the building of talent team. Moreover we should push forward international co-operations for TCM health care, education, researches and trade. At the Conference, representatives from the health departments of Jiangsu, Henan, Sichuan and China-CDC had exchanges with each other. Around 150 representatives attended the Conference. They were from the Ministry of Foreign Affairs, the Ministry of Commerce, the State Food and Drug Administration, the State Administration of Traditional Chinese Medicine, Health Departments (Bureaus) of the provinces, autonomous regions, municipalities, and cities with independent planning, institutions directly under the Ministry of Health and departments within the Ministry. The Conference was organized by Health, Population and Family Planning Commission of Shenzhen.

(Shan Yongxiang)

Section 6 Collaborations with Hong Kong, Macao and Taiwan

1. Deputy Health Minister Yin Li met with 2011 Beijing Visit Delegation of Hong Kong Internet Industry

On January 14, 2011, Deputy Health Minister Yin Li met with Beijing visit delegation of Hong Kong Internet Professional Association attending the 2011 Digital Summit. Yin Li told the guests about the size and development of inland medical and health services as well as the development history of inland construction of health informationization. Finally, he hoped that both sides would strengthen the collaboration in improving health services capacity to promote the management and regulation of health information construction.

(Shan Yongxiang)

2. The 9th and 10th Inland China-Hong Kong-Macao Health Administration High-Level Joint Meeting was held in Hong Kong and Beijing

On January 27-30 and November 3-6, 2011, the 9th and 10th Inland China-Hong Kong-Macao Health Administration High-Level Joint Meeting was held in Hong Kong and Beijing. Deputy Health Minister Huang Jiefu and officials from the Food and Health Bureau of Hong Kong SAR and the Secretariat for Social and Cultural Affairs of Macao SAR attended the Meeting. At the two sessions, new measures for 2010 and 2011 Inland China-Hong Kong-Macao health reform development were discussed. Experiences in the following areas were shared: the prevention and control of contagious diseases and chronic diseases, innovations and development of health science and technology, development of AIDS vaccine, research collaboration for chronic diseases, public hospital reform, tobacco control, quality review of hospitals, control of chronic diseases, and trainings of general practitioners and specialists. An agreement on strengthening the collaboration in tobacco control legislation and quality review of hospitals was reached.

(Shan Yongxiang)

Section 7 Work Progress of Center for International Exchanges and Co-operations

1. Philips (China) Investment Co., Ltd. Phase II Collaborative Project for Training of Breast Cancer Screening of Rural Women

In 2011, to coordinate the focus of medical reform and improve the basic screening for breast cancer, under the specific guidance of the Ministry of Health, the Center for International Exchanges and Co-operations under the Ministry of Health proceeded with Philips (China) Investment Co., Ltd. Phase II Collaborative Project for Training of Breast Cancer Screening of Rural Women, with the funds raised through private channels. Twelve training workshops for ultrasonic technology and four training workshops for X-ray technology were completed, with 1,256 people attended.

(Shan Yongxiang)

2. Colgate-Palmolive (China) Co., Ltd. Collaborative Project for Dental Services in Qinghai Disaster Area

To help with post-disaster reconstruction in Qinghai and promote the post-disaster reconstruction of dental care service system and residents' oral health in the quake-hit area, in 2011, the Center for International Exchanges and Co-operations under the Ministry of Health established Colgate-Palmolive (China) Co., Ltd. Collaborative Project for Dental Services in Qinghai Disaster Area under the guidance of the Ministry of Health through private channels. Meanwhile the modality of prevention and control for dental disease was explored.

(Shan Yongxiang)

Section 8 Work Progress of the Service Center for Regulation of Project-Funding

The Completion of World Bank Grants Phase II Project of the Capability Construction of Prevention and Control for China Highly Pathogenic Avian Influenza and Human Influenza Pandemic

The World Bank Grants Phase II Project of the Capability Construction of Prevention and Control for China Highly Pathogenic Avian Influenza and Human Influenza Pandemic was completed as scheduled on November 30. The Project explored a path for "transforming the international concept of preparedness and response to influenza pandemic into practice at primary levels in China". The project goal was achieved: to improve the national strategy for prevention and control of avian flu, to improve the readiness of flu pandemic at primary levels and to improve early-warning, surveillance and quick response at primary levels. That provided the country with demonstrative experience.

(Shan Yongxiang)

Chapter XIX The Construction of Spiritual Civilization

2011 Working Conference on Discipline Inspection and the Checking of Unhealthy Tendencies and Malpractices in National Health System

From Jan. 13 to 14, Working Conference on Discipline Inspection and the Checking of Unhealthy Tendencies and Malpractices in National Health System was held in Beijing. At the conference, the important contents of the speech given by Hu Jintao, General Secretary of the Communist Party of China at the 17th Session of the 6th Plenary Session of the Central Commission for Discipline Inspection, and the contents of the work statement by He Guoqiang, Secretary of the Central Commission for Discipline Inspection were transmitted, the work of combating corruption and upholding integrity was summarized and the tasks in 2011 were assigned. Chen Zhu, Minister of Ministry of Health, attended the conference and made a speech. Li Xi, a member of the Central Commission for Discipline Inspection, member of the Party Group of Ministry of Health and the leader of ministerial discipline inspection team, made a working report. The responsible leaders from the relevant departments of the Central Commission for Discipline Inspection and organs of Ministry of Supervision were invited to the conference.

Chen Zhu fully confirmed the achievements in checking unhealthy tendencies and malpractices of national health system in the past year and he said that the activity of "Three Goods and One Satisfaction" of "Good Service, Good Quality, Good Medical Ethics and Satisfaction from the Masses" should be extensively conducted in national health system in 2011, the cases of pharmaceutical purchase and sale and those of unhealthy tendency in medical service must be investigated and treated to make professional discipline strict, and the convenient and beneficial measures for people must be implemented with the deepening of the reform on medical health system, democratic appraisal on health practice should be carried out comprehensively to satisfy the society, the centralized procurement of medicines must be promoted continuously and the internal and external supervision and restriction mechanism should be established and perfected.

Chen Zhu required that health administrative departments and medical health units at each level must feasibly reinforce the organization and leadership of the checking of unhealthy tendencies and malpractices, and further perfect work responsibility system for checking unhealthy tendencies and malpractices to ensure the implementation of responsibility. And the organizations for checking unhealthy tendencies and malpractices must be feasibly enhanced to improve the organizations and replenish forces.

Li Xi summarized the checking of unhealthy tendencies and malpractices of national health system in 2010. He required that health administrative departments, medical health units and organizations for health discipline inspection at each level must further improve the responsibility system for the construction of the working style of the honest and clean Party and work responsibility system for checking unhealthy tendencies and malpractices so as to feasibly form the overall force to promote anti-corruption. The effective ways to strengthen the construction of the working style of the honest and clean Party and the checking of unhealthy tendencies and malpractices must be energetically explored.

(Ji Chenglian)

Part IV Academic and Civil Societies

Chapter I Chinese Medical Association

Work of Chinese Medical Association in 2011

I. Organize and Host Association Democratically

The Standing Council of Chinese Medical Association (hereinafter referred to as Association) has held meetings for 6 times in 2011 (including communication meeting) according to the newly revised rules of procedure to make repeated studies and discussions on *The Five-year Plan of the 24th Session of the Council of Chinese Medical Association*, deliberations on *Management Methods for Specialized Branch of Chinese Medical Association, Project Management Approach for Continuing Medical Education of Chinese Medical Association* and other rules and regulations, which were included in *Minutes of the Standing Council*, and mailed them to all the council members. Many conferences of working committees of organizations, academy, popular science and continuing education were held successively to give review and approval to the important work items. The new leading body of the Association established the important matters of the work, especially the subjects under discussion involving "Three Importances and One Largeness", which must keep to the discussing principles of collective study and democratic decision-making. The system of joint conference of the Party and the government was established. In 2011, more than 20 times of administrative office meetings, office meetings of secretary general and the joint meetings of the Party and government were held.

II. Organization and Construction

In order to promote the development and management of the members, the Association keeps and strengthens the connection with local medical associations. On April 25th, 2011, Meeting of Local Medical Association and Seminar of Organizational Work of Chinese Medical Association were held in Ningbo City, Zhejiang Province. At the meeting, all local medical associations carried out extensive and deep-going exchanges on challenges and opportunities for associations and special topics on active involvement in medical reform, and they also carried out the discussions on the enhanced management of the members and reached consensus. In 2011, the Association further perfected the transitional program of office term for specialized branches, *Management Methods for Specialized Branch of Chinese Medical Association* and other rules and regulations, which were approved in principle at the 9th meeting of the Standing Council. The Association changed the term of office by sticking to organizational structure of "former, current and designated chairman of committee", completed the changes of office term in 15 specialized branches, the establishment and office term changes in youth assemblies of 19 specialized branches, and 82 professional groups in 18 specialized branches. In 2011, 580 members of specialized branches were enrolled and the accumulative number of the members in specialized branches was 3,038. Examined and approved by China Association for Science and Technology and recorded for reference by Ministry of Civil Affairs, the establishment of the first committee of Clinical Pharmacy Branch and Medical Disaster Branch of Chinese Medical Association was officially completed in 2011 and the number of the branches increased to 85.

III. Academic Exchange

In 2011, Chinese Medical Association revised and improved *Management Methods for Academic Conference of Specialized Branch of Chinese Medical Association* and a series of managerial methods relating to academic exchanges. 357 academic conferences of various kinds were held and as many as 52 specialized branches held academic conferences on a regular basis. The academic level, scale and benefits of the conferences were obviously improved. 61 national academic conferences or annual academic conferences, 17 international, prefectural and bilateral academic conferences, 15 academic meetings for the young and middle-aged and 158 symposiums were hosted by the specialized branches, of which 78 large-scale annual academic conferences of national academic conferences were organized with direct responsibility of the Association. Totally, the number of the representatives was

105,955, the number of the theses received was 73,640 and 80 books of the theses were edited and assembled. More than half of the conferences with more than one thousand representatives were large-scale annual academic meetings or national academic meetings, which attracted some representatives from abroad. The number of the representatives to The 13th Academic Conference of Orthopedics & The 6th COA International Academic Conference held by Chinese Medical Association was more than 11,000 and more than 300 representatives (the greatest number of all previous meetings) came from orthopedics associations of more than 47 countries and regions. More than 12,000 theses were received, including 500 ones in English. The number of the conference reports was 1,500 and nearly a hundred lectures on continuing education were organized.

IV. Publication and Distribution

The publication and distribution of series journals. In 2011, the total number of journals sponsored by Chinese Medical Association was 125, in which China Association for Science and Technology was responsible for 86 magazines and Ministry of Health was in charge of 39 magazines distributed in 18 provinces, cities and autonomous regions around the country. 1,393 issues of magazines are published in a year, of which there is one weekly publication, three periodicals in every 10 days, six publications in every 15 days, 65 monthly, 47 bimonthly and 3 quarterly publications. According to the statistics on 21 periodicals with the base locations generally in the Association Building (excluding *Information Guides of China Medicine*), about 1,684,000 volumes were published in 2011, 1.9% lower than that of 2010. The total circulation in 2011 was 1,670,000 volumes, which was 1.75% lower than that of 2010.

The publication and distribution of electronic audio and video products. In 2011, 140 edition numbers of electronic audio and video products as well as 26 copies of 162 issues of serial electronic publications (electronic magazines) were published. 21 kinds of books were jointly published with other publishing houses and 517,745 disks were made for publication.

V. International Exchange and Cooperation

In 2011, Chinese Medical Association paid visits in groups to foreign countries for 17 times successively, attending working conference of West Pacific Ocean of WHO, the 188th Council Meeting of World Medical Association and other important meetings of international organizations. The international representatives and those from organizations of medical profession in Hong Kong, Macao and Taiwan were received for 10 times for the important activities of organizing and holding "Sino-France Week of Medicine" and "Medical Exchange between Beijing and Hong Kong".

VI. Active Launch of Science Popularization

In 2011, Chinese Medical Association launched various kinds of propagandas in grassroots communities and west areas by focusing on *Action Plan Outline for National Scientific Literacy* and basing on the requirements of the reform on medical health and the demands of the public. In order to improve diagnosis, treatment and management of diabetes in our country, Chinese Medical Association and the center for clinical examination of Ministry of Health, basing on the joint start of "China Plan for Education of Glycosylated Hemoglobin", launched 18 trainings for more than 6,200 physicians of secretion and test in 8 provincial capitals of Xining, Qinghai Province, Yinchuan, Ningxia Hui Autonomous Region, Hohhot, Inner Mongolia Autonomous Region and Urumchi, Xinjiang Uygur Autonomous Region and continued the cooperation with Johnson & Johnson by launching activities *of Chinese Medical Association and Johnson & Johnson Academic Lecture in West Areas, Grassroots Training Classes for West Areas by Science Popularization Department of Chinese Medical Association* for 5 times in grassroots of West Areas.

VII. Undertake Government Function Transfers and Entrusted Tasks

Awards for science and technology. In 2011, Chinese Medical Association appraised and selected prize winning items by means of formal examination, preliminary examination, public announcement, and final judgment on the recommended projects. They are 85 winning projects of the "Award for China Medical Science and Technology in 2011": 7 items of the first prize, 25 of the second, 48 of the third, 2 items of health management, 2 items of popularization of medical science, and 1 item of international cooperation of science and technology. As the direct recommending unit for National Award for Progress in Science and Technology, Chinese Medical Association recommended 8 items of the first and second prizes of "China Medical Science and Technology in 2010" by merits, of which 5 items won the second prize of China Medical Science and Technology in 2011.

Continuing education. In 2011, Chinese Medical Association performed functions of national office for continuing medical education committee, continued the report acceptance on national continuing medical education programs, organized and appraised the reports, made centralized appraisal on 7,869 reported projects of national continuing medical education programs in 2012 by means of remote network, printed and issued more than 800,000 books of national credit certificates, more than 70,000 books of electronic credit certificates of continuing medical education programs of Chinese Medical Association and about 160,000 books of credit certificates of national continuing medical education programs. In December, 2011, entrusted by Finance Planning Department of Ministry of Health, Chinese Medical Association continued professional proficiency assessment on the personnel of medical equipment in 2011. The registration number exceeded 30,000 around the country. Besides, Chinese Medical Association launched the continuing education projects of "Qualification Training for Specialized Critical Medicine" and "Training for Clinical Researchers".

Technical appraisal for medical negligence. In 2011, Chinese Medical Association accepted the letters of entrustment and completed 166 cases of technical appraisal for medical accidents entrusted by superior people's courts and provincial health administrative departments in various places. 128 cases were not handled after the demonstration by the experts and 39 cases were handled, of which 2 cases of technical consultation were completed and totally 30 cases of technical appraisal for medical negligence were organized (19 cases were entrusted by courts of justice and 11 ones by health departments), which accounted for 96.7%. 5 times of written replies to clients' consultation letters were done and the appraisal conclusions given by Chinese Medical Association entrusted by courts of justice and health administrative departments were admitted.

The rest of work entrusted by government. In 2011, Chinese Medical Association completed more than 10 items of tasks of project appraisal, technology demonstration and consultation, plan formulation and revision for diagnosis and treatment entrusted by government. In 2011, entrusted by Medical Administrative Department of Ministry of Health, Chinese Medical Association took charge of assessment on the construction of national key clinical specialty. From July 3 to 15, 2011, the conference on the assessment of national key clinical specialty construction was held in Beijing International Conference Center. Chinese Medical Association organized 996 experts (times) to make appraisals on 1,155 construction projects of 21 specialties in accordance with the principles and procedures specified by Ministry of Health, which lasted 13 days and all work entrusted by Ministry of Health was completed successfully. In 2011, after the printing and distribution of *Instructions on General Practitioner System Establishment by the State Council*, on July 15, Chinese Medical Association and Chinese Medical Doctor Association invited the leaders from health administrative departments, medical education field, and experts from general medical branches and news media to have a forum on the implementation of *Instructions on General Practitioner System Establishment by the State Council*. At the forum, the responsible person of Chinese Medical Association read out initial written proposal on *Implementation of Instructions on General Practitioner System Establishment by the State Council*, and called on all medical workers to make a positive contribution to creating general practitioner system with Chinese characteristics. Xinhua News Agency, People's Network, other mainstream media and times of periodicals published the initial written proposal and reported the contents of the forum.

(Ji Chenglian)

Chapter II Chinese Association of Preventive Medicine

Work of Chinese Association of Preventive Medicine in 2011

I. Construction of Organization

In 2011, 8 times of the meetings of general secretary and 3 times of the Standing Council meetings were organized and held by Chinese Association of Preventive Medicine. All preparations were done for the 5th Session of National Members of Congress.

By the end of 2011, office term of 9 branches has expired, of which 2 specialized committees have changed the term of office, 4 branches established academic groups and 7 branches admitted new members. Chinese Association of Preventive Medicine received application reports for establishment from 4 branches, which were approved by the Standing Council of Chinese Association of Preventive Medicine and reported to China Association for Science and Technology.

The specialized committee of health risk assessment and control, and the specialized committee of apoplexy prevention and control did pilot work of member development for specialized committees. More than 200 persons were made the members of specialized committees.

II. Academic Exchange

In 2011, 207 academic conferences were held, of which 5 were international academic conferences and the ones on Hong Kong, Macao and Taiwan regions. 28,315 scholars attended the conferences and 2,980 theses were exchanged.

Rewarding Methods for Scientific and Technical Awards of Chinese Association of Preventive Medicine and the relevant documents were revised. Totally, 94 units recommended 134 items of scientific research projects for Scientific and Technical Awards of Chinese Association of Preventive Medicine. The 12th Session of the 4th Standing Council examined and discussed the items and formally approved 127 items. The committee for final examination made appraisals on 62 items, of which 4 items were given the first prize, 16 items the second and 29, the third.

The supporting project of "Funds for Application and Research of Public Health & Scientific Research on Diseases Preventable with Vaccine", started in November, 2010, was continued. 21 items of "Research on Strategy System of Chickenpox Vaccine Immunization" were given strict mid-term examination and appraisal. Generally, all items were well completed. Most of the items were in the phase of project completion, inspection and acceptance at the end of 2011.

To carry out national planning policy for extensive immunization, Chinese Association of Preventive Medicine held many seminars and exchange activities to different groups of people in different places, such as seminars on new progress in polio prevention, forums on pentavaccine use, meetings on dengue fever prevention and control & its vaccine use, new era summit meetings on combined vaccine, and seminars on immunization strategy of the four places across the strait and others. More than 3,000 persons attended the gatherings.

Ⅲ. Continuing Medical Education

In 2011, 51 national programs and 178 programs of continuing education at association level were ratified by Ministry of Health. By November, 2011, 161 programs of continuing education, that is, 25 national programs of continuing education and 136 programs of continuing education at Association level had been completed. More than 63,000 persons were trained.

In 2011, the Association, GlaxoSmithKline, Pfizer Pharmaceuticals Ltd. and other companies cooperated for the launch of "Training Conference on Strengthening Standardized Immunization Management", "Training Classes for Public Health at County Level", "Seminar on Immunization, Disease and Vaccine", "2011 Seminar on Immunization of Hepatitis B Vaccine for College Students", "2011 Academic Seminar on Seasonal Influenza Prevention and Control" and other symposiums, and jointly held "Training Class for the Development and Management of Public Health" with Tsinghua University, which was sponsored by Pfizer Pharmaceuticals Ltd. In August, sponsored by United States-China Medical Board, Chinese Association of Preventive Medicine and Chinese Center for Disease Prevention and Control jointly held "Training Class for 'Double Ten' Action of Medical Workers' Tobacco Control Ability" and "Training Class for Leadership Ability of Creating Smoke-free Medical

Health Institutions" in Liuzhou City, Guangxi Zhuang Autonomous Region. Nearly 150 responsible leaders and professional staff from the units launching "'Double Ten' Action of Medical Workers' Tobacco Control Ability" and health bureaus in all cities and prefectures of Guangxi Province, patriotic sanitation offices, centers for disease prevention and control and other institutions attended the trainings. More than 20 rounds of training classes were held in fields of "food safety, occupational-disease protection, radiological health, performance appraisal in disease prevention and control system, AIDS testing, and tuberculosis prevention and treatment. And about 700 persons attended the trainings.

IV. Propaganda of Science Popularization

In accordance with the project requirements of "Technical Key Point Screening of Common and Frequently-occurring Infectious Disease" covered in "the Eleventh-five-year" national supporting plan, and *Criteria for Demonstration Bases of Popular Health Science by Chinese Association of Preventive Medicine,* Yongning County Health Bureau in Ningxia Hui Autonomous Region, Health Service Center in Beiguan, Datong City, Shanxi Province, and College of Public Health of Jining Medical College were appraised by the experts as the first batch of "Demonstration Base of Science Popularization" of Chinese Association of Preventive Medicine.

Technical Key Point Screening of Common and Frequently-occurring Infectious Disease and Research Project by China Association for Science and Technology was completed and passed financial audit, acceptance check, and project acceptance.

In April, in response to "No Smoking in Indoor Public Places" covered in *Implementation Rules for Health Management Regulations in Public Places,* Chinese Association of Preventive Medicine organized 10 medical mass organizations of Chinese Medical Association and Chinese Association on Tobacco Control, and made an initiative to medical mass organizations of all levels around China to fully implement laws and regulations on non-smoking in all indoor public places, including offices, and support the implementation of the 80th Order by Ministry of Health with practical action. People's Network and other media reported on it.

To fully reflect the achievements in "the Eleventh-five-year" national supporting plan, Chinese Association of Preventive Medicine showed the project of Technical Key Point Screening of Common and Frequently-occurring Infectious Disease and Research in Achievement Exhibition of Science and Technology jointly held by Ministry of Science and Technology, Organization Department of CCCPC and other relevant units.

V. Work Entrusted by China Association for Science and Technology and Governmental Departments

The pilot work of *Management Standards for Infectious Diseases in Medical Institutions and Criteria for Examination and Appraisal* was launched (hereinafter referred to as *Standards and Criteria*). The pilot work in Beijing, Hunan Province and Gansu Province was run and the pilot units were required to put forward opinions and suggestions in the operation of *Standards and Criteria* and improve their management of infectious diseases.

Entrusted by Health Emergency Office of Ministry of Health, Chinese Association of Preventive Medicine undertook secretariat work of "Health Emergency Expert Advisory Committee of Ministry of Health", organized the experts for "Seminar on Health Emergency Work Development in Public Health Service System during 'the Twelfth-Five-Year' Period", and provided consultation for the formulation of "the Twelfth-Five-Year Plan for Health Emergency by Health Emergency Office.

Chinese Association of Preventive Medicine organized the relevant branches and the experts to put forward modification suggestions on *Amendment of the Occupational Disease Prevention Law of the People's Republic of China (Draft)* and report to the superiors.

VI. International and Regional Exchange and Cooperation

12 batches of more than 30 persons/times of groups visiting of foreign countries, Hong Kong, Macao and Taiwan were attended to. 15 experts and scholars from British Health Unlimited, Asia-Pacific AIDS Business Alliance, Japan National Science Academy of Health Care and Medicine to China were received.

All activities of Chinese Association of Preventive Medicine and four consecutive terms of executive committee member. In 2011, the Union Commission, insisting on the principle of one China, took Taiwan in as the supporting member of Union Commission, assisted Indonesia Public Health Association in the preparations for the conference on public health in West Pacific Region and hosting the 3rd working conference of coordination committee in West Pacific Region, and established the website of liaison office in West Pacific Region affiliated to World Federation of Public Health Associations. In August, 2011, Chinese Association of Preventive Medicine helped The UN Commission on Life and Health Counselor of China Association for Science and Technology (hereinafter referred to as CCLH) attend The 10th International AIDS Conference in Asia-Pacific Region (ICAAP10) held in Pusan、International Conference Center of South Korea.

VII. Cooperative Implementation of AIDS and Chronic Diseases

(1) AIDS Program of the Global Fund

In 2011, Chinese Association of Preventive Medicine undertook AIDS Program of the Global Fund, took the charge of the training for social organizations in 5 provinces and regions of Ningxia, Inner Mongolia, Gansu, Shaanxi and Xinjiang in Northwest Areas, and held 3 times of trainings for the establishment of AIDS prevention and treatment of social organizations. After the trainings, the return visits were paid to 22 organizations in 4 provinces and regions. The development of social organizations in northwest areas and the training results were assessed. The suggestions on training were reported back to national program office of AIDS Program of the Global Fund.

(2) China-Gates AIDS Program

In 2011, Chinese Association of Preventive Medicine adjusted strategy priorities of China-Gates AIDS Program, formulated program plan based on the suggestions of community organizations and held the annual conference of China-Gates AIDS Program in Haikou City of Hainan Province, and the non-governmental meeting on the Program during the period of this annual conference, for which Chinese Association of Preventive Medicine was responsible, was held. Chinese Association of Preventive Medicine launched training for management change in Beijing, organized 10 administrative staff of the Program at provincial and municipal levels to practice in Hong Kong AIDS Foundation. Chinese Association of Preventive Medicine organized the practice taken part in by administrative staff of the Program at provincial and municipal levels and delegations of social organizations in Tianjin City, and did supervision, investigation and research in Shenyang, Guangzhou, Changsha, Hainan, Chongqing and other places.

(3) Online Education Program of Sino-German AIDS Prevention and Treatment

The total funds for the program was 890,000 RMB Yuan and the assorting funds of Chinese Association of Preventive Medicine was 300,000 RMB Yuan. Two issues of trainings of online AIDS education were held in Haikou City, Hainan Province and Changsha City, Hunan Province. And 50 students graduated from the trainings. In June, 2011, the training of management change for the students was developed and 11 outstanding students from 6 provinces were invited to the training. In December, the 11th Seminar on Policy Development of AIDS Prevention and Treatment was held in Haikou City, Hainan Province.

(4) Social Mobilization Program for National AIDS Prevention and Treatment

Social mobilization programs of "Exploitation into Ability Establishment Mode and the Practice of Ability Establishment with Community Team as the Core" and "Risk Research on AIDS Infection and Intervention Programs for MSM Sex Workers of Cross-dressing in Beijing Area" were approved with 240,000 RMB Yuan as the supporting funds. The working contents covered in these two programs have been completed.

(5) Burden of Main Chronic Diseases of the People in China's Western Rural Areas and Program for Strategies of Prevention and Control

In 2011, Chinese Association of Preventive Medicine and Center for Chronic Disease Prevention and Treatment of China's Center for Disease Prevention and Control jointly launched the program of "Burden of Main Chronic Diseases of the People in China's Western Rural Areas and Program for Strategies of Prevention and Control" and intervention activities against unhealthy life habits with on-the-spot investigation and baseline survey, carried out health education lectures for the focused groups of people, like housewives and pupils by means of broadcast, pamphlet and trainings for clerks at grassroots and the anticipated goal was reached.

VIII. Journal Management and Network Construction

Chinese Association of Preventive Medicine hosts 69 kinds of journals and 1 kind of newspaper, of which 45 kinds of magazines were included in "Journals of Statistic Source" of China science and technology papers by selection, and 22 kinds were in "Chinese Core Periodicals". Some of the journals are cited frequently with the factor of influence among the top professional journals and a certain percentage of journals are included into the six world famous retrieve institutions. *Chinese Journal of Nosocomiology, Chinese Journal of Parasitology and Parasitic Diseases, and China Public Health* were rewarded "One Hundred Kinds of Outstanding Academic Journals" in 2010. 10 articles in series of magazines hosted by Chinese Association of Preventive Medicine were rewarded "China's One Hundred Academic Papers with the Most International Influence". Chinese Association of Preventive Medicine was included into the important indicators of CSTPCD, and the average times of citation and factor of influence were higher than the national average. *Chinese Journal of Schistosomiasis Prevention and Treatment* was included into MEDLINE data base of National Library of Medicine (NLM) of the United States. *Chinese Journal of Viral Disease* was included into Journals of Statistic Source of China science and technology papers (CSTPCD). *Chinese Journal of Viral Disease* was given the second prize and *Chinese Journal of Preventive Medicine* was given Editor Choice of excellent journal.

Since the revision of website of the Association at the end of 2009, the click rate was constantly rising. By October, 2011, the number of clicks has broken through 960,000. The websites of "Knowledge Base for Common and Frequently-occurring Infectious Disease Prevention and Treatment" and "Liaison Office of World Public

Health Alliance in West Pacific Region" were established. In 2011, 8 issues of *Work Communication of Chinese Association of Preventive Medicine* fully covered the key work of Chinese Association of Preventive Medicine.

(Ji Chenglian)

Part V
Health Work Chronicle

2011 Health Work Chronicle

January 3, Ministry of Health printed and issued T*he Key Points of Health Work of 2011*.

January 5, Ministry of Health printed and issued Guiding *Opinions of Evaluation Mechanism Establishment of Social Stability Risks for Major Affairs of Health System (trial edition)*.

On the same day, Ministry of Health printed and issued *The Provisional Methods of Warning System of Conversation for Safety of Medical Quality*.

January 6-7, Ministry of Health convened 2011 National Health Working Conference in Beijing. At the conference, the achievements of health development of the Eleventh-five-year Plan and health work in 2010 were summed up and the tasks of health development of the Twelfth-five-year Plan and the health work in 2011 were deployed. Chen Zhu, Minister of Ministry of Health, made a working report entitled *Rouse Ourselves and Work Hard, Carry forward the Cause and Forge ahead into the Future, and Create a New Aspect of Scientific Development of Health Undertaking*. At the same time, Ministry of Health conducted commendation to the representatives of the excellent village doctors nationwide and awarded Wang Shaoming and other 200 village doctors with the honorable title of National Excellent Village Doctors of 2011. Zhang Mao, Secretary of the Party Group and Vice-minister of Ministry of Health made the summing-up report.

January 11-12, 2011 National Conference of Food Safety and Health Supervision Work of Health System was held in Wuxi of Jiangsu Province. Chen Zhu, Minister of Ministry of Health made video speech and Chen Xiaohong, Vice-minister of Ministry of Health presented the conference and made the main report.

January 11-19, Zhang Mao, Secretary of the Party Group and Vice-minister of Ministry of Health, with his delegation, paid a visit to India and Yemen, investigating the health system and hospital management of the two countries, attended the unveiling inauguration ceremony of Sino-Yemen Ophthalmology Cooperative Center, visiting and saluting our aid medical team to Yemen.

January 13-14, The National Conference of Supervisory Discipline Inspection and Style-rectifying Work of Health System was convened in Beijing. At the conference, the summing-up and review of promoting the counter-corruption and honest administration work of health system in 2010 was conducted and the working tasks of 2011 deployed. Minister of Ministry of Health, Chen Zhu, was present at the conference and made a speech.

January 14, Wang Zhenyi, Academician of Chinese Engineering Academy and lifelong professor of Ruijin Hopsital Affiliated to Medical College of Shanghai Communication University and honorary rector of the Research Institute of Hematology of Shanghai was gained the state highest award of science and technology of 2010. Ministry of Health decided to launch an activity of learning from Wang Zhenyi widely in the health system.

On the same day, Ministry of Health printed and issued *The Provisional Regulations of Report of the Safety Events of Medical Quality.*

January 17, Chen Zhu, Minister of Ministry of Health signed and issued No. 79 of Minister Order: *Administrative Standards of the Quality of Medical Production* (revised edition of 2010), which will be effective from March 1 of 2011.

On the same day, the General Office of Ministry of Health printed and issued *Guidance to the Technique of Prevention and Control of the Infections by Multiple Drug-fast Bacteria in Hospital (trial edition).*

January 21, Ministry of Health, jointly with Ministry of Agriculture printed and issued *The Largest Limited Amount of Residues of Agricultural Chemicals Including Paraquat and other 53 Kinds*, which will come into effect on April 1 of 2011.

On the same day, Ministry of Health printed and issued the national standards of *Vocational Health Standardization of Guardian Technique for the Radiation Working Personnel*, implemented from August 1 of 2011.

January 24, Ministry of Health held video-tele conference for learning from the Advanced Achievements of Wang Zhenyi. Chen Zhu, Minister of Ministry of Health, presided over the conference and Zhang Mao, Secretary of the Party Group and Vice-minister of Ministry of Health attended the conference and made a speech.

January 28, the Office of Ministry of Health printed and issued *The Sentinel Monitoring Scheme for Hospitalized Acute Cases of Infection of Respiratory Tract* (2011 edition).

January 30, The 58th Anniversary Day of Prevention and Treatment of Leprosy. The theme was "Remove the Harm of Leprosy and Protect the Legal Rights of Health".

On the same day, Minister of Ministry of Health signed and issued No. 80 of Minister Order of Ministry of Health: *Detailed Rules and Regulations of Implementation of*

Health Management in Public Places, which will be implemented from May 1 of 2011.

On the same day, Minister of Ministry of Public Security, Meng Jianzhu and Minister of Ministry of Health, Chen Zhu, jointly signed and issued the 115th Minister Order: The Method of Affirmation of Drug Addiction, which shall come into force from April 11 of 2011.

On the same day, Ministry of Health printed and issued *Regulations of Management of Medicinal Affairs in Medical Institutions*.

January 31, Ministry of Health and Ministry of Human Power Resources & Social Safeguard jointly established Examination Committee of the Practice Qualification of Nurses.

February 4, The Day of the World Cancer. The theme is "Cancer Is a Preventible Disease.

February 11, Ministry of Health printed and issued *Diagnostic and Therapeutic Scheme of Plague (trial edition)*.

February 11-12, The Second Session of Sino-Africa Health Cooperation International Seminar was held in Beijing.

The China South-South Cooperative Research Alliance was established so as to strengthen the exchange and cooperation between China and the countries in the realm of health of the south part, and promote continuously the effect of China in the international society, especially in the South-South cooperation. Han Qide, Vice-committee Director of the Standing Committee of People's Congress and Chen Zhu, Minister of Ministry of Health presented at the seminar and made speeches.

February 12, Ministry of Health printed and issued *The Mid-term and Long-term Development Plan for Talents of Medical and Health (2011-2020)*. On the same day, the General Office of Ministry of Health printed and issued *The Implementation Scheme for the Prevention of Baby and Mother Transmission of AIDS, Syphilis and Hepatitis B*.

February 13, the General Office of the State Council printed and issued *The Five Key Points of Systemic Reform of Medical and Health and Arrangement of 2011*.

February14, Wang Wanqing, former Director Doctor of Surgery Department in People's Hospital of Maqu County, Gansu Province, was selected as one of the Top 10 Great Figures of Moving China.

February 15-16, Li Keqiang, member of the Standing Committee of Political Bureau of the Central Party Group, Vice Premier of the State Council, leader of the Leading Group of Medical and Health Systemic Reform attended National Working Conference on Medical and Health Systemic Reform and made a speech. Minister of Ministry of Health, Chen Zhu, attended the conference.

February 16, the General Office of Ministry of Health printed and issued *Directive Principles for Clinical Application of Glucocorticoid Medicines, Standardizations of Diagnosis and Treatment of Gastric Cancer (2011 edition) and Standardizations of Diagnosis and Treatment of Primary Pulmonary Cancer (2011 edition).*

February 17, the General Office of Ministry of Health printed and issued *Guidance to the Diagnosis and Treatment of Epidemic Influenza (2011 edition).*

February 22, Ministry of Health, China General Association of Red Cross and the Department of Health of General Logistic Ministry held the Large National Commendation Meeting of Gratis Blood Donation (2008-2009) in Beijing. Han Qide, Vice-director of the Standing Committee of People's Congress and Chen Zhu, Minister of Minister of Health were present at the meeting.

February 28, the General Office of the State Council printed and issued *Arrangement of the Pilot Reform Work of Public Hospital of 2011.*

On the same day, Ministry of Health and National General Bureau of Supervision and Inspection of Quality and Quarentine jointly printed and issued *Standard of Food Additives.*

March 2, Ministry of Health and the Section of WHO representatives stationed in China jointly held a meeting of "Giving Some Relevant Information on Chinese Medical Reform Development". Chen Zhu, Minister of Ministry of Health introduced the condition of progress of deepened Chinese medical and health systemic reform to all the institutions of UN systems, relevant international organizations and officers of the relevant embassies stationed in China.

On the same day, Ministry of Health printed and issued *Administrative Method for Local Standards of Food Safety.*

March 3, The 12th Day of State Loving Ears. The theme was "Rehabilitation Begins from Discovery — Energetically Promote Hearing Ability Screening for the Newborn.

On the same day, Ministry of Health printed and issued *National Working Standardizations for Prevention and Control of Chronic Diseases (trial edition).*

March 9, Chen Zhu, Minister of Ministry of Health, Sun Zhigang, Vice-director of the State Development and Reform Commission and director of Medical Reform Office of the State Council, Wang Jun, Vice-minister of Ministry of Finance and Hu Xiaoyi, Vice-minister of Ministry of Human Power Resources and Social Safeguard replied the questions about the deepening medical and health reform of Chinese and foreign reporters.

March 10, The 6th World Day of Kidney. The theme is "Protect Kidney, Save the Heart".

One the same day, Ministry of Health decided to establish the Expert Council Committee of Health Response to the Emergent Events, printed and issued *The Management Method for the Expert Council Committee of Health Response to the Emergent Events by Ministry of Health.*

March 11, Minister of Ministry of Health Chen Zhu, and the Chairman of Shandong People's Government, Jiang Daming, jointly signed *The Cooperation Agreement of Promoting Medical and Health Undertaking Development of Shandong Province between Ministry of Health and Shandong People's Government*. Yin Li, Vice-minister of Ministry of Health and Wang Suilian, Vice-chairman of Shandong People's Government jointly signed *The Agreement of Joint Project Cooperation of Salt-reduction and the Prevention and Control of High Blood Pressure between Ministry of Health and Shandong People's Government*. Zhang Mao, Secretary of the Party Group and Vice-minister of Ministry of Health and Wang Min, the Standing Committee member and General Secretary of Shandong Province attended the signature ceremony.

On the same day, the General Office of Ministry of Health printed and issued *The Implementation Opinions about the Assessment of Performance Work of Township Health Centers and Village Health Rooms*.

March 14, China Influenza Center held the unveiling ceremony for Global Influenza Participation in Comparison and Cooperation Research Center of WHO in Beijing. Chen Zhu, Minister of Ministry of Health, Shin Young-soo, Director of West Pacific Region of WHO and health experts and officers from 16 countries were presented at the ceremony.

March 15, Minister of Ministry of Health, Chen Zhu wrote to the Minister of Japanese Ministry of Health and Labor, on behalf of Ministry of Health and himself to express heartful sympathy and solicitude for the Japanese people, especially the afflicted in the calamity of the serious earthquake and tsunami and their relatives. Ministry of Health of China showed special attention to the rescue and treatment work for the sufferers in the calamity and were ready and willingly at any time to provide necessary medical and health assistance.

On the same day, Chen Zhu, Minister of Ministry of Health and Zhao Ke-zhi, Chairman of Guizhou People's Government jointly signed *The Cooperative Agreement of the Promotion of the Strategic Striding-across Development of Guizhou Medical and Health Undertakings between Ministry of Health and Guizhou People's Government*.

On the same day, Ministry of Health printed and issued *The Basic Standards of Nursing Institute (2011 edition)*.

March 17, Ministry of Health convened the grassroots health and new agricultural cooperation work conference. Chen Zhu, Minister of Ministry of Health and Zhang Mao, Secretary of the Party Group and Vice-minister of Ministry of Health were present at the conference and made speeches respectively. The conference was presided over by Liu Qian, Vice-minister of Ministry of Health.

On the same day, Ministry of Health printed and issued *Basic Standards of Out-patient Section of Clinical Psychology Department of Medical Institutes (trial edition)*.

On the same day, the General Office of Ministry of Health printed and issued *The Management Method for the Demonstrative Districts of Comprehensive Prevention and Control of Chronical Non-infectious Diseases.*

(Wang Dian)

March 21 The 10th World Sleep Day with the theme of "Concerning the Sleep for the Middle-aged and the Old".

March 23 MOH printed and issued *Working Plan on Promoting High Quality Nursing Services.*

March 24 The 16th World Tuberculosis Day with the theme of "On the move against TB: Transforming the fight towards elimination"

On the same day, MOH printed and issued *Measures for Administration of Medical Equipment of Medical and Health institutions and Provisions on Administration of Administrative Licensing for New Varieties of food-related Products.*

March 26-30 A delegation led by Minister of Health Chen Zhu visited France to attend the Seventh BioVision- the World Life Sciences Forum and the Sixth Session of Sino-French Guiding Committee on the Cooperative Program on the Prevention and Control of Newly Detected Infectious Diseases and communicated on further strengthening cooperation on health with France.

March 28 The general office of MOH printed and issued *Detailed Rules for the Implementation of the Regulations on Administration of Sanitation in Public Places and Technical Operation Specifications for Blood Plasma Stations (2011 edition).*

March 30 National Development and Reform Commission jointly printed and issued *Circular on Issues Related to Carrying out Pilot on Payment by Diagnosis Related Groups.*

April 6 MOH printed and issued *Plan for Campaign of "Long March of Medical Quality" in 2011.* On the same day, MOH printed and issued *Scoring Criteria for National Clinical Key Specialties including Cardiovascular Medicine (trial edition).*

On the same day, MOH printed and issued *Testing Specifications for the Imaging Quality Control of Medical Regular X Ray Diagnosing Devices,* which should come into force on September 30, 2011.

April 7 The 62nd World Health Day, with the theme of "Antimicrobial resistance: no action today, no cure tomorrow".

April 11 MOH printed and issued *Circular on Launching the Campaign of "Three Excellent and One Satisfactory" in Medical and Health System Nationwide.*

April 12, MOH held a video conference on launching the campaign of "Three Excellent and One Satisfactory" in medical and health system nationwide to deploy activities of "Three Excellent and One Satisfactory", which the Minister of Health, Chen Zhu, and Vice Minister of Health, Ma Xiaowei attended and addressed.

On the same day, MOH printed and issued *Requirements of Mycobactericidal Evaluation for Disinfectant in Laboratory*, which should come into force on September 30, 2011.

April 13 MOH printed and issued *Diagnosis of Occupational Leukoderma*, which should come into force on October 1, 2011.

April 14 MOH printed and issued *Guide on the Construction and Administration of the Department of Rehabilitation Medicine in General Hospitals.*

April 15 MOH printed and issued *Interim Provisions on the Administration of Interior Prices for Medical Institutions.*

On the same day, the General Office of MOH printed and issued *Measures for the Implementation of Performance Evaluation for Health Supervisory Institutions (trial edition).*

April 15-21 The 17th National Tumor Prevention and Treatment Week with the theme of "Combating Cancer Scientifically, Caring for Lives".

April 18 The first Sino-Australian Talk on Health Policies was held in Beijing. Chen Zhu, Minister of Health, and Nicola Roxon, Minister for Health and Ageing of Australia, attended the conference together, delivered keynote speeches respectively and jointly signed Sino-Australian Executive Plan for Health Cooperation 2011-2014.

On the same day, Zhang Mao, Secretary of Party Group of MOH and Vice Minister of Health, published an article entitled *Exploration and Practice on the Reform and Development of Medical Health in the County Regions in Health News.*

On the same day, MOH printed and issued *Evaluation and Examination Criteria for Tertiary General Hospitals (2011 edition).*

April 20 MOH printed and issued *Criteria for the Use of Food Additives.*

April 20-29 Ma Xiaowei, Vice Minister of Health, led a delegation to visit Hungary and Montenegro and signed *Sino-Hungarian 2011-2013 Executive Plan for Cooperation in the Field of Health and Medical Science.*

April 21 MOH printed and issued *Diagnosis Criteria of Acute Occupational Phosgene Poisoning*, which should come into force on November 1, 2011.

April 25 The 25th National Vaccination Day, with the theme of "Vaccine Jabs, Healthy Babies"

On the same day, Li Keqiang, Member of CPC Political Bureau Standing Committee, Vice Premier of the State Council and Director of Leading Group for Deepening Reform on Medical and Health Care System of the State Council, participated in the activities of 2011 National Vaccination Day for Children.

On the same day, Chen Zhu, Minister of Health, met Didier Burkhalter, member of Swiss Federal Council and Head of the Department of Home Affairs. Both parties jointly issued *Joint Announcement on Bilateral Cooperation in the Field of Health* and started the health policy cooperation between four pairs of cities (states) in China and Swiss, especially the partnership on the reform of public hospitals.

On the same day, MOH printed and issued *Emergency Pre-plan on Issues Related to Imported Epidemics of Wild Poliovirus and Vaccine Derived Poliovirus (For Trial Implementation).*

April 25-May 1 2011 Pblicity week for *Law on the Prevention and Control of Occupational Diseases* with the theme of "Caring for the occupational health of migrant workers".

April 26 The 4th National Malaria Day with the theme of "Eliminating malaria and fulfilling the commitments".

On the same day, MOH printed and issued the recommended standard of *Diagnostic Standard for Keshan Disease*, which should come into force on November 1, 2011.

April 28-29 MOH held 2011 National work Conference on Health Talents in Beijing. Chen Zhu, Minister of Health, chaired the conference. Zhang Mao, Party Group Secretary of MOH and Vice Minister of Health, delivered a speech, and Liu Qian and Yin Li, Vice Ministers of Health, attended the conference. Liu Qian, Vice Minister of Health announced *Decision on Granting 80 Comrades Including Ma Xin etc. the Titles of "2009-2010 Middle-aged and Young Experts with Extinguished Contribution of MOH" by MOH, SFDA and SATCM.*

May 3 MOH announced the list of excellent hospitals, wards and individuals in the evaluations for excellent nursing service in 2010.

May 4 Chen Zhu, Minister of Health, signed and issued No. 81 Decree of the Ministry of Health entitled *Measures for the Reporting and Monitoring of Adverse Drug Reactions, which should come into force on July 1, 2011.*

May 7 The General Office of MOH printed and issued *Working Pre-plan for Risk Communication on Emergent Public Incidents in the Field of Health.*

May 10 MOH held a video conference to celebrate International Nurses' Day and promote excellent nursing service nationwide. Ma Xiaowei, Vice Minister of Health, transmitted the essence of the important instructions made by Comrade Li Keqiang, Member of the Standing Committee of CPC Political Bureau and Vice Premier of the State Council, and delivered a speech entitled *Taking Advantage of the Opportunities and Sparing No efforts to Promote the Sustainable and Sound Development of Excellent Nursing Service.*

On the same day, MOH held the national video and teleconference on improving the system of people's meditation for medical disputes and on sustaining the normal order for diagnosis and treatment. Ma Xiaowei, Vice Minister of Health, attended and addressed the conference.

May 11 The General Office of the Ministry of Health printed and issued *Standards for the Evaluation on Transparent Hospital Information in County Level Hospitals and Township Health Centers (For Trial Implementation).*

May 12 International Nurses Day with the theme of "Closing The Gap: Increasing Access and Equity".

On the same day, MOH printed and issued *MHO Health Emergency Pre-plan for Emergent Poisoning Events and Detailed Rules for the Designated Work of Preservation Institutions for the Human Pathogenic Bacteria (virus) Strains.*

May 15 The 18th Preventing and Treating Iodine Deficiency Day with the theme of "Adhering to scientific Iodine Supplement, Prevent Iodine Deficiency."

May 16-24 The 64th World Health Conference was held in Geneva, at which a series of WHO policies and issues on public health were discussed. Chen Zhu, Minister of Health, led a delegation to the conference and delivered an address entitled Urgency in Preventing and Controlling Chronic Noninfectious Diseases. At the conference, Wang Dechen, Director of Health Education Institute in Ningxia Hui Autonomous Region, was awarded 2011 Kuwait Prize on Health Promotion.

May 18 MOH printed and issued the announcement of *Authenticating Maca Powder as a New Resource Food.*

May 19 MOH printed and issued *Basic Criteria for the Rehabilitation Department in General Hospitals (For Trial Implementation).*

May 20 Chinese Students Nutrition Day with the theme of "All-round, Balanced, Appropriated-Developing Healthful Diet".

On the same day, Minister of Health Chen Zhu signed No 82 Decree of the Ministry of Health entitled *Measures for Administration of Recalling Medical Apparatuses (For Trial Implementation)*, which should come into force on July 1.

May 23 *Agreement on Sino-Japanese Cooperation Program on Telemedicine* was signed at the Ministry of Health and Vice Minister of Health Ma Xiaowei attended the signing ceremony.

On the same day, the Ministry of Health, the Ministry of Industry and Information Technology, the Ministry of Commerce, General Administration of Industry and Commerce, General Administration of Quality Inspection and State Food and Drug Administration jointly issued *Decree on Banning BPA (bisphenol A) in Infant Feeding Bottles.*

May 31 World No Tobacco Day with the theme of "The WHO Framework Convention on Tobacco Control".

On the same day, MOH printed and issued *Implementation Plan on National Health and Medical Talents Engineering.*

On the same day, General Office of MOH printed and issued *Clinical Norms for the Diagnosis and Treatment of Breast Cancer (2011 Edition).*

June 1 MOH printed and issued *Name List for Non-edible Substances and Abusive Food Additives Liable to Be Added in Food (Sixth Batch).*

June 2 An Evening was held in Beijing to celebrate the 90th anniversary for the founding of the Communist Party of China by the national medical and health system named For the Entrustment of Life. At the Evening were Minister of Health Chen Zhu, Secretary of Party Group of MOH and Vice Minister of Health Zhang Mao, Vice Ministers of Health Wang Guoqiang, Chen Xiaohong, Shao Mingli and Liu Qian, Director of Discipline Inspection Group of the Central Discipline Inspection Commission at MOH Li Xi, leaders from the Work Committee of Central Government Departments, Health Department of General Logistics, State Commission Office for Public Sector Reform, Ministry of Commerce, Population and Family Planning Commission, State Council Research Office and All-China Federation of Trade Unions as well as hundreds of medical stuff members.

June 3 WHO Director-General Dr Margaret Chan appointed the famous Chinese soprano and actress Peng Li Yuan as WHO Goodwill Ambassador for Tuberculosis and HIV/AIDS at the headquarters of WHO in Geneva. Vice Minister of Health Yin Li attended the ceremony.

June 6 The 16th National Eye Care Day with the theme of "Caring for the Patients with Poor Eyesight, Improving the Quality of Rehabilitation".

June 8-10 The 65th UN General Assembly on AIDS was held at the headquarters of the United Nations in New York. Vice Minister of Health Yin Li led a delegation to the conference and delivered an address entitled Taking Vigorous Actions and Improving Cooperation to Achieve the New Goals for Prevention and Control of AIDS. At the conference an outcome document was adopted entitled *Political Declaration on HIV/AIDS: Intensifying Our Efforts and Eliminating HIV/AIDS.*

June 13-14 MOH held the 2011 national coordination and promotion conference on health system counterpart assisting Xinjiang in Urumqi. Minister of Health Chen Zhu attended and addressed the conference. The conference was chaired by Chen Xiaohong, the administrative vice director of working group on Ministry of Health counterpart assisting Xinjiang and Vice Minister of Health.

June 14 The 8th World Blood Donor Day with the theme of "More Blood, More Life."

June 16 MOH printed and issued *Guidelines on Clinical Nursing Practices (2011 edition).*

June 15-24 Li Xi, Director of Discipline Inspection Group of the Central Discipline Inspection Commission at MOH, led a Chinese delegation to visit the Bolivarian

Republic of Venezuela and the Republic of Ecuador. Li Xi talked with the Minister of Health of Venezuela and jointly signed *Memorandum of Understanding on Cooperation in the Field of Health between the Ministry of Health of People's Republic of China and the Ministry of Health of the Bolivarian Republic of Venezuela*. Besides, he also talked with the Vice Minister of Health of Ecuador and jointly signed *Agreement on Cooperation in the Field of Health between the Ministry of Health of the People's Republic of China and the Ministry of Health of the Republic of Ecuador*.

June 17-July 6 National Knowledge Contest on *Food Safety Laws* was held by Office of Food Safety Committee of the State Council together with Ministry of Health, Ministry of Agriculture, State Administration of Industry and Commerce, Administration of Quality Supervision, Inspection and Quarantine, and State Food and Drug Administration.

June 22-July 1 Vice Minister of Health Chen Xiaohong led a delegation to visit Italy and Albania. Chen Xiaohong talked with Italian Minister of Health Ferruccio Fazio, jointly signed *2011-2014 Implementation Plan for the Memorandum of Understanding on Cooperation in the Field of Health and Medical Science between Chinese and Italian Ministries of Health* and witnessed the signing of *Memorandum of Understanding on Conducting Scientific Research and Academic Cooperation in the Field of Medicine and Health between MOH Research Center on Development of Health and Italian Senior Research Institute on Health*. Besides, he also talked with Albanian Minister of Health Petrit Vasili and jointly signed *2011-2015 Implementation Plan for Cooperation in the Filed of Health between MOH and Ministry of Health of Albania*.

June 23 Minister of Health Chen Zhu signed No.83 Decree of the Ministry of the People' Republic of China, which decided to annul the following rules: *Criteria and Requirements for Quality of Prenatal Care in Urban and Rural Areas Nationwide, Staffing Principles for Research Institutes of Medical Science Affiliated to MOH (for Trial Implementation), Organization Staffing Principles for Maternity Hospitals (for Trial Implementation), Measures for the Administration of Urban Perinatal Care Nationwide (for Trial Implementation), Measures for the Administration of Systematic Care for Rural Pregnant and Lying-in Women (for Trial Implementation), Rules for Home Delivery (for Trial Implementation)*, and *Measures for the Supervision on Collective Dinning Hygiene for Students*.

On the same day, MOH printed and issued *Measures for the Administration of Prenatal Care and Specifications for Prenatal Care*.

June 27, MOH printed and issued *Guidelines on the Diagnosis and Treatment of EHEC O 104: H4 (for Trial Implementation)*.

June 28 Premier Wen Jiabao and Chancellor Merkel of German held the first round of government consultation between the two governments in Berlin, German. Zhang

Mao, Secretary of Party Group of MOH and Vice Minister of Health, who was also a member of the Chinese delegation, talked with Daniel Bahr, the German Minister of Health, and jointly signed *Joint Statement on Establishing Cooperative Partnership for Administration of Hospitals*, which would promote the hospitals in the two countries to establish long and stable partnership directly.

June 30 The foundation-laying ceremony of National High Security Biosafety Laboratory was held in Wuhan. Chen Zhu, Minister of Health and Chairperson of the Chinese side of Sino-French Guiding Commission of Cooperative Program on the Prevention and Control of Emerging Infectious Diseases, attended and addressed the ceremony.

On the same day in Wuhan, Minister of Health Chen Zhu granted Chinese Health Award to Alain Merieux, President of French Merieux Research Institute.

July 1 MOH printed and issued standards for health industry: *Cervical Artificial Disk Replacement, Standard for Anesthesia Record, Diagnosis of Polycystic Ovarian Syndrome, Diagnosis of Gestational Diabetes Mellitus, Diagnosis of Acute Appendicitis, Diagnosis of Pancreatic Cancer, Diagnosis of Cervical Cancer, Artificial Total Kneel, Hip Replacement, Diagnosis of Prostatic Cancer*, all of which should come into force on December 1, 2011.

July 3 In Shanghai, MOH and Shanghai municipal government held the consultation conference between the ministry and the municipality and the signing ceremony for the agreement on further deepening cooperation between the ministry and the municipality. Minister of Health Chen Zhu and Mayor of Shanghai Municipal Government Han Zheng jointly signed *Agreement on Further Deepening Cooperation between MOH and Shanghai Municipal Government and Complementary Agreement on Jointly Building and Administrating Health Administrative Units in Shanghai.*

July 4 MOH printed and issued *The Sixth Five-Year Program of Health System on Conducting Law Publicity and Education (2011-2015) and Technical Specifications for Residents' Health Cards.*

On the same day, MOH printed and issued *Working Specifications for Comprehensive Intervention Program on Children's Oral Diseases in the Middle and Western Regions (2011 edition).*

July 5 MOH printed and issued *General Rules for Compound Food Additives.*

July 6 General Office of MOH printed and issued *Technical Plan for the Health Emergency Handling of Emergent Poisoning Accidents.*

July 7 MOH printed and issued *Measures for the Administration of Township Health Centers (for trial implementation).*

July 11 The first BRICS Health Ministers' Meeting was held in Beijing. The theme of the meeting was "Global Health-Access to Medicine". At the meeting, discussion was carried out around the theme and *the First BRICS Health Ministers" Meeting Beijing Declaration* was issued. The meeting was hosted by Minister of Health Chen Zhu.

July 12 MOH printed and issued *Decision on Naming 2009-2010 National Youth Civilization and Young Expert at Post of the Health System.*

July 15 The 70th anniversary of the publication of Mao Zedong's inscription "Heal the wounded, rescue the dying, and practice revolutionary humanitarianism." MOH, State Administration of Traditional Chinese Medicine and the Health Department of the General Logistics held a symposium at the Grand Hall of the People to commemorate the 70th anniversary of the publication of the inscription. Minister of Health Chen Zhu attended and addressed the symposium, which was hosted by Zhang Mao, the Secretary of Party Group of MOH and Vice Minister of Health.

July 20 MOH printed and issued *Regulations on the Administration of Reports on Health Supervision Information (2011 revised edition).*

July 22 MOH printed and issued *Standards for 27 Food Additive Products Including Potassium Nitrate.*

July 23 On the very night of 7.23 train crash on the Yongtaiwen railway line, Minister of Health Chen Zhu and Secretary of the Party Group of MOH and Vice Minister of Health Zhang Mao made deployments on rescuing and curing the wounded and experts at the national level were sent to provide technical support. Vice Minister of Health Chen Xiaohong followed Vice Premier Zhang Dejiang to Wenzhou to guide rescuing.

July 28 World Health Organization declared the 28th July as World Hepatitis Day. The slogan for this first year is "Know it. Confront it. Hepatitis affects everyone, everywhere".

July30 The State Council printed and issued *Program for the Development of Chinese Women (2011-2020)* and *Program for the Development of Chinese Children (2011-2020).*

August 1 MOH posthumously awarded Lan Yun the honor of Guard for People's Health.

August 1-7 World Breast-Feeding Week, with the theme of "Breast-Feeding: Listening, Talking, and Sharing".

August 2 MOH printed and issued compulsory standards for health industry: *Health Data Element Dictionary, Classification and Coding for Value Domain of Health Data Element, Basic Dataset of Health Record for Residents,* all of which should come into force on February 1, 2012.

August 3-5 MOH held a training workshop for the directors of health bureaus in Ordos, Inner Mongolia. Minister of Health Chen Zhu delivered a speech on some important issues concerning the present situation of medical and health reform and deepening medical and health reform during the 12th Five-Year-Plan period. The

Secretary of Party Group and Vice Minister of Health Zhang Mao made a report on improving the executive ability of health administrative departments and working well on the development of health reform in the second half of the year.

August 10-19 Delegated by MOH, Jilin Department of Health sent a medical team of 15 doctors to the People's Republic of Korea to conduct free clinic. They conducted cataract surgery and provided stomatological and medical treatment in Chongpyong Hospital, South Hamgyong, Korea, and donated medicine worth one million RMB Yuan to Korean Health Ministry.

August 11 MOH founded National Cancer Center and National Center for Cardiovascular Diseases.

August 12 General Office of MOH printed and issued *Management Standards for Interventional Treatment of Cardiovascular Diseases (2011 edition)* and *Standards for the Diagnosis and Treatment of Chronic Obstructive Pulmonary Disease (2011 edition).*

On the same day, MOH printed and issued compulsory industry standard *Diagnosis of Esophagus Cancer.*

August 16 MOH held a symposium on the handling of key proposals. Minister of Health Chen Zhu attended and addressed the symposium.

On the same day, National Committee of Population and Family Planning, Ministry of Public Security, Ministry of Health, State Administration of Traditional Chinese Medicine, Health Department of General Logistic Department Of PLA, and All-China Women's Federation jointly held a video and teleconference on the national special campaign to rectify identifying the gender of a fetus and aborting the pregnancy based on gender without medical needs. Vice Minister of Health Liu Qian required that the health administrative departments strengthen the responsibility of supervision and administration, the medical and health care institutions at all levels work well on the normalized management of routine work and focus on the two key links of gender identification of fetus and induction of labor.

August 18 General Office of MOH printed and issued *Circular on Strengthening the Administration of Clinical Drug Use for Pregnant Women and Children.*

August 18-19 Co-hosted by Ministry of Health, P. R. China, State Food and Drug Administration, and State Administration of Traditional Chinese Medicine, the second China Health Forum was held in China National Convention Center in Beijing. The theme of the forum was "*Sustainable Health Development*", around which the participants discussed the reform and development of health. Han Qide, Vice Chairman of the Standing Committee of National People's Congress, attended the forum. Chen Zhu, who is Minister of Health and the Chairman of China Health Forum, attended the forum and delivered a speech. Speeches on the theme were made by Sun Zhigang, the vice chairman of the National Development and Reform

Commission, Hu Xiaoyi, Vice Minister of Human Resources and Social Security Ministry, Chen Chuanshu, Vice director of National Committee on Ageing, Dr Shin Young-soo, WHO Regional Director for the Western Pacific, Xavier Bertrand, Minister of Labor, Employment and Health, France, and José Angel Córdova Villalobos, Minister of Health, Mexico.

August 19 MOH printed and issued *28 Recommended National Standards for Occupational Health*, which should come into force on March 1, 2012.

August 23 Secretary of Party Group of MOH and Vice Minister of Health Zhang Mao attended and addressed the reporting conference for the campaign of Investigation in A Hundred Villages by the young civil servants from the administrative organ of MOH.

August 23-September 1 Vice Minister of Health Huang Jiefu led a delegation to visit Azerbaijan and Israel. Huang Jiefu talked with Vice Minister of Health of Israel Yakov Litzman and signed *2011-2015 Program for the Cooperation on Health and Medical Science between the Ministry of Health of the People's Republic of China and the Ministry of Health of Israel.*

August 24 MOH established MOH expert committee on biosafety for pathogenic microorganism laboratory, and formulated *Administrative Measures for MOH Expert Committee on Biosafety for Pathogenic Microorganism Laboratory.*

August 26 The awarding ceremony for the 43rd Nightingale Florence Medal was held in the Great Hall of the People in Beijing. General Secretary of CPC Central Committee, President of PRC and Chairman of Central Military Committee Hu Jintao, who is also the honorary president of the Red Cross Society of China (RCSC), presented the medals to the eight winners of the medals. Member of the Standing Committee of the Political Bureau of the CPC Central Committee and Vice Premier Li Keqiang attended the ceremony.

August 26-27 National work conference on health informationization was held in Hangzhou, Zhejiang province. Minister of Health Chen Zhu and Vice Minister of Health Yin Li attended and addressed the conference.

August 28-30 Dr Shin Young-soo, WHO Regional Director for the Western Pacific, visited Shanghai and attended the naming ceremony for the WHO Cooperation Center for Healthy City.

August 30 General Office of MOH printed and issued *Measures for Performance Evaluation in Health Education Institutions (for trial implementation).*

September 1 The fifth National Healthy Lifestyle Day, with the slogan of "I Am Acting, I Am Healthy and I Am Happy," and the theme of "Reducing Salt to Prevent Hypertension."

(Zhao Xuemei)

图书在版编目（CIP）数据

中国卫生年鉴. 2012 = 2012 Year book of health in the people's republic of china : 英文 / 陈竺主编 . —北京: 人民卫生出版社，2013

ISBN 978-7-117-18161-7

Ⅰ. ①中… Ⅱ. ①陈… Ⅲ. ①卫生工作 – 中国 –2012– 年鉴 – 英文 Ⅳ. ① R199. 2-54

中国版本图书馆 CIP 数据核字（2013）第 227907 号

2012 中国卫生年鉴(英文)

主　　编: 陈　竺
出版发行: 人民卫生出版社（中继线 010-59780011）
地　　址: 中国北京市朝阳区潘家园南里 19 号
世界医药图书大厦 B 座
邮　　编: 100021
网　　址: http://www.pmph.com
E - mail: pmph @ pmph.com
购书热线: 010-59787592　010-59787584　010-65264830
开　　本: 787 × 1092　1/16
版　　次: 2013 年 12 月第 1 版　2013 年 12 月第 1 版第 1 次印刷
标准书号: ISBN 978-7-117-18161-7/R · 18162